Kawasaki Disease

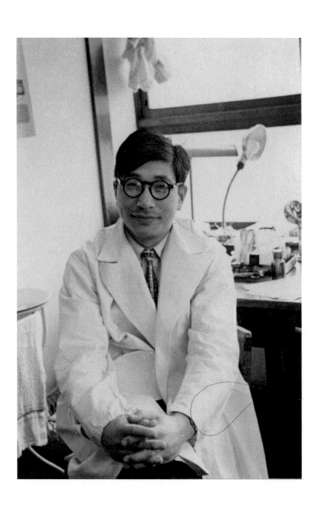

Ben Tsutomu Saji • Jane W. Newburger •
Jane C. Burns • Masato Takahashi

Editors

Kawasaki Disease

Current Understanding of the Mechanism
and Evidence-Based Treatment

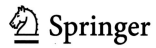 Springer

Editors
Ben Tsutomu Saji
Advanced and Integrated Cardiovascular
   Research Course in the Young and
   Adolescence
Toho University
Tokyo, Japan

Jane W. Newburger
Harvard Medical School,
   Department of Cardiology
Boston Children's Hospital
Boston, USA

Jane C. Burns
Department of Pediatrics,
   Rady Children's Hospital
University of California San Diego
   School of Medicine
La Jolla, USA

Masato Takahashi
Heart Center
Seattle Children's Hospital
Seattle, USA

ISBN 978-4-431-56037-1   ISBN 978-4-431-56039-5   (eBook)
DOI 10.1007/978-4-431-56039-5

Library of Congress Control Number: 2016940912

Printed on acid-free paper

This Springer imprint is published by Springer Nature
The registered company is Springer Japan KK

Dedication

It was almost 45 years ago, in November 1969, when I met Dr. Kawasaki. I was working in the Department of Pathology at the Japanese Red Cross Medical Center (formerly: Red Cross Central Hospital). I had little knowledge of Kawasaki disease but suddenly became interested when I conducted autopsies of Kawasaki disease patients. I have been deeply involved with this mysterious disease ever since.

Dr. Kawasaki is a great doctor, who proved from daily observations of patients that Kawasaki disease has very peculiar features. He has always been straightforward, like an innocent child, and I have been on friendly terms with this "Extraordinary child" for a long time.

Admiring the Glory of Dr. Tomisaku Kawasaki and his family.

Shiro Naoe, M.D., Ph.D.
Professor Emeritus
Toho University

***

I feel greatly privileged to have the opportunity to write this dedication to honor Dr. Tomisaku Kawasaki, my dear friend for the past 31 years. Tomi has devoted his life to the care of children as Pediatrician Extraordinaire! *This is one of life's greatest opportunities and responsibilities. In addition, Tomi's outstanding clinical skills led him in the 1960s to recognize the important illness that should forever bear his name. For many decades Dr. Kawasaki has tirelessly and effectively devoted himself to fostering research within Japan and internationally to help solve the mysteries surrounding this disorder, always being most supportive, gracious, and collaborative, focusing on advancing understanding of the disease to improve patient care and outcomes.*

My wife Claire and I have been so fortunate for the friendship of Reiko and Tomi Kawasaki since the First US–Japan Workshop on Kawasaki Disease at Makaha, Hawaii, organized by Marian Melish in January 1984. We have traveled together in Kyushu, Honshu, Hawaii, Pisa, Amsterdam, Taiwan, Manila, Chicago, and other locales.

The French embryologist Jean Rostand stated: "What a profession this is—this daily inhalation of wonder." Since caring for his first Kawasaki patient in 1961, Tomisaku Kawasaki has lived by these words.

Stanford T. Shulman, M.D.
Virginia H. Rogers
Professor of Pediatric Infectious Diseases
Northwestern University's Feinberg
School of Medicine

Chief, Division of Infectious Diseases

Ann & Robert H. Lurie
Children's Hospital of Chicago

***

When the first research committee on MCLS [Kawasaki disease was called Muco-Cutaneous Lymph Node Syndrome (MCLS) at that time] was organized in 1970, the first nationwide epidemiologic survey of Kawasaki disease was conducted with the collaboration of the late Professor Itsuzo Shigematsu, Head of the Department of Epidemiology at the National Institute of Public Health. Since the first survey, I was in charge of the surveys until handing over responsibility to my successor, Professor Yoshikazu Nakamura, Department of Public Health, Jichi Medical University.

I met Professor Tomisaku Kawasaki when I was a young staff member in the department and was assigned to the survey by Professor Shigematsu. I feel quite fortunate to have had this unexpected encounter with Professor Kawasaki and to have had the chance to come into contact with his personality.

He has always said, "Be strict in medical research and be warm in medical practice." His attitudes in clinical practice and in scientific research have always been consistent with his principles. I am convinced that the discovery of Kawasaki disease was a logical consequence of his serious attitude.

I firmly believe that Professor Kawasaki is the most important person in the support and leadership for those involved with research on Kawasaki disease. I sincerely hope for his continued good health and happiness.

Hiroshi Yanagawa, M.D., Dr. Med. Sci.
Professor Emeritus
Jichi Medical University
Tochigi-ken
Japan

***

Almost half a century has passed Prof. Tomisaku Kawasaki's first description of a unique disease. He saw the first 4-year-old patient with fever and rash in 1961. At that time he described the diagnosis "unknown". This "unknown diagnosis" may be an important key to his serendipitous discovery of this new disease, based on his deep insight into clinical observations and scientific considerations. His first English article reported the detailed clinical findings, and the epidemiology of Kawasaki disease (KD) in Japan and was surprising because it described the very small number of patients who died from myocardial infarction (Kawasaki: Pediatrics 1974). In 1973, I introduced coronary angiography for patients who recovered from acute KD and found that a certain number of them had silent coronary aneurysms even if they were free from cardiac symptoms or normal ECG findings (Kato: J Pediatr 1975). Prof. Kawasaki appreciated our study and since then has always encouraged our research. My personal communication with Prof. Kawasaki started and then, and I resolved to continue KD research at that time. During 40 years of contact with Prof. Kawasaki, I have been honored to learn from him the clinician's careful observations and deep considerations, the pediatrician's warm and gentle way with children, and the scientist's deep insight and careful discretion.

KD is not only great interest in pediatric medicine but also has a great impact in various fields of clinical medicine. In pediatric cardiology, KD is now a leading cause of acquired heart disease among children in Japan and North America. In the past, pediatric cardiologists knew little about the coronary arteries, but now must learn about coronary artery disease. Furthermore, patients in an earlier era already carried the disease to adulthood, and for a certain number of them coronary artery sequelae developed into adult coronary artery disease manifesting as a new coronary syndrome and premature atherosclerosis. These presented long-term problems in the areas of adult cardiology and vascular biology.

The incidence of KD rapidly increased since 1960s and continuing to increase, particularly in Japan? This mystery likely depends on the etiology of the disease. The epidemiology suggests that KD develops in susceptible children exposed to a common infectious agent or agents. However, the question remains as to why KD has rapidly increased in incidence in Japan. Some additional environmental factor(s) may be involved. Elucidation of the etiology of the disease is an urgent issue, and must certainly be Prof. Kawasaki's wish.

Hirohisa Kato, MD, PhD, FACC
Emeritus Professor of Pediatrics
Honorary President of the Cardiovascular Research Institute
Kurume University, Japan

Foreword

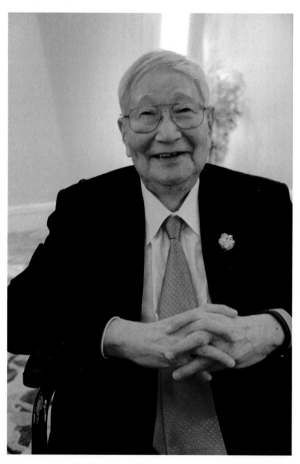

In January 1961, I saw my first case of what is now known as typical Kawasaki disease. The 4-year-old boy had unique symptom complexes, ones that I had never experienced in my 10-year pediatric career. I could not help but classify it as "diagnosis unknown" when he was released from the hospital. In February 1962, one year later, a 2-year-old boy with suspected sepsis was admitted to the emergency room of our hospital. When I saw him, I immediately remembered the undiagnosed case I had seen the previous year. By the end of 1966, I had experienced 50 cases that fell into the same category. I reported these cases in an article, "Acute Febrile Muco-Cutaneous Lymph Node Syndrome: Clinical Observation of 50 cases," which was published in the Japanese journal *Allergy* in 1967.

With research funds obtained from the Ministry of Health and Welfare in 1970, we organized a research committee, drew up a diagnostic guideline, and conducted the first nationwide survey. Although the committee had thought that the prognosis for the disease was favorable, cases of sudden death had been reported. Kawasaki disease is now classified as a systemic vasculitis that can result in coronary artery lesions. It requires not only the services of pediatric internists but also those of professionals from a wide range of disciplines, from the basic sciences to social medicine.

One of four untreated patients develops coronary artery aneurysms, which can persist after the acute period and result in myocardial infarction or sudden death. Although intravenous immunoglobulin therapy, the standard therapy for acute Kawasaki disease, has reduced the incidence of coronary artery aneurysms, some patients are resistant to this therapy. Effective therapy is necessary for these patients. Unfortunately, the etiology of Kawasaki disease remains unknown despite the efforts of many researchers.

It has been 53 years since I saw my first KD case, and 47 years have passed since the original paper on Kawasaki disease was published in Japanese. This is the first reference work on Kawasaki disease and provides current information regarding basic research, epidemiology, medical treatment, diagnosis, examination, interventions, and surgical treatment of Kawasaki disease. I hope it will be useful for all medical professionals, from those in basic research to those in clinical practice.

                                                                                Tomisaku Kawasaki

Preface

Kawasaki Disease: Current Understanding of the Mechanism and Evidence-Based Treatment has been a monumental undertaking and is an appropriate tribute to the genius of Dr. Tomisaku Kawasaki.

Many are familiar with the story of his first encounter with mucocutaneous lymph node syndrome, later renamed Kawasaki Disease, as told by Dr. Kawasaki himself. In January 1961 he encountered a 4-year-old boy who presented with what we now recognize as the classic clinical signs. After meticulously recording and pondering the child's presentation and laboratory test results, Dr. Kawasaki could not recognize the clinical signs as those of any known childhood illness. Nevertheless, with improvised treatments of intravenous hydration, penicillin, and a few doses of prednisone, the child's condition improved over a few weeks and he was discharged without a specific diagnosis. It was not until Dr. Kawasaki saw the second patient with similar clinical features a year later that he suspected that he was seeing a new disease. Over the next 6 years, he made meticulous notes on 50 similar cases that formed the basis of his landmark Japanese publication in 1967 [1]. It was not until a committee convened by the Japanese Ministry of Health conducted a nationwide survey that it was recognized that the "benign, self-limited syndrome" could be associated with coronary artery aneurysms, thrombosis, and myocardial infarction in a subset of children. The expanded syndrome was first presented to Western audiences in the 1974 publication in *Pediatrics* entitled "A new infantile acute mucocutaneous lymph node syndrome prevailing in Japan" [2].

In 2001, the Japan Kawasaki Disease Research Center re-published his original 1967 paper in booklet form with a side-by-side, page-by-page English translation. In its Preface, Dr. Kawasaki quoted a message from Dennis Burkitt (of lymphoma fame) to his medical students: "You should not despair if you do not have access to sufficient research funds or facilities: what is most important in conducting outstanding studies are steady observation and logical deduction." Like Burkitt before him, Dr. Kawasaki has a penchant for detailed observation and intellectual honesty that has earned universal respect from scholars and clinicians throughout the world. And yet Dr. Kawasaki remains genuinely friendly and humble. He always addresses himself as *boku* (僕) ("servant"), and lends his ear to anyone with any topic. He attributes his success to having able co-workers and being at the right place at the right time. Without Dr. Kawasaki's missionary zeal to influence so many scholars from infectious disease to cardiology, from epidemiology to pathology, from all corners of the globe, we could not have made such strides in research efforts in the areas of genetics, pathology, pathogenesis, treatment, and psychosocial concerns, and certainly this kind of book could not have been written.

We, the undersigned, join all the contributors to this book in saying a heart-felt "Thank you" to our friend and *sen-sei* ("teacher"), Dr. Tomisaku Kawasaki.

Seattle, WA, USA   Masato Takahashi
San Diego, CA, USA   Jane C. Burn
Boston, MA, USA   Jane W. Newburger
Tokyo, Japan   Ben Tsutomu Saji

References

1. Kawasaki, T. Acute febrile mucocutaneous syndrome with lymphoid involvement with specific desquamation of the fingers and toes in children. Arerugi. 1967;16(3):178–222.
2. Kawasaki, T, et al. A new infantile acute febrile mucocutaneous lymph node syndrome (MLNS) prevailing in Japan. Pediatrics. 1974;54(3):271–6.

Contents

Part I
Basic Research

The History of Kawasaki Disease: A Personal Perspective

Marian E. Melish

Abstract To understand the history of Kawasaki Disease (KD) one has to examine three periods of time: (A) the period from 1960 through the mid-1980s, (B) back to the 1870s, and (C) forward to the present. Dr. Kawasaki's seminal paper, published in the Japanese-language journal *Arerugi* (Japanese Journal of Allergy) (Kawasaki, Arerugi [Japanese J Allergy] 16:178–222, 1967) in 1967, is the best starting point, because of its remarkably complete delineation of the clinical features of KD in living children, which is the basis for the diagnostic criteria we use today. The more than 100 years of pathologic records from the first description of fatal KD, by Samuel Gee in 1871, (Gee, St Barth Hosp Rep 7:148, 1871) to Kawasaki's report includes the era of growing interest in and elegant description of the autopsy diagnosis that came to be called "infantile periarteritis nodosa". (Munro-Faure, Pediatrics 23:914–926, 1959; Roberts and Fetterman, J Pediatr 63:519–529, 1963) The most recent period, from the mid-1980s to the present, marks the period of international cooperation, heightened interest, and scientific progress in the understanding of this still enigmatic disease. The following chapters will outline the many areas of scientific progress. The history of KD is very personal to me as I have had the special privilege to be a participant in all these eras of discovery.

Keywords Tomisaku Kawasaki • Infantile periarteritis nodosa • Mucocutaneous lymph node syndrome • Mucocutaneous ocular syndrome

Introduction

To understand the history of Kawasaki Disease (KD) one has to go through three periods of time: (A) the period from 1960 through the mid-1980s, (B) back to the 1870s, and (C) forward to the present. Dr. Kawasaki's seminal paper, published in the Japanese-language journal *Arerugi* (Japanese Journal of Allergy) [1] in 1967, is the best starting point, because of its remarkably complete delineation of the

---

M.E. Melish (✉)
Tropical Medicine and Medical Microbiology, John A. Burns School of Medicine, University of Hawaii, 651 Ilalo St, Honolulu, HI 96813, USA
e-mail: marianm@kapiolani.org

© Springer Japan 2017   3
B.T. Saji et al. (eds.), *Kawasaki Disease*, DOI 10.1007/978-4-431-56039-5_1

clinical features of the disease in living children, which is the basis for the diagnostic criteria we use today. The more than 100 years of pathologic records from the first description of fatal KD, by Gee in 1871, [2] to Kawasaki's report includes the era of growing interest in and elegant description of the autopsy diagnosis that came to be called "infantile periarteritis nodosa" (IPN). [3, 4] The most recent period, from the mid-1980s to the present, marks the era of international cooperation, heightened interest, and scientific progress in the understanding of this still enigmatic disease. The following chapters will outline the many areas of scientific progress. The history of KD is very personal to me as I have had the special privilege to be a participant in all these eras of discovery.

The Era of Clinical Description and Pathologic Recognition: 1960–1984

I came of age in medicine in the 1960s, already fascinated by the elegant case series of IPN presented by Munro–Faure, and Roberts and Fetterman, when I saw my first two patients with KD in 1967, as a pediatric resident in Rochester, New York. Unable to reach a diagnosis, we presented the first case at Grand Rounds to a fascinated audience. Our colleagues were as puzzled as we were, so, like Kawasaki when he saw his first case in 1960, we filed these two cases away in our minds under "God only knows". [5] I had the good fortune to come to Hawai'i as an Assistant Professor in 1972. I began to see more puzzling cases and met my rheumatologist colleague, Dr. Raquel Hicks, at the bedside of febrile children with persistent fever, conjunctivitis without exudate, stomatitis, rash, arthritis, and urethritis. As newly minted academic physicians we had trouble believing that we were seeing a new or previously undescribed disease. We were sure that these children had the same unique disease and were toying with the idea that they might have a childhood version of Reiter syndrome, because of the triad of conjunctival involvement, arthritis, and urethritis common to most of our patients. We also became aware that our pathologist colleague, Dr. Eunice Larson, had diagnosed IPN in a child who died in our Children's Hospital in the year before our arrival. The clinical features he had before his sudden death—bilateral thrombosed aneurysms on the 22nd day of illness—were very similar to those in the children we were seeing. In 1973, at the time of our 12th case, we had lunch with Dr. Fumio Kosaki, a colleague of Dr. Kawasaki at the Japan Red Cross Hospital, who was on the final stop of a personal tour of North American Children's Hospitals. He showed us photographs of children with mucocutaneous lymph node syndrome (MCLS). He had shown these photographs and described Kawasaki's diagnostic criteria at all the medical centers he had visited and no one recalled seeing any similar cases. We said that we were not only very familiar with the symptom complex but indeed had a compatible patient in the hospital on that same day. Dr. Kosaki visited the patient with us and agreed that it was Kawasaki's MCLS. We were momentarily chagrined that we were not the first to recognize a new disease but pleased to know that we were correct in our suspicion that it was a unique entity. We began corresponding with Dr. Kawasaki in Japanese, grateful that we had many nurse and housekeeper colleagues who were fluent in Japanese. We presented our experience at the May 1974 meeting of the North American Society for Pediatric Research and published our series of 16 cases in 1976 [6].

Meanwhile, events had been progressing rapidly in Japan since 1967. Kawasaki's presentations and publication were initially met with skepticism as to whether his cases were a newly recognized disease entity or a variant of scarlet fever, Stevens-Johnson syndrome, or erythema multiforme. There were reports and small case series from other Japanese physicians of what was called mucocutaneous ocular syndrome (MCOS), which did not fully match Kawasaki's criteria but would now fall under the expanded KD umbrella. The pathologist at the Japan Red Cross Hospital, Dr. Noboru Tanaka, autopsied a child who Kawasaki had diagnosed as having MCOS. That child died suddenly and unexpectedly and had post-mortem findings of coronary thrombosis [7].

The presence of cardiac involvement in living children meeting MCLS and MCOS characteristics at another Tokyo hospital was reported in a paper published in 1968 by Takajiro Yamamoto [8]. The controversy and interest regarding MCLS/MCOS led to the formation of a research group and the First National Survey of MCLS just 3 years after Kawasaki's first paper. This survey was supported by the Japanese Ministry of Health and was headed by an epidemiologist, Dr. Itsuzo Shigematsu. A questionnaire using Kawasaki's diagnostic guidelines and photographs of the major features in a brochure were sent to children's hospitals with over 100 beds. It included questions about cardiac complications encountered.

The First National Survey validated Kawasaki's description of a new clinical entity and demonstrated an astonishing prevalence for a previously unrecognized entity: 415 hospitals (43 % response rate) reported 3140 cases during the decade 1961–1970. There was a monomodal age distribution with a peak in the second year of life, a male:female ratio of 1.5–1, and a seasonal distribution of cases, with clusters in winter and spring [9].

Until that time Kawasaki believed that MCLS was severe and often prolonged but ultimately benign and self-limited. He was surprised by the results of the First National Survey, which reported 10 cases of sudden death in children meeting his diagnostic criteria [10] The first two national surveys demonstrated an annual case-fatality rate of 1.7 %. Four of the first 10 cases were autopsied; all had thrombosed coronary artery aneurysms. The histologic appearance was similar to the pathologic diagnosis generally reported as infantile periarteritis (or polyarteritis) nodosa (IPN) [11]. Initially, Japanese pathologists disagreed about how similar these cases of fatal MCLS were to IPN. Controversy aside, the reports of sudden death due to coronary disease focused attention on the cardiovascular system of all children with MCLS. This was explored elegantly by the coronary angiography studies of Dr. Hirohisa Kato, which revealed coronary dilation and aneurysms in 12/20 MCLS patients with no cardiac symptoms [12]. The period 1970–1984 was one of active research and discovery in Japan with ever increasing yearly KD incidence, introduction of noninvasive echocardiography allowing for universal screening and monitoring of coronary abnormalities, more complete discovery of the natural history of KD (namely, the findings that coronary aneurysms occur in 20–25 % of patients and peripheral aneurysms in 5 % of patients), and the first nationwide epidemics, in 1979 and 1982 [13]. Japanese physicians and scientists held regular research meetings and established collaborations. Because of the usefulness of anti-inflammatory doses of aspirin in acute rheumatic fever, this therapy became standard for KD. Toward the end of this period came the seminal collaborative study of Dr. Kensi Furusho and colleagues from several institutions, which demonstrated that 1.6 g of intravenous immunoglobulin (IVIG) plus aspirin (n = 40) was more effective than aspirin alone (n = 45) in reducing transient (incidence: 15 % vs. 42 %, respectively) and persistent (31 % vs. 8 %) coronary artery abnormalities [14].

During this period interest in KD was building in North America and Europe but active investigation in those regions was far less robust than in Japan. The opportunity for investigators to meet and collaborate was very limited. Review of the histories and pathologic findings of cases diagnosed as IPN in continental North America and fatal KD cases in Hawai'i and Japan confirmed that they were indistinguishable but different from adult or classical periarteritis nodosa [15]. Echocardiography and angiography findings became established and reported [16, 17]. Community-wide epidemics were reported in several regions [18, 19]. A racial difference in incidence was established: children of Japanese ancestry had a markedly elevated risk as compared with children of European ancestry living in the same multiethnic community [19, 20].

Back to the Future: 1871–1984 and Other Riddles of KD

Disease is very old, and nothing about it has changed. It is we who change, as we learn to recognize what was formerly imperceptible. *(De l'expectation en médecine.* Jean Marie Charcot 1825–93)

Gee's report of the death, in 1871, of an English boy with thrombosed coronary aneurysms and Malet's report in the Lancet in 1887 show that fatal KD was present in Europe in the nineteenth century [2]. At its emergence in Japan in the 1960s, KD had a case fatality rate of 1.7 %. But where were the 98 % of non-fatal cases? Starting in the 1930s there were many single case reports of IPN in the United States, all diagnosed at autopsy and most with clinical features we would now recognize as KD. Roberts and Fetterman were able to develop an autopsy series, but no clinician had encountered and followed more than one IPN patient in his/her lifetime. Monro–Faure, and Roberts and Fetterman, recognized, and very nearly described, the principal diagnostic features of KD retrospectively from the case reports [3, 4]. While alive these patients had received diagnoses of Stevens–Johnson syndrome, erythema multiforme, scarlet fever, and hypersensitivity reaction, as had the early KD patients identified in the First National Survey in Japan. It seems likely that KD had sometimes been misdiagnosed as measles, adenovirus, or enterovirus infection among patients in North America [21]. The presence of these confounding conditions explains how KD was "hiding in plain sight" in North America and Europe, where we know it existed from reports of fatal cases in the pathologic record. In Japan, however, KD may have emerged, as both a pathologic and clinical entity, in the 1950s. The search for evidence of convincing KD autopsy and clinical cases before 1950 has been unrewarding [22]. Fatal cases with autopsy findings consistent with KD were seen in the Annual of Pathologic Autopsy Cases from 1960 to 1970, and had received varied clinical diagnoses. From 1970 through 1982 there was a striking increase in the number of autopsy KD cases, and a steady fall from the mid-1980s, due to better diagnosis and treatment. Unfortunately, the autopsy registry began in 1958 [23]. A review of clinical records at Tokyo University Hospital from 1940 to 1965 identified diagnoses that could mimic KD and revealed 10 apparent KD cases from 1950 to 1967 but no convincing cases from 1940 to 1950 [24, 25]. Among the many unsolved mysteries of KD is the microbial or environmental agent that may have triggered the sudden emergence of the still expanding epidemic of KD cases among the uniquely susceptible child population of Japan [26].

The Era of Enhanced Discovery and International Collaboration: 1984–2015

In contrast to their colleagues in Japan, the relatively small number of clinicians and researchers interested in KD in North America and Europe were isolated and not fully aware of the progress being made in Japan. I organized what would become the First International Kawasaki Disease Symposium (IKDS), which was held at Makaha Hawaii in January of 1984. At that meeting the North American colleagues learned much more from the leading Japanese researchers than we contributed. Nevertheless, we established productive and personal relationships that have endured and produced many advances in the understanding of KD. Members of the US contingent organized the first US Multicenter Trial of the Efficacy of IVIG in the Treatment of Kawasaki Syndrome at that meeting [27]. The following IKDS conferences have been held in Asia or the US every 3–4 years, most recently, the 11th IKDS in Honolulu Hawai'i in February 2015. These meetings invite abstracts and have research poster and oral presentations with invited lectures focusing on new directions. The major sessions at the 11th IKDS were on epidemiology, genetics, etiology and pathogenesis, animal models, clinical studies in diagnosis/biomarkers, therapy, imaging, natural history, and long-term prognosis, with invited lectures on the conduct of clinical trials and a session on collaborative research. KD is now recognized among children of all racial and ethnic groups in all continents. Major advances in clinical care have reduced the mortality rate and severity of vascular disease, helped define the natural history and long-term prognosis, and increased interest in the genetics of susceptibility in various populations. KD cases are seen worldwide, but the disease remains underdiagnosed and undertreated in most areas with low prevalences and in locations where it has only recently been diagnosed for the first time. The etiologic agent has not been discovered, and a sensitive and specific diagnostic test is not available. IVIG, the current standard therapy, is expensive, requires hospitalization for administration, and fails to control inflammation in 15–20 % of cases. Serious coronary vascular lesions still develop, with no proven effective adjunctive therapy. Despite our historical progress there is much work to be done to remove this threat to the children of the world.

References

1. Kawasaki T. Pediatric acute febrile mucocutaneous lymph node syndrome: clinical observation of 50 cases. Arerugi [Japanese J Allergy]. 1967;16:178–222. PMID:6062087.
2. Gee S. Aneurysms of coronary arteries in a boy. St Barth Hosp Rep. 1871;7:148.
3. Munro-Faure H. Necrotizing arteritis of the coronary vessels in infancy; case report and review of the literature. Pediatrics. 1959;23(5):914–26. PMID:13645127.
4. Roberts FB, Fetterman GH. Polyarteritis nodosa in infancy. J Pediatr. 1963;63(4):519–29. http://dx.doi.org/10.1016/S0022-3476(63)80361-3 PMID:14074409.
5. Kawasaki T. Personal communication. May 4, 1974.
6. Melish ME, Hicks RM, Larson EJ. Mucocutaneous lymph node syndrome in the United States. Am J Dis Child. 1976;130(6):599–607. PMID:7134.
7. Burns JC, Kushner HI, Bastian JF, Shike H, Shimizu C, Matsubara T, et al. Kawasaki disease: A brief history. Pediatrics. 2000;106(2), E27. http://dx.doi.org/10.1542/peds.106.2.e27 PMID:10920183.
8. Yamamoto T, Kimura J. Acute febrile mucocutaneous, lymph node Syndrome (Kawasaki) subtype of mucocutaneous ocular syndrome of erythema multiforme complicated with carditis. Shonka Rinsho [Japanese J Pediatr]. 1968;21:336–9.
9. Shigematsu I. Epidemiology of mucocutaneous lymph node syndrome MCLS. Nippon Shonika Gakkai Zasshi [Acta Pediatr Jpn]. 1972;76:695–6.
10. Kawasaki T, Naoe S. History of Kawasaki disease. Clin Exp Nephrol. 2014;18(2):301–4. http://dx.doi.org/10.1007/s10157-013-0877-6 PMID:24595558.
11. Kawasaki T, Kosaki F, Okawa S, Shigematsu I, Yanagawa H. A new infantile acute febrile mucocutaneous lymph node syndrome (MLNS) prevailing in Japan. Pediatrics. 1974;54 (3):271–6. PMID:4153258.
12. Kato H, Koike S, Yamamoto M, Ito Y, Yano E. Coronary aneurysms in infants and young children with acute febrile mucocutaneous lymph node syndrome. J Pediatr. 1975;86 (6):892–8. http://dx.doi.org/10.1016/S0022-3476(75)80220-4 PMID:236368.
13. Yanagawa H, Ohgane H, Nagai M. Space-time clustering of Kawasaki disease—with special reference to the 1979 and 1982 incidences. Nihon Rinsho. 1983;41(9):1987–93. PMID:6663736.
14. Furusho K, Kamiya T, Nakano H, Kiyosawa N, Shinomiya K, Hayashidera T, et al. High-dose intravenous gammaglobulin for Kawasaki disease. Lancet. 1984;2(8411):1055–8. http://dx. doi.org/10.1016/S0140-6736(84)91504-6 PMID:6209513.
15. Landing BH, Larson EJ. Are infantile periarteritis nodosa with coronary artery involvement and fatal mucocutaneous lymph node syndrome the same? Comparison of 20 patients from North America with patients from Hawaii and Japan. Pediatrics. 1977;59(5):651–62. PMID:16242.

16. Takahashi M, Schieber RA, Wishner SH, Ritchie GW, Francis PS. Selective coronary arteriography in infants and children. Circulation. 1983;68(5):1021–8. http://dx.doi.org/10.1161/01. CIR.68.5.1021 PMID:6616785.

17. Chung KJ, Brandt L, Fulton DR, Kreidberg MB. Cardiac and coronary arterial involvement in infants and children from New England with mucocutaneous lymph node syndrome (Kawasaki disease). Angiocardiographic-echocardiographic correlations. Am J Cardiol. 1982;50 (1):136–42. http://dx.doi.org/10.1016/0002-9149(82)90019-4 PMID:7090996.

18. Patriarca PA, Rogers MF, Morens DM, Schonberger LB, Kaminski RM, Burns JC, et al. Kawasaki syndrome: association with the application of rug shampoo. Lancet. 1982;2 (8298):578–80. http://dx.doi.org/10.1016/S0140-6736(82)90660-2 PMID:6125730.

19. Dean AG, Melish ME, Hicks R, Palumbo NE. An epidemic of Kawasaki syndrome in Hawaii. J Pediatr. 1982;100(4):552–7. http://dx.doi.org/10.1016/S0022-3476(82)80751-8 PMID:7062202.

20. Shulman ST, McAuley JB, Pachman LM, Miller ML, Ruschhaupt DG. Risk of coronary abnormalities due to Kawasaki disease in urban area with small Asian population. Am J Dis Child. 1987;141(4):420–5. PMID:3565328.

21. Rose V, Lightfoot NE, Fournier A, Gibbons JE. The descriptive epidemiology of Kawasaki syndrome in Canada, 1979–1985. Prog Clin Biol Res. 1987;250:45–53. PMID:3423054.

22. Kushner HI, Bastian JF, Turner CL, Burns JC. The two emergences of Kawasaki syndrome and the implications for the developing world. Pediatr Infect Dis J. 2008;27(5):377–83.

23. Takahashi K, Oharaseki T, Yokouchi Y, Yamada H, Shibuya K, Naoe S. A half-century of autopsy results—incidence of pediatric vasculitis syndromes, especially Kawasaki disease. Circ J. 2012;76(4):964–70. http://dx.doi.org/10.1253/circj.CJ-11-0928 PMID:22313802.

24. Shibuya N, Shibuya K, Kato H, Yanagisawa M. Kawasaki disease before kawasaki at Tokyo university hospital. Pediatrics. 2002;110(2 Pt 1):e17. http://dx.doi.org/10.1542/peds.110.2.e17 PMID:12165616.

25. Kato H, Inoue O, Kawasaki T, Fujiwara H, Watanabe T, Toshima H. Adult coronary artery disease probably due to childhood Kawasaki disease. Lancet. 1992;340(8828):1127–9. http://dx.doi.org/10.1016/0140-6736(92)93152-D PMID:1359212.

26. Burns JC, Kushner HI, Bastian JF, Shike H, Shimizu C, Matsubara T, Turner CL. Kawasaki disease: a brief history. Pediatrics. 2000;106:e27.

27. Newburger JW, Takahashi M, Burns JC, Beiser AS, Chung KJ, Duffy CE, et al. The treatment of Kawasaki syndrome with intravenous gamma globulin. N Engl J Med. 1986;315(6):341–7. http://dx.doi.org/10.1056/NEJM198608073150601 PMID:2426590.

Histopathology of Coronary Arteritis in Acute Kawasaki Disease and Murine Systemic Vasculitis Induced by *Candida Albicans* Cell Wall Polysaccharide

Toshiaki Oharaseki, Yuki Yokouchi, Yasunori Enomoto, and Kei Takahashi

Abstract This chapter describes the characteristics of Kawasaki disease vasculitis and a *Candida albicans* cell wall polysaccharide–induced murine vasculitis model. Kawasaki disease vasculitis and murine vasculitis have a number of similarities, namely, (1) vasculitis readily develops at bifurcations of medium-sized arteries, (2) inflammatory cell infiltrate mainly comprises neutrophils and macrophages; fibrinoid necrosis is rare, (3) vasculitis follows the typical course of acute inflammation, (4) proinflammatory cytokines such as tumor necrosis factor α are closely associated with vasculitis onset, and (5) vasculitis shows some response to IVIG therapy and anti–tumor necrosis factor α therapy.

Keywords Kawasaki disease • Arteritis • Pathology • *Candida albicans* • Pathogen-associated molecular patterns (PAMPs)

Introduction

Kawasaki disease (KD) is an acute febrile disease of children and is classified as a vasculitis syndrome. Relapse and recurrence are rare, but most cases follow the typical course of acute inflammation. This is a major difference between KD and other types of vasculitis, such as polyarteritis nodosa and Takayasu arteritis.

This chapter outlines the histopathological features of coronary arteritis in acute KD, describes the characteristics of a KD vasculitis model, and explains the similarities between this model and KD vasculitis.

T. Oharaseki (✉) • Y. Yokouchi • Y. Enomoto • K. Takahashi
Department of Pathology, Toho University Ohashi Medical Center, 2-17-6, Ohashi,
Meguro-ku, Tokyo 153-8515, Japan
e-mail: oharasek@oha.toho-u.ac.jp

© Springer Japan 2017
B.T. Saji et al. (eds.), *Kawasaki Disease*, DOI 10.1007/978-4-431-56039-5_2

Histopathological Characteristics of Coronary Arteritis in Acute KD

KD is characterized by a high incidence of infiltration of epicardial coronary arteries. The origins of coronary arteries are particularly prone to aneurysm development. Occasionally, a bead-like aneurysm forms along the entire length of the coronary artery outside the muscle layer, starting at the origin [1–4].

Histologically, the earliest changes are seen on the sixth to eighth day of illness, starting with edematous changes in the media and progressing to neutrophil and macrophage infiltration of the intima and adventitia. By the 10th day of illness, inflammation in the intima and adventitia merges, forming panvasculitis across all layers of the vessel wall. The lesion exhibits inflammatory cell infiltration by macrophages and neutrophils and proliferative changes of fibroblasts, among other changes [5]. Inflammation rapidly worsens and becomes panvasculitis involving all layers of the vessel wall. Even at the peak of inflammation, fibrinoid necrosis like that seen in polyarteritis nodosa is rare. If the internal and external elastic lamina and smooth muscle cells in media are damaged by severe inflammation, the artery becomes unable to withstand the pressure of the blood and dilates; thus, aneurysm formation is complete by about the 12th day of illness. Thrombi readily form inside the aneurysm and are a cause of ischemic heart disease (Fig. 1). Therefore, completion of treatment by the 10th disease day is important in preventing aneurysm formation.

Severe inflammatory cell infiltration persists until around the 25th day of illness, after which it usually gradually subsides. Infiltration is usually almost gone by about the 40th day of illness. Therefore, KD vasculitis generally exhibits the typical course of acute inflammation. Scarring remains if the vessel wall undergoes a certain degree of destruction. If a giant aneurysm persists, long-term antithrombotic and anticoagulant therapy is required.

A recent study of KD vasculitis histology reported findings that differed from previously reported results [6]. The authors described a subacute/chronic vasculitis

Fig. 1 Histology of coronary aneurysm with thrombotic occlusion in acute KD

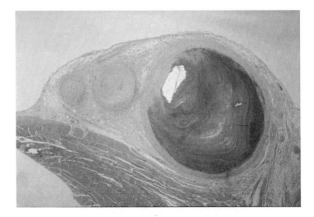

that is usually observed several months to years after KD onset. Although this may represent a new disease pattern, it is necessary to clarify the clinical characteristics of the patients studied. Our group has examined more than 100 KD autopsy cases but has never found evidence of chronic vasculitis.

The *C. Albicans* Cell Wall Polysaccharide–Induced Murine Vasculitis Model

Mice [7–9], rabbits [10], and swine [11] have been used as models of KD vasculitis. Here, we describe systemic vasculitis induced in mice by a *C. albicans* cell wall polysaccharide.

Model Development and Description of the Vasculitis-Inducing Agent

This vasculitis model was originally reported by Murata, in 1979 [7]. He ascertained that the amount of *Candida* in stool was significantly greater in children with KD than in healthy control children and that anti–*Candida* antibody titers were higher than in patients with scarlet fever. As an inflammatory agent, Murata initially used a polysaccharide component extracted from *C. albicans* with alkali. However, it was later found that a similar vasculitis could be induced with a polysaccharide released into the supernatant when *Candida* was cultured in a completely synthetic medium [12]. The inflammatory agent is a complex of mannan, beta-glucan, and protein [13]. Interestingly, the structure of the polysaccharide varies with the culture conditions, resulting in differences in vasculitis-inducing activity [14]. The receptor for the inflammatory substance was identified as dectin-2, which is believed to be involved in innate immunity in the onset of vasculitis [15].

Histopathological Characteristics of C. **Albicans** *Polysaccharide–Induced Murine Vasculitis*

In this model, the coronary bifurcation and aortic root are the most frequent sites of vasculitis (Fig. 2a). In addition to the coronary arteries, vasculitis develops in renal arteries, common iliac arteries, at bifurcations of medium-sized arteries such as the intercostal arteries, and the aorta. In all vascular lesions, the main infiltrating inflammatory cells are neutrophils and macrophages (Fig. 2b) [16]. Small numbers of T lymphocytes are seen in the adventitia but almost no B lymphocytes. This

Fig. 2 Histology of murine
coronary arteritis induced
by polysaccharide extracted
from *Candida albicans* with
alkali. (**a**) Low-power view
(elastica van Gieson stain),
(**b**) High-power view
(hematoxylin and eosin
stain)

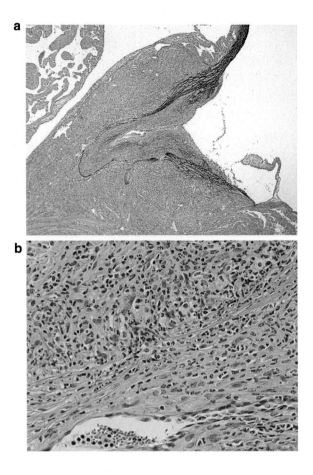

vasculitis follows a typical course of acute inflammation, ie, inflammation gradually disappears and lesions become scar tissue.

Relationship of Mouse Genetic Background to Cytokines and Vasculitis

The incidence of vasculitis development in this model differs among mouse strains,
which indicates that genetic factors are involved in vasculitis development
[16]. Although the disease-associated genes have not yet been identified, two
chromosomal regions have been reported to be associated with vasculitis
[17]. Numerous genes related to inflammation are clustered in those regions.

Cytokine production in response to exposure to *Candida*-derived polysaccharide
also differs between mouse strains. Splenocytes obtained from a high-incidence
mouse strain produced proinflammatory cytokines such as IL-1β, IL-6, and TNF-α,

whereas low-incidence-strain cells did not and instead produced IL-10, an anti-inflammatory cytokine [18].

Response of C. Albicans *Polysaccharide–Induced Vasculitis to Treatment*

The vasculitis in this model was suppressed by administration of a high-dose human immunoglobulin [19].

In recent years, anti-TNF-α agents have been used as additional therapy for IVIG nonresponders. Anti-TNF-α agents potently suppress vasculitis in this murine *C. albicans* polysaccharide–induced vasculitis model, and TNF-α is thus believed to be closely associated with vasculitis development [20].

There is still no animal model that exhibits all the clinical symptoms of KD. However, the *C. albicans* cell wall polysaccharide–induced murine vasculitis model described here is similar to KD vasculitis in histopathological characteristics and vasculitis course, the principal feature of KD.

References

1. Tanaka N, Naoe S, Masuda H, Ueno T. Pathological study of sequelae of Kawasaki disease (MCLS). With special reference to the heart and coronary arterial lesions. Acta Pathol Jpn. 1986;36(10):1513–27. PMID:3799188.
2. Naoe S, Takahashi K, Masuda H, Tanaka N. Kawasaki disease. With particular emphasis on arterial lesions. Acta Pathol Jpn. 1991;41(11):785–97. PMID:1785339.
3. Fujiwara H, Hamashima Y. Pathology of the heart in Kawasaki disease. Pediatrics. 1978;61 (1):100–7. PMID:263836.
4. Landing BH, Larson EJ. Are infantile periarteritis nodosa with coronary artery involvement and fatal mucocutaneous lymph node syndrome the same? Comparison of 20 patients from North America with patients from Hawaii and Japan. Pediatrics. 1977;59(5):651–62. PMID:16242.
5. Takahashi K, Oharaseki T, Naoe S, Wakayama M, Yokouchi Y. Neutrophilic involvement in the damage to coronary arteries in acute stage of Kawasaki disease. Pediatr Int. 2005;47 (3):305–10. http://dx.doi.org/10.1111/j.1442-200x.2005.02049.x PMID:15910456.
6. Orenstein JM, Shulman ST, Fox LM, Baker SC, Takahashi M, Bhatti TR, et al. Three linked vasculopathic processes characterize Kawasaki disease: a light and transmission electron microscopic study. PLoS One. 2012;7(6):e38998. http://dx.doi.org/10.1371/journal.pone. 0038998 PMID:22723916.
7. Murata H. Experimental candida-induced arteritis in mice. Relation to arteritis in the muco-cutaneous lymph node syndrome. Microbiol Immunol. 1979;23(9):825–31. http://dx.doi.org/ 10.1111/j.1348-0421.1979.tb02815.x PMID:395420.
8. Lehman TJ, Walker SM, Mahnovski V, McCurdy D. Coronary arteritis in mice following the systemic injection of group B Lactobacillus casei cell walls in aqueous suspension. Arthritis Rheum. 1985;28(6):652–9. http://dx.doi.org/10.1002/art.1780280609 PMID:3924060.

9. Nishio H, Kanno S, Onoyama S, Ikeda K, Tanaka T, Kusuhara K, et al. Nod1 ligands induce site-specific vascular inflammation. Arterioscler Thromb Vasc Biol. 2011;31(5):1093–9. http://dx.doi.org/10.1161/ATVBAHA.110.216325 PMID:21330608.

10. Onouchi Z, Ikuta K, Nagamatsu K, Tamiya H, Sakakibara Y, Ando M. Coronary artery aneurysms develop in weanling rabbits with serum sickness but not in mature rabbits. An experimental model for Kawasaki disease in humans. Angiology. 1995;46(8):679–87. http://dx.doi.org/10.1177/000331979504600806 PMID:7639414.

11. Philip S, Lee WC, Liu SK, Wu MH, Lue HC. A swine model of horse serum-induced coronary vasculitis: an implication for Kawasaki disease. Pediatr Res. 2004;55(2):211–19. http://dx.doi.org/10.1203/01.PDR.0000104151.26375.E5 PMID:14630987.

12. Ohno N. Chemistry and biology of angiitis inducer, Candida albicans water-soluble mannoprotein-beta-glucan complex (CAWS). Microbiol Immunol. 2003;47(7):479–90. http://dx.doi.org/10.1111/j.1348-0421.2003.tb03409.x PMID:12953841.

13. Uchiyama M, Ohno N, Miura NN, Adachi Y, Aizawa MW, Tamura H, et al. Chemical and immunochemical characterization of limulus factor G-activating substance of Candida spp. FEMS Immunol Med Microbiol. 1999;24(4):411–20. http://dx.doi.org/10.1111/j.1574-695X.1999.tb01313.x PMID:10435760.

14. Tada R, Nagi-Miura N, Adachi Y, Ohno N. The influence of culture conditions on vasculitis and anaphylactoid shock induced by fungal pathogen Candida albicans cell wall extract in mice. Microb Pathog. 2008;44(5):379–88. http://dx.doi.org/10.1016/j.micpath.2007.10.013 PMID:18065191.

15. Hirata N, Ishibashi K, Sato W, Nagi-Miura N, Adachi Y, Ohta S, et al. β-mannosyl linkages inhibit CAWS arteritis by negatively regulating dectin-2-dependent signaling in spleen and dendritic cells. Immunopharmacol Immunotoxicol. 2013;35(5):594–604. http://dx.doi.org/10.3109/08923973.2013.830124 PMID:23981001.

16. Takahashi K, Oharaseki T, Wakayama M, Yokouchi Y, Naoe S, Murata H. Histopathological features of murine systemic vasculitis caused by Candida albicans extract—an animal model of Kawasaki disease. Inflamm Res. 2004;53(2):72–7. http://dx.doi.org/10.1007/s00011-003-1225-1 PMID:15021972.

17. Oharaseki T, Kameoka Y, Kura F, Persad AS, Suzuki K, Naoe S. Susceptibility loci to coronary arteritis in animal model of Kawasaki disease induced with Candida albicans -derived substances. Microbiol Immunol. 2005;49(2):181–9. http://dx.doi.org/10.1111/j.1348-0421.2005.tb03708.x PMID:15722603.

18. Nagi-Miura N, Shingo Y, Adachi Y, Ishida-Okawara A, Oharaseki T, Takahashi K, et al. Induction of coronary arteritis with administration of CAWS (Candida albicans water-soluble fraction) depending on mouse strains. Immunopharmacol Immunotoxicol. 2004;26 (4):527–43. http://dx.doi.org/10.1081/IPH-200042295 PMID:15658603.

19. Takahashi K, Oharaseki T, Yokouchi Y, Miura NN, Ohno N, Okawara AI, et al. Administration of human immunoglobulin suppresses development of murine systemic vasculitis induced with Candida albicans water-soluble fraction: an animal model of Kawasaki disease. Mod Rheumatol. 2010;20(2):160–7. http://dx.doi.org/10.3109/s10165-009-0250-5 PMID:19943075.

20. Oharaseki T, Yokouchi Y, Yamada H, Mamada H, Muto S, Sadamoto K, et al. The role of TNF-α in a murine model of Kawasaki disease arteritis induced with a Candida albicans cell wall polysaccharide. Mod Rheumatol. 2014;24(1):120–8. http://dx.doi.org/10.3109/14397595.2013.854061 PMID:24261768.

Histopathological Characteristics of Noncardiac Organs in Kawasaki Disease

Kei Takahashi, Toshiaki Oharaseki, Yuki Yokouchi, and Yoshinori Enomoto

Abstract Kawasaki disease (KD) causes inflammation in medium-sized muscular arteries throughout the body, including the coronary artery, and is thus classified as a systemic vasculitis syndrome. In this chapter we review the histopathology of noncardiac organs, with a focus on vascular lesions. The main histopathological characteristic of KD vasculitis is proliferative inflammation consisting of marked accumulation of monocytes/macrophages. Vasculitis throughout the body starts at disease onset, rapidly reaches an inflammatory peak, and then slowly subsides and heals with scarring. KD vasculitis is thus a monophasic inflammatory process.

Keywords Kawasaki disease • Systemic vasculitis syndrome • Pathology • Macrophages

Introduction

Histopathological observation of Kawasaki disease (KD) has focused on the coronary artery because coronary arterial lesions are directly associated with mortality and long-term outcomes. However, noncardiac lesions must also be considered when describing KD pathology and etiology. In this chapter, we review the histopathology of noncardiac organs in KD, with a focus on vascular lesions.

Brief Overview of Systemic Vascular Lesions in KD

In the 1980s systemic vasculitis in KD was histologically evaluated in the body by Amano et al. [1], Hamashima et al. [2], Naoe et al. [3], and Landing et al. [4]. They reported that, although the incidence was highest for coronary arteritis, vasculitis developed at various other sites in the body (Table 1). Amano et al. [1] and

K. Takahashi (✉) • T. Oharaseki • Y. Yokouchi • Y. Enomoto
Department of Pathology, Toho University Ohashi Medical Center, 2-17-6 Ohashi, Meguro, Tokyo 153-8515, Japan
e-mail: keitak@oha.toho-u.ac.jp; opatho@oha.toho-u.ac.jp

© Springer Japan 2017   17
B.T. Saji et al. (eds.), *Kawasaki Disease*, DOI 10.1007/978-4-431-56039-5_3

Hamashima et al. [2] reported that vasculitis started in arterioles, venules, and capillaries, and inflammation disseminated to larger arteries, including the coronary artery. Naoe et al. [3] reported that KD vascular lesions started in the tunica interna and externa of medium-sized muscular arteries, such as the coronary artery. The size of vessels in which inflammation starts is unclear, but researchers agree that the histological characteristic of KD vasculitis is proliferative inflammation consisting of markedly accumulating monocytes/macrophages—fibrinoid necrosis is rare— and that vasculitis in KD starts at disease onset, rapidly reaches an inflammatory peak, and then slowly subsides and heals with scarring. Thus, KD vasculitis is a monophasic inflammatory process. However, Landing et al. [4] observed vasculitis scars in about one-third of arteries in patients who died during the acute stage (within 2 weeks after onset) and acute inflammation in about half of arteries even at 3 months after onset. These findings show that vasculitis during the acute and cicatricial phases is mixed in KD. Our observations indicate that the course of KD vasculitis is synchronous throughout the body [5]. The mixed presence of acute-phase and cicatrical-phase vasculitis is a histological feature of polyarteritis nodosa (PAN). Patients with PAN during childhood might have been included in the survey reported by Landing et al.

Histological Changes in Noncardiac Organs in KD

Kidney   The incidence of panarteritis in kidney varies [6–8]. Asaji et al. [6] observed panangiitis or its resultant scarring in kidney arteries during autopsy in 75 % of KD patients who died 6 days to 11 years after KD onset. Arteritis developed in a patient who died on the 13th illness day, and proliferative inflammation was noted in patients who died on days 17–28. Inflammation resolved after day 30. Panangiitis is localized in the interlobar arteries and rarely develops in arcuate and interlobular arteries [Fig. 1]. Renal aneurysm is a known complication, and renal hypertension due to renal arterial stenosis has been reported [9]. Regarding glomerular lesions, the presence of segmental or global glomerulosclerosis has been frequently reported, but such changes are considered to be physiological changes occurring with childhood development, ie, infantile glomerulosclerosis. Focal segmental mesangial proliferation is another reported glomerular change in KD [7, 10]. Tubular changes were reported in 8 % of cases [6].

Liver   Liver dysfunction is a frequent complication of acute KD. Tanaka et al. [11] performed liver biopsies of 19 patients at 7–36 days after KD onset and observed fatty and edematous degeneration of hepatocytes and severe inflammatory cell infiltration in the portal area in most of them. Vascular inflammation in the portal area was unclear, and hepatic changes were assumed to be caused by toxicity rather than by circulatory impairment. Ohshio et al. [12] reported frequent inflammatory cell infiltration in the portal area during acute KD and that, in the portal area, cholangitis and pericholangitis were more noticeable than vasculitis.

Table 1 Incidence of arteritis in various organs

	Amano [1]	Hamashima [2]	Naoe [3]	Landing [4]
Aorta	100 %	82 %	+	41 %
Carotid A	75 %		+	23 %
Subclavian A	71 %	67 %	+	
Celiac A	79 %	63 %	+	
Iliac A	100 %	93 %	+	
Coronary A	**100 %**	**95 %**	**95 %**	**100 %**
Renal A	80 %	64 %	73 %	55 %
Mesenteric A	79 %	86 %	+	27 %
Hepatic A	76 %	44 %	+	23 %
Intercostal A	58 %	60 %	+	
Spleen	50 %		11 %	50 %
Gastrointestinal tract			10 %	18 %
Paratrachea			+	36 %
Pancreas/peripancreas			31 %	36 %
Adrenal/periadrenal			+	32 %
Spermatic cord			+	41 %
Testis		67 %	15 %	18 %
Vagina			+	9 %
Uterus			+	5 %
Skeletal muscle				27 %
Meninges		36 %	1 %	5 %
Pulmonary A	71 %	50 %	59 %	32 %

Pancreas and Spleen Vascular lesions in the pancreas developed in 30 % of autopsy patients examined. The lesions were located at sites up to the pancreatic interlobular arteries. Vasculitis started on the 10th illness day, reached an inflammatory peak at about day 28, and then healed, although fibrous intimal thickening remained [13]. Yoshioka et al. [14] reported that inflammatory cell infiltration of the pancreatic duct and surrounding tissue and vasculitis were characteristic findings and that inflammation was marked in the pancreatic duct during acute KD. Regarding the spleen, arteritis was noted in the hilar and trabecular regions of arteries, and histological changes were similar to those in the pancreas [13].

Gallbladder Masuda et al. [15] histopathologically investigated gallbladders that were surgically excised after a diagnosis of cholecystitis in four patients with acute KD and observed characteristic nonspecific acalculous cholecystitis. Regarding vascular changes, perivascular cell infiltration was present, but panangiitis was noted in only one of the four patients, and panangiitis was noted in an artery in the subserosal layer. Gallbladder inflammation improved as KD resolved, which indicates that surgical excision of a swollen gallbladder is unnecessary in patients with KD.

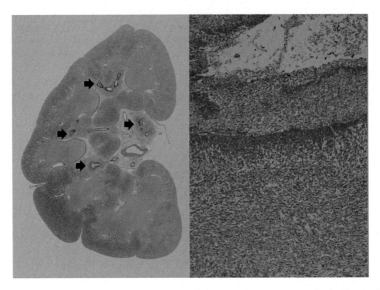

Fig. 1 Arteritis in the kidney. Panarteritis is localized in the interlobar arteries in the renal hilar region (*arrow*). The lesions show proliferative inflammation consisting of markedly accumulating macrophages. (*left*: Azan-Mallory stain; *right*: H & E stain)

Gastrointestinal Tract Vasculitis was noted in 10 % of KD patients at autopsy [16] but was exclusively localized in arteries in the subserosa and not present between the mucosal and muscular layers. Ulcers were present in three patients, and reactive hyperplasia of lymphoid follicles was often noted in mucosa at the end of the ileum. Nagata et al. [17] immunohistochemically investigated biopsy specimens of small-intestinal mucosa and hypothesized that the antigen that activates CD4-positive cells in intestinal mucosa and intestinal epithelial cells is associated with KD development.

Skin Changes in the skin are a principal clinical finding in KD diagnostic guidelines, and many pathological observations have been reported. These reports can be summarized as follows [18, 19]: (1) skin lesions are characterized by markedly inflammatory edema accompanied by vasodilatation in the dermal papillary layer and fibrin exudation; (2) endothelial cells are enlarged and surrounded by infiltrating monocytes/macrophages and CD4-positive T cells, although very few neutrophils and B cells were present; and (3) panangiitis is absent. Immunohistological studies showed that IL-1α and TNF-α are strongly positive in the acute phase but negative during recovery [20]. These changes are marked in BCG vaccination scars, and granulomatous inflammation was noted in some patients [21].

Lymph Nodes Cervical lymph node swelling is also a principal clinical finding in KD diagnostic guidelines and is present in 70 % of acute cases. Yokouchi et al. [22] reported that histological changes occur not only in the cervical region but also in lymph nodes throughout the body. Most lymphadenopathy is nonspecific and is caused by sinus expansion and paracortical zone enlargement, but there are also necrotic lesions of various sizes that are likely due to ischemic changes in some lymph nodes. Necrotic foci start to develop immediately below the capsule and are accompanied by fibrin thrombi in small vessels and perivascular nuclear debris. Especially in cases of cervical lymph nodes with necrosis, a high degree of nonpurulent inflammation develops in the lymph node capsule and surrounding connective tissue.

Lung Panvasculitis developed in the pulmonary artery in 59 % of patients within 60 days after onset, and inflammation was localized to the elastic pulmonary artery at sites up to the fourth branching [23]. The earliest change in the pulmonary artery was edematous dissociation of the tunica media in a patient who died on the 13th illness day. The condition progressed to severe panarteritis on the 25th–30th illness day. After day 30, inflammation started to subside, and scars formed in patients who died at 3 months. No aneurysm or arterial dilatation was noted in the pulmonary artery, perhaps due to low blood pressure. During acute KD, some patients have interstitial lung shadows. On autopsy, interstitial changes were observed in 31 % of patients who died on the 29th–57th illness day. Histologically, the changes corresponded to diffuse alveolar damage [24].

Central Nervous System Aseptic choriomeningitis and/or leptomeningitis was noted in about half of KD autopsy cases, and mild or moderate inflammatory cell infiltration by lymphocytes, monocytes/macrophages, and a few neutrophils was observed. Edema in perivascular or perineuronal areas and a localized spongy state were occasionally noted. Regarding cerebral blood vessels, perivascular inflammatory cell infiltration was observed, but panangiitis was not [25].

References

1. Amano S, Hazama F, Kubagawa H, Tasaka K, Haebara H, Hamashima Y. General pathology of Kawasaki disease. On the morphological alterations corresponding to the clinical manifestations. Acta Pathol Jpn. 1980;30(5):681–94. PMID:7446109.
2. Hamashima Y. Kawasaki disease [in Japanese]. Tr Soc Path Jap. 1977;66:59–92.
3. Naoe S. Pathology of Kawasaki disease, excluding cardiac changes. J Soc Kinki Area Kawasaki Dis Res. 1987;9:1–3 (in Japanese).
4. Landing BH, Larson EJ. Pathological features of Kawasaki disease (mucocutaneous lymph node syndrome). Am J Cardiovasc Pathol. 1987;1(2):218–29. PMID:3333141.
5. Takahashi K, Oharaseki T, Yokouchi Y, Naoe S, Jennette JC. Kawasaki disease arteries and polyarteritis nodosa. Pathol Case Rev. 2007;12(5):193–9. http://dx.doi.org/10.1097/PCR.0b013e3181557eeb.
6. Asaji A, Shibuya H, Masuda H, Tanaka N. The histological study on the kidney involved with Kawasaki disease – with a comparative study on the coronary aerterial lesions. J [in Japanese] Jap Cool Angiol. 1989;29:453–60.
7. Ogawa H. Kidney pathology in muco-cutaneous lymphnode syndrome. Nihon Jinzo Gakkai Shi. 1985;27(9):1229–37. PMID:4087543.
8. Takeuchi E, Ohshio G, Shimizu J, et al. Pathology of the kidney in Kawasaki disease. J Soc Kinki Area Kawasaki Dis Res. 1987;9:26–9 (in Japanese).

22

K. Takahashi et al.

9. Morishita S, Mawatari K, Yoshimi K, et al. Catheter intervention and surgical treatment of renovascular hypertension due to Kawasaki disease. In: Kato H, editor. Kawasaki disease. Amsterdam: Elsevier; 1995.

10. Salcedo JR, Greenberg L, Kapur S. Renal histology of mucocutaneous lymph node syndrome (Kawasaki disease). Clin Nephrol. 1988;29(1):47–51. PMID:3289806.

11. Tanaka T, Koike M, Minami Y. Pathology of liver injury in Kawasaki disease [in Japanese]. Shoni-Naika. 1984;16:2393–7.

12. Ohshio G, Furukawa F, Fujiwara H, Hamashima Y. Hepatomegaly and splenomegaly in Kawasaki disease. Pediatr Pathol. 1985;4(3–4):257–64. http://dx.doi.org/10.3109/15513818509026899 PMID:3835550.

13. Ando M, Asaji A, Naoe S, Masuda H, Tanaka N: Pathology of pancreatic arterial lesions in Kawasaki disease. Research committee of intractable vasculitis syndromes of the ministry of health and welfare of Japan, annual report for 1985. 1986;117–122.(in Japanese).

14. Yoshioka H, Miyake T, Oshio G, Shimizu J, et al. Clinicopathological study on the pancreas in 26 autopsy cases of Kawasaki disease. J Soc Kinki Area Kawasaki Dis Res. 1986;8:30–3.

15. Masuda H, Naoe S, Tanaka N: Pathological study on initial arterial lesions of Kawasaki disease, observation of removed gallbladders. Research committee of intractable vasculitis syndromes of the ministry of health and welfare of Japan, annual report for 1981. 1982;274–279. (in Japanese).

16. Kurashige M, Naoe S, Masuda H, Tanaka N. A morphological study of the digestive tract in Kawasaki disease – 31 autopsies. J Jap [in Japanese] Coll Angiol. 1984;24:407–18.

17. Nagata S, Yamashiro Y, Ohtsuka Y, Shimizu T, Sakurai Y, Misawa S, et al. Heat shock proteins and superantigenic properties of bacteria from the gastrointestinal tract of patients with Kawasaki disease. Immunology. 2009;128(4):511–20. http://dx.doi.org/10.1111/j.1365-2567.2009.03135.x PMID:19950419.

18. Hirose S, Hamashima Y. Morphological observations on the vasculitis in the mucocutaneous lymph node syndrome. A skin biopsy study of 27 patients. Eur J Pediatr. 1978;129(1):17–27. http://dx.doi.org/10.1007/BF00441370 PMID:679953.

19. Sugawara T, Hattori S, Hirose S, Furukawa S, Yabuta K, Shirai T. Immunopathology of the skin lesion of Kawasaki disease. Prog Clin Biol Res. 1987;250:185–92. PMID:3321075.

20. Sato N, Sagawa K, Sasaguri Y, Inoue O, Kato H. Immunopathology and cytokine detection in the skin lesions of patients with Kawasaki disease. J Pediatr. 1993;122(2):198–203. http://dx.doi.org/10.1016/S0022-3476(06)80113-7 PMID:8094096.

21. Kuniyuki S, Asada M. An ulcerated lesion at the BCG vaccination site during the course of Kawasaki disease. J Am Acad Dermatol. 1997;37(2 Pt 2):303–4. http://dx.doi.org/10.1016/S0190-9622(97)80376-3 PMID:9270532.

22. Yokouchi Y, Oharaseki T, Harada M, Ihara F, Naoe S, Takahashi K. Histopathological study of lymph node lesions in the acute phase of Kawasaki disease. Histopathology. 2012. http://dx.doi.org/10.1111/his.12007 PMID:23020240.

23. Shibuya K, Atobe T, Masuda H, Tanaka N. The histological study on pulmonary vascular lesions in Kawasaki disease [in Japanese]. J Jap Coll Angiol. 1987;27:293–304.

24. Shibuya K, Atobe T, Naoe S, Masuda H, Tanaka N, Kusawaka S. The histological study on pulmonary lesions in autopsy cases of Kawasaki disease [in Japanese]. Prog Med. 1986;6:35–42.

25. Amano S, Hazama F. Neutral involvement in kawasaki disease. Acta Pathol Jpn. 1980;30(3):365–73. PMID:7395511.

Identification of Novel Kawasaki Disease Susceptibility Genes by Genome-Wide Association Studies

Yoshihiro Onouchi

Abstract Completion of the Human Genome Project has helped in identifying disease genes, particularly with regard to mapping high-density single nucleotide polymorphisms and development of high-throughput genotyping platforms, which have considerably advanced research on complex disorders. Genome-wide searches are now practical and led to identification of genetic variations within previously unexamined genes relevant to diseases. In a genome-wide linkage study, the author and colleagues discovered that *ITPKC* and *CASP3* are common susceptibility genes for Kawasaki disease. This prompted examination of the Ca^{2+}/NFAT pathway and a subsequent continuous series of newly identified Kawasaki disease susceptibility genes. The recent identification of the *FCGR2A*, *BLK*, *CD40*, and *HLA class II* gene regions in genome-wide association studies has shed new light on the pathogenesis of Kawasaki disease.

Keywords Kawasaki disease • Susceptibility gene • Single nucleotide polymorphism • Genome-wide association study

Introduction

Although clinical and epidemiological features suggest the presence of infectious triggers in Kawasaki disease (KD) pathogenesis, genetic components appear to have important roles. KD is thus a multifactorial disease, and its pathogenesis involves both environmental and genetic factors. These two elements must therefore be unraveled before the cause of KD is fully understood.

Y. Onouchi (✉)
Department of Public Health, Graduate School of Medicine, Chiba University, 1-8-1 Inohana, Chuo, Chiba 260-8670, Japan

Laboratory for Cardiovascular Diseases, Center for Integrated Medical Science, RIKEN, 1-7-22, Suehiro, Tsurumi, Yokohama, Kanagawa 230-0045, Japan
e-mail: onouchy@chiba-u.jp; onouchi@riken.jp

© Springer Japan 2017
B.T. Saji et al. (eds.), *Kawasaki Disease*, DOI 10.1007/978-4-431-56039-5_4

History of the Genetic Study of KD

Until the draft sequence of the human genome was released, genetic studies of complex diseases were based on limited information of sequence variation in genes of interest. Most studies investigated several known polymorphisms in candidate genes (e.g., human leukocyte antigen [HLA] and cytokine genes) [1]. Unfortunately, these candidate gene studies could not identify a susceptibility gene that was repeatedly found to be associated with KD.

Genomic Studies of KD in the Post-Genomic era

Completion of the Human Genome Project, along with single nucleotide polymorphism (SNP) and haplotype mapping by the International HapMap project and the development of high-throughput genotyping platforms, has enabled genome-wide scans for susceptibility genes of complex diseases. In particular, establishment of a method for genome-wide association studies (GWAS) has dramatically improved such studies. Today, six susceptibility genes/loci for KD were found to have significant associations in GWAS (Table 1).

ITPKC

A SNP located in intron 1 of the inositol 1,4,5-trisphosphate 3-kinase C (*ITPKC*) gene, in the 19q13.2 region, was found to be significantly associated with KD susceptibility [2]. A positive linkage signal had been identified in an earlier genome-wide linkage study [3]. ITPKC is a kinase of inositol 1,4,5-trisphosphate, the second messenger molecule in the Ca^{2+}/NFAT signaling pathway, which transduces signals from various surface receptors (Fig. 1). ITPKC is believed to negatively regulate this pathway, and the associated SNP allele (C allele of rs28493229) reduces expression of *ITPKC* mRNA in peripheral blood mononuclear cells (PBMCs). The association of rs28493229 with KD has been replicated in several populations [4, 5].

CASP3

A positional candidate gene study of the 4q34–35 region, where a positive linkage signal was reported [3], identified SNPs around the caspase-3 (*CASP3*) gene that were significantly associated with KD [6]. CASP3 is an effector caspase that directly cleaves cellular proteins and triggers apoptosis. rs113420705, one of the

Table 1 Functions of KD susceptibility genes and possible roles in disease pathogenesis

Location	Gene	Gene product function	Effect of susceptibility allele on gene function	Possible influence of susceptibility allele on KD pathogenesis
1q23	FCGR2A[a]	IgG Fc receptor	Increased binding affinity of the protein to IgG2 isotype	Enhanced neutrophil/macrophage activation
4q34–q35	CASP3	Executioner of cellular apoptosis	Decreased mRNA expression	Increased longevity of activated immune cells
6p21.3	Undetermined (HLA or non-HLA genes)	Antigen presentation (HLA)	Unknown	Unknown
8p23–p22	BLK or FAM167A	BLK: nonreceptor protein tyrosine kinase FAM167A: function unknown	Decreased (BLK) or increased (FAM167A) mRNA expression[b]	Unknown
19q13.2	ITPKC	Kinase of inositol 1,4,5-trisphosphate	Decreased mRNA expression	Enhanced activation of inflammatory cells and vascular endothelial/smooth muscle cells
20q12–q13.2	CD40	Receptor of CD40L	Increased protein expression	Enhanced activation of inflammatory cells and vascular endothelial/smooth muscle cells

[a]It is possible that other variants within neighboring FCGR genes confer KD susceptibility
[b]Observation in B lymphoblastoid cell lines from a European population [14]

associated SNPs located in exon 1 of *CASP3*, affects *CASP3* mRNA expression, and the risk allele (A) expresses less *CASP3* mRNA, as compared with the opposite allele (G), in PBMCs [6]. CASP3 is pivotal in the apoptosis of immune cells; thus, reduced CASP3 expression likely facilitates sustained activation of immune cells and progression of KD inflammation. The results of several replication studies and a meta-analysis of these studies support an association of rs113420705 with KD [7].

FCGR2A

SNPs near the Fc gamma receptor (*FCGR*) gene cluster on chromosome 1q23 were associated with KD in a GWAS of a European population [5]. The strongest significant association was for a functional SNP of the Fc fragment of IgG, low affinity IIa, receptor (*FCGR2A*) gene, and this association has been confirmed in different ethnic groups [8, 9]. FCGR2A is expressed on neutrophils and

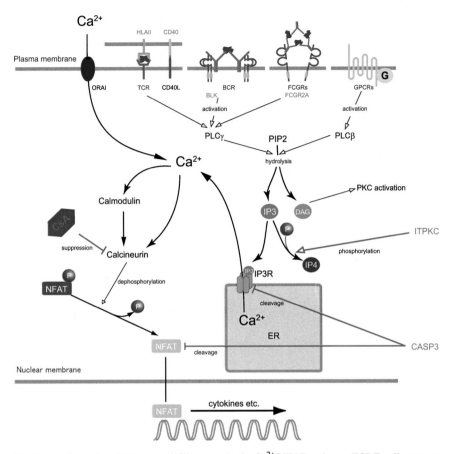

Fig. 1 Possible roles of KD susceptibility genes in the Ca^{2+}/NFAT pathway. *TCR* T-cell receptor, *BCR* B-cell receptor, *FCGRs* Fc gamma receptors, *GPCRs* G-protein-coupled receptors, *PLC* phospholipase C, *PIP2* phosphatidylinositol 4,5-bisphosphate, *IP3* inositol 1,4,5-trisphosphate, *IP3R* inositol 1,4,5-trisphosphate receptor, *IP4* inositol 1,3,4,5-tetrakisphosphate, *DAG* diacylglycerol, *PKC* protein kinase C, *ITPKC* inositol 1,4,5-trisphosphate 3-kinase C, *CASP3* caspase-3, *ER* endoplasmic reticulum, *NFAT* nuclear factor of activated T-cells, *CsA* cyclosporine A

macrophages and transduces the activation signal when ligated with immune complexes and clustered on the cell surface. The associated allele (A) of the SNP (rs1801274 A/G) changes the 131st amino acid from arginine to histidine and enhances its binding affinity to the IgG2 subclass.

BLK

Two independent GWAS, in Japan [9] and Taiwan [10], identified significant associations of SNPs in the 8p23–p22 region. The association peak at this locus was located in the intergenic region between the B lymphoid kinase (*BLK*) and family with sequence similarity 167, member A (*FAM167A*) genes. SNPs in this area have been associated with multiple autoimmune diseases. Because BLK is expressed mainly in B cells and is involved in B cell receptor signaling, *BLK*, but not *FAM167A* (which has not been characterized functionally), is considered a susceptibility gene because of the pivotal roles of B cells in autoimmunity.

CD40

CD40, also known as TNF receptor superfamily member 5 (*TNFRSF5*), is located on chromosome 20q12–q13.2. It is expressed on the cell surface of antigen-presenting cells and vascular endothelial cells and is stimulated when ligated with CD40L, which is expressed on activated CD4 T cells and platelets and transmits activation or differentiation signals into cells. A significant association of the SNPs around *CD40* with KD susceptibility was reported in the abovementioned two GWAS [9, 10]. The associated SNPs were in linkage disequilibrium with a known functional SNP that alters the efficiency of CD40 protein translation (rs1883832 C/T), and the C allele, which corresponds to higher CD40 protein expression, is linked with the SNP alleles conferring susceptibility to KD in this area. As with *BLK*, *CD40* is a common autoimmune disease susceptibility gene.

HLA class II

SNPs in the HLA class region were significantly associated with KD in a GWAS of Japanese KD patients [9]. This association peaked in the intergenic region between *HLA-DQB2* and *HLA-DOB*. Unfortunately, extended linkage disequilibrium and numerous genes with high sequence homology and densely distributed variations in this area complicate identification of the true susceptibility gene and variant. However, a better understanding of this association might help elucidate the contribution of HLA to KD susceptibility, which has long been controversial.

Current Understandings and Recognition

Although a number of the identified susceptibility genes appear to be related to immune function (Table 1), many have not been investigated as potential candidate genes in KD, and the exact functions of their products in KD pathogenesis are not understood. However, the existing evidence has provided several new insights. The association of the SNPs of *ITPKC* and *CASP3* (described in the next section "Recent Advances") has shed light on a new treatment strategy that targets the Ca $^{2+}$/NFAT signaling pathway [11, 12]. The robust association of the SNP in the *FCGR* gene cluster suggests the involvement of immune complexes in KD pathogenesis. Although the involvement of autoimmunity in KD has not been conclusively demonstrated, genetic components (*BLK* and *CD40*) shared with systemic lupus erythematosus and rheumatoid arthritis suggest a common pathophysiological mechanism between KD and other diseases. However, *ITPKC* and *CASP3* variants have not been associated with any other inflammatory/infectious disorders in GWAS and might reflect conditions highly specific to KD. It is clear there are many more unidentified susceptibility genes because the present evidence cannot fully account for differences in incidence rates among ethnic groups or for observed familial aggregation.

Recent Advances

Onouchi et al. reported that KD patients with susceptibility alleles of both *ITPKC* and *CASP3* had an increased risk for resistance to intravenous immunoglobulin therapy and coronary artery lesion formation [13]. This finding, together with previous knowledge of IP3R and NFATc2 cleavage in T cells by CASP3, suggests that CASP3 also acts as a negative regulator of the Ca^{2+}/NFAT pathway in KD pathophysiology (Fig. 1). Cyclosporine, a calcineurin inhibitor that specifically suppresses this signal transduction pathway, has received attention as an effective drug for refractory KD [11, 12].

References

1. Onouchi Y. Molecular genetics of Kawasaki disease. Pediatr Res. 2009;65(5 Pt 2):46R–54. http://dx.doi.org/10.1203/PDR.0b013e31819dba60 PMID:19190534.
2. Onouchi Y, Gunji T, Burns JC, Shimizu C, Newburger JW, Yashiro M, et al. ITPKC functional polymorphism associated with Kawasaki disease susceptibility and formation of coronary artery aneurysms. Nat Genet. 2008;40(1):35–42. http://dx.doi.org/10.1038/ng.2007.59 PMID:18084290.
3. Onouchi Y, Tamari M, Takahashi A, Tsunoda T, Yashiro M, Nakamura Y, et al. A genomewide linkage analysis of Kawasaki disease: evidence for linkage to chromosome 12.

J Hum Genet. 2007;52(2):179–90. http://dx.doi.org/10.1007/s10038-006-0092-3 PMID:17160344.

4. Lou J, Xu S, Zou L, Zhong R, Zhang T, Sun Y, et al. A functional polymorphism, rs28493229, in ITPKC and risk of Kawasaki disease: an integrated meta-analysis. Mol Biol Rep. 2012;39 (12):11137–44. http://dx.doi.org/10.1007/s11033-012-2022-0 PMID:23065250.

5. Khor CC, Davila S, Breunis WB, Lee YC, Shimizu C, Wright VJ, Hong Kong–Shanghai Kawasaki Disease Genetics Consortium, Korean Kawasaki Disease Genetics Consortium, Taiwan Kawasaki Disease Genetics Consortium, International Kawasaki Disease Genetics Consortium, US Kawasaki Disease Genetics Consortium, Blue Mountains Eye Study, et al. Genome-wide association study identifies FCGR2A as a susceptibility locus for Kawasaki disease. Nat Genet. 2011;43(12):1241–6. http://dx.doi.org/10.1038/ng.981 PMID:22081228.

6. Onouchi Y, Ozaki K, Buns JC, Shimizu C, Hamada H, Honda T, et al. Common variants in CASP3 confer susceptibility to Kawasaki disease. Hum Mol Genet. 2010;19(14):2898–906. http://dx.doi.org/10.1093/hmg/ddq176 PMID:20423928.

7. Xing Y, Wang H, Liu X, Yu X, Chen R, Wang C, et al. Meta-analysis of the relationship between single nucleotide polymorphism rs72689236 of caspase-3 and Kawasaki disease. Mol Biol Rep. 2014;41(10):6377–81. http://dx.doi.org/10.1007/s11033-014-3517-7 PMID:24990693.

8. Duan J, Lou J, Zhang Q, Ke J, Qi Y, Shen N, et al. A genetic variant rs1801274 in FCGR2A as a potential risk marker for Kawasaki disease: a case-control study and meta-analysis. PLoS One. 2014;9(8):e103329. http://dx.doi.org/10.1371/journal.pone.0103329 PMID:25093412.

9. Onouchi Y, Ozaki K, Burns JC, Shimizu C, Terai M, Hamada H, Japan Kawasaki Disease Genome Consortium, US Kawasaki Disease Genetics Consortium, et al. A genome-wide association study identifies three new risk loci for Kawasaki disease. Nat Genet. 2012;44 (5):517–21. http://dx.doi.org/10.1038/ng.2220 PMID:22446962.

10. Lee YC, Kuo HC, Chang JS, Chang LY, Huang LM, Chen MR, Taiwan Pediatric ID Alliance, et al. Two new susceptibility loci for Kawasaki disease identified through genome-wide association analysis. Nat Genet. 2012;44(5):522–5. http://dx.doi.org/10.1038/ng.2227 PMID:22446961.

11. Suzuki H, Terai M, Hamada H, Honda T, Suenaga T, Takeuchi T, et al. Cyclosporin A treatment for Kawasaki disease refractory to initial and additional intravenous immunoglobulin. Pediatr Infect Dis J. 2011;30(10):871–6. http://dx.doi.org/10.1097/INF. 0b013e318220c3cf PMID:21587094.

12. Tremoulet AH, Pancoast P, Franco A, Bujold M, Shimizu C, Onouchi Y, et al. Calcineurin inhibitor treatment of intravenous immunoglobulin-resistant Kawasaki disease. J Pediatr. 2012;161(3):506–12 e1.

13. Onouchi Y, Suzuki Y, Suzuki H, Terai M, Yasukawa K, Hamada H, et al. ITPKC and CASP3 polymorphisms and risks for IVIG unresponsiveness and coronary artery lesion formation in Kawasaki disease. Pharmacogenomics J. 2013;13(1):52–9. http://dx.doi.org/10.1038/tpj.2011. 45 PMID:21987091.

14. Hom G, Graham RR, Modrek B, Taylor KE, Ortmann W, Garnier S, et al. Association of systemic lupus erythematosus with C8orf13-BLK and ITGAM-ITGAX. N Engl J Med. 2008;358(9):900–9. http://dx.doi.org/10.1056/NEJMoa0707865 PMID:18204098.

Immunological Abnormalities and Use of Biomarkers and Cytokines to Predict the Severity of Kawasaki Disease

Jun Abe

Abstract Although the cause of KD remains unknown, understanding of its pathogenesis has increased. An overt immune reaction triggered by unknown infectious agents may cause systemic vasculitis. The mediators of this reaction are mainly inflammatory cytokines such as TNF-α, IL-1β, and IFN-γ. Several genetic factors differentially affect susceptibility to KD in various ethnic groups. However, the mechanisms of overt immune reaction during acute KD and the cytokines/biomarkers that are best able to predict KD severity are not well understood. Knowledge of the systems biology of complex cytokine networks is essential for the development of new diagnostic and therapeutic strategies to prevent CAL formation in KD.

Keywords Biomarkers • Proinflammatory cytokines • Interleukins • G-CSF • Systems biology

Introduction

Kawasaki disease (KD) is an acute systemic vasculitis associated with fever, cervical lymphadenopathy, skin rash, conjunctival injection, strawberry tongue, and induration of hands and feet. Although the cause of KD remains unknown, evidence regarding its pathogenesis is increasing. It is now known that an overt immune reaction triggered by unknown infectious agents is responsible for systemic vasculitis. The mediators of this reaction are mainly inflammatory cytokines such as tumor necrosis factor (TNF)-α, interleukin (IL)-1β, and interferon (IFN)-γ. In addition, genetic factors differentially influence susceptibility to KD in various ethnic groups. The recent success of biologic therapy, such as infliximab, in the treatment of intravenous immunoglobulin (IVIG)-nonresponsive KD suggests that TNF-α has a central role in KD pathogenesis [1].

J. Abe (✉)
Department of Allergy and Immunology, National Research Center for Child Health and Development, 2-10-1 Ohkura Setagaya-ku, Tokyo, Japan
e-mail: abe-j@ncchd.go.jp

© Springer Japan 2017
B.T. Saji et al. (eds.), *Kawasaki Disease*, DOI 10.1007/978-4-431-56039-5_5

IVIG, the standard initial therapy for KD, reduces systemic inflammation and the incidence of coronary artery lesions (CAL). However, when KD is suspected in patients with fewer clinical symptoms, clinicians must weigh the possibility of unnecessary IVIG treatment against that of delayed diagnosis of KD. In addition, about 20–30 % of KD patients do not respond to IVIG, and develop CAL more frequently than do IVIG responders. Therefore, it is essential to identify risk factors associated with IVIG nonresponse, to allow rescue therapy to be started before coronary artery aneurysms develop.

This review will provide a current overview of cytokine storm, an important immunological abnormality in KD, and discuss the possibility of using cytokines and the other biomarkers as prognostic indicators of IVIG responsiveness and the risk of CAL formation.

KD and Hypercytokinemia

Cytokines are small proteins released by cells. They affect other cells by means of transfer signals relating to proliferation, differentiation, metabolism, and motility of the target cells. Cytokines include interleukins, chemokines, colony-stimulating factors, and interferons. The inflammatory cytokines, which have roles in innate immune response, have received most of the attention in KD pathogenesis. A pioneering study by Leung et al. noted that the monokines IL-1 and TNF made cultured vascular endothelial cells more susceptible to lysis by antibodies circulating during KD [2]. Later, researchers thought that overt secretion and consumption of inflammatory cytokines such as TNF-α and IFN-γ by T cells were important in KD pathogenesis because of the resemblance of clinical symptoms in KD and toxic shock syndrome, which is caused by *Staphylococcus aureus* infection. Such infection produces a superantigen, TSST-1, and is associated with cytokine storm [3]. Subsequently, a variety of cytokine and chemokine genes, such as IL-6, IL-8, monocyte chemotactic protein-1 (MCP-1), and vascular endothelial growth factor (VEGF), were cloned and measured in the plasma of KD patients, using ELISA [4, 5]. Today, the plasma levels of more than 30 cytokines are known to be elevated in KD (Table 1).

A characteristic of hypercytokinemia in KD is that innate immune cells such as neutrophils, macrophages, and dendritic cells—as well as endo/epithelial cells—are important in the production of inflammatory cytokines. In innate immune response, a variety of cells recognize and respond to infection by pathogens, and to injuries caused by burns, irradiation, and chemical exposures, and release inflammatory mediators responsible for acute inflammation (Fig. 1). These cytokines induce or suppress their own synthesis or that of other cytokines in other target cells and regulate the extent of inflammatory responses, so as to limit injury to the host, reduce inflammation, and eventually re-establish immune homeostasis (cytokine network). On the basis of this homeostatic perspective, cytokines are often classified as pro- and anti-inflammatory. Plasma levels of pro- and anti-inflammatory

Table 1 Hypercytokinemia reported in Kawasaki disease

Year of publication	Cytokine/Chemokine
1988	Tumor necrosis factor (TNF)-α, interleukin (IL)-1β, interferon (IFN)-γ
1989	IL-6
1990	Soluble IL-2 receptor-α
1991	IL-2
1992	IL-8
1994	Soluble TNF-α receptors
1996	IL-4, IL-10
1997	Regulated on activation, normal T cell expressed and secreted (RANTES), monocyte chemotactic protein (MCP)-1, macrophage inflammatory protein (MIP)-1β
1998	Thrombopoietin, vascular endothelial growth factor (VEGF)
1999	Macrophage-colony stimulating factor (M-CSF), granulocyte-colony stimulating factor (G-CSF)
2002	Hepatocyte growth factor (HGF)
2003	IL-15, IL-17, CD40 ligand, IP-10, S100A12
2004	IL-18
2005	S100A8, S100A9
2006	Stromal cell-derived factor (SDF-1)
2007	Macrophage migration inhibitory factor (MIF)
2008	High mobility group box 1(HMGB1)
2010	IL-23, Transforming growth factor (TGF)-β[a]
2011	Brain natriuretic peptide (BNP)
2012	Resistin, hepcidin
2013	B-cell activating factor (BAFF)

[a]Decreased level

cytokines are elevated during acute KD [6]. Neonatal innate responses differ from those in adults. In response to most TLR ligands, neonatal immune cells produce less IL-12p70, IFN-γ, and TNF-α and more IL-1β, IL-6, IL-23, and IL-10 [7, 8]. This may explain the simultaneous elevation of TNF-α, IL-6, and IL-10 levels in the very early phase of KD inflammation.

Which Cytokines/Biomarkers Best Predict KD Severity?

The introduction of IVIG has led to better control of systemic inflammation in KD and decreased the prevalence of CAL from 20 to <5 %. However, fever and KD symptoms persist after IVIG in some patients, and this is associated with increased risk for CAL. Numerous studies have attempted to identify risk factors associated with IVIG nonresponse and have investigated patient baseline clinical and laboratory parameters. Among the factors studied, sex, age, white blood cell and

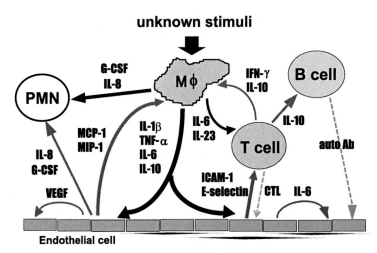

Fig. 1 Interactions between immune cells and endothelial cells in KD (Abbreviations: *PMN* polymorphonuclear leukocyte, *ICAM* intercellular adhesion molecules; *auto Ab* auto-antibody)

neutrophil counts, and serum aspartate aminotransferase and C-reactive protein (CRP) levels were frequently shown to be useful in devising a risk classification instrument [9–11]. (For a detailed review of risk scoring methods, see chapter "Scoring Systems to Predict Coronary Artery Lesions and Nonresponse to Initial Intravenous Immunoglobulin Therapy".) However, because these factors were selected by retrospective statistical analysis of medical records, the precise mechanisms underlying the relations of these factors with clinical outcomes remain uncertain. Moreover, it is unclear whether a particular risk classification is valid in all populations. Sleeper et al. reported that the sensitivity of three risk scoring systems used to predict IVIG resistance in Japan was low (33–42 %) in patients from North America [12]. They and another research group suggested that genetic differences between cohorts influence the effectiveness of these scoring systems.

Despite these limitations, some laboratory variables, such as neutrophil count and percent bands and plasma concentrations of CRP, appear to be higher in patients with severe KD. Tremoulet et al. reported that higher percent bands and CRP were strongly associated with IVIG nonresponse in 362 patients in San Diego [13]. In addition, DNA microarray studies conducted by the present author and colleagues and another group showed that neutrophils in IVIG nonresponders were more numerous and qualitatively different in their expression of an immature granulocyte-specific marker, polycythemia rubra vera 1 (PRV-1, CD177) [14, 15]. Similarly, serum granulocyte colony-stimulating factor (G-CSF) levels were higher in IVIG nonresponders than in responders. These findings suggest that G-CSF is overproduced by inflamed vascular endothelial cells in patients with severe KD and is involved in the expansion and premature egress of granulocytes from bone marrow. In addition, high-dose IgG specifically and completely inhibited overproduction of inflammatory cytokines such as G-CSF, IL-6, and IL-1β by cultured human coronary artery endothelial cells [16].

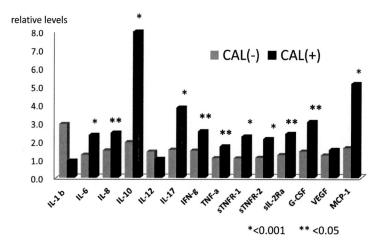

Fig. 2 Cytokines and chemokines that are elevated in IVIG-nonresponsive KD patients

In addition to G-CSF, a variety of pro- and anti-inflammatory cytokines (see Table 1) are overproduced in patients with KD. Moreover, plasma levels of most of these cytokines are higher in patients with more severe KD. However, it is not clear which of these cytokines can be used as clinical biomarkers to predict IVIG response and risk of CAL formation. Recently developed techniques in quantitative suspension array may help answer this question by analyzing patterns and correlations among cytokines/chemokines (cytokine profiling). In 2012, Wang et al. used this type of assay to analyze serum levels of IL-2, IL-4, IL-6, IL-10, TNF-α, and IFN-γ in 143 KD patients [17]. They found that IL-6 and IL-10 were particularly elevated, before and after IVIG treatment, in patients who later developed CAL. Our preliminary analysis using a multiplex bead assay system indicated that, among 14 cytokines studied in 273 KD patients before IVIG treatment, 8 proinflammatory cytokines (TNF-α, IL-6, IL-8, IL-17, IFN-γ, G-CSF, MCP-1, and sIL-2Rα) and 3 anti-inflammatory cytokines (IL-10, sTNFR1, and sTNFR2) were simultaneously elevated in patients who later developed CAL (Fig. 2) [18]. Moreover, levels of some of these cytokines were strongly correlated, particularly TNF-α, IL-10, sIL-2Rα, sTNFR1, and sTNFR2. These results suggest that both pro- and anti-inflammatory cytokines are relevant to KD severity and prognosis.

Conclusions

The use of newly developed methods such as quantitative suspension array technology and proteomics analysis of blood and urine is increasing our nascent understanding of the immune pathogenic mechanisms of KD [19, 20]. However, we have not yet identified the cytokines and biomarkers best suited for predicting

KD severity. Cytokine profiling shows that pro- and anti-inflammatory cytokine levels are simultaneously elevated in patients with more severe KD, which indicates that not every biomarker is an appropriate therapeutic target. An improved understanding of the systems biology of the complex cytokine networks is essential to the development of new diagnostic and therapeutic strategies to prevent CAL formation in KD.

References

1. Son MB, Gauvreau K, Burns JC, Corinaldesi E, Tremoulet AH, Watson VE, et al. Infliximab for intravenous immunoglobulin resistance in Kawasaki disease: a retrospective study. J Pediatr. 2011;158(4):644–9.e1. http://dx.doi.org/10.1016/j.jpeds.2010.10.012 PMID:2112 9756.
2. Leung DY, Geha RS, Newburger JW, Burns JC, Fiers W, Lapierre LA, et al. Two monokines, interleukin 1 and tumor necrosis factor, render cultured vascular endothelial cells susceptible to lysis by antibodies circulating during Kawasaki syndrome. J Exp Med. 1986;164 (6):1958–72. http://dx.doi.org/10.1084/jem.164.6.1958 PMID:3491174.
3. Miethke T, Duschek K, Wahl C, Heeg K, Wagner H. Pathogenesis of the toxic shock syndrome: T cell mediated lethal shock caused by the superantigen TSST-1. Eur J Immunol. 1993;23(7):1494–500. http://dx.doi.org/10.1002/eji.1830230715 PMID:8325325.
4. Ueno Y, Takano N, Kanegane H, Yokoi T, Yachie A, Miyawaki T, et al. The acute phase nature of interleukin 6: studies in Kawasaki disease and other febrile illnesses. Clin Exp Immunol. 1989;76(3):337–42. PMID:2473858.
5. Terai M, Jibiki T, Harada A, Terashima Y, Yasukawa K, Tateno S, et al. Dramatic decrease of circulating levels of monocyte chemoattractant protein-1 in Kawasaki disease after gamma globulin treatment. J Leukoc Biol. 1999;65(5):566–72. PMID:10331483.
6. Hamada H, Suzuki H, Abe J, Suzuki Y, Suenaga T, Takeuchi T, et al. Inflammatory cytokine profiles during Cyclosporin treatment for immunoglobulin-resistant Kawasaki disease. Cytokine. 2012;60(3):681–5. http://dx.doi.org/10.1016/j.cyto.2012.08.006 PMID:22944461.
7. Angelone DF, Wessels MR, Coughlin M, Suter EE, Valentini P, Kalish LA, et al. Innate immunity of the human newborn is polarized toward a high ratio of IL-6/TNF-alpha production in vitro and in vivo. Pediatr Res. 2006;60(2):205–9. http://dx.doi.org/10.1203/01.pdr. 0000228319.10481.ea PMID:16864705.
8. Kollmann TR, Crabtree J, Rein-Weston A, Blimkie D, Thommai F, Wang XY, et al. Neonatal innate TLR-mediated responses are distinct from those of adults. J Immunol. 2009;183 (11):7150–60. http://dx.doi.org/10.4049/jimmunol.0901481 PMID:19917677.
9. Kobayashi T, Inoue Y, Takeuchi K, Okada Y, Tamura K, Tomomasa T, et al. Prediction of intravenous immunoglobulin unresponsiveness in patients with Kawasaki disease. Circulation. 2006;113(22):2606–12.   http://dx.doi.org/10.1161/CIRCULATIONAHA.105.592865 PMID:16735679.
10. Egami K, Muta H, Ishii M, Suda K, Sugahara Y, Iemura M, et al. Prediction of resistance to intravenous immunoglobulin treatment in patients with Kawasaki disease. J Pediatr. 2006;149 (2):237–40. http://dx.doi.org/10.1016/j.jpeds.2006.03.050 PMID:16887442.
11. Sano T, Kurotobi S, Matsuzaki K, Yamamoto T, Maki I, Miki K, et al. Prediction of non-responsiveness to standard high-dose gamma-globulin therapy in patients with acute Kawasaki disease before starting initial treatment. Eur J Pediatr. 2007;166(2):131–7. http:// dx.doi.org/10.1007/s00431-006-0223-z PMID:16896641.
12. Sleeper LA, Minich LL, McCrindle BM, Li JS, Mason W, Colan SD, Pediatric Heart Network Investigators, et al. Evaluation of Kawasaki disease risk-scoring systems for intravenous

immunoglobulin resistance. J Pediatr. 2011;158(5):831–5.e3. http://dx.doi.org/10.1016/j.jpeds.2010.10.031 PMID:21168857.

13. Tremoulet AH, Best BM, Song S, Wang S, Corinaldesi E, Eichenfield JR, et al. Resistance to intravenous immunoglobulin in children with Kawasaki disease. J Pediatr. 2008;153 (1):117–21. http://dx.doi.org/10.1016/j.jpeds.2007.12.021 PMID:18571548.

14. Abe J, Ebata R, Jibiki T, Yasukawa K, Saito H, Terai M. Elevated granulocyte colony-stimulating factor levels predict treatment failure in patients with Kawasaki disease. J Allergy Clin Immunol. 2008;122(5):1008–13.e8. http://dx.doi.org/10.1016/j.jaci.2008.09.011 PMID:18930517.

15. Popper SJ, Shimizu C, Shike H, Kanegaye JT, Newburger JW, Sundel RP, et al. Gene-expression patterns reveal underlying biological processes in Kawasaki disease. Genome Biol. 2007;8(12):R261. http://dx.doi.org/10.1186/gb-2007-8-12-r261 PMID:18067656.

16. Matsuda A, Morita H, Unno H, Saito H, Matsumoto K, Hirao Y, et al. Anti-inflammatory effects of high-dose IgG on TNF-α-activated human coronary artery endothelial cells. Eur J Immunol. 2012;42(8):2121–31. http://dx.doi.org/10.1002/eji.201242398 PMID:22585560.

17. Wang Y, Wang W, Gong F, Fu S, Zhang Q, Hu J, et al. Evaluation of intravenous immuno-globulin resistance and coronary artery lesions in relation to Th1/Th2 cytokine profiles in patients with Kawasaki disease. Arthritis Rheum. 2013;65(3):805–14. http://dx.doi.org/10.1002/art.37815 PMID:23440694.

18. Abe J. Cytokines in Kawasaki disease [Japanese]. Nippon Rinsho. 2014;72:2014–19.

19. Kentsis A, Shulman A, Ahmed S, Brennan E, Monuteaux MC, Lee YH, et al. Urine proteomics for discovery of improved diagnostic markers of Kawasaki disease. EMBO Mol Med. 2013;5 (2):210–20. http://dx.doi.org/10.1002/emmm.201201494 PMID:23281308.

20. Ogata S, Shimizu C, Franco A, Touma R, Kanegaye JT, Choudhury BP, et al. Treatment response in Kawasaki disease is associated with sialylation levels of endogenous but not therapeutic intravenous immunoglobulin G. PLoS One. 2013;8(12), e81448. http://dx.doi.org/10.1371/journal.pone.0081448 PMID:24324693.

Pathophysiology of Kawasaki Disease

Anne H. Rowley, Stanford T. Shulman, and Jan M. Orenstein

Abstract Kawasaki Disease (KD) vasculopathy, which most significantly affects the coronary arteries, is characterized by three linked pathological processes: necrotizing arteritis, subacute/chronic (SA/C) vasculitis, and luminal myofibroblastic proliferation (LMP). Necrotizing arteritis (NA), initiated at the endothelial luminal surface, leads to giant aneurysms that can rupture or thrombose. SA/C vasculitis begins in the adventitia and is closely associated with LMP. LMP consists of actively proliferating smooth muscle cell-derived myofibroblasts and their matrix products, and can result in progressive arterial luminal stenosis. All three processes begin in the first 2 weeks after fever onset. NA subsides in the first 2 weeks, while subacute/chronic vasculitis and LMP can persist for months or years. The clinical and epidemiological features of KD are best explained by infection with an as-yet-unidentified ubiquitous agent, likely a virus entering via the respiratory route. Recent advances in genomics and RNA sequencing are beginning to reveal specific immune response dysfunction in KD that could lead to new diagnostics and therapeutics for this important childhood illness.

Keywords Necrotizing arteritis • Subacute/chronic vasculitis • Luminal myofibroblastic proliferation • Pathology • Gene expression

A.H. Rowley, M.D. (✉) • S.T. Shulman
Feinberg School of Medicine, Northwestern University, 310 E Superior Street, Morton 4-685B, Chicago, IL 60611, USA

The Division of Infectious Diseases, The Ann & Robert H. Lurie Children's Hospital of Chicago, Chicago, IL, USA
e-mail: a-rowley@northwestern.edu

J.M. Orenstein
Research Emeritus Professor of Pathology, The George Washington University School of Medicine, Washington, DC, USA

© Springer Japan 2017
B.T. Saji et al. (eds.), *Kawasaki Disease*, DOI 10.1007/978-4-431-56039-5_6

Introduction

A complete understanding of the pathogenesis of Kawasaki Disease (KD) awaits identification of the etiological agent(s). However, with the new description of the three linked pathological processes of KD and their sequelae [1], our understanding of the pathological basis for potential adverse outcomes in KD patients has improved. Previous descriptions of "regression" or "resolution" of coronary artery (CA) aneurysms by echocardiography and/or angiography likely represent reductions in luminal diameter as a result of thrombosis or from subacute/chronic arteritis with luminal myofibroblastic proliferation (LMP) [1], and therefore likely do not indicate that CAs have returned to normal structure and function. These new pathological findings should change approaches to long-term evaluation and management of KD patients with coronary arteritis.

History

Early KD pathological studies proposed a model of KD vasculitis as a self-limited, staged process of early neutrophil infiltration into medium-sized muscular arteries, particularly the CAs, with subsequent evolution of the inflammatory infiltrate to large mononuclear cells after the first week, and cessation of vascular inflammation within 2 months after onset of fever [2, 3]. Stenoses of CAs in KD patients who died months or years after onset in these studies were attributed to scar formation (implying an inactive, nonproliferative process). This model failed to explain the following subsequent clinical observations in KD patients: (1) reports of patients who died months or years after onset with inflammatory cell infiltrates and luminal myofibroblastic proliferation in CAs at autopsy [4–7], (2) reports of patients with apparent worsening of CA aneurysms over the course of months or years [8–11], and (3) reports of patients who had normal CA angiographic findings months or years after onset but who then developed myocardial infarction years later [12, 13]. Because early pathological studies indicated resolution of CA inflammation within 2 months after onset, and because C-reactive protein level and erythrocyte sedimentation rate in KD children typically normalize within 2 months after onset of fever, children with CA abnormalities persisting for more than 2 months after KD onset have been historically considered to have an inactive, noninflammatory condition. Our recent extensive light and electron microscopic study of the pathology of KD vasculopathy in 41 cases significantly challenges this previously held model and suggests that a re-evaluation of the clinical approach to KD children with persistent CA abnormalities is needed [1]. Our three-processes model of KD vasculopathy accurately predicts the potential for the above clinical outcomes [4–13], which were not explained by the previous model of KD vasculopathy.

The Three Linked Pathological Processes of KD Vasculopathy

The three linked vasculopathic processes are necrotizing arteritis (NA), subacute/chronic vasculitis (SA/C), and LMP [1]. NA is a synchronous neutrophilic process that starts at the endothelium of medium-sized muscular arteries, most critically the CAs. It begins and ends in the first 2 weeks after fever onset and progressively destroys the arterial wall into the adventitia, with the potential to result in large saccular or giant aneurysms that can rupture or thrombose. Rupture may occur when NA is transmural. SA/C, which can cause mild inflammation of the veins but primarily affects medium-sized muscular arteries such as the CAs, is an asynchronous process that begins in the first 2 weeks after fever onset but can persist for months or years. It is comprised of lymphocytes (including CD8 T lymphocytes) [14], plasma cells (including IgA plasma cells) [15, 16], eosinophils, and fewer macrophages. SA/C starts focally in the adventitia and progresses circumferentially and toward the lumen—damaging the media, elastic laminae, and intima—and is closely associated with the third process, LMP. LMP is a unique proliferative process of smooth muscle cell-derived pleomorphic myofibroblasts and their matrix products, including collagens, fibronectin, and external lamina, and can cause progressive stenosis of the arterial lumen. The LMP process is not synchronous, and although it may begin focally it eventually becomes circumferential and can unpredictably progress to the point that only a slit-like lumen remains. Persistent or worsening CA abnormalities after the second week are likely the result of SA/C. Myocardial ischemia leading to infarction months or years after an apparently normal angiographic study (which can assess lumen diameter but not the presence of arterial wall thickening due to thromboses or LMP) is likely to be caused by ongoing thrombosis and/or progressive LMP.

These pathological findings have significant clinical implications. At present, long-term follow-up of KD patients with significant CA abnormalities consists of evaluation of the arteries for luminal dilation by echocardiography, with periodic assessments of cardiac function in selected patients. Assessment of CA wall thickness, which would provide insight into the extent of thromboses or LMP, is not routinely performed. While it is probable that inflammation in the CAs of KD patients who develop no or only very mild dilation will resolve without long-term complications, it is likely that patients with more significant abnormalities are at risk of subsequent complications from subacute/chronic arteritis, LMP, and thrombosis as children or young adults. It may be incorrect to conclude that a KD patient who developed significant CA abnormalities is not at risk of future myocardial ischemia on the basis of reduction in CA luminal diameter to the normal range, normal angiographic findings at 1–2 years after onset, or a study showing normal cardiac function in patients who have layers of thrombi or ongoing LMP in the CAs [12, 13]. Decreases in CA lumen diameter in KD patients with significant CA abnormalities are often viewed as "remodeling", "regression", or "healing", partly because of early pathology models that suggested a lack of ongoing inflammation or cellular proliferation after the second month. However, our pathological findings indicate that saccular aneurysms with severe damage to the media do not appear to regenerate smooth muscle cells or elastic lamina, and that apparent "regression" represents filling of the aneurysmal cavity by thrombi that can obliterate the lumen over time, although some re-canalization can occur. We observed that calcification occurred in the oldest, most peripheral thrombi rather than in the remaining arterial wall. The lumen of fusiform aneurysms that have some preserved media can appear to "regress" when medial smooth muscle cells transition to the myofibroblasts of LMP, with concentric filling of the lumen by LMP and/or thrombus. Our recent pathological study and the clinical outcomes described above suggest that a readjustment in the approach to long-term follow-up of KD children with significant CA disease is warranted. New technologies that enable assessment of CA wall thickness may provide a better evaluation of the presence of ongoing thrombosis or LMP in the CAs in the future [17], which could assist clinicians in determining the most appropriate long-term follow-up and management.

Recent Advances in Etiological, Genomic, and Gene Expression Studies

The leading theory of KD etiology, based on the clinical and epidemiological features of the illness, is that a ubiquitous infectious agent acquired in early childhood, usually after loss of maternal antibody, results in KD in a genetically susceptible host [18]. Our studies support the hypothesis of a "new" virus as the cause of KD [19]. It is hoped that deep sequencing of KD tissues will ultimately result in identification of this agent, which would allow for great advances in diagnosis, therapy, and prevention. The higher attack rate in Asian children and increased prevalence of KD in siblings and parents provide strong support for genetic susceptibility to the disease [20]. Polymorphisms in several immune response genes, such as *ITPKC, FCGR2A,* and *CASP3*, are associated with KD. Nevertheless, the genes identified to date, even in combination, do not explain increased Asian susceptibility [20]. Improved techniques for determining gene expression in formalin-fixed, paraffin-embedded tissue samples are providing new information about dysregulated genes in KD coronary arteries, including *POSTN, ITGA4,* and *CD84* [21–23]. Hopefully, more comprehensive analyses of gene expression in KD CAs will provide key information about dysregulated immune pathways in KD vasculitis, which could lead to new therapeutic targets and disease biomarkers.

Conclusions

The three linked pathological processes model of KD requires a reassessment of the clinical management of children who develop coronary arteritis. Children with persistent CA abnormalities may have ongoing subacute/chronic arteritis for months or years. Biomarkers to identify such children are urgently needed in order to facilitate future therapeutic trials of additional immunomodulatory agents. LMP is an actively proliferative process that can lead to progressive arterial stenosis. Diagnostic methods and therapies to treat or prevent LMP are needed but presently unavailable. The evidence indicates that we should discard the widely held notion that children with KD who develop aneurysms but subsequently have non-dilated CA luminal diameter on echocardiography or angiography are no longer at risk [12, 13]. New imaging modalities that can provide an assessment of CA wall thickening may be helpful in identifying children with progressive CA thrombosis or LMP [17]. Although identification of the etiological agent(s) of KD is the best means to elucidate its pathogenesis, genetic analyses, including gene expression analyses of KD CAs, may guide future diagnostic and therapeutic strategies.

References

1. Orenstein JM, Shulman ST, Fox LM, Baker SC, Takahashi M, Bhatti TR, et al. Three linked vasculopathic processes characterize Kawasaki disease: a light and transmission electron microscopic study. PLoS One. 2012;7(6):e38998. http://dx.doi.org/10.1371/journal.pone. 0038998 PMID:22723916.
2. Fujiwara H, Hamashima Y. Pathology of the heart in Kawasaki disease. Pediatrics. 1978;61 (1):100–7. PMID:263836.
3. Amano S, Hazama F, Hamashima Y. Pathology of Kawasaki disease: I. Pathology and morphogenesis of the vascular changes. Jpn Circ J. 1979;43(7):633–43. http://dx.doi.org/10. 1253/jcj.43.633 PMID:41111.
4. Kuijpers TW, Biezeveld M, Achterhuis A, Kuipers I, Lam J, Hack CE, et al. Longstanding obliterative panarteritis in Kawasaki disease: lack of cyclosporin A effect. Pediatrics. 2003;112(4):986–92. http://dx.doi.org/10.1542/peds.112.4.986 PMID:14523200.
5. Burke AP, Virmani R, Perry LW, Li L, King TM, Smialek J. Fatal Kawasaki disease with coronary arteritis and no coronary aneurysms. Pediatrics. 1998;101(1 Pt 1):108–12. http://dx. doi.org/10.1542/peds.101.1.108 PMID:9417162.
6. Satoda M, Tatsukawa H, Katoh S. Images in cardiovascular medicine. Sudden death due to rupture of coronary aneurysm in a 26-year-old man. Circulation. 1998;97(7):705–6. http://dx. doi.org/10.1161/01.CIR.97.7.705 PMID:9495308.
7. Heaton P, Wilson N. Fatal Kawasaki disease caused by early occlusive coronary artery disease. Arch Dis Child. 2002;87(2):145–6. http://dx.doi.org/10.1136/adc.87.2.145 PMID:12138067.
8. Ozawa J, Suzuki H, Hasegawa S, Numano F, Haniu H, Watanabe K, et al. Two cases of new coronary aneurysms that developed in the late period after Kawasaki disease. Pediatr Cardiol. 2013;34(8):1992–5. http://dx.doi.org/10.1007/s00246-012-0543-x PMID:23052675.

9. Toyono M, Shimada S, Aoki-Okazaki M, Kubota H, Oyamada J, Tamura M, et al. Expanding coronary aneurysm in the late phase of Kawasaki disease. Pediatr Int. 2012;54(1):155–8. http://dx.doi.org/10.1111/j.1442-200X.2011.03403.x PMID:22335330.
10. Tsuda E, Kamiya T, Ono Y, Kimura K, Echigo S. Dilated coronary arterial lesions in the late period after Kawasaki disease. Heart. 2005;91(2):177–82. http://dx.doi.org/10.1136/hrt.2003.025338 PMID:15657227.
11. Kobayashi T, Sone K, Shinohara M, Kosuda T, Kobayashi T. Images in cardiovascular medicine. Giant coronary aneurysm of Kawasaki disease developing during postacute phase. Circulation. 1998;98(1):92–3. http://dx.doi.org/10.1161/01.CIR.98.1.92 PMID:9665066.
12. Kawai H, Takakuwa Y, Naruse H, Sarai M, Motoyama S, Ito H, et al. Two cases with past Kawasaki disease developing acute myocardial infarction in their thirties, despite being regarded as at low risk for coronary events. Heart Vessels. 2014. http://dx.doi.org/10.1007/s00380-014-0541-4 PMID:24985931.
13. Tsuda E, Hanatani A, Kurosaki K, Naito H, Echigo S. Two young adults who had acute coronary syndrome after regression of coronary aneurysms caused by Kawasaki disease in infancy. Pediatr Cardiol. 2006;27(3):372–5. http://dx.doi.org/10.1007/s00246-005-1233-8 PMID:16565902.
14. Brown TJ, Crawford SE, Cornwall ML, Garcia F, Shulman ST, Rowley AH. CD8 T lymphocytes and macrophages infiltrate coronary artery aneurysms in acute Kawasaki disease. J Infect Dis. 2001;184(7):940–3. http://dx.doi.org/10.1086/323155 PMID:11528596.
15. Rowley AH, Eckerley CA, Jäck HM, Shulman ST, Baker SC. IgA plasma cells in vascular tissue of patients with Kawasaki syndrome. J Immunol. 1997;159(12):5946–55. PMID:9550392.
16. Rowley AH, Shulman ST, Mask CA, Finn LS, Terai M, Baker SC, et al. IgA plasma cell infiltration of proximal respiratory tract, pancreas, kidney, and coronary artery in acute Kawasaki disease. J Infect Dis. 2000;182(4):1183–91. http://dx.doi.org/10.1086/315832 PMID:10979916.
17. Greil GF, Seeger A, Miller S, Claussen CD, Hofbeck M, Botnar RM, et al. Coronary magnetic resonance angiography and vessel wall imaging in children with Kawasaki disease. Pediatr Radiol. 2007;37(7):666–73. http://dx.doi.org/10.1007/s00247-007-0498-x PMID:17541574.
18. Rowley AH, Baker SC, Orenstein JM, Shulman ST. Searching for the cause of Kawasaki disease–cytoplasmic inclusion bodies provide new insight. Nat Rev Microbiol. 2008;6 (5):394–401. http://dx.doi.org/10.1038/nrmicro1853 PMID:18364728.
19. Rowley AH, Baker SC, Shulman ST, Rand KH, Tretiakova MS, Perlman EJ, et al. Ultrastructural, immunofluorescence, and RNA evidence support the hypothesis of a "new" virus associated with Kawasaki disease. J Infect Dis. 2011;203(7):1021–30. http://dx.doi.org/10.1093/infdis/jiq136 PMID:21402552.
20. Onouchi Y. Genetics of Kawasaki disease: what we know and don't know. Circ J. 2012;76 (7):1581–6. http://dx.doi.org/10.1253/circj.CJ-12-0568 PMID:22789975.
21. Reindel R, Baker SC, Kim KY, Rowley CA, Shulman ST, Orenstein JM, et al. Integrins α4 and αM, collagen1A1, and matrix metalloproteinase 7 are upregulated in acute Kawasaki disease vasculopathy. Pediatr Res. 2013;73(3):332–6. http://dx.doi.org/10.1038/pr.2012.185 PMID:23344661.
22. Reindel R, Bischof J, Kim KY, Orenstein JM, Soares MB, Baker SC, et al. CD84 is markedly up-regulated in Kawasaki disease arteriopathy. Clin Exp Immunol. 2014;177(1):203–11. http://dx.doi.org/10.1111/cei.12327 PMID:24635044.
23. Reindel R, Kim KY, Baker SC, Shulman ST, Perlman EJ, Lingen MW, et al. Periostin is upregulated in coronary arteriopathy in Kawasaki disease and is a potential diagnostic biomarker. Pediatr Infect Dis J. 2014;33(6):659–61. http://dx.doi.org/10.1097/INF.0000000000000233 PMID:24476956.

Update on Pathogenesis: Lessons Learned from Animal Models of Disease

Trang T. Duong and Rae S.M. Yeung

Abstract Independent approaches in mouse and human have identified regulation of T-cell activation as the critical factor in determining Kawasaki disease susceptibility and severity in children and suggest a final common pathway of T-cell activation and persistence in disease pathogenesis. This chapter will review evidence that the critical interplay of innate and adaptive immune response leads to enhanced costimulation, survival of pathogenic T-cells, and, ultimately, coronary artery inflammation in Kawasaki disease.

Keywords Kawasaki disease • Pathogenesis • Animal models

Introduction

Genetically determined dysregulation of the immune response is an integral factor in the pathogenesis of Kawasaki disease (KD). Independent approaches in mouse and human have identified regulation of T-cell activation as the critical factor in determining KD susceptibility and severity in children and suggest the presence of a final common pathway in disease pathogenesis. First, a genetic association study of Japanese sib pairs showed that a polymorphism in the *ITPKC* gene—which encodes a kinase (inositol 1,4,5-triphosphate 3-kinase C) that regulates T-cell activation—is associated with susceptibility to and increased severity of KD [1]. A second independent approach, which used an animal model of KD, also identified regulation of T-cell activation and survival as the critical determinant of coronary disease and confirmed the importance of ITPKC in disease pathogenesis. Costimulation, the second signal regulating optimal T-cell activation, has been identified as the critical regulator of susceptibility to and severity of vascular inflammation [2].

T.T. Duong
The Hospital for Sick Children, Cell Biology Research Program, Toronto, ON, Canada

R.S.M. Yeung, M.D., Ph.D., FRCPC (✉)
The Hospital for Sick Children, Cell Biology Research Program, Toronto, ON, Canada

Departments of Paediatrics, Immunology and Institute of Medical Science, University of Toronto, 555 University Avenue, Toronto, ON M5G 1X8, Canada
e-mail: rae.yeung@sickkids.ca

© Springer Japan 2017
B.T. Saji et al. (eds.), *Kawasaki Disease*, DOI 10.1007/978-4-431-56039-5_7

45

T-Cell Activation and Survival and the Role of Costimulation

Optimal T-cell activation requires engagement of the T-cell receptor (TCR) (signal one) and a costimulatory signal (signal two). The second signal is dependent on soluble factors such as interleukin (IL)-2 and ligation of cell surface molecules. Most T-cell surface costimulatory molecules are members of the immunoglobulin and tumor necrosis factor (TNF) superfamilies and are important components of the immunologic synapse. The simultaneous occurrence of signals one and two leads to optimal T-cell activation, as evidenced by IL-2 production and T-cell survival. CD28 and 4-1BB are examples of positive costimulatory receptors. Positive second signals (co-stimulators) enhance and sustain T-cell responses, and co-inhibitors (or negative costimulatory molecules) inhibit TCR mediated responses. Initial T-cell activation is usually dependent on CD28/B7 interaction [3]. The CD28 pathway has a critical role in regulating the development of coronary inflammation in KD and in animal models of the disease [2]. CD28 costimulation promotes survival of TCR-mediated activation of T-cells by up-regulating expression of anti-apoptotic factors such as MCL1, Bcl-x_L, and cFLIP [4]. Indeed, dysregulated lymphocyte survival is a critical factor contributing to autoimmunity, as members of the TNFR family of costimulatory molecules have been identified as risk genes for various autoimmune diseases in multiple, well powered, genetic case-control studies.

The innate immune system, namely, the professional antigen-presenting cells (APCs) such as macrophages and dendritic cells, is important in providing costimulation to T-cells. Danger signals lead to stimulation and maturation of these cells into professional APCs with increased expression of costimulatory molecules. Accumulating evidence in mouse and human indicates that interplay between the innate and adaptive immune system leads to survival of pathogenic T-cells and therefore is an important underlying theme in KD pathogenesis.

A challenge in understanding the immunopathogenesis of KD is the lack of affected tissue from children with KD. To answer questions about immunopathogenesis, we need immune cells and affected heart tissue. However, this is a significant obstacle in KD, as many patients are very young children and it is thus not possible to procure enough biospecimens and affected heart tissue. Disease models are therefore necessary. No animal model completely mimics human disease, but such models have proven to be powerful tools in investigating immunopathology in the context of the whole organism. Use of transgenic or knockout strains, together with newer technologies (CRISPR/Cas9), facilitates identification of key genes that contribute to disease susceptibility or pathogenesis, and animal models can be used to test novel therapeutic concepts and serve as pre-clinical models for drug testing. Although non-murine models of KD exist, including dog [5], rabbit [6], and pig [7] models, this review will focus on lessons learned from murine models and how the results complement findings in affected children.

Murine Models of KD

The three major murine models most commonly used in KD studies are the *Lactobacillus casei, Candida albican*, and Nod1 ligand models. Other models include administration of polysaccharide-peptidoglycan isolated from the cell wall of *Streptococcus pyogenes* [8] and inoculation of bacillus Calmette-Guerin followed by a crude extract of *Mycobacterium intracellulare* [9]. In this review, we will focus on the three most commonly used models, which have greatly illuminated the underlying molecular pathogenic mechanisms of KD and contributed to identification of new drug targets and inception of clinical trials.

The *L. casei* cell wall extract (LCWE)-induced coronary arteritis model of KD was pioneered by Lehman and his group in the mid-1980s [10]. Inbred mouse strains develop coronary arteritis in response to a single intraperitoneal injection of LCWE. A superantigen present in LCWE is responsible for disease induction [11]. The resultant vasculitis is histopathologically very similarly to KD and has a predilection for affecting the coronary arteries and aneurysm formation [10, 11]. This model closely mimics KD and exhibits many of the important features seen in KD patients, including an infectious trigger leading to massive immune involvement, disease susceptibility in the young, a similar disease time course, and the pathology of coronary arteritis. Furthermore, LCWE-induced coronary arteritis is responsive to intravenous immunoglobulin (IVIG), the gold standard therapy for children with KD [12, 13]. After LCWE injection, massive immune activation occurs in the periphery, followed by local infiltration into cardiac tissue by day 3–7. The inflammatory infiltrate is mainly composed of T-cells and intensifies and peaks by day 21–28 [11, 14]. Elastin breakdown, the hallmark of aneurysm formation, and disruption of the intima and media, are detectable by day 42 [15].

This model demonstrated that, whereas IFNγ is not required, TNFα is a critical pro-inflammatory mediator leading to heart disease [16, 17] and that treatment with the TNF-blocking agent etanercept ameliorates disease. These findings provide further support and corroboration for two current clinical trials of TNFα inhibition in children with acute KD [18, 19].

The role of innate immunity has also been demonstrated in this model [14, 20]. Intact innate immune signaling via TLR2 and MyD88 is necessary for development of coronary arteritis [21], which is consistent with detection of augmented TLR2 expression on monocytes in human KD and in the LCWE mouse model [22].

A unique feature of the LCWE model is the development of aneurysm formation, as demonstrated by elastin breakdown of the vessel wall [11, 17]. Subsequent studies using this model revealed involvement of matrix metalloproteinase-9 (MMP9) in this process [23] and that its inhibition leads to better coronary outcomes, suggesting that MMP inhibition is a promising therapeutic strategy for management of KD in children. Conversely, TGFβ suppresses elastin degradation by inhibiting MMP9 activation, and TGFβ inhibition thus worsens elastin breakdown [24], an important clinical lesson regarding the risk of TGFβ inhibition in KD. Furthermore, atorvastatin has the therapeutic potential to modulate T-cell activation and MMP9 production in response to LCWE and TNFα, respectively [25].

IL-1β is crucial in the induction of coronary artery inflammation in the LCWE mouse model, which suggests another potential therapeutic target [20]. In response to LCWE, bone marrow-derived macrophages secrete high levels of IL-1β, which is processed from pro-IL-1β by caspase-1 through the NLRP3 inflammasome. More importantly, LCWE-induced coronary arteritis can be blocked by an IL-1 receptor antagonist. Interestingly, a recent study showed that activation of endothelial inflammasome by LCWE is associated with endothelial dysfunction [26].

Another model of KD was introduced in 1979 by Murata and colleagues [27]. *C. albicans* alkaline extract or *C. albicans* water-soluble fraction (CAWS), when repeatedly given intraperitoneally to certain inbred strains of mice, induces systemic arteritis with a predilection for the coronary artery and aortic root [27–29]. Diseased mice share some histologic features with KD and respond to IVIG treatment [30]. Immune activation was evidenced by the presence of neutrophil activation and elevated levels of pro-inflammatory cytokines such as IL-1β, IL-6, and IL-12 [31, 32]. As is the case for the LCWE murine model, TNFα is important in vasculitis development in this model, and etanercept treatment thus reduces the incidence and severity of CAWS-induced vasculitis [33]. As in the LCWE model, evidence for a role of innate immunity in coronary vasculitis is supported by the finding that CAWS-induced vasculitis is reduced in mice deficient in CC chemokine receptor 2 [34].

Nod1 ligand-mediated coronary arteritis is the most recently described murine model [35]. Nod1 is an intracellular pattern recognition receptor for bacterial peptidoglycan fragments and is important in mediating danger signals in innate immune response. Several synthetic Nod1 ligands, such as γ-D-glutamyl-meso-diaminopimelic acid, FK156, and FK565, induce coronary arteritis at various potencies in mice previously primed with lipopolysaccharide (LPS) for 24 h. When mice are given 4 weekly subacute injections of FK565 with LPS priming each time, they develop panarteritis with dense inflammatory infiltrate consisting mainly of neutrophils and macrophages. The mice do not develop coronary aneurysms, but rupture of elastic fibers in coronary artery is present [35]. A unique feature of this model is that multiple oral administrations of FK565 and LPS priming lead to coronary arteritis and valvulitis in mice. Furthermore, a recent study found that accumulated CD11c+MHC II+ macrophages in the heart play a pathogenic role in this model of coronary arteritis, as disease severity is significantly reduced in CD11c-depleted mice [36]. Arteritis is also reduced in mice lacking CCR2, suggesting that Nod1L stimulates production of chemokines to recruit pathogenic cells to the heart.

In summary, convergence of data from human and mouse suggest that the critical interplay of innate and adaptive immune response leads to T-cell activation and persistence, the final common pathway leading to coronary artery inflammation in KD. This hypothesis is supported by data showing cooperation between the innate and adaptive arms of the immune system in three murine models of KD.

References

1. Onouchi Y, Gunji T, Burns JC, Shimizu C, Newburger JW, Yashiro M, et al. ITPKC functional polymorphism associated with Kawasaki disease susceptibility and formation of coronary artery aneurysms. Nat Genet. 2008;40(1):35–42. http://dx.doi.org/10.1038/ng.2007.59 PMID:18084290.
2. Moolani YD, Yeung RS. The role of co-stimulation in sustaining the immune response in Kawasaki disease. Arthritis Rheum. 2008;58(9):S502.
3. Watts TH. TNF/TNFR family members in costimulation of T cell responses. Annu Rev Immunol. 2005;23(1):23–68. http://dx.doi.org/10.1146/annurev.immunol.23.021704.115839 PMID:15771565.
4. Boise LH, Minn AJ, Noel PJ, June CH, Accavitti MA, Lindsten T, et al. CD28 costimulation can promote T cell survival by enhancing the expression of Bcl-XL. Immunity. 1995;3 (1):87–98. http://dx.doi.org/10.1016/1074-7613(95)90161-2 PMID:7621080.
5. Felsburg PJ, HogenEsch H, Somberg RL, Snyder PW, Glickman LT. Immunologic abnormalities in canine juvenile polyarteritis syndrome: A naturally occurring animal model of Kawasaki disease. Clin Immunol Immunopathol. 1992;65(2):110–18. http://dx.doi.org/10.1016/0090-1229(92)90213-8 PMID:1395127.
6. Onouchi Z, Ikuta K, Nagamatsu K, Tamiya H, Sakakibara Y, Ando M. Coronary artery aneurysms develop in weanling rabbits with serum sickness but not in mature rabbits. An experimental model for Kawasaki disease in humans. Angiology. 1995;46(8):679–87. http://dx.doi.org/10.1177/000331979504600806PMID:7639414.
7. Philip S, Lee WC, Liu SK, Wu MH, Lue HC. A swine model of horse serum-induced coronary vasculitis: an implication for Kawasaki disease. Pediatr Res. 2004;55(2):211–19. http://dx.doi.org/10.1203/01.PDR.0000104151.26375.E5 PMID:14630987.
8. Ohkuni H, Todome Y, Yokomuro K, Kimura Y, Ishizaki M, Fukuda Y, et al. Coronary arteritis in mice after systemic injection of bacterial cell wall peptidoglycan. Jpn Circ J. 1987;51 (12):1357–61. http://dx.doi.org/10.1253/jcj.51.1357PMID:3327953.
9. Nakamura T, Yamamura J, Sato H, Kakinuma H, Takahashi H. Vasculitis induced by immunization with Bacillus Calmette-Guérin followed by atypical mycobacterium antigen: a new mouse model for Kawasaki disease. FEMS Immunol Med Microbiol. 2007;49(3):391–7. http://dx.doi.org/10.1111/j.1574-695X.2007.00217.x PMID:17298582.
10. Lehman TJ, Walker SM, Mahnovski V, McCurdy D. Coronary arteritis in mice following the systemic injection of group B Lactobacillus casei cell walls in aqueous suspension. Arthritis Rheum. 1985;28(6):652–9. http://dx.doi.org/10.1002/art.1780280609 PMID:3924060.
11. Duong TT, Silverman ED, Bissessar MV, Yeung RS. Superantigenic activity is responsible for induction of coronary arteritis in mice: an animal model of Kawasaki disease. Int Immunol. 2003;15(1):79–89. http://dx.doi.org/10.1093/intimm/dxg007 PMID:12502728.
12. Myones BL, Bathoria JM, Lehman TJ, Shulman ST. Human IVIG inhibits Lactobacillus casei-inducible coronary arteritis in a murine model. In: Kato H, editor. The 5th International Kawasaki Disease Symposium. Fukuoka: Elsevier Science; 1995.
13. Lau AC, Duong TT, Ito S, Yeung RS. Intravenous immunoglobulin and salicylate differentially modulate pathogenic processes leading to vascular damage in a model of Kawasaki disease. Arthritis Rheum. 2009;60(7):2131–41. http://dx.doi.org/10.1002/art.24660 PMID:19565485.
14. Schulte DJ, Yilmaz A, Shimada K, Fishbein MC, Lowe EL, Chen S, et al. Involvement of innate and adaptive immunity in a murine model of coronary arteritis mimicking Kawasaki

disease. J Immunol. 2009;183(8):5311–18. http://dx.doi.org/10.4049/jimmunol.
0901395PMID:19786535.

15. Lau AC, Duong TT, Ito S, Yeung RS. Matrix metalloproteinase 9 activity leads to elastin
breakdown in an animal model of Kawasaki disease. Arthritis Rheum. 2008;58(3):854–63.
http://dx.doi.org/10.1002/art.23225 PMID:18311803.

16. Chan WC, Duong TT, Yeung RS. Presence of IFN-gamma does not indicate its necessity for
induction of coronary arteritis in an animal model of Kawasaki disease. J Immunol. 2004;173
(5):3492–503. http://dx.doi.org/10.4049/jimmunol.173.5.3492 PMID:15322214.

17. Hui-Yuen JS, Duong TT, Yeung RS. TNF-alpha is necessary for induction of coronary artery
inflammation and aneurysm formation in an animal model of Kawasaki disease. J Immunol.
2006;176(10):6294–301. http://dx.doi.org/10.4049/jimmunol.176.10.6294PMID:16670341.

18. Burns JC, Best BM, Mejias A, Mahony L, Fixler DE, Jafri HS, et al. Infliximab treatment of
intravenous immunoglobulin-resistant Kawasaki disease. J Pediatr. 2008;153(6):833–8. http://
dx.doi.org/10.1016/j.jpeds.2008.06.011 PMID:18672254.

19. Portman MA, Olson A, Soriano B, Dahdah N, Williams R, Kirkpatrick E. Etanercept as
adjunctive treatment for acute Kawasaki disease: Study design and rationale. Am Heart
J. 2011;161(3):494–9. http://dx.doi.org/10.1016/j.ahj.2010.12.003 PMID:21392603.

20. Lee Y, Schulte DJ, Shimada K, Chen S, Crother TR, Chiba N, et al. Interleukin-1β is crucial for
the induction of coronary artery inflammation in a mouse model of Kawasaki disease.
Circulation. 2012;125(12):1542–50. http://dx.doi.org/10.1161/CIRCULATIONAHA.111.
072769 PMID:22361326.

21. Rosenkranz ME, Schulte DJ, Agle LM, Wong MH, Zhang W, Ivashkiv L, et al. TLR2 and
MyD88 contribute to Lactobacillus casei extract-induced focal coronary arteritis in a mouse
model of Kawasaki disease. Circulation. 2005;112(19):2966–73. PMID:16275884.

22. Lin IC, Kuo HC, Lin YJ, Wang FS, Wang L, Huang SC, et al. Augmented TLR2 expression on
monocytes in both human Kawasaki disease and a mouse model of coronary arteritis. PLoS
One. 2012;7(6), e38635. http://dx.doi.org/10.1371/journal.pone.0038635 PMID:22737215.

23. Lau AC, Duong TT, Ito S, Wilson GJ, Yeung RS. Inhibition of matrix metalloproteinase-9
activity improves coronary outcome in an animal model of Kawasaki disease. Clin Exp
Immunol. 2009;157(2):300–9. http://dx.doi.org/10.1111/j.1365-2249.2009.03949.x
PMID:19604270.

24. Alvira CM, Guignabert C, Kim YM, Chen C, Wang L, Duong TT, et al. Inhibition of
transforming growth factor β worsens elastin degradation in a murine model of Kawasaki
disease. Am J Pathol. 2011;178(3):1210–20. http://dx.doi.org/10.1016/j.ajpath.2010.11.054
PMID:21356372.

25. Blankier S, Lau AC, McCrindle B, Ito S, Yeung RS. HMG-CoA reductase inhibition reduces
T-cell proliferation and MMP-9 gene expression in a superantigenic mouse model of Kawasaki
disease. Arthritis Rheum. 2007;56:S677.

26. Chen Y, Li X, Boini KM, Pitzer AL, Gulbins E, Zhang Y, et al. Endothelial Nlrp3
inflammasome activation associated with lysosomal destabilization during coronary arteritis.
Biochim Biophys Acta. 2015;1853(2):396–408. http://dx.doi.org/10.1016/j.bbamcr.2014.11.
012 PMID:25450976.

27. Murata H. Experimental candida-induced arteritis in mice. Relation to arteritis in the mucocutaneous lymph node syndrome. Microbiol Immunol. 1979;23(9):825–31. http://dx.doi.org/
10.1111/j.1348-0421.1979.tb02815.x PMID:395420.

28. Takahashi K, Oharaseki T, Wakayama M, Yokouchi Y, Naoe S, Murata H. Histopathological
features of murine systemic vasculitis caused by Candida albicans extract—an animal model
of Kawasaki disease. Inflamm Res. 2004;53(2):72–7. http://dx.doi.org/10.1007/s00011-003-
1225-1 PMID:15021972.

29. Ohno N. Murine model of Kawasaki disease induced by mannoprotein-beta-glucan complex,
CAWS, obtained from Candida albicans. Jpn J Infect Dis. 2004;57(5):S9–10.
PMID:15507772.

30. Takahashi K, Oharaseki T, Yokouchi Y, Miura NN, Ohno N, Okawara AI, et al. Administration of human immunoglobulin suppresses development of murine systemic vasculitis induced with Candida albicans water-soluble fraction: an animal model of Kawasaki disease. Mod Rheumatol. 2010;20(2):160–7. http://dx.doi.org/10.3109/s10165-009-0250-5 PMID:19943075.

31. Ishida-Okawara A, Nagi-Miura N, Oharaseki T, Takahashi K, Okumura A, Tachikawa H, et al. Neutrophil activation and arteritis induced by C. albicans water-soluble mannoprotein-beta-glucan complex (CAWS) [CAWS]. Exp Mol Pathol. 2007;82(2):220–6. http://dx.doi.org/10.1016/j.yexmp.2006.05.006 PMID:17208225.

32. Miura NN, Komai M, Adachi Y, Osada N, Kameoka Y, Suzuki K, et al. IL-10 is a negative regulatory factor of CAWS-vasculitis in CBA/J mice as assessed by comparison with Bruton's tyrosine kinase-deficient CBA/N mice. J Immunol. 2009;183(5):3417–24. http://dx.doi.org/10.4049/jimmunol.0802484 PMID:19675170.

33. Oharaseki T, Yokouchi Y, Yamada H, Mamada H, Muto S, Sadamoto K, et al. The role of TNF-α in a murine model of Kawasaki disease arteritis induced with a Candida albicans cell wall polysaccharide. Mod Rheumatol. 2014;24(1):120–8. http://dx.doi.org/10.3109/14397595.2013.854061 PMID:24261768.

34. Martinez HG, Quinones MP, Jimenez F, Estrada C, Clark KM, Suzuki K, et al. Important role of CCR2 in a murine model of coronary vasculitis. BMC Immunol. 2012;13(1):56. http://dx.doi.org/10.1186/1471-2172-13-56 PMID:23074996.

35. Nishio H, Kanno S, Onoyama S, Ikeda K, Tanaka T, Kusuhara K, et al. Nod1 ligands induce site-specific vascular inflammation. Arterioscler Thromb Vasc Biol. 2011;31(5):1093–9. http://dx.doi.org/10.1161/ATVBAHA.110.216325 PMID:21330608.

36. Motomura Y, Kanno S, Asano K, Tanaka M, Hasegawa Y, Katagiri H, et al. Identification of pathogenic cardiac CD11c+ Macrophages in Nod1-Mediated acute coronary arteritis. Arterioscler Thromb Vasc Biol. 2015;35(6):1423–33. http://dx.doi.org/10.1161/ATVBAHA.114.304846 PMID:25838430.

The Climate–KD Link

Jane C. Burns and Daniel R. Cayan

Abstract The agent of Kawasaki disease (KD) remains unknown after more than 40 years of intensive research, but new information from analyses of KD time series from locations worldwide suggests that KD activity is modulated by weather and climate processes. Most Northern Hemisphere locations with a sufficient number of KD cases to allow for analysis exhibit seasonal fluctuations in KD incidence. Analyses of climate variables have linked seasonal and shorter period variations of KD with fluctuations in large-scale tropospheric wind patterns. A recent set of analyses suggests that the KD agent is transported to particular regions by distinct wind flow patterns and that a potential source region for Japan is upstream over northeast China. Analysis of aerosol samples from peak and trough periods of KD activity in Japan is ongoing and will likely yield further insights into the nature of the causative agent.

Keywords Epidemiology • Climate • Tropospheric winds

In an analysis of KD cases in Japan, Nakamura and colleagues were the first to recognize that KD cases cluster spatially over a given region, which suggests that a broad-scale environmental mechanism might be involved [1]. Seasonal fluctuations of KD had been observed in different regions of the world, but it was not until Cayan and colleagues analyzed the entire KD time series of more than 135,000 cases from Japan that a statistically robust analysis revealed the strong seasonality of KD in Japan with two distinct peaks: one in winter and a lesser peak in mid-summer [2]. Later analyses of KD records from a global collection of available KD records revealed that most Northern Hemisphere locations with a sufficient

J.C. Burns, M.D. (✉)
Department of Pediatrics, University of California San Diego School of Medicine,
9500 Gilman Dr., La Jolla, CA 92093-0641, USA

Rady Children's Hospital San Diego, San Diego, CA 92123, USA
e-mail: jcburns@ucsd.edu

D.R. Cayan, Ph.D.
Scripps Institution of Oceanography, University of California San Diego, La Jolla, CA 92093,
USA

© Springer Japan 2017
B.T. Saji et al. (eds.), *Kawasaki Disease*, DOI 10.1007/978-4-431-56039-5_8

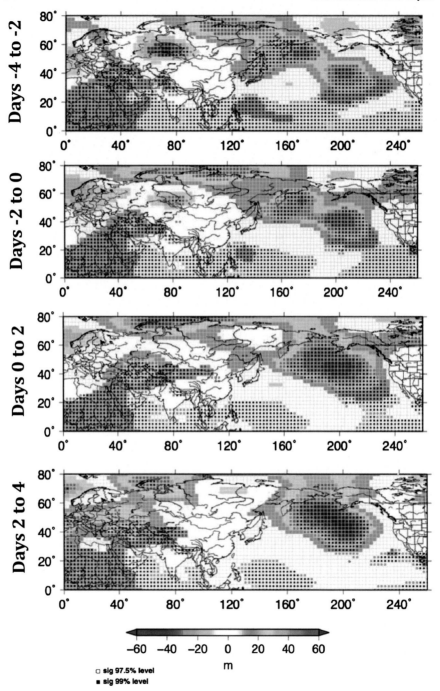

Fig. 1 Analysis of San Diego time series from 2004–2013 revealed 27 periods of at least 10 days duration with no KD patients ("dry spells"). The maps above show a composite of the evolution of the 700-mb height anomaly pattern for these 27 dry spells, averaged over 3 days beginning 4 days

number of KD cases to allow for time-series analyses exhibit seasonal fluctuations in KD incidence [3].

Records of KD cases in San Diego County were used to formally analyze geospatial clustering of cases in a small time series, using the Knox statistic. After the index case, a second case was more likely to be diagnosed within 3–5 days and to have a primary place of residence within a radius of 3 km from the index case [4].

Recent analyses of seasonal variation in KD revealed an association between fluctuations in KD case numbers and large-scale wind patterns in the troposphere, 1–3 km above the Earth's surface [5, 6]. Two seasonal wind patterns were associated with increases in KD cases: (1) a northwesterly flow originating in the mainland of central/eastern Asia that sweeps over Japan and (2) a zonal wind pattern that traverses the North Pacific, spanning from Japan to Hawaii and ultimately reaching the US mainland. The window for both of these wind patterns tended to close each year in early spring, which coincided with a decline in KD cases. An enhanced version of these wind patterns also appeared to operate at interannual time scales in association with periods with exceptionally high numbers of KD cases. These results suggest that the environmental trigger for KD may be transported through winds and that bursts of anomalously high numbers of KD cases may be linked via long-range wind transport across oceans. Conversely, distinctly different flow patterns were associated with periods of low numbers of KD cases across Japan.

A recent analysis of composite atmospheric circulation patterns leading up to periods with low numbers of KD cases ("dry spells") observed in San Diego from 2004–2013 indicates that the "dry spells" are strongly associated with periods after a persistent, anomalously high pressure pattern offshore and over the coast of California. (Fig. 1) This high pressure pattern would block onshore circulation coming from the North Pacific.

We now have further evidence of the link between tropospheric wind patterns and fluctuations in KD cases in Japan and have identified a source region in northeastern China for the aerosols carried by these disease-associated winds [7]. Rodó and colleagues performed back-tracing of the wind using Lagrangian analysis of FLEXPART data and identified a potential source region in northeastern China. Their analysis suggested an extremely short incubation time between

---

Fig. 1 (continued) before the onset of the dry spell (*top panel*). Day 0 is the first day of the dry spell composite. The maps show anomalously high pressure over the eastern North Pacific and offshore of California, which would interrupt the west-to-east airflow that would normally ventilate the southern California region with air masses crossing from the North Pacific. Note that the anomalous high pressure pattern from the composite sequence persists for several days, which is consistent with a long dry spell that lasts at least 10 days. *Yellow/red colors* indicate higher than normal pressures, and *blue/purple colors* indicate lower than normal pressures. Significance is indicated at the 97.5 % level (*open black squares*) and 99 % level (*filled black squares*)

putative exposure and onset of fever, which suggests that a toxin or microbial antigen exposure is more likely than infection with a replicating agent. No relationship to chemicals, industrial pollutants, pollens, or heavy metals was found. Analysis of aerosols collected by research aircraft over Japan in March 2011, before the Tohoku earthquake, identified many microbial species, but Candida sp. were most prominent. Further analysis of aerosols trapped on filters collected during peak and trough periods of disease activity in Japan is in progress. Given the proposed short incubation period, it is possible that an antigenic trigger rather than an infectious agent is the cause of KD. In support of this hypothesis, an analysis of age-incidence patterns indicated that KD was unlikely to be caused by a single, acute, immunizing infection [8].

There is no known disease of humans caused by organisms lofted into the wind on one continent, carried across a large body of water, and inhaled by persons in a distant region who then develop disease. Although studies have documented a rich microbiome in the troposphere, little is known about how these organisms or their toxins may impact human health. [9]. As a proof-of-principle example, analysis of large-scale wind patterns and microbiologic sampling of air currents revealed long-range transport over the Atlantic Ocean of fungal spores of *Aspergillus sydowii*, which lofted into tropospheric wind currents during Saharan dust storms [10]. These spores carried within dust particles were then deposited into the Caribbean and caused a fatal infection in *Gorgonia* fan coral [11]. Similarly, long-distance aerial dispersal has been shown for pathogens of crop plants, with transport of fungal spores by the wind and spreading of plant diseases between continents [12]. The recent publication of an analysis of intercontinental transport of over 10,000 different microbial species on tropospheric wind currents has led us to consider the possibility that the troposphere is a new ecologic niche inhabited by a rich and diverse microbiome [13]. The extent to which pathogenic organisms that cause diseases in humans, animals, and plants may be transported around the globe is unknown. Another large unknown is whether chemical processing of molecules in aerosols as they pass through clouds can create toxins from previously benign molecules. In addition, heavy metals such as zinc and mercury can be transported on aerosolized particles and act as haptens that render antigenic the proteins to which they bind. The implications for human health may be highly significant, and KD may be the first human disease to be linked to inhaled aerosols transported on tropospheric wind currents from distant sites.

References

1. Nakamura Y, Yanagawa I, Kawasaki T. Temporal and geographical clustering of Kawasaki disease in Japan. Prog Clin Biol Res. 1987;250:19–32. PMID:3423038.
2. Burns JC, Cayan DR, Tong G, Bainto EV, Turner CL, Shike H, et al. Seasonality and temporal clustering of Kawasaki syndrome. Epidemiology. 2005;16(2):220–5. http://dx.doi.org/10. 1097/01.ede.0000152901.06689.d4 PMID:15703537.

3. Burns JC, Herzog L, Fabri O, Tremoulet AH, Rodó X, Uehara R, et al. Kawasaki Disease Global Climate Consortium. Seasonality of Kawasaki disease: a global perspective. PLoS One. 2013;8(9), e74529. http://dx.doi.org/10.1371/journal.pone.0074529 PMID:24058585.

4. Kao AS, Getis A, Brodine S, Burns JC. Spatial and temporal clustering of Kawasaki syndrome cases. Pediatr Infect Dis J. 2008;27(11):981–5. http://dx.doi.org/10.1097/INF. 0b013e31817acf4f PMID:18852687.

5. Rodó X, Ballester J, Cayan D, Melish ME, Nakamura Y, Uehara R, et al. Association of Kawasaki disease with tropospheric wind patterns. Sci Rep. 2011;1:152. http://dx.doi.org/10. 1038/srep00152 PMID:22355668.

6. Frazer J. Infectious disease: blowing in the wind. Nature. 2012;484(7392):21–3. http://dx.doi. org/10.1038/484021a PMID:22481336.

7. Rodó X, Curcoll R, Robinson M, Ballester J, Burns JC, Cayan DR, et al. Tropospheric winds from northeastern China carry the etiologic agent of Kawasaki disease from its source to Japan. Proc Natl Acad Sci U S A. 2014;111(22):7952–7. http://dx.doi.org/10.1073/pnas.1400380111 PMID:24843117.

8. Pitzer VE, Burgner D, Viboud C, Simonsen L, Andreasen V, Steiner CA, et al. Modelling seasonal variations in the age and incidence of Kawasaki disease to explore possible infectious aetiologies. Proc Biol Sci. 2012;279(1739):2736–43. http://dx.doi.org/10.1098/rspb.2011. 2464 PMID:22398170.

9. DeLeon-Rodriguez N, Lathem TL, Rodriguez-R LM, Barazesh JM, Anderson BE, Beyersdorf AJ, et al. Microbiome of the upper troposphere: species composition and prevalence, effects of tropical storms, and atmospheric implications. Proc Natl Acad Sci U S A. 2013;110 (7):2575–80. http://dx.doi.org/10.1073/pnas.1212089110 PMID:23359712.

10. Fujino Y, Attizzani GF, Tahara S, Takagi K, Bezerra HG, Nakamura S, et al. Frequency-domain optical coherence tomography evaluation of a patient with Kawasaki disease and severely calcified plaque. Int J Cardiol. 2014;171(2):281–3. http://dx.doi.org/10.1016/j.ijcard. 2013.11.084 PMID:24365617.

11. Zhang X, Sun J, Zhai S, Yang S. Kawasaki disease in two sets of monozygotic twins: is the etiology genetic or environmental? Pak J Med Sci. 2013;29(1):227–30. PMID:24353547.

12. Liu F, Ding Y, Yin W. Expression of sICAM-1 in children with intravenous immunoglobulin-resistant Kawasaki disease. Zhongguo Dang Dai Er Ke Za Zhi. 2013;15(12):1109–12. PMID:24342209.

13. Smith DJ, Timonen HJ, Jaffe DA, Griffin DW, Birmele MN, Perry KD, et al. Intercontinental dispersal of bacteria and archaea by transpacific winds. Appl Environ Microbiol. 2013;79 (4):1134–9. http://dx.doi.org/10.1128/AEM.03029-12 PMID:23220959.

Kawasaki Disease Shock Syndrome

Ming-Tai Lin and Mei-Hwan Wu

Abstract Hemodynamic instability is relatively uncommon during the acute phase of Kawasaki disease. This condition is referred to as Kawasaki disease shock syndrome (KDSS), and in this chapter we review the epidemiology, proposed mechanisms, clinical course, and treatment of KDSS. Differential diagnosis of KDSS and toxic shock syndrome is also discussed. The overlap between these two disease entities may provide clues for future studies.

Keywords Kawasaki disease • Shock • Risk factors

Introduction

In the acute phase of Kawasaki disease (KD), hemodynamic instability is less common than development of coronary artery complications. Hemodynamic instability, such as hypotension or clinical signs of poor perfusion, is referred to as KD shock syndrome (KDSS). KDSS is defined as an episode during acute KD of hypotension or shock requiring volume expanders, infusion of vasoactive agents, or transfer to intensive care units [1].

Incidence and Demographics

The incidence of KDSS varied among study cohorts. Kanegaye et al. [1] reported that approximately 7 % of KD patients admitted to Rady Children's Hospital developed KDSS. Gamez-Gonzalez et al. [2] studied 214 Mexican children with KD and found that 11 (5.1 %) met the definition of KDSS. In a study of the national health insurance database of Taiwan for the period 2000–2009, Lin et al. [3] found that the incidence of KDSS was 1.45 per 100 KD cases (range in annual incidence,

M.-T. Lin, M.D., Ph.D. • M.-H. Wu, M.D., Ph.D. (✉)
Department of Pediatrics, National Taiwan University Hospital, No. 8, Chung-Shan South Road, Taipei 100, Taiwan
e-mail: mingtailin@ntu.edu.tw; wumh@ntu.edu.tw

© Springer Japan 2017
B.T. Saji et al. (eds.), *Kawasaki Disease*, DOI 10.1007/978-4-431-56039-5_9

Table 1 Demographic characteristics of Kawasaki disease (KD) patients with and without KD shock syndrome[a]

	All KD (n = 9488)	Subgroups		
		KD without shock (n = 9350)	KDSS (n = 138)	P value
Male gender	61.9%	61.8%	69.6%	.061
Age in months, median (IQR)	17.87 (9.16–34.9)	17.78 (9.17–34.78)	23.2 (10.4–45.9)	.031
Hospitalization duration, in days, median (IQR)	5 (3–7)	5 (3–7)	8 (6–14)	<.001
Coronary artery lesions (%)	679 (7.1%)	657 (7.0%)	22 (15.9%)	<.001

Among 9488 patients with KD, 138 developed KD shock syndrome
IQR interquartile range
[a]Modified from a table by Lin et al. [3]

0.9–1.98%). The incidence of KDSS seems to be higher in Western countries than in Asia.

The demographics of patients with KDSS and a comparison of KD patients with and without KDSS are shown in Table 1, which is modified from our previous study [3]. KDSS patients had a higher risk of coronary artery lesions (CALs) and longer hospital stays. Several studies reported that KDSS patients were more likely than KD patients without hemodynamic instability to be resistant to intravenous immunoglobulin (up to 46–60%) and to develop CALs (15.9–62.7%) [1, 2, 4]. In addition, KDSS patients were more likely to develop gallop and mitral regurgitation and had lower left ventricular ejection fractions during the acute stage [4, 5]. With regard to laboratory data, KDSS patients tend to have lower hemoglobin concentrations, larger proportions of bands, lower platelet counts, higher C-reactive protein levels, and a greater risk of consumptive coagulopathy [4, 5].

Mechanisms

The causes, risk factors, and pathophysiological mechanism of KDSS are unclear. Laboratory data suggest that KDSS is associated with increased underlying inflammation. The higher frequency of consumptive coagulopathy in patients with KDSS indicates that vasculitis is more severe. Associated myocardial dysfunction could also contribute to hemodynamic instability. Echocardiographic studies often show impaired ventricular relaxation, elevation of left ventricular end-diastolic pressure, and decreased ventricular compliance, which are uncommon in KD patients without KDSS [1]. Therefore, shock in KD can be cardiogenic and/or distributive.

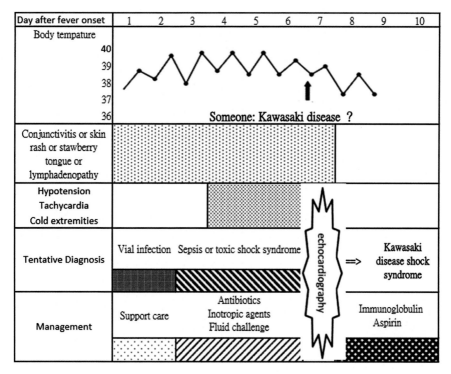

Fig. 1 Typical clinical presentation of patients with Kawasaki disease shock syndrome

Clinical Course and Treatment

The typical clinical course is shown in Fig. 1. Hemodynamic instability usually occurs within 1 week after fever onset. It is sometimes difficult to differentiate between toxic shock syndrome (TSS) and KDSS, although echocardiographic evaluation is helpful for this purpose. In addition to intravenous immunoglobulin, supportive management for shock is important. Because vasculitis and myocardial dysfunction contribute to KDSS development, patients with these conditions usually need vasoactive agents such as dopamine. Patients with KDSS require close monitoring and might need hemodynamic support in an intensive care unit. Use of fluid resuscitation and inodilator therapy (eg, milrinone) should be based on cautious monitoring of cardiac output, central venous pressure, and systemic vascular resistance. As yet, there are no randomized controlled studies of the effects of concurrent use of steroids in this subgroup of KD patients.

Table 2 Differences in the clinical presentation of Kawasaki disease shock syndrome and toxic shock syndrome

	Kawasaki disease shock syndrome	Toxic shock syndrome
Usual age [7]	<5 years	>10 years
Fever	Indistinguishable	
Oral mucosa		
Extremities		
Skin rash		
Lymphadenopathy [7]	More frequent	Less frequent
End organ involvement [8]	More coronary involvement	More renal and central nervous system involvement
Identifiable focus	Rare	Frequent

Differential Diagnosis

Toxic shock syndrome (TSS) is also an acute multisystem disease characterized by fever, hypotension, erythematous rash with subsequent desquamation on the hands and feet, and multisystem involvement (i.e., ≥ 3 of the following clinical features: involvement of mucous membranes [conjunctiva and/or tongue], vomiting and/or diarrhea, liver or renal dysfunction, myalgia, and nonfocal neurologic abnormalities) [6].

The clinical presentation of KDSS closely resembles that of TSS. Differential diagnosis may be difficult and can be aided by the following differences in clinical presentation. First, nonmenstrual TSS in children is usually associated with an identifiable focus of *Staphylococcus* or *Streptococcus* infection, such as wound infection, sinusitis, empyema, and pneumonia [7]. The clinical course of TSS is usually rapidly progressive, with abrupt onset of high fever [7]. A diffuse erythematous macular rash appears within 24 h in TSS. Renal involvement, together with elevation of creatinine phosphokinase, is quite common in TSS but rare in KDSS [7]. Although myocardial involvement is characteristic of both TSS and KDSS, coronary vasculitis is more specific for a diagnosis of KD. We summarize the differences in the clinical presentation of KDSS and TSS in Table 2.

Future Perspectives

Hemodynamic instability during acute KD, which may be less common than the development of CAL, should be regarded as a distinct disease entity. Prompt recognition and proper cardiac and fluid support are essential. The pathophysiology and genetic susceptibility to this condition are unclear. However, the overlap between KDSS and TSS provides intriguing clues for future studies.

References

1. Kanegaye JT, Wilder MS, Molkara D, Frazer JR, Pancheri J, Tremoulet AH, et al. Recognition of a Kawasaki disease shock syndrome. Pediatrics. 2009;123(5):e783–9. http://dx.doi.org/10.1542/peds.2008-1871 PMID:19403470.
2. Gámez-González LB, Murata C, Muñoz-Ramírez M, Yamazaki-Nakashimada M. Clinical manifestations associated with Kawasaki disease shock syndrome in Mexican children. Eur J Pediatr. 2013;172(3):337–42. http://dx.doi.org/10.1007/s00431-012-1879-1 PMID:23152158.
3. Lin MT, Fu CM, Huang SK, Huang SC, Wu MH. Population-based study of Kawasaki disease shock syndrome in Taiwan. Pediatr Infect Dis J. 2013;32(12):1384–6. http://dx.doi.org/10.1097/INF.0b013e31829efae6 PMID:23748909.
4. Dominguez SR, Friedman K, Seewald R, Anderson MS, Willis L, Glodé MP. Kawasaki disease in a pediatric intensive care unit: a case-control study. Pediatrics. 2008;122(4):e786–90. http://dx.doi.org/10.1542/peds.2008-1275 PMID:18809597.
5. Luca NJ, Yeung RS. Epidemiology and management of Kawasaki disease. Drugs. 2012;72(8):1029–38. http://dx.doi.org/10.2165/11631440-000000000-00000 PMID:22621692.
6. Todd JK. Toxic shock syndrome. Nelson textbook of pediatrics. 19th ed. Chap 174. 2.
7. Yanagihara R, Todd JK. Acute febrile mucocutaneous lymph node syndrome. Am J Dis Child. 1980;134(6):603–14. PMID:6104439.
8. Rowley AH, Shulman ST. Kawasaki syndrome. Clin Microbiol Rev. 1998;11(3):405–14. PMID:9665974.

Future Directions in Kawasaki Disease Research

Jane C. Burns

Abstract After almost five decades since the publication of Dr. Kawasaki's land-mark paper in 1967, the etiology of Kawasaki disease (KD) and many aspects of its pathophysiology remain obscure [1, 2]. Although there are over 5000 articles in the English-language, peer-reviewed literature on various aspects of KD, there remain many important unanswered questions. To discover the best path forward, it may be instructive to look at how progress has been achieved in the past.

Keywords Treatment • Genetics • Epidemiology • Research

Advances in Treatment

A major breakthrough in the care of KD patients was the discovery that intravenous immunoglobulin (IVIG) was an effective therapy for reducing the risk of coronary artery aneurysms. This major advance in the care of KD patients came from observations by investigators at a single center in Japan, which were further tested in a large, randomized clinical trial by a collaborative group of investigators in the United States [3, 4]. This large-scale collaboration enrolled adequate numbers of subjects and had sufficient statistical power to test the hypotheses and led to a definitive trial that firmly established IVIG as the treatment of choice for KD. The necessary ingredients for success were strict adherence to best practices for modern clinical trials and securing adequate funding to conduct the trial. More than two decades later, the RAISE trial in Japan studied a subset of patients at highest risk for aneurysm development, as determined by risk scoring, and demonstrated a benefit in reduction in aneurysm rate for the group receiving an extended period of steroid therapy in addition to IVIG and moderate-dose aspirin [5]. Again, the trial required the collaboration of multiple investigators and sufficient funding to provide oversight and standardization of procedures across all the clinical sites.

J.C. Burns, M.D. (✉)
Department of Pediatrics, Rady Children's Hospital San Diego, San Diego, CA, USA

University of California San Diego School of Medicine, 9500 Gilman Dr., La Jolla, CA 92093-0641, USA
e-mail: jcburns@ucsd.edu

© Springer Japan 2017

65

B.T. Saji et al. (eds.), *Kawasaki Disease*, DOI 10.1007/978-4-431-56039-5_10

The key to both of these successful trials was enrollment of sufficient numbers of subjects to test the hypotheses proposed. This was only possible through collaboration of sufficient numbers of sites, which allowed timely completion of the trials. Now, in an era of reduced funding for biomedical research, how will we continue to make progress in devising new therapies for our patients? Will we be able to secure funding for the "gold standard" randomized, placebo-controlled, double-blind clinical trial? What other options might be explored? Perhaps we could learn from the advances in pediatric oncology that were achieved through the use of standardized protocols across large numbers of clinical centers with centralized clinical trial design and standardized implementation across all participating sites. This type of grand vision might be difficult to achieve in an environment of constrained funding. However, the protocol-driven care of all KD patients could be a goal to which we can aspire.

Another option could be the standardization of care using a strict protocol within a given center followed by comparison of outcomes across sites using different therapies but all following strict protocols. This could be implemented for therapies for which there is currently clinical equipoise, such as the choice between second IVIG and infliximab for IVIG-resistant patients. Each center would need to have Investigational Review Board approval and signed consent forms from participants, but the consents would only cover sharing of data rather than the actual treatment, since the treatment administered at that site would be the local standard of care. Even retrospective studies across centers with protocol-driven care could provide useful information, as in a study that compared treatments for IVIG-resistance between two US sites [6]. For studies examining treatments and coronary artery outcomes, acquisition of images could be standardized and a core lab could be designated to interpret all echocardiograms across sites. With the wide adoption of the electronic medical record, there should be new opportunities for data mining across centers that follow protocol-driven care of KD patients.

Advances in Genetics

Another success of the last several decades has been the discovery of variants that influence genetic susceptibility to disease in both Asian and non-Asian populations [7, 8]. These efforts were possible only through collaborations that spanned not only countries but also continents [9]. The gold standard of genotyping in a discovery cohort, followed by validation in an independent cohort, requires thousands of DNA samples from both cases and controls. This effort, by definition, requires collaboration among large numbers of investigators [10, 11]. The successes to date have suggested new therapeutic approaches, including the use of calcineurin inhibitors to block the calcium signaling pathway and statins to block the TGFβ signaling pathway [12–16]. To make further progress in this area, it is necessary for more clinicians to join established groups in collecting DNA from carefully phenotyped KD patients. Concomitant collection of acute and convalescent whole-blood RNA samples allows assessment of the impact of the proposed variant on gene expression [17]. Coordinated efforts across populations in different countries and the creation of carefully curated banks of DNA and RNA samples with appropriate patient permission for the sharing of samples will accelerate discovery in defining the genetic patterns responsible for susceptibility to KD, response to therapy, and coronary artery outcomes. In addition, all genomic and genetic data should be deposited into databanks, such as the iDASH data repository, so that investigators could apply for access and use of data for future studies in collaboration with the group that originally generated the data. Unfortunately, many of these datasets are currently locked behind firewalls and not available to other groups. This clearly has impeded the pace of discovery in this arena.

Advances in Biomarkers and Diagnostic Tests

A major limitation in the discovery of biomarkers and aids to diagnosis and clinical prognostication has been the failure to utilize appropriate control samples. For a biomarker for KD diagnosis, the relevant control group must be young children with fever and at least one of the mucocutaneous signs of KD. It is not relevant to use patients with primary gastrointestinal or respiratory disease as a control group for these types of studies. Because so many of the diseases in the differential diagnosis of KD share inflammation and activation of coagulation as features of the disease process, candidate single-protein biomarkers in these pathways are unlikely to be sufficiently robust in separating KD patients from controls. Failure to use proper statistical techniques to evaluate proposed biomarkers has also hampered progress in this field. Moving forward, collaboration should be improved with colleagues in clinics, emergency departments, and urgent care settings who can collect relevant controls samples. Biostatisticians must be incorporated into the research team to provide direction in both study design from the outset and statistical analysis of the data at the end of the study. Again, collaboration across sites is needed in order to ensure adequate numbers of subjects for these studies.

Advances in Understanding Long-Term Outcomes

Without national and international patient registries that provide longitudinal data on long-term patient outcomes, we will continue to lack adequate answers to the question most frequently posed by parents: What does this mean for my child in the future? In Japan, a large cohort study of over 6000 subjects was initiated in 1992, to follow these patients longitudinally [18]. In the United States, a recent initiative through the Coordination of Rare Diseases at Sanford (CoRDS) research group and the parent-based KD Foundation will offer a web-based registry for families and individuals with KD to help track patients over time. Another initiative, from The

Adult KD Collaborative Study at the University of California San Diego (adultkd@ucsd.edu), will track health trends in adult KD patients over time. In India, where KD is newly emergent, there as been a call to establish a registry [19]. These efforts should be applauded, and creation of such registries should be expanded to allow tracking of patient outcomes over time.

In summary, the first five decades of KD research have taught us that significant progress can only be made through large-scale collaboration, sharing of data, and standardization of patient care protocols. Funding for such efforts will continue to be a challenge, and creative approaches to using the electronic medical record and data mining and analysis should be considered in order to circumvent the need for the gold standard, but expensive, randomized, placebo-controlled clinical trial. Sharing of data in a usable format should be mandated and enforced by funding agencies to accelerate the process of discovery. More collaboration and data sharing and better tracking of patient outcomes will take us to the next level in KD research.

References

1. Shike H, Burns JC, Shimizu C. English translation of Dr. Tomisaku Kawasaki's original report of fifty patients in 1967 (in Japanese). Pediatr Infect Dis J. 2002;21:993. http://dx.doi.org/10. 1097/00006454-200211000-00002 PMID:12442017.
2. Kawasaki T. Acute febrile mucocutaneous syndrome with lymphoid involvement with specific desquamation of the fingers and toes in children. Arerugi. 1967;16(3):178–222. PMID:6062087.
3. Furusho K, Kamiya T, Nakano H, Kiyosawa N, Shinomiya K, Hayashidera T, et al. High-dose intravenous gammaglobulin for Kawasaki disease. Lancet. 1984;2(8411):1055–8. http://dx. doi.org/10.1016/S0140-6736(84)91504-6 PMID:6209513.
4. Newburger JW, Takahashi M, Burns JC, Beiser AS, Chung KJ, Duffy CE, et al. The treatment of Kawasaki syndrome with intravenous gamma globulin. N Engl J Med. 1986;315(6):341–7. http://dx.doi.org/10.1056/NEJM198608073150601 PMID:2426590.
5. Kobayashi T, Saji T, Otani T, Takeuchi K, Nakamura T, Arakawa H, et al. RAISE study group investigators. Efficacy of immunoglobulin plus prednisolone for prevention of coronary artery abnormalities in severe Kawasaki disease (RAISE study): a randomised, open-label, blinded-endpoints trial. Lancet. 2012;379(9826):1613–20. http://dx.doi.org/10.1016/S0140-6736(11) 61930-2 PMID:22405251.
6. Son MB, Gauvreau K, Burns JC, Corinaldesi E, Tremoulet AH, Watson VE, et al. Infliximab for intravenous immunoglobulin resistance in Kawasaki disease: a retrospective study. J Pediatr. 2011;158(4):644–9 e1. http://dx.doi.org/10.1016/j.jpeds.2010.10.012.
7. Onouchi Y. Genetics of Kawasaki disease: what we know and don't know. Circ J. 2012;76 (7):1581–6. http://dx.doi.org/10.1253/circj.CJ-12-0568 PMID:22789975.
8. Onouchi Y. Molecular genetics of Kawasaki disease. Pediatr Res. 2009;65(5 Pt 2):46R–54R. http://dx.doi.org/10.1203/PDR.0b013e31819dba60 PMID:19190534.
9. Khor CC, Davila S, Breunis WB, Lee YC, Shimizu C, Wright VJ, et al. Hong Kong–shanghai Kawasaki disease genetics consortium; Korean Kawasaki disease genetics consortium; Taiwan Kawasaki disease genetics consortium; international Kawasaki disease genetics consortium; US Kawasaki disease genetics consortium; blue mountains Eye study. Genome-wide association study identifies FCGR2A as a susceptibility locus for Kawasaki disease. Nat Genet. 2011;43(12)):1241–6. http://dx.doi.org/10.1038/ng.981 PMID:22081228.

10. Kuo HC, Hsu YW, Wu CM, Chen SH, Hung KS, Chang WP, et al. A replication study for association of ITPKC and CASP3 two-locus analysis in IVIG unresponsiveness and coronary artery lesion in Kawasaki disease. PLoS One. 2013;8(7), e69685. http://dx.doi.org/10.1371/journal.pone.0069685 PMID:23894522.

11. Shrestha S, Wiener H, Shendre A, Kaslow RA, Wu J, Olson A, et al. Role of activating FcγR gene polymorphisms in Kawasaki disease susceptibility and intravenous immunoglobulin response. Circ Cardiovasc Genet. 2012;5(3):309–16. http://dx.doi.org/10.1161/CIRCGENETICS.111.962464 PMID:22565545.

12. Onouchi Y, Gunji T, Burns JC, Shimizu C, Newburger JW, Yashiro M, et al. ITPKC functional polymorphism associated with Kawasaki disease susceptibility and formation of coronary artery aneurysms. Nat Genet. 2008;40(1):35–42. http://dx.doi.org/10.1038/ng.2007.59 PMID:18084290.

13. Tremoulet AH, Pancoast P, Franco A, Bujold M, Shimizu C, Onouchi Y, et al. Calcineurin inhibitor treatment of intravenous immunoglobulin-resistant Kawasaki disease. J Pediatr. 2012;161(3):506–12 e1.

14. Suzuki H, Terai M, Hamada H, Honda T, Suenaga T, Takeuchi T, et al. Cyclosporin a treatment for Kawasaki disease refractory to initial and additional intravenous immunoglobulin. Pediatr Infect Dis J. 2011;30(10):871–6. http://dx.doi.org/10.1097/INF.0b013e318220c3cf PMID:21587094.

15. Kuo HC, Onouchi Y, Hsu YW, Chen WC, Huang JD, Huang YH, et al. Polymorphisms of transforming growth factor-β signaling pathway and Kawasaki disease in the Taiwanese population. J Hum Genet. 2011;56(12):840–5. http://dx.doi.org/10.1038/jhg.2011.113 PMID:22011813.

16. Shimizu C, Oharaseki T, Takahashi K, Kottek A, Franco A, Burns JC. The role of TGF-β and myofibroblasts in the arteritis of Kawasaki disease. Hum Pathol. 2013;44(2):189–98. http://dx.doi.org/10.1016/j.humpath.2012.05.004 PMID:22955109.

17. Burgner D, Davila S, Breunis WB, Ng SB, Li Y, Bonnard C, et al. International Kawasaki disease genetics consortium. A genome-wide association study identifies novel and functionally related susceptibility loci for Kawasaki disease. PLoS Genet. 2009;5(1):e1000319. http://dx.doi.org/10.1371/journal.pgen.1000319 PMID:19132087.

18. Nakamura Y, Yanagawa H, Kato H. Kawasaki T; Kawasaki disease follow-up group. Mortality rates for patients with a history of Kawasaki disease in Japan. J Pediatr. 1996;128(1):75–81. http://dx.doi.org/10.1016/S0022-3476(96)70430-4 PMID:8551424.

19. Khubchandani R. Kawasaki disease--call for a national registry for India. Indian Pediatr. 2010;47(2):200. PMID:20228443.

Part II
Epidemiology

Epidemiologic Perspectives

Jane C. Burns

Abstract Epidemiology is the branch of medical science that deals with the incidence, distribution, and control of disease in a population. It has long been the hope that epidemiologic research would provide clues to the central mystery of Kawasaki disease: its etiology. New insights regarding the seasonality of KD and the relationship to wind patterns may now indeed lead us to the answer.

Keywords Race • Ethnicity • Epidemiology • Research

Historical Perspective

There has been considerable debate as to whether KD is a new or old disease. Most current opinion regards KD as an old but rare disease in the West and a new disease in the East [1–4]. The emergence of KD in India is a fascinating case study of the apparent introduction of a new disease into a population with a high incidence of many other pediatric illnesses characterized by rash and fever, including rheumatic fever, rubella, rubeola, and varicella. Current estimates indicate that the number of KD cases in India has surpassed the number of cases of rheumatic fever [5]. KD has now been described on every continent and in all races and ethnicities. Careful tracking of cases in time and space has led to important new hypotheses about etiology. But if we are to make further progress in the future, worldwide KD surveillance must be improved.

J.C. Burns, M.D. (✉)
Department of Pediatrics, Rady Children's Hospital San Diego, San Diego, CA, USA

University of California San Diego School of Medicine, 9500 Gilman Dr., La Jolla, CA 92093-0641, USA
e-mail: jcburns@ucsd.edu

© Springer Japan 2017
B.T. Saji et al. (eds.), *Kawasaki Disease*, DOI 10.1007/978-4-431-56039-5_11

KD Surveillance: Moving Forward

The Japanese dataset of KD cases, which was initiated in the first national survey in 1970, remains the most robust resource for KD research [6]. The systematic, questionnaire-based surveys, which are conducted every 2 years, have become a model for many other countries around the world, including China, Korea, and Taiwan[7–9]. Detailed epidemiologic investigation is facilitated in countries with national health care systems linked to patient databases, such as Taiwan and countries in Northern Europe, and many interesting studies have emerged [10, 11]. Unfortunately, the one country that is a major outlier in tracking KD cases over time is the United States. There is no systematic, mandated reporting of U.S. KD cases. Thus, epidemiologic surveys have relied on single-center active surveillance, passive national reporting to the Centers for Disease Control and Prevention, or insurance and other administrative databases that were not created for the purposes of epidemiologic research [12–14]. In an era of decreasing funds for public health surveillance and research, other strategies must be devised to create robust datasets for epidemiologic research.

One such strategy could take advantage of the electronic medical record and International Classification of Disease (ICD) codes. The ICD-9 code for KD is 446.1, and the ICD-10 code is M30.3. These codes are not shared with any other disease, making this a robust tool for tracking KD patients. Currently, U.S. databases, such as the Pediatric Hospital Information Service, which tracks detailed hospitalization charges and associated codes from 44 pediatric hospitals across the United States, have been used to perform epidemiologic surveys [15]. However, the distribution of hospitals is uneven across the United States, and the sampling only captures patients hospitalized in the 44 member institutions. A better method would be a query of all hospitals using an electronic medical record (EMR) system across a given geographic region or even the entire country. As the EMR is further developed as a research tool, this should become possible in the future for collection of de-identified data about KD patients.

KD Surveillance: Prescription for the Future

In a recent effort to develop a snapshot of KD worldwide, time series from 25 countries were collected and analyzed for seasonality [16] (Fig. 1). The presence of seasonal variation in KD at individual locations was evaluated using three different tests: time series modeling, spectral analysis, and a Monte Carlo technique. The study found a broad coherence in fluctuations in KD cases across the Northern Hemisphere extra-tropical latitudes, where KD case numbers were highest in January through March and approximately 40 % higher than in the months with the lowest case numbers, namely, August through October (Fig. 1). The time series for locations in the tropics and extra-tropical Southern Hemisphere

KD Seasonality
Strength indicted by circle size and month of max/min indicated by color

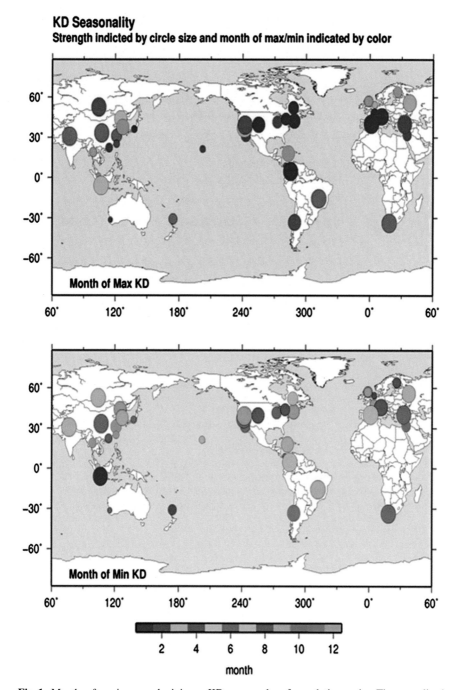

Fig. 1 Months of maximum and minimum KD case numbers for each time series. The normalized amplitude of the seasonal difference (maximum case numbers minus minimum case numbers) is indicated by *circle size*. The month of maximum case numbers (*upper map*) and month of minimum case numbers (*lower map*) are indicated by *circle color*. The number of Northern hemisphere cases was 40 % higher in January through March than in August through October

were sparse, and no robust statistical conclusion regarding seasonal coherence could be drawn. However, the analysis for the Southern Hemisphere suggested a maximum in May through June, with an approximately 30 % higher number of cases than in the least active months of February, March, and October. This was the first attempt at a global analysis of KD cases. Going forward, collection of comprehensive time series will allow a more robust analysis of seasonality, clustering of cases, and changes in KD trends over time. Use of national health system databases and individual hospital EMRs should yield a detailed snapshot of global KD activity. Analysis of global KD time series will allow testing of hypotheses about etiology and should be actively pursued.

References

1. Burns JC, Kushner HI, Bastian JF, Shike H, Shimizu C, Matsubara T, et al. Kawasaki disease: a brief history. Pediatrics. 2000;106(2), E27. http://dx.doi.org/10.1542/peds.106.2.e27 PMID:10920183.
2. Kushner HI, Bastian JF, Turner CL, Burns JC. The two emergencies of Kawasaki syndrome and the implications for the developing world. Pediatr Infect Dis J. 2008;27(5):377–83. http://dx.doi.org/10.1097/INF.0b013e318166d795 PMID:18398382.
3. Kushner HI, Macnee RP, Burns JC. Kawasaki disease in India: increasing awareness or increased incidence? Perspect Biol Med. 2009;52(1):17–29. http://dx.doi.org/10.1353/pbm.0.0062 PMID:19168941.
4. Kushner HI, Abramowsky CR. An old autopsy report sheds light on a "new" disease: infantile polyarteritis nodosa and Kawasaki disease. Pediatr Cardiol. 2010;31(4):490–6. http://dx.doi.org/10.1007/s00246-009-9625-9 PMID:20054530.
5. Singh S, Aulakh R, Bhalla AK, Suri D, Manojkumar R, Narula N, et al. Is Kawasaki disease incidence rising in Chandigarh, north India? Arch Dis Child. 2011;96(2):137–40. http://dx.doi.org/10.1136/adc.2010.194001 PMID:20923951.
6. Yanagawa H, Nakamura Y, Yashiro M, Fujita Y, Nagai M, Kawasaki T, et al. A nationwide incidence survey of Kawasaki disease in 1985–1986 in Japan. J Infect Dis. 1988;158(6):1296–301. http://dx.doi.org/10.1093/infdis/158.6.1296 PMID:3198940.
7. Jiao F, Yang L, Li Y, Qiao J, Guo X, Zhang T, et al. Epidemiologic and clinical characteristics of Kawasaki disease in Shaanxi province, China, 1993–1997. J Trop Pediatr. 2001;47(1):54–6. http://dx.doi.org/10.1093/tropej/47.1.54 PMID:11245353.
8. Park YW, Park IS, Kim CH, Ma JS, Lee SB, Kim CH, et al. Epidemiologic study of Kawasaki disease in Korea, 1997–1999: comparison with previous studies during 1991–1996. J Korean Med Sci. 2002;17(4):453–6. http://dx.doi.org/10.3346/jkms.2002.17.4.453 PMID:12172037.
9. Lue HC, Chen LR, Lin MT, Chang LY, Wang JK, Lee CY, et al. Epidemiological features of Kawasaki disease in Taiwan, 1976–2007: results of five nationwide questionnaire hospital surveys. Pediatr Neonatol. 2014;55(2):92–6. http://dx.doi.org/10.1016/j.pedneo.2013.07.010 PMID:24120536.
10. Woon PY, Chang WC, Liang CC, Hsu CH, Klahan S, Huang YH, et al. Increased risk of atopic dermatitis in preschool children with Kawasaki disease: a population-based study in Taiwan. Evid Based Complement Alternat Med. 2013;2013:605123. http://dx.doi.org/10.1155/2013/605123.
11. Salo E, Griffiths EP, Farstad T, Schiller B, Nakamura Y, Yashiro M, et al. Incidence of Kawasaki disease in northern European countries. Pediatr Int. 2012;54(6):770–2. http://dx.doi.org/10.1111/j.1442-200X.2012.03692.x PMID:22726311.

12. Holman RC, Belay ED, Christensen KY, Folkema AM, Steiner CA, Schonberger LB. Hospitalizations for Kawasaki syndrome among children in the United States, 1997–2007. Pediatr Infect Dis J. 2010;29(6):483–8. PMID:20104198.
13. Belay ED, Maddox RA, Holman RC, Curns AT, Ballah K, Schonberger LB. Kawasaki syndrome and risk factors for coronary artery abnormalities: United States, 1994–2003. Pediatr Infect Dis J. 2006;25(3):245–9. http://dx.doi.org/10.1097/01.inf.0000202068.30956.16 PMID:16511388.
14. Bronstein DE, Dille AN, Austin JP, Williams CM, Palinkas LA, Burns JC. Relationship of climate, ethnicity and socioeconomic status to Kawasaki disease in San Diego county, 1994 through 1998. Pediatr Infect Dis J. 2000;19(11):1087–91. http://dx.doi.org/10.1097/00006454-200011000-00012 PMID:11099092.
15. Son MB, Gauvreau K, Ma L, Baker AL, Sundel RP, Fulton DR, et al. Treatment of Kawasaki disease: analysis of 27 US pediatric hospitals from 2001 to 2006. Pediatrics. 2009;124(1):1–8. http://dx.doi.org/10.1542/peds.2008-0730 PMID:19564276.
16. Burns JC, Herzog L, Fabri O, Tremoulet AH, Rodó X, Uehara R, et al. Kawasaki disease global climate consortium. Seasonality of Kawasaki disease: a global perspective. PLoS One. 2013;8(9), e74529. http://dx.doi.org/10.1371/journal.pone.0074529 PMID:24058585.

Update on Nationwide Surveys and Epidemiologic Characteristics of Kawasaki Disease in Japan

Yosikazu Nakamura

Abstract Twenty-two biennial nationwide surveys of Kawasaki disease have been conducted in Japan since 1970. The surveys reveal the epidemiologic features of the disease, such as the number of patients and incidence rates, age- and sex-specific incidence rates, seasonal trends, geographic distributions, status of cardiac lesions, and treatment. The descriptive epidemiologic features suggest that an infectious agent(s) is related to disease onset. However, sibling cases, parent and child cases, and differences in incidence rate among races suggest that host factors are important in disease onset.

Keywords Mucocutaneous lymph node syndrome • Epidemiology • Epidemics • Incidence rate • Cardiovascular diseases

Introduction

The Kawasaki Disease Research Committee was established in 1970, 3 years after Dr. Tomisaku Kawasaki first described Kawasaki disease (KD) as mucocutaneous lymph node syndrome [1]. Since then, nationwide epidemiologic surveys have been conducted every 2 years, to reveal the epidemiologic features of the disease in Japan. This chapter presents the results of these surveys and describes the epidemiologic features of KD.

Methods of the Nationwide Surveys

Twenty-two nationwide surveys have been conducted in Japan since 1970 [2]. Although the surveys differ in detail, the main methods of the surveys have been identical. This section will describe the methods for the 22nd survey [3].

Y. Nakamura (✉)
Department of Public Health, Jichi Medical University, 3311-1 Yakushiji, Shimotsuke, Tochigi 329-0498, Japan
e-mail: nakamuyk@jichi.ac.jp

© Springer Japan 2017

79

B.T. Saji et al. (eds.), *Kawasaki Disease*, DOI 10.1007/978-4-431-56039-5_12

The 22nd Nationwide Survey of KD was conducted in 2013, mainly by post. The target patients were those with KD who first visited hospitals for treatment of KD in 2011 and 2012. All hospitals with a pediatric department and 100 or more beds and all children's hospitals with fewer than 100 beds were sent an invitation letter, questionnaire forms, and disease diagnostic guidelines with color figures. In total, 1983 hospitals were targeted, and 1420 (71.6 %) replied.

Patient data requested on the questionnaire were name (initials only), address (municipality), sex, date of birth, date and day of illness at first hospital visit, diagnosis (typical definite, atypical definite, or incomplete), intravenous immuno-globulin (IVIG) therapy, IVIG response status, additional therapy (if administered), recurrences, history of KD among patients' siblings and parents, cardiac lesions (at the first visit, during the acute phase, and as sequelae), and blood tests (white blood cell count, platelet count, albumin level, and C-reactive protein level). Acute cardiac lesions were defined as those that developed within 1 month of disease onset, and cardiac sequelae were defined as those that persisted beyond 1 month after onset. Almost all patients underwent two-dimensional echocardiographic evaluation for cardiac lesions. Incidence rates were calculated using population data from vital statistics in Japan.

Results of Nationwide Surveys

Of the 2006 target hospitals, 23 had closed or closed their pediatric department at the time they received the survey. Of the 1983 remaining hospitals, 1420 (71.6 %) returned the questionnaire. A total of 26,691 patients (12,774 in 2011 and 13,917 in 2012) were reported: 15,442 males and 11,249 females. Annual incidence rates were 243.1/100,000 population aged 0–4 years in 2011 (275.2 for males; 209.4 for females), and 264.8/100,000 population in 2012 (298.6 for males; 229.4 for females). The incidence rate in 2012 was the highest ever recorded in Japan. As shown in Fig. 1, three nationwide epidemics in Japan were observed—in 1979, 1982, and 1986. In 1979, the epidemic wave of the disease moved from the west of the country to the northeast during spring and early summer. The epidemics in 1982 and 1986 started in large cities, including Tokyo and Osaka, and propagated to surrounding areas. There has been no further nationwide epidemic after these three epidemics, but the number of patients started to increase in the mid-1990s. Since then, the annual number of patients has increased gradually, and the incidence rate has increased even more rapidly because of the decreased number of children in the country, i.e., the denominator of the incidence rate.

The seasonal pattern is specific: the largest number of patients is in January, small peaks are observed in summer, and the lowest number is in October, as shown in Fig. 2.

Among the patients, 66.2 % were younger than age 3 years. The age-specific incidence rate was the highest for infants aged 9–11 months (409.8/100,000 population).

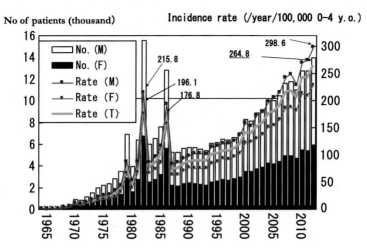

Fig. 1 Numbers of patients and incidence rate, by calendar year and sex

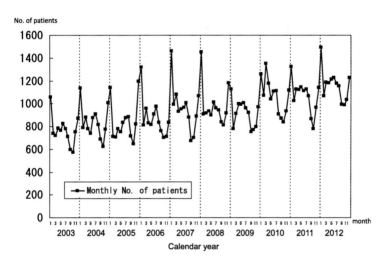

Fig. 2 Monthly numbers of patients, by sex (the previous 10 years)

Of the patients reported in the 22nd survey, 78.4 % were typical definite cases (with five or six principal symptoms), 1.8 % were atypical definite cases (with four symptoms and cardiac lesions), and 19.8 % were incomplete cases (with four symptoms and no cardiac lesions, or three or fewer symptoms).

The number of patients with one or more siblings affected by KD was 408 (1.5 %), and 237 patients (0.89 %) had at least one parent with a history of the disease. There were 946 (3.5 %) recurrent cases.

Of the 26,691 patients reported in the 22nd survey, 1241 patients (4.6 %) had one or more cardiac lesions due to KD at the first visit to hospital, namely, coronary dilatation (3.59 %), valvular lesions (0.91 %), coronary aneurysms (0.25 %), giant coronary aneurysms >8 mm in diameter (0.04 %), coronary stenosis (0.01 %), and no myocardial infarction. During the acute phase, 2487 patients (9.3 %) had cardiac lesions, namely, coronary dilatation (6.99 %), valvular lesions (1.66 %, coronary aneurysms (0.91 %), giant coronary aneurysms (0.18 %), coronary stenosis (0.02 %), and myocardial infarction (0.004 %). One month after onset of KD, 754 patients (2.8 %) had cardiac sequelae, namely, coronary dilatation (1.75 %), valvular lesions (0.37 %, coronary aneurysms (0.72 %), giant coronary aneurysms (0.18 %), coronary stenosis (0.02 %), and myocardial infarction (0.004 %). Cardiac lesions were more prevalent among males. The prevalence of cardiac lesions was high among patients younger than 1 year and those older than 5 years. Fortunately, lesion frequency is decreasing year by year.

Overall, 24,346 (91.2 %) patients received IVIG therapy. Of these, 20,954 (86.1 %) underwent IVIG therapy before the sixth day of illness and 1279 (5.3 %) received steroid therapy with IVIG therapy. However, 4150 (17.0 %) of the 24,346 patients treated with IVIG did not respond to the treatment; 3798 of these (91.5 % of nonresponders) received additional IVIG therapy, 1245 (30.0 %) steroids, 179 (4.31 %) infliximab, 155 (3.73 %) immunosuppressants, and 93 (2.24 %) were treated with plasmapheresis.

What We Have Learned from the Descriptive Epidemiology

Table 1 summarizes the descriptive epidemiologic features of KD from the three perspectives of descriptive epidemiology—person, time, and place. These epidemiologic features suggest the following hypothesis regarding the etiology of KD:

Table 1 Results of descriptive epidemiology

Person	
Sex ratio	M/F = 1.4
Age	Peak at age 0 year; 80 % of patients <4 year
Race	Prevalent among Japanese
	In USA: Japanese > Asians > African-Americans > whites
Sibling cases	
Parental history of KD	
Time	
Nationwide epidemics (1979, 1982, and 1986)	
Many patients in January, small peaks in summer, and lower incidence in autumn	
Place	
60+ countries and regions in the world	
Epidemics in Japan and foreign countries such as Korea and Taiwan	
Movement of epidemics	
Epidemics in small areas	

the disease develops in susceptible children after being triggered by an infectious agent(s).

First, seasonal change in the number of patients, as shown in Fig. 2, appears to be related to an infectious agent(s). Otherwise, such seasonal changes occur by allergic reaction to seasonal allergens such as cider pollinosis, which is prevalent in spring in Japan; however, the probability of an allergic reaction is not very high. Other epidemiologic features of KD support the trigger hypothesis. In addition to the occurrence of the disease in all seasons in Japan, spikes in January and gently sloping peaks in summer have been observed. If three infectious agents are triggers of KD, one of which is present in all seasons, one of which is prevalent in January, and the last of which is present in summer, the seasonal change in KD in Japan could be explained. In addition, the seasonal patterns differ by country and region globally. For example, KD is prevalent in May and June in Korea and Taiwan [4]. If the triggers differ among countries and areas, these phenomena are reasonable. KD has been reported in tropical countries and in countries close to the poles. Thus, it makes sense that KD is related to several different agents.

Age-specific incidence rate also suggests the presence of infectious agents. The rate is quite low among infants younger than 6 months, perhaps because of passive natural immunity from mothers.

Three nationwide epidemics in Japan, movement of epidemics, and temporal and geographic clustering in small areas [5] also suggest an infectious origin. Sibling cases support an infectious hypothesis as well as susceptible host factors. Detailed observations from sibling cases show that the frequency of KD was about ten times higher if a sibling was affected by the disease [6]. In addition, the distribution of intervals to onset of two sibling cases had small peaks for same-day onset and a 1-week interval. The former suggests simultaneous infection, and the latter might be the incubation period.

Sibling cases and parent–child cases support a susceptible host hypothesis. Incidence rates differ by race; incidence is highest among Japanese, followed by Asians, African-Americans, and whites. Although the number of patients and incidence rate have increased in Japan during the past two decades, the frequency is not as high as those for measles and varicella before the era of vaccination. This also supports the susceptible host hypothesis.

Conclusions

The epidemiologic features of KD support the hypothesis that infectious agents trigger KD onset in susceptible children.

References

1. Kawasaki T. Febrile oculo-oro-cutaneo-acrodesquamatous syndrome with or without acute non-suppurative cervical lymphadenitis in infancy and childhood: clinical observations of 50 cases. Arerugi. 1967;16:178–222. Available from: http://www.jskd.jp/info/pdf/kawasaki.pdf PMID:6062087.
2. Yanagawa H, Nakamura Y, Yashiro M, Kawasaki T, editors. Epidemiology of Kawasaki disease: a 30-year achievement. Tokyo: Shindan-To-Chiryosha Co., Ltd.; 2004.
3. Nakamura Y, Yashiro M, Uehara R, Sadakane A, Tsuboi S, Aoyama Y, et al. Epidemiologic features of Kawasaki disease in Japan: results of the 2009–2010 nationwide survey. J Epidemiol. 2012;22(3):216–21. http://dx.doi.org/10.2188/jea.JE20110126 PMID:22447211.
4. Wu MH, Nakamura Y, Burns JC, Rowley AH, Takahashi K, Newburger JW, et al. State-of-the-art basic and clinical science of Kawasaki disease: the 9th international Kawasaki disease symposium 10–12 April 2008, Taipei. Taiwan Ped Health. 2008;2(4):405–9. http://dx.doi.org/10.2217/17455111.2.4.405.
5. Nakamura Y, Yanagawa I, Kawasaki T. Temporal and geographical clustering of Kawasaki disease in Japan. Prog Clin Biol Res. 1987;250:19–32. PMID:3423038.
6. Fujita Y, Nakamura Y, Sakata K, Hara N, Kobayashi M, Nagai M, et al. Kawasaki disease in families. Pediatrics. 1989;84(4):666–9. PMID:2780128.

Kawasaki Disease Epidemiology in Europe

Eeva Salo

Abstract The epidemiology of Kawasaki disease (KD) has not been well described in Europe. In many European countries, annual incidence increased during the 1990s and then plateaued. Current annual incidence is about 5–10 per 100,000 children younger than 5 years. The highest incidence is in Ireland (15.2 per 100,000). Discrepancies in incidence rates may reflect differences in disease recognition rather than true variation in incidence.

Keywords Epidemiology • Kawasaki disease • Europe

History

In 1870 a 7-year-old boy in London was treated at St. Bartholomew Hospital for a disease called "scarlatinal dropsy". He died, and an autopsy was performed by Dr. Samuel Gee, who described the findings in the hospital's journal [1]. The heart was preserved, and a histological examination 130 years later showed aneurysms of the coronary arteries, with clots, and pathological changes consistent with KD and infantile periarteritis nodosa. This is probably the first known case of KD. Additional cases of fatal coronary arteritis and infantile periarteritis nodosa were described in the medical literature in the nineteenth century [2], and the symptoms were compatible with what we now know as KD. However, diagnosis was by pathologists and was only possible after death. Cases resulting in clinical recovery went undiagnosed and were camouflaged among diseases like measles, scarlet fever, and rheumatic fever.

KD existed in Europe before Kawasaki's original description in English, in 1974 [3], but the clinical syndrome was not recognized. Kawasaki's article in Pediatrics explained these enigmatic cases and enabled clinicians to diagnose new cases of KD. Case reports and editorials alerted pediatricians to a new and fascinating

E. Salo, M.D. (✉)
Helsinki University Children's Hospital, PB 281, Stenbäckinkatu 11, 00029 HUS Helsinki, Finland
e-mail: eeva.salo@hus.fi

© Springer Japan 2017
B.T. Saji et al. (eds.), *Kawasaki Disease*, DOI 10.1007/978-4-431-56039-5_13

disease. Still, for a long time, KD was often perceived as rare, almost exotic—a disease common in Japan but seldom encountered in Europe.

Incidence

The epidemiology of KD has not been well described in Europe. The published findings of nationwide surveys are mainly from northern and northwestern Europe (Table 1) [4–15]. The rates reported in these studies should be compared with caution because of differences in methodology and study period.

In Finland, a sharp increase in KD diagnoses prompted national surveillance in 1981. An outbreak was observed [16]. During the busiest 3 months, the attack rate was equivalent to the annual incidence of 60 per 100,000 children younger than 5 years. After the outbreak the incidence fell to about 5 per 100,000, then increased steadily to about 10 per 100,000 toward the end of the millennium (Fig. 1). In England a doubling of KD incidence was reported during the 1990s, from 4.0 per 100,000 in 1991–1992 to 8.1 in 1999–2000 [8], after which it seemed to reach a plateau at 8.4 [12]. Similarly, the incidence in Denmark appeared to increase throughout the 1980s and 1990s and stabilized after 1999 [11]. An earlier French study reported an incidence of 3.0 per 100,000 [7]. A prospective study conducted in northern France in 2005–2006 reported a KD incidence of 9 per 100,000 children

Table 1 Reported Kawasaki disease incidence rates in Europe (after the year 2000)

Country	Period	Incidence	Method	Reference
Czech Republic	1997–1999	1.6	Prospective, questionnaires about vasculitides	Dolezalova et al. (2004) [10]
Denmark	1999–2004	4.9	Hospital discharge records	Fischer et al. (2007) [11]
England	1998–2003	8.4	Hospital admissions data	Harnden et al. (2009) [12]
Finland	1998–2009	11.4	Hospital discharge records	Salo et al. (2012) [14]
Iceland	1996–2005	10.7	Hospital chart review	Olafsdottir (2012) [13]
Ireland	1996–2000	15.2	Hospital discharge records	Lynch et al. (2003) [9]
Northern France	2005–2006	9	Prospective, hospital-based	Heuclin et al. (2009) [17]
Netherlands	2008–2012	5.8	Prospective electronic questionnaires	Tacke et al. (2014) [15]
Norway	1998–2009	5.4	Hospital discharge records	Salo et al. (2012) [14]
Sweden	1998–2009	7.4	Hospital discharge records	Salo et al. (2012) [14]

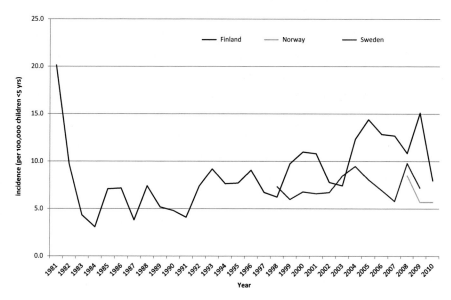

Fig. 1 Incidence of Kawasaki disease in three Nordic countries, 1981–2010

[17]. These figures are lower than those reported in North American white children [4].

A substantial proportion of the increased incidence in KD is probably attributable to increased recognition and correct diagnosis of the disease. Availability of treatment increased the need for prompt recognition and increased physician awareness in the 1990s. It is also possible that the reported increase in these studies is partly due to a real rise in incidence.

In Ireland, the incidence during 1996–2000 was 15.2 per 100,000 children younger than 5 years [9], the highest annual incidence reported in Europe. Similar incidences have been reported from regional surveys. A recent study from the Netherlands revealed a lower mean annual incidence of 5.8 [15], which is similar to the incidence of 5.4 in Norway [14] and 4.9 in Denmark [11].

The only national incidence study outside these countries, in the Czech Republic in 1997–1999, reported an incidence as low as 1.6 per 100,000 children younger than 5 years [10]. That study used questionnaires to enquire about vasculitides. The pediatric consultants answering the questions may have been more familiar with rheumatological diseases than with hands-on observation and treatment in acute wards; thus, the study method may have influenced the results. The French study that reported an incidence of 9 per 100,000 had pediatricians monitoring every hospital [17]. Studies using data from national hospital registers differ in regard to whether the country's privacy policy allows for identification of individual patients in registers, as is the case in the Nordic countries [6, 11, 14]. If such identification is not possible, all hospital entries can be included and patients may therefore be counted twice [8] if interhospital transfers are not excluded [9].

Age

KD patients in Europe are older than those in Japan [14]. The proportion of KD patients younger than 5 years ranges from 67 %, in Sweden, to 79 %, in the Netherlands [14]. Incidence is consistently higher among boys.

Seasonality

KD is a winter disease in Europe, and starts earlier in colder, Northern climates. In Finland and Ireland monthly numbers start to increase in November; in Denmark, England, and the Netherlands the months of highest incidence are December through February [18]. In southern Greece February and March are the months with the most cases [19].

Cardiac Sequelae

The proportion of reported coronary abnormalities differs depending on the methods, population, and study period. The Dutch nationwide study reported that 5.6 % of KD patients had coronary artery abnormalities persisting longer than 8 weeks [14]. A recent Greek tertiary care referral center reported coronary artery lesions in 33 % of KD patients [20].

Way Ahead

It is possible that KD is still under-recognized in Europe, leading to late diagnosis and treatment. Better awareness and suspicion of the diagnosis were called for in two recent articles [19, 20].

References

1. Gee SJ. Cases of morbid anatomy. St Bartholomew's Hosp Rep. 1871;7:141–8.
2. Kryszkovski J. Periarteritis nodosa. Przegl post nauk lek. 1899;38:30.
3. Kawasaki T, Kosaki F, Okawa S, Shigematsu I, Yanagawa H. A new infantile acute febrile mucocutaneous lymph node syndrome (MLNS) prevailing in Japan. Pediatrics. 1974;54 (3):271–6. PMID:4153258.
4. Uehara R, Belay ED. Epidemiology of Kawasaki disease in Asia, Europe, and the United States. J Epidemiol. 2012;22(2):79–85. http://dx.doi.org/10.2188/jea.JE20110131 PMID:22307434.

5. Salo E. Kawasaki disease in Finland in 1982–1992. Scand J Infect Dis. 1993;25(4):497–502. http://dx.doi.org/10.3109/00365549309008532 PMID:8248750.

6. Schiller B, Fasth A, Björkhem G, Elinder G. Kawasaki disease in Sweden: incidence and clinical features. Acta Paediatr. 1995;84(7):769–74. http://dx.doi.org/10.1111/j.1651-2227. 1995.tb13753.x PMID:7549295.

7. Borderon JC, Grimprel E, Begue P. Le syndrome de Kawasaki en France. Enquête prospective sur 1 an. Med Mal Infect. 1998;28(6):550–9. http://dx.doi.org/10.1016/S0399-077X(98) 90002-6.

8. Harnden A, Alves B, Sheikh A. Rising incidence of Kawasaki disease in England: analysis of hospital admission data. BMJ. 2002;324(7351):1424–5. http://dx.doi.org/10.1136/bmj.324. 7351.1424 PMID:12065266.

9. Lynch M, Holman RC, Mulligan A, Belay ED, Schonberger LB. Kawasaki syndrome hospitalizations in Ireland, 1996 through 2000. Pediatr Infect Dis J. 2003;22(11):959–63. http://dx. doi.org/10.1097/01.inf.0000095194.83814.ee PMID:14614367.

10. Dolezalová P, Telekesová P, Nemcová D, Hoza J. Incidence of vasculitis in children in the Czech Republic: 2-year prospective epidemiology survey. J Rheumatol. 2004;31(11):2295–9. PMID:15517648.

11. Fischer TK, Holman RC, Yorita KL, Belay ED, Melbye M, Koch A. Kawasaki syndrome in Denmark. Pediatr Infect Dis J. 2007;26(5):411–5. http://dx.doi.org/10.1097/01.inf. 0000259964.47941.00 PMID:17468651.

12. Harnden A, Mayon-White R, Perera R, Yeates D, Goldacre M, Burgner D. Kawasaki disease in England: ethnicity, deprivation, and respiratory pathogens. Pediatr Infect Dis J. 2009;28 (1):21–4. http://dx.doi.org/10.1097/INF.0b013e3181812ca4 PMID:19145710.

13. Olafsdottir HS, Oskarsson G, Haraldsson Á. Kawasaki disease in Iceland 1996–2005, epidemiology and complications. Laeknabladid. 2012;98(2):91–5. PMID:22314510.

14. Salo E, Griffiths EP, Farstad T, Schiller B, Nakamura Y, Yashiro M, et al. Incidence of Kawasaki disease in northern European countries. Pediatr Int. 2012;54(6):770–2. http://dx.doi. org/10.1111/j.1442-200X.2012.03692.x PMID:22726311.

15. Tacke CE, Breunis WB, Pereira RR, Breur JM, Kuipers IM, Kuijpers TW. Five years of Kawasaki disease in the Netherlands: a national surveillance study. Pediatr Infect Dis J. 2014;33(8):793–7. http://dx.doi.org/10.1097/INF.0000000000000271.

16. Salo E, Pelkonen P, Pettay O. Outbreak of Kawasaki syndrome in Finland. Acta Paediatr Scand. 1986;75(1):75–80. http://dx.doi.org/10.1111/j.1651-2227.1986.tb10160.x PMID:3953281.

17. Heuclin T, Dubos F, Hue V, Godart F, Francart C, Vincent P, et al. Hospital network for evaluating the management of common childhood diseases. Increased detection rate of Kawasaki disease using new diagnostic algorithm, including early use of echocardiography. J Pediatr. 2009;155(5):695–9.e1. http://dx.doi.org/10.1016/j.jpeds.2009.04.058 PMID:19595368.

18. Burns JC, Herzog L, Fabri O, Tremoulet AH, Rodó X, Uehara R, et al. Kawasaki disease global climate consortium. Seasonality of Kawasaki disease: a global perspective. PLoS One. 2013;8(9), e74529. http://dx.doi.org/10.1371/journal.pone.0074529 PMID:24058585.

19. Giannouli G, Tzoumaka-Bakoula C, Kopsidas I, Papadogeorgou P, Chrousos GP, Michos A. Epidemiology and risk factors for coronary artery abnormalities in children with complete and incomplete Kawasaki disease during a 10-year period. Pediatr Cardiol. 2013;34 (6):1476–81. http://dx.doi.org/10.1007/s00246-013-0673-9 PMID:23463134.

20. Patel A, Holman RC, Callinan LS, Sreenivasan N, Schonberger LB, Fischer TK, et al. Evaluation of clinical characteristics of Kawasaki syndrome and risk factors for coronary artery abnormalities among children in Denmark. Acta Paediatr. 2013;102(4):385–90. http:// dx.doi.org/10.1111/apa.12142 PMID:23278838.

Recent Topics in the Epidemiology of Kawasaki Disease

Ritei Uehara

Abstract The incidence rates of Kawasaki disease (KD) in Northeast Asians are almost 20 times those of whites. Incidence is higher among Japanese Americans than among other Asian Americans living in Hawaii, which indicates that genetic factors rather than environmental factors have the predominant role in the occurrence of KD in these populations. Approximately 10–15 % of KD patients have persistent or recrudescent fever more than 36 h after the end of initial intravenous immunoglobulin infusion. KD is uncommon in adults, although the prevalences of specific diagnostic criteria are roughly similar in adults and children. The prevalence of coronary aneurysms is lower in adults than in children. Dr. Kawasaki saw the first case of typical KD in 1961. After he treated several more similar cases, the first epidemiologic survey of KD was conducted in 1970.

Keywords Epidemiology • Incidence • Immunoglobulin • Adult

Kawasaki Disease in Japan and Other Countries

Nationwide epidemiologic surveys of Kawasaki disease (KD) in Japan have been conducted almost every 2 years since 1970 [1]. The most recent published study was for the survey conducted in 2011 and included patients who visited hospitals during 2009–2010. The total number of KD patients who visited hospitals during the 2-year period was 23,730 (13,515 boys; 10,215 girls). The average annual KD incidence rate during the 2-year period was 222.9 per 100,000 children younger than 5 years (boys, 247.6; girls, 196.9). The male-to-female ratio in incidence was 1.26. The average annual incidence rate for KD in Korea was 113.1 per 100,000 children younger than 5 years during 2006–2008 [2], which was the second highest rate in the world. During 2003–2006, the annual incidence rate of KD in Taiwan was 69 per 100,000 for children younger than 5 years during 2003–2006. The male-to-female ratio was 1.62. In Beijing, China, the average annual incidence rate of KD

R. Uehara (✉)
Utsunomiya City Public Health Center, Takebayashi 972, Utsunomiya City, Tochigi 321-0974, Japan
e-mail: u-ritei@ksf.biglobe.ne.jp

© Springer Japan 2017   91
B.T. Saji et al. (eds.), *Kawasaki Disease*, DOI 10.1007/978-4-431-56039-5_14

during 2000–2004 was 49.4 per 100,000 children younger than 5 years. A significant increasing trend in KD incidence was observed during 1995–2004. In Shanghai, the average annual incidence rate during 1998–2002 was 27.3 per 100,000 children younger than 5 years. The incidence rate of KD was 2.12–3.43 per 100,000 children younger than 5 years in 1998–2002 in Thailand. The incidence of KD showed an increasing trend during the 15-year period 1994–2008 in India. In the United States, the hospitalization rate per 100,000 children younger than 5 years was 20.8 in 2006, as reported using data from the Kids Inpatient Database.

KD incidence varies by race/ethnicity. Among children younger than 5 years living in Hawaii during 1996–2006, Japanese Americans had the highest incidence rate (210.5 per 100,000), followed by Native Hawaiians (86.9 per 100,000) and Chinese Americans (83.2 per 100,000). Children classified in the census as "Other Asian" (predominantly Korean Americans and Vietnamese Americans) had a KD incidence of 84.9 per 100,000. The incidence rate among Japanese-American children living in Hawaii was slightly higher than that for Japanese children living in Japan (184.6 per 100,000 for 2005–2006). This higher incidence among Japanese Americans relative to other Asian Americans living in Hawaii indicates that genetic factors rather than environmental factors have a predominant role in the occurrence of KD among these populations. In the province of Ontario, Canada, KD incidence among children younger than 5 years increased from 14.4 during 1995–1997 to 26.2 during 2004–2006. The KD incidence rate appears to have reached a plateau around 8.4 per 100,000 children younger than 5 years in England. KD incidence was 15.2 per 100,000 children younger than 5 years in Ireland for 1996–2000. For a 1-year period during 2005–2006, KD incidence was 9 per 100,000 children in northern France. KD incidence was 4.9 per 100,000 children younger than 5 years for Denmark (1999–2004), 6.2 for Sweden (1990–1992), and 7.2 for Finland (1982–1992). Australia has one of the lowest reported rates (3.7 per 100,000 children younger than 5 years of age) [3]. Incidence in New Zealand is also low (8 per 100,000 children younger than 5 years of age).

Seasonal variation in incidence rates is well recognized. The monthly number of KD patients peaks during the winter and spring months, and lower peaks were noted during summer months [1]. The United States, England, and Australia reported higher incidences in winter and spring, whereas peaks in spring or summer were seen in China [3].

Epidemiologic Characteristics of Intravenous Immunoglobulin Nonresponders

Approximately 10–15 % of KD patients have a persistent or recrudescent fever more than 36 h after the end of initial intravenous immunoglobulin (IVIG) infusion [4]. Nonresponse to initial IVIG infusion is associated with increased risk of coronary artery complications [5], especially giant coronary aneurysms [4]. Risk factors for poor response include male sex, age younger than 12 months, delayed initiation of treatment (more than day 10 days after symptom onset), and abnormal laboratory findings such as increased numbers of neutrophils and bands, low platelet levels, elevated levels of aspartate aminotransferase, alanine aminotransferase, C-reactive protein (CRP), total bilirubin, and lactate dehydrogenase, and low albumin, hemoglobin, and sodium levels [5].

Epidemiology of Adult-Onset KD

KD is uncommon in adults. A review of over 50 adult-onset KD patients [6] found that the male-to-female ratio was 1.56. Mean (SD) age was 27.6 (10.3) years (range, 18–68 years), and 74 % of reported patients were younger than 30 years. Conjunctival congestion was noted in 93 % of adult patients. Bilateral anterior uveitis was also reported. All patients had exanthema, variously described as diffuse erythematous, macular, maculopapular, or scarlatiniform. Enanthema was present in almost all adult patients: 80 % of patients had strawberry tongue, 60 % had dry fissured lips, and 80 % had marked oropharyngeal erythema. Changes in palms or soles were noted in 89 % of patients. Desquamation was noted in all but two patients at some point during the clinical course. Cervical lymphadenopathy occurred in most cases and was painful, symmetrical, and sometimes unilateral. Axillary, subclavicular, and inguinal adenopathy was also reported.

Incomplete KD is diagnosed in patients with fever, at least two of the clinical criteria for KD, and laboratory data showing systemic inflammation. Incomplete KD is rare in adults [7]. The prevalences of specific diagnostic criteria were roughly similar in adults and children [6]. Cheilitis and meningitis seemed to occur less frequently in adults (60 % and 11 % of cases, respectively) than in children (90 % and 44 % of cases, respectively). In contrast, articular involvement and adenopathy were more frequent in adults (61 % and 93 % of cases, respectively) than in children (24–38 % and 75 % of cases, respectively). Thrombocytosis was less frequent in adults (56 %) than in children (100 %) with KD, whereas elevated liver enzyme levels were more frequent in adults (65 %) than in children (10 %). Cardiac complications are the most severe manifestations of KD. Coronary aneurysms were detected in relatively few adult patients. The prevalence of coronary aneurysms was lower in adults (5 %) than in children (20 %). Myocarditis and tricuspid regurgitation were also reported.

Forty-Five Years After the First Report of KD

Kawasaki et al. described the history of KD in detail [8] and saw the first case of typical KD in 1961. After treating several similar cases, he helped conduct the first epidemiologic survey of KD, in 1970, with research funds from the Japanese

Ministry of Health and Welfare. Hospitals with a pediatrics department and more than 100 beds were asked to participate in the survey. The research committee developed a diagnostic guideline, which was sent to those hospitals, along with a questionnaire asking about the number of cases meeting the diagnostic criteria, dates of presentation, and diagnoses. After this first survey, nationwide epidemiologic surveys of KD have been conducted in Japan nearly every 2 years, and several features of the disease have been revealed [1]. KD cases were reported in both Japan and the United States in the 1970s. Burns et al. provided a detailed history of KD in the United States [9].

References

1. Nakamura Y, Yashiro M, Uehara R, Sadakane A, Tsuboi S, Aoyama Y, et al. Epidemiologic features of Kawasaki disease in Japan: results of the 2009–2010 nationwide survey. J Epidemiol. 2012;22(3):216–21. http://dx.doi.org/10.2188/jea.JE20110126 PMID:22447211.
2. Uehara R, Belay ED. Epidemiology of Kawasaki disease in Asia, Europe, and the United States. J Epidemiol. 2012;22(2):79–85. http://dx.doi.org/10.2188/jea.JE20110131 PMID:22307434.
3. Yim D, Curtis N, Cheung M, Burgner D. Update on Kawasaki disease: epidemiology, aetiology and pathogenesis. J Paediatr Child Health. 2013;49(9):704–8. http://dx.doi.org/10.1111/jpc.12172 PMID:23560706.
4. Yim D, Curtis N, Cheung M, Burgner D. An update on Kawasaki disease II: clinical features, diagnosis, treatment and outcomes. J Paediatr Child Health. 2013;49(8):614–23. http://dx.doi.org/10.1111/jpc.12221 PMID:23647873.
5. Bayers S, Shulman ST, Paller AS. Kawasaki disease: part II. Complications and treatment. J Am Acad Dermatol. 2013;69(4):513 e1–8. http://dx.doi.org/10.1016/j.jaad.2013.06.040.
6. Sève P, Stankovic K, Smail A, Durand DV, Marchand G, Broussolle C. Adult Kawasaki disease: report of two cases and literature review. Semin Arthritis Rheum. 2005;34(6):785–92. http://dx.doi.org/10.1016/j.semarthrit.2005.01.012 PMID:15942913.
7. Gomard-Mennesson E, Landron C, Dauphin C, Epaulard O, Petit C, Green L, et al. Kawasaki disease in adults: report of 10 cases. Medicine (Baltimore). 2010;89(3):149–58. http://dx.doi.org/10.1097/MD.0b013e3181df193c PMID:20453601.
8. Kawasaki T, Naoe S. History of Kawasaki disease. Clin Exp Nephrol. 2014;18(2):301–4. http://dx.doi.org/10.1007/s10157-013-0877-6 PMID:24595558.
9. Burns JC, Kushner HI, Bastian JF, Shike H, Shimizu C, Matsubara T, et al. Kawasaki disease: a brief history. Pediatrics. 2000;106(2), E27. http://dx.doi.org/10.1542/peds.106.2.e27 PMID:10920183.

Part III
Medical Treatment

Overview of Medical Treatment

Jane W. Newburger

Abstract Kawasaki disease is an acute childhood vasculitis syndrome of uncertain etiology that results in coronary artery aneurysms in one of five children who are not treated in the acute phase of illness. The standard therapy for acute Kawasaki disease is high-dose intravenous immunoglobulin (IVIG), 2 g/kg, over 8–12 h, together with aspirin, for its anti-inflammatory and then anti-platelet effects. Despite such treatment, however, up to 5 % of children will develop coronary artery aneurysms. Adjunctive anti-inflammatory therapies for such patients may be given as primary therapy, together with initial IVIG; aggressive primary therapy would ideally be targeted to those identified by a risk score as being most likely to develop coronary artery aneurysms. Alternatively, rescue therapy can be given to children with persistent or recrudescent fever. Adjunctive therapies have included additional IVIG therapy, corticosteroids, tumor necrosis factor (TNF)-α blockers (e.g., infliximab, etanercept), calcineurin inhibitors (e.g., cyclosporine), interleukin-1 receptor antagonist (IL1RA) agents (e.g., anakinra), methotrexate, and cyclophosphamide. Among these adjunctive therapies, only corticosteroids have been proven to be effective in reducing the incidence of coronary artery aneurysms, in a phase III randomized trial in a high-risk Japanese population. Further research is needed in order to improve understanding of the pathobiology of Kawasaki disease arteritis and to develop and test more targeted and cost-effective therapies.

Keyword Kawasaki disease • Mucocutaneous lymph node syndrome • Intravenous immunoglobulin • Vascular medicine • Acquired heart disease

J.W. Newburger, M.D., M.P.H. (✉)
Harvard Medical School, Boston, MA, USA

Department of Cardiology, Children's Hospital, 300 Longwood Ave., Boston, MA 02115, USA
e-mail: jane.newburger@cardio.chboston.org

© Springer Japan 2017
B.T. Saji et al. (eds.), *Kawasaki Disease*, DOI 10.1007/978-4-431-56039-5_15

Introduction

The goal of medical therapy for acute Kawasaki disease (KD) is to reduce the systemic inflammatory response, prevent coronary aneurysms, and, if aneurysms are already present, to minimize the peak dimensions reached and prevent coronary thrombosis. Management of KD late after onset is targeted at prevention of coronary ischemia and myocardial infarction in patients who have coronary artery aneurysms. The current chapter will focus on anti-inflammatory therapies in the acute phase.

Intravenous Immunoglobulin Therapy

Recommended therapy for all KD patients in the acute phase includes intravenous immunoglobulin (IVIG), 2 g/kg over 8–12 h, together with aspirin in first anti-pyretic and then anti-platelet dosages [1]. First reported in the English literature by Furosho et al. in the Lancet in 1984, IVIG has been shown in many subsequent randomized clinical trials to be effective in reducing the incidence of coronary aneurysms [1]. IVIG is made from pooled immunoglobulin G (IgG) purified from the plasma of more than 1000 donors per lot.

The exact mechanism of action by which IVIG exerts its dramatic therapeutic effect in children with KD remains uncertain. High doses of IVIG are required for efficacy, suggesting that the mechanism of action is unlikely to be neutralization of an etiologic agent. Rather, its immunomodulatory actions are thought to mediate efficacy in immune disorders [2–5]. IVIG may block activating Fcγ receptors or stimulate the inhibitory FcγRIIb receptor, induce neutrophil apoptosis, bind activated components C3b and C4b of the complement system, neutralize anti-idiotypic or anti-cytokine antibodies, and/or suppress other acute inflammatory responses, including chemokines and metalloproteinases [2–5]. Recently, Burns and Franco have posited that the mechanism of action of IVIG in modulating the inflammatory response in KD may also relate to stimulation of an immature myeloid population of dendritic cells secreting interleukin (IL)-10 and/or to its effects on Fc-specific natural regulatory T cells [5].

Moreover, IVIG appears to have a dose-response effect on aneurysm incidence; 2 g/kg is more effective than smaller doses [6]. This dose-response effect was the rationale for the 2004 American Heart Association recommendation that IVIG retreatment be given to children with recrudescent or recurrent fever at least 36 h after cessation of initial IVIG, in the absence of an alternative explanation for fever. However, there has never been a randomized trial on the efficacy of IVIG retreatment. The rising incidence of severe hemolysis after IVIG retreatment in individuals with blood type A, together with accumulating data on the use of other anti-inflammatory agents, has increased interest in alternative rescue therapies for those with IVIG resistance [7].

Corticosteroid Therapy

The least expensive and best studied anti-inflammatory agents for treatment of KD are corticosteroids. They are widely used in therapy for other forms of vasculitis and are powerful anti-inflammatory agents, due to their effects on a multitude of inflammatory genes. Corticosteroid therapy has been reported to be effective as "rescue" therapy for patients with recurrent or recrudescent fever after IVIG; the most compelling multicenter study used the so-called RAISE regimen of a tapering dose of prednisolone over several weeks [8]. Corticosteroids have also been used as primary therapy for patients who are judged to be at high risk for coronary artery aneurysms at the time of first presentation, as best demonstrated in a randomized controlled trial of IVIG plus prednisolone (RAISE regimen) conducted at 74 institutions in Japan, which used the Kobayashi score to identify participants at high risk for IVIG resistance [9]. Children treated with both IVIG and a course of prednisolone therapy were less likely than those treated with IVIG alone to develop coronary artery aneurysms at any time during the study period and also specifically at week 4. In addition, children treated with the RAISE regimen of corticosteroids were less likely to receive additional rescue therapy.

Other Anti-inflammatory Therapies

The rationale for use of tumor necrosis factor (TNF)-α inhibitors began with the observation that patients with acute KD had high levels of the pro-inflammatory cytokine TNF-α, and that the levels were highest in those who developed coronary aneurysms [10]. Infliximab is a chimeric monoclonal antibody that binds with high affinity to TNF-α. In a randomized double-blind, placebo-controlled trial, infliximab together with conventional therapy including IVIG resulted in shorter fever duration and faster normalization of inflammatory markers [11]. A retrospective study of rescue therapy with infliximab compared with IVIG retreatment similarly showed that use of infliximab was associated with fewer days of fever; coronary outcomes did not differ [12]. Use of etanercept, a recombinant soluble TNF receptor, has also been reported in KD; [13] a randomized trial of primary therapy with this agent is ongoing.

Small studies have reported possible efficacy of the calcineurin inhibitor cyclosporine in rescue therapy for KD [14, 15]. The rationale for its use includes the observation that T cells have a role in mediating damage to the coronary artery wall. In addition, genetic studies have shown that activation of the nuclear factor of activated T cells (NFAT)–calcineurin signaling pathway is associated with susceptibility to KD, as well as with development of coronary artery aneurysms.

Recent interest in the use of statin agents, particularly atorvastatin, stems from the association of coronary artery aneurysms with polymorphisms in the transforming growth factor (TGF)-β signaling pathway. In particular, single-nucleotide polymorphisms in TGF-β2, TGF-βR2, and SMAD3, as well as in a gene encoding Caspase 3, appear to heighten the risk of aneurysms [16]. These fundamental observations resulted in a randomized clinical trial of atorvastatin in children with acute KD and coronary ectasia (www.clinicaltrials.gov; unique identifier: NCT 01431105), which is ongoing.

Conclusions

In summary, outcomes for children with KD have dramatically improved since the disease was first described. However, even with timely diagnosis and treatment, an important subset of these children continues to develop coronary aneurysms. In the future, improved understanding of the pathobiology of KD arteritis may be translated into more targeted and cost-effective therapies.

References

1. Newburger JW, Takahashi M, Gerber MA, Gewitz MH, Tani LY, Burns JC et al. Committee on Rheumatic Fever, Endocarditis and Kawasaki Disease; Council on Cardiovascular Disease in the Young; American Heart Association; American Academy of Pediatrics. Diagnosis, treatment, and long-term management of Kawasaki disease: a statement for health professionals from the Committee on Rheumatic Fever, Endocarditis and Kawasaki Disease, Council on Cardiovascular Disease in the Young, American Heart Association. Circulation 2004;110:2747–71. http://dx.doi.org/10.1161/01.CIR.0000145143.19711.78 PMID:15505111.
2. Kazatchkine MD, Kaveri SV. Immunomodulation of autoimmune and inflammatory diseases with intravenous immune globulin [Medline]. N Engl J Med. 2001;345(10):747–55. http://dx.doi.org/10.1056/NEJMra993360 PMID:11547745.
3. Yi QJ, Li CR, Yang XQ. Effect of intravenous immunoglobulin on inhibiting peripheral blood lymphocyte apoptosis in acute Kawasaki disease. Acta Paediatr. 2001;90(6):623–7. http://dx.doi.org/10.1080/080352501750258667 PMID:11440093.
4. Dalakas MC. Mechanisms of action of IVIg and therapeutic considerations in the treatment of acute and chronic demyelinating neuropathies. Neurology. 2002;59(12 Suppl 6):S13–21. http://dx.doi.org/10.1212/WNL.59.12_suppl_6.S13 PMID:12499466.
5. Burns JC, Franco A. The immunomodulatory effects of intravenous immunoglobulin therapy in Kawasaki disease. Expert Rev Clin Immunol. 2015;11(7):819–25. http://dx.doi.org/10.1586/1744666X.2015.1044980 PMID:26099344.
6. Terai M, Shulman ST. Prevalence of coronary artery abnormalities in Kawasaki disease is highly dependent on gamma globulin dose but independent of salicylate dose. J Pediatr. 1997;131(6):888–93. http://dx.doi.org/10.1016/S0022-3476(97)70038-6 PMID:9427895.
7. http://www.fda.gov/downloads/BiologicsBloodVaccines/NewsEvents/WorkshopsMeetingsConferences/UCM387078.pdf.
8. Kobayashi T, Kobayashi T, Morikawa A, Ikeda K, Seki M, Shimoyama S, et al. Efficacy of intravenous immunoglobulin combined with prednisolone following resistance to initial intravenous immunoglobulin treatment of acute Kawasaki disease. J Pediatr. 2013;163(2):521–6. http://dx.doi.org/10.1016/j.jpeds.2013.01.022 PMID:23485027.

9. Kobayashi T, Saji T, Otani T, Takeuchi K, Nakamura T, Arakawa H, et al. RAISE study group investigators. Efficacy of immunoglobulin plus prednisolone for prevention of coronary artery abnormalities in severe Kawasaki disease (RAISE study): a randomised, open-label, blinded-endpoints trial. Lancet. 2012;379(9826):1613–20. http://dx.doi.org/10.1016/S0140-6736(11)61930-2 PMID:22405251.

10. Matsubara T, Furukawa S, Yabuta K. Serum levels of tumor necrosis factor, interleukin 2 receptor, and interferon-gamma in Kawasaki disease involved coronary-artery lesions. Clin Immunol Immunopathol. 1990;56(1):29–36. http://dx.doi.org/10.1016/0090-1229(90)90166-N PMID:2113446.

11. Tremoulet AH, Jain S, Jaggi P, Jimenez-Fernandez S, Pancheri JM, Sun X, et al. Infliximab for intensification of primary therapy for Kawasaki disease: a phase 3 randomised, double-blind, placebo-controlled trial. Lancet. 2014;383(9930):1731–8. http://dx.doi.org/10.1016/S0140-6736(13)62298-9 PMID:24572997.

12. Son MB, Gauvreau K, et al. Infliximab for intravenous immunoglobulin resistance in Kawasaki disease: a retrospective study. J Pediatr. 2011;158(4):644–649 e41. http://dx.doi.org/10.1016/j.jpeds.2010.10.012.

13. Choueiter NF, Olson AK, Shen DD, Portman MA. Prospective open-label trial of etanercept as adjunctive therapy for kawasaki disease. J Pediatr. 2010;157(6):960–966.e1. http://dx.doi.org/10.1016/j.jpeds.2010.06.014 PMID:20667551.

14. Tremoulet AH, Pancoast P, Franco A, Bujold M, Shimizu C, Onouchi Y, Tamamoto A, Erdem G, Dodd D, Burns JC. Calcineurin inhibitor treatment of intravenous immunoglobulin-resistant Kawasaki disease. J Pediatr. 2012;161(3):506–512 e501.

15. Suzuki H, Terai M, Hamada H, Honda T, Suenaga T, Takeuchi T, et al. Cyclosporin A treatment for Kawasaki disease refractory to initial and additional intravenous immunoglobulin. Pediatr Infect Dis J. 2011;30(10):871–6. http://dx.doi.org/10.1097/INF.0b013e318220c3cf PMID:21587094.

16. Burns JC, Newburger JW. Genetics insights into the pathogenesis of Kawasaki disease. Circ Cardiovasc Genet. 2012;5(3):277–8. http://dx.doi.org/10.1161/CIRCGENETICS.112.963710 PMID:22715279.

Overview of the New Japanese Guideline2012 for the Medical Treatment of Acute Stage of Kawasaki Disease

Ben Tsutomu Saji and Tohru Kobayashi

Abstract In the research of the treatment of acute stage of Kawasaki disease, only small case series of initial treatment were reported in decades ago. However recently, more reliable results with high-evidenced outcomes from well-designed and with high quality clinical trials like RAISE study have been increasingly reported. We here introduce the revised guideline of the medical treatment of acute phase of KD in 2012 (KDGL 2012), organized by the Japanese Society of Pediatric Cardiology and Cardiac Surgery (Pediatr Int 56:135–58, 2014).

Keywords RAISE study • KDGL • Guidelines for medical treatment of acute Kawasaki disease

Introduction

In the research of the treatment of acute stage of Kawasaki disease, only small case series of initial treatment were reported in decades ago. However recently, more reliable results with high-evidenced outcomes from well-designed and with high quality clinical trials like RAISE study have been increasingly reported. We here introduce the revised guideline of the medical treatment of acute phase of KD in 2012 (KDGL 2012), organized by the Japanese Society of Pediatric Cardiology and Cardiac Surgery [1].

The guidelines in this chapter are reprinted with permission from *Pediatrics International*, John Wiley & Sons, Inc., 2014.

B.T. Saji (✉)
Department of Pediatrics, Toho University, Medical Center Omori Hospital, 6-11-1, Omori-nishi, Ota-ku, Tokyo 143-8541, Japan
e-mail: saji34ben@med.toho-u.ac.jp

T. Kobayashi
Department of Pediatrics, Gunma University, 3-39-15 Showa-machi, Maebashi, Gunma 377-8511, Japan

© Springer Japan 2017
B.T. Saji et al. (eds.), *Kawasaki Disease*, DOI 10.1007/978-4-431-56039-5_16

Fundamentals of New Guideline 2012

Essentially, the guideline must be prepared on the academic basis and organized with recommendations for supporting clinicians and patients at clinical decision makings. It can be used for the treatment options and special medications. But, it should not deny their valuable experiences or can't always be adapted for every case. An attending physician should determine a therapeutic strategy in the guideline by discussing with patients, their parents, or tutelary guardians. Most important discussion is how reliable the GL to them.

Previous Guideline 2003

JSPCCS published first KDGL in 2003, when the single infusion of IVIG 1–2 g/kg/dose was recommended and replaced the divided dose of IVIG 200–400 mg/kg/dose for 3–5 days, which became a standard regimen as an initial treatment.

Currently, IVIG 1–2 g/kg/dose is established as a standard regimen for initial treatment in 98.2 % of patients reported by biannual Japanese Survey 2009–2010, which was around 86 % in survey 2003–2004. Coincidentally, the incidence of coronary artery abnormality at 1 month (CAA) was 3.83 % in 2003–2004, decreased to 2.47 % in 2011–2012.

After the first KDGL 2003 published, the new regimen of single infusion of IVIG 1–2 g/kg/dose was approved by Japanese Pharmaceutical and Medical Devices Agency (PMDA). The regimen of IVIG 1–2 g/kg/dose was established almost 20 years after the first in human report of 100 mg/kg/dose for initial treatment reported in 1982 by Kondo et al. Then IVIG 400 mg/kg divided dose reported by Furusho, et al. in 1983 gave a historical step after conventional treatment with ASA.

General Principles of the New Guideline 2012

The philosophy of the new KDGL for acute treatment includes,

1. Assessment of the evidence level and recommendation grade of the drug therapy
2. Stratification for IVIG non-responsiveness by the risk score
3. Set the treatment algorithm for 1st line IVIG non-responder and 2nd line non-responder
4. Recommendation of upgrade therapy ex, IVIG plus prednisolone or pulse methylprednisolone (iMP) as an initial therapy on 2nd line treatment for suspected 1st line IVIG non-responder predicted by the risk score
5. Recommendation of upgrade of 3rd line treatment when 2nd line treatment is ineffective.

6. No recommendation on the treatment selection for incomplete form or order of priority of each treatment

What to Do When the Child is Admitted

First, we calculate the risk score and stratify the high-risk and low risk for 1st line IVIG treatment. If the patient is suspected as 1st line IVIG non-responder, we select IVIG plus predonisolone or IVIG plus iMP, basically listed in the 2nd line treatment. Twenty four hours after the conclusion of 1st line treatment, we assess the response. When fever is ≦37.5 °C, it is assessed as a responder.

When you recognize that the 1st line treatment is not effective, you immediately select the 2nd line treatment from one of the candidates for the 3rd line treatment

Guidelines for medical treatment of acute Kawasaki disease: Report of the Research Committee of the Japanese Society of Pediatric Cardiology and Cardiac Surgery (2012 revised version)

Authors

Research Committee of the Japanese Society of Pediatric Cardiology,
Cardiac Surgery Committee for Development of Guidelines for Medical Treatment
  of Acute Kawasaki Disease

Principal Author

Tsutomu Saji, Department of Pediatrics, Toho University Omori Medical Center,
  Tokyo, Japan

Section Authors

Mamoru Ayusawa, Department of Pediatrics and Child Health, Nihon University
  School of Medicine, Tokyo, Japan
Masaru Miura, Division of Cardiology, Tokyo Metropolitan Children's Medical
  Center, Tokyo, Japan
Tohru Kobayashi, Department of Pediatrics, Gunma University Graduate School of
  Medicine, Maebashi, Gunma, Japan
Hiroyuki Suzuki, Department of Pediatrics, Wakayama Medical University, Waka-
  yama, Japan
Masaaki Mori, Department of Pediatrics, Yokohama City University Medical
  Center, Yokohama, Kanagawa, Japan
Masaru Terai, Department of Pediatrics, Yachiyo Medical Center, Tokyo Women's
  Medical University, Tokyo, Japan
Shunichi Ogawa, Department of Pediatrics, Nippon Medical School, Tokyo, Japan

Associate Member

Hiroyuki Matsuura, Department of Pediatrics, Toho University Omori Medical
  Center, Tokyo, Japan

External Evaluation Committee

Tomoyoshi Sonobe, Department of Pediatrics, Japan Red Cross Medical Center,
  Tokyo, Japan
Shigeru Uemura, Cardiovascular Center, Showa University Northern Yokohama
  Hospital, Yokohama, Kanagawa, Japan
Kenji Hamaoka, Pediatric Cardiology and Nephrology, Kyoto Prefectural Univer-
  sity of Medicine Graduate School of Medical Science, Kyoto, Japan
Hirotaro Ogino, Department of Pediatrics, Kansai Medical University, Osaka,
  Japan

Masahiro Ishii, Department of Pediatrics, Kitasato University School of Medicine, Tokyo, Japan

Correspondence Tsutomu Saji, MD, First Department of Pediatrics, Toho University, 6-11-1 Omori-Nishi, Ota-Ku, Tokyo 143-8541, Japan. Email: saji34ben@med.toho-u.ac.jp

The primary purpose of practical guidelines is to contribute to timely and appropriate diagnosis and treatment of a given disease or condition, in addition to providing current medical information on pathogenesis and treatment, as determined by specialists in the field. Guidelines, however, should not be considered procedure manuals that limit the treatment options of practitioners, because treatment modalities other than those recommended in such guidelines are often required. Such treatment choices are the result of comprehensive analysis of all medical circumstances, including patient condition, treatment option, and disease severity. Furthermore, certain drugs shown to be useful in studies conducted in other countries may not yet have been approved for use here in Japan. The results of clinical research (including randomized controlled trials) must be verified in subsequent research, and the safety and effectiveness of a particular treatment may take several months to confirm.

Evidence classification
Recent clinical guidelines typically provide evidence levels based on study design and reported effectiveness.

Level (class) based on study design

These are defined as follows: class Ia, systematic reviews, meta-analyses; class Ib, randomized controlled trials; class IIa, non-randomized controlled trials; class IIb, other quasi-experimental studies; class III, non-experimental reports (comparative studies, correlation studies, case studies); and class IV, opinions of committees of experts and authorities.

Classification (grade) based on efficacy

These are given as follows: grade A, highly recommended; grade B, recommended; grade C, recommended, but evidence is uncertain; and grade D, contraindicated.

The present guidelines will use these classification systems in reviewing the available evidence for the various treatments.

Background of the present revision of the treatment guidelines
In July 2003, the Scientific Committee of the Japanese Society of Pediatric Cardiology and Cardiac Surgery published its Treatment Guidelines for Acute Kawasaki Disease (KD). These guidelines were designed to present, in a clinically relevant manner, the findings of Ministry of Health research done from 1998 through 2000 by the Onishi group at Kagawa Medical University (working under the official title, "The Pediatric Pharmaceutical Investigation Research Group"). This research had been published as "Research designed to identify and solve problems in the suitable use of pharmaceuticals for pediatric medical treatment: pharmaceuticals in

cardiology" and had originally been conducted to provide clinical data for the approval of single-use i.v. immunoglobulin (IVIG).

During the 9 years that have passed since the publication of the previous guideline, new data have been collected, and reports on new drug treatments have been published. Members of the International Kawasaki disease Symposium have been waiting for a revision of the previous Japanese guideline. Thus, the Scientific Committee was restructured and assigned the task of revising the guideline.

Purpose and methods

Data on IVIG that have accumulated since it was approved and first marketed have confirmed the efficacy and safety of single-use IVIG therapy. In addition, the incidence of coronary artery lesions (CAL) has gradually decreased every year since IVIG treatment was introduced in Japan. [1] The incidence of giant coronary artery aneurysms (CAA), however, has remained almost unchanged, which highlights the importance of timely use of second- and third-line treatments for IVIG-resistant patients.

In developing the present guideline, we carefully reviewed the most recent available literature, classified evidence and efficacy, and revised suggested treatment methods, including procedures for selecting first-, second- and third-line medications, with a special focus on off-label uses. For example, the previous guideline did not mention new therapeutic agents such as infliximab (IFX), cyclosporin A (CsA), or methotrexate (MTX). In the present edition, risk/benefit considerations are also clearly presented, based on data collected in and outside Japan. Despite the publication of almost 200 reports every year on KD, there is still no universally accepted treatment for IVIG resistance. This is also the case, however, for many other disorders, such as autoimmune disease and rheumatoid conditions, given that no single medication will benefit all patients in the same way. Thus, to ensure optimal outcome, physicians must treat each patient individually.

Diagnosis and treatment of incomplete KD

In the published results of the 21st Nationwide Survey of KD by Jichi Medical School a total of 23 730 cases of KD were reported in Japan during the 2 year period 2009–2010.[1] Diagnosis of KD follows the criteria outlined in the fifth edition of the diagnosis guidelines for KD, [2] which requires that at least five of the following six principal symptoms are present: (i) fever persisting ≥ 5 days (including fever that subsides before the fifth day in response to therapy); (ii) bilateral conjunctival congestion; (iii) changes in lips and oral cavity: reddening of lips, strawberry tongue, diffuse injection of oral and pharyngeal mucosa; (iv) polymorphous exanthema; (v) changes in peripheral extremities: reddening of palms and soles, indurative edema (initial stage); membranous desquamation from fingertips (convalescent stage); and (vi) acute non-purulent cervical lymphadenopathy.

Kawasaki disease, however, may also be diagnosed when only four of the aforementioned symptoms are present, if during the period of illness either 2-D echocardiography or coronary angiography shows CAA, including dilation of coronary artery, and other causes of CAA can be excluded. A diagnosis of KD is possible even if five or more of the principal symptoms are not present, if other conditions can be excluded and KD is suspected – a condition known as incomplete

KD. Indeed, approximately 15–20 % of KD patients have incomplete KD. But, even if a patient has four or fewer of the principal symptoms, the illness should not be regarded as less severe, because cardiovascular abnormalities are not rare in patients with incomplete KD. For this reason, even patients with fewer than five of the aforementioned symptoms should be evaluated for KD. Early treatment is essential, particularly when fever is present, because CAL development in such cases is not uncommon. Diagnosis of incomplete KD is not a simple matter of adding up the number of overt KD symptoms: the importance and individual characteristics of each symptom of the illness must be correctly assessed. For example, redness and crusting at a bacille Calmette–Guérin (BCG) inoculation site in infants younger than 1 year and multilocular cervical lymphadenopathy in children aged ≥4 years are characteristic features of KD.

Basic pathology

The 2012 Revised International Chapel Hill Consensus Conference Nomenclature of Vasculitides defines KD as an arteritis associated with mucocutaneous lymph node syndrome, predominantly affecting medium and small arteries.[3] There is very little damage to veins. The location of pathological changes clearly differentiates KD from other vasculitis syndromes, given that the principal danger of KD is inflammatory vasculitis of the coronary arteries. Edematous lesions develop in the intima media, and vascular fragility increases due to partial rupture of the internal and external elastic lamina. As a result, the arterial wall can no longer withstand its internal pressure, particularly diastolic pressure, and becomes distended and deformed, leading in severe cases to aneurysm formation. Only a few other diseases cause distension of coronary arteries. These include vasculitis resulting from Epstein–Barr virus infection, lupus, classical periarteritis nodosa, and atherosclerotic lesions. Calcification can also occur in rare cases and affect coronary arteries, for example in cases of renal dialysis in adults and herpes infection in newborns.

Patients with KD may develop multiple lesions in the proximal region and vessels branching out from it. As aneurysms begin to calcify, further pathological distension or development of aneurysms and intimal thickening may develop 2–3 years later in areas with previously disrupted internal and external elastic lamina.[4]

Coronary artery lesions

The principal characteristics of KD are dilation of coronary arteries and CAA. Most CAA occur in the proximal region and its branches, and arteries with a CAA measuring ≥8 mm in diameter are very unlikely to regain their normal morphology. Right CAA may lead to occlusion or recanalization, and left CAA may progress to stenotic lesions.

Rupture of the internal elastic lamina in the intima media of the dilated area weakens the artery wall, and coronary arterial pressure then becomes the direct mechanical cause of distension. In rare cases, aneurysms may develop in branches of the axillary or celiac arteries. During acute KD, vasculitis worsens during the first 7 days after disease onset. In patients with mild illness, the vasculature returns to normal by the second or third week.

Suitable pharmaceuticals for treating KD

Treatment of acute KD

The principal objective in treating acute KD is minimizing the risk of developing CAL. In practice, this means quickly suppressing the acute-phase inflammatory reaction caused by KD. Except in cases of very mild KD, IVIG should be started before illness day 7. Histological studies have shown that arteritis typically develops by 8 or 9 days after KD onset. Therefore, treatment should begin before this point, to suppress arteritis and hasten resolution of fever and normalization of inflammation markers. In patients with incomplete KD, IVIG should also be begun as soon as possible after a diagnosis of KD, especially if fever is present. In approximately 80 % of cases, fever should be lowered to $\leq$37.5 °C within 48 h of starting IVIG. In 40 % of IVIG-resistant patients, fever can be reduced to $\leq$37.5 °C with additional IVIG of 1 g/kg. Persistent fever after 48 h of starting IVIG should be regarded as evidence of IVIG-resistant KD. Prevention of CAA in such patients may largely depend on the selection of subsequent treatment.

In addition to CAL, other cardiovascular complications may develop in patients with acute KD, including myocarditis, pericardial effusion, valvular regurgitation, and, rarely, arrhythmia. Specific treatment may be required for these sequelae, as well as for cardiac dysfunction or heart failure. Furthermore, other symptom-specific treatment may be required for systemic complications such as edema, hypoalbuminemia, electrolyte imbalances (i.e. hyponatremia), paralytic ileus, hepatic dysfunction, cholecystitis, impaired consciousness, convulsions, anemia, diarrhea, vomiting, and dehydration. Particularly during high-dose IVIG infusion, care must be taken to prevent volume overload so as to protect the patient from complications such as heart failure.

There is currently no universally accepted classification system to evaluate KD severity and need for IVIG use, although many such scoring systems have been proposed. Initial attempts were made by Asai and Kusakawa,[5] which were followed by the Iwasa score[6] and Harada score.[7] More recently, predictive models designed to evaluate the possibility of IVIG resistance were proposed, including the Kobayashi score,[8] Egami score,[9] and Sano score.[10] In general, such predictive models consider factors such as age, gender, days of illness, white blood cell count, %neutrophils, hematocrit, platelet count, C-reactive protein (CRP), aspartate aminotransferase (AST), alanine aminotransferase (ALT), total bilirubin, sodium, and albumin. Recently, a randomized controlled trial found that IVIG plus steroid as initial therapy for patients predicted to be at high risk for IVIG resistance improved clinical and coronary arterial outcomes.[11-13] The effectiveness of such predictive models, however, has not been confirmed in large-scale prospective cohort studies or meta-analyses, and controversy remains as to whether initial therapy with IVIG plus steroids is the optimal treatment.

Choice of treatment for IVIG-resistant patients

Several second-line treatment options are available if fever persists or has reappeared at 24 h after first-line treatment. The efficacy of these second-line treatments for resistance to first-line treatment is currently being investigated by researchers in many countries, but evidence remains limited due to the lack of randomized controlled trials.

Options for second-line treatment include additional IVIG, i.v. methylprednisolone pulse (IVMP), prednisolone (PSL), IFX, ulinastatin (UTI), CsA, MTX, and plasma exchange (PE). The decision to use any of these treatments requires careful consideration of patient characteristics. At present, the most commonly used second-line treatment is additional IVIG,[1] which is sometimes given in combination with other medications. As for steroids, a retrospective study noted a high incidence of giant aneurysms.[14] That small uncontrolled case study reported that several patients had received steroids before rupture of coronary arteries, which suggests that physicians should carefully consider the decision to use steroids for patients with KD if CAA are already present. When steroids, biologics, or immunosuppressants are given to infants, there is also a risk of long-term side-effects, and questions remain regarding the general safety of such medications. Thus, a careful risk/benefit evaluation should be done to consider the likelihood of such adverse effects versus the possibility of CAA formation.

Algorithm for selecting optimal treatment

To decrease the risks of first-line IVIG resistance and CAA, it seems reasonable to consider risk stratification using predictive models and to select more-aggressive initial treatment for patients at high risk of IVIG resistance. Such patients should be treated with 2 g/kg of IVIG in combination with either 2 mg/kg per day PSL or 30 mg/kg per day IVMP. If the patients fail to respond to these treatments, a third-line treatment will be upgraded to a second-line treatment.

Because few studies have assessed the efficacy of medications other than IVIG retreatment, it is impossible at this time to assign an objective order of these treatment options. The present guidelines, however, offer evidence levels and grades to assist physicians in selecting appropriate alternatives. Various methods of calculating KD patient risk scores and, thereby, estimating KD severity have been developed at a number of institutions by different physicians, based on their particular experience with KD.[8-10] The Japanese Society of Pediatric Cardiology and Cardiac Surgery does not intend to limit the treatment options available to clinicians, especially when such options have already received ethics committee approval at their institution. Instead, the judgment of physicians in selecting treatments should be respected, for practical reasons as well. Such treatments may be given after a physician has established a sufficient basis for selecting a given treatment and received informed consent/assent from the family/patient (Fig. 1).

Immunoglobulin

Purpose

Currently, the most effective anti-inflammatory treatment for KD is early IVIG. [15-17] The latest systematic review by the Cochrane Collaboration states that CAL development can be reduced by a single dose of 2 g/kg IVIG given before the 10th day after onset.[18]

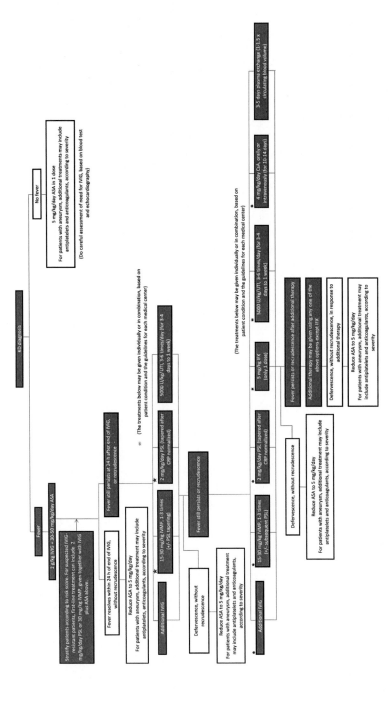

Fig. 1 Algorithm for the treatment of acute Kawasaki disease (*KD*). If patient risk score indicates severe KD (i.e., suspected IVIG resistance), the starred 2nd-line therapies may be used as 1st-line therapies, and 3rd-line asterisked options may be used as 2nd-line therapies, as required. *ASA* acetyl salicylic acid, *CRP* C-reactive protein, *IFX* infliximab, *IVIG* i.v. immunoglobulin, *IVMP* i.v. methylprednisolone pulse, *PSL* prednisolone, *UTI* ulinastatin

Table 1 Immunoregulatory effects of IVIG[19–22]

I. Fc receptor-mediated effects
Blockade of Fc receptors on macrophages and effector cells
Antibody-dependent cellular cytotoxicity
Induction of inhibitory FcγRIIB receptors
Promotes clearance of antibodies that block FcRn
II. Anti-inflammatory effects
Attenuation of complement-mediated damage
Decrease in immune complex-mediated inflammation
Induction of anti-inflammatory cytokines
Inhibition of activation of endothelial cells
Neutralization of microbial toxins
Reduction in steroid requirements
Modulation of matrix metalloproteinases
II. Effect on B cells and antibodies
Control of emergent bone marrow B-cell repertoires
Negative signaling through Fcγ receptor
Selective downregulation/upregulation of antibody production
Neutralization of circulating autoantibodies by anti-idiotypes
V. Effect on T cells
Regulation of T-helper cell cytokine production
Neutralization of T-cell superantigens
Regulation of apoptosis
V. Effect on dendritic cells
Inhibition of differentiation and maturation
Regulation of inflammatory cytokine production
VI. Other
Mutually interacts with immunological molecules
Suppression of autoantibody production against vascular endothelial cells
Acceleration of phagocytosis arising from binding of neutrophils and macrophages (opsonin effect)
Suppression of inflammation-related gene S100 mRNA
Suppression of MCP-1 receptor CCR2 gene expression produced by macrophages

CCR2, C-C chemokine receptor type 2; FcγRIIB, Fc gamma receptor IIB; FcRn, neonatal Fc receptor; IVIG, i.v. immunoglobulin; MCP-1, monocyte chemotactic protein-1

Mechanism of action

Because the causes of KD are unknown, the mechanisms underlying the therapeutic benefits of IVIG remain speculative. Table 1 lists the hypothesized mechanisms of action.[19-22]

Indications

I.v. immunoglobulin is suitable for almost all cases of typical acute KD, that is, when KD is diagnosed based on the presence of the principal symptoms specified in the criteria of the diagnostic guideline for KD[2] and the patient is at risk for CAL. For patients with symptoms that only partially fulfill the diagnostic criteria, incomplete KD may be diagnosed – if other diseases or conditions can be excluded – after which IVIG should be started as quickly as possible due to the risk of CAL.[17]

In cases of less severe KD or spontaneous defervescence, clinicians may refrain from IVIG, in accordance with the considerations detailed in the Ministry of Health Group Committee guidelines for IVIG (Harada score)[7] and disease severity standards established at the physician's institution.

Data from the 21st Nationwide Survey of KD show that IVIG was given to 89.5 % of patients.[1]

Treatment method and dosage

Period of treatment

I.v. immunoglobulin should be started on or before the seventh day after KD onset. It is essential to quickly reduce inflammation and duration of fever, definitely before illness day 8 or 9, when CAL begin to appear. Markers of systemic inflammation, for example CRP and neutrophil count, should be lowered as well.

One study compared patients receiving IVIG on the fifth of illness day or earlier with those who received IVIG on the sixth through ninth days of illness. Although duration from treatment onset to defervescence was slightly longer overall among those receiving IVIG earlier, total duration of fever was shorter. Moreover, the groups did not differ in incidence of fever recurrence or additional IVIG treatment, or in number of days of hospitalization. Furthermore, 1 year after appearance of symptoms, those who had received IVIG earlier had a lower incidence of CAL.[23]

Dosage

The suggested IVIG dosage for acute KD is 2 g/kg per day (single use), 1 g/kg per day for 1 or 2 days continuously (modified single use), or 200–400 mg/kg per day, over 3–5 days (divided dosing).

Studies in a number of countries have shown that, as compared with divided-dose regimens, a single dose of 2 g/kg per day significantly reduced CAL incidence, more quickly normalized inflammation markers, and was more effective in reducing fever.[4, 5] As for 1 g/kg/day use, if clinical efficacy is seen on the first day, it might not be necessary to continue treatment into the second day.

The 21st Nationwide Survey of KD found that a single dose of 2 g/kg per day IVIG was used in 85 % of reported cases and that 1 g/kg per day was given for 1 or 2 days in 6.2 % and in 7.7 % of cases, respectively.[1]

There is no consensus in Japan as to whether older/larger children should be treated with 2 g/kg IVIG or a lower dose.

As for 2 g/kg regimen, the treatment rate varies slightly for different products, although IVIG is typically given over a period of approximately 12 h in North America. In Japan, one product permits use within a similar 12 h period, but the total volume of 2 g/kg IVIG is usually given over a period of 24 h. Because volume overload might occur when the treatment rate is too fast, which can lead to cardiac dysfunction, it is important to adhere to the recommended treatment rate and carefully observe patient hemodynamics.

Product types and directions for use

At present, four brands of IVIG are approved for KD in Japan (Table 2): two are processed with polyethylene glycol (PEG), one is sulfonated, and one is processed to ensure a pH of 4 (acidic). No major differences in efficacy have been reported. Table 2 lists the characteristics of these products, as described in their respective product inserts.

The principal differences are as follows.

(1) The sulfonated product (Kenketsu Venilon-I; Teijin, Tokyo, Japan) contains serum albumin, and its sodium concentration is identical to that of saline (154 mEq/L).

(2) The two products processed with PEG come in freeze-dried (Kenketsu Glovenin-I; Nihon Shinyaku, Kyoto, Japan) and liquid (Venoglobulin IH; Japan Blood Products Organization, Tokyo, Japan) form. The suggested infusion rate for PEG-processed IG is slightly slower than that of the sulfonated product. Kenketsu Glovenin-I has a sodium concentration of 154 mEq/L. Because liquid preparations are usually refrigerated until use, they must be warmed to at least room temperature beforehand.

(3) The pH 4-processed IG (Nisseki Polyglobin-N; Japan Red Cross Society, Tokyo, Japan) comes in liquid form and should also be warmed to at least room temperature before use. During injection, it is essential that the liquid does not leak out of the vein, because this may cause necrosis of the skin. Furthermore, because the preparation contains maltose, the plasma glucose dehydrogenase method should not be used to measure blood sugar after injection, given that this method can be affected by the presence of maltose.

Close monitoring and a slower infusion rate are required during the first 30–60 min, given that all the aforementioned products might result in anaphylaxis during treatment. If no adverse reactions occur during the first hour of treatment (rate, 0.01 mg/kg per min), the maximum rate (<0.03 mg/kg per min) of 2 g/kg may then be used over a course of 12–20 h.

116 B.T. Saji and T. Kobayashi

Table 2 IVIG medications

Product name	Kenketsu Venilon-I (for i.v. use)		Kenketu Glovenin-I (for i.v. use)		Kenketu Venoglobulin IH (for i.v. use)		Nisseki Polyglobin N (for i.v. use)	
Generic name	Freeze-dried sulfonated human normal immunoglobulin		Freeze-dried polyethylene glycol-treated human normal immunoglobulin		Polyethylene glycol-treated human normal immunoglobulin		pH 4-treated acidic human normal immunoglobulin	
Company (manufacturer/distributor)	Kaketsuken-Teijin Pharma Limited		Nihon Pharmaceutical–Takeda Pharmaceutical		Japan Blood Products Organization-Mitsubishi Tanabe Pharma		Japan Blood Products Organization-Japan Red Cross Society	
Form of medication	Freeze-dried preparation		Freeze-dried preparation		Liquid medication		Liquid medication	
Constituents (in 2.5 g of product)	Sulfonated human immunoglobulin G	2500 mg	Polyethylene glycol treated human immunoglobulin G	2500 mg	Human immuno-globulin G	2500 mg	Human immuno-globulin G	2500 mg
	Glycin	1125 mg	D-mannitol	750 mg	D-sorbitol	2500 mg	Maltose hydrate	5000 mg
	Human plasma albumin	125 mg	Glycin	225 mg	Sodium hydroxide	Suitable amount	Hydrochloric acid	Suitable amount
	D-mannitol	500 mg	Sodium chloride	450 mg	Hydrochloric acid	Suitable amount	Sodium hydroxide	Suitable amount
	Sodium chloride	450 mg						
Treatment route and dosing	Normally given as sulfonated human immunoglobulin G either i.v. or by direct i.v. infusion, at 200 mg (4 mL)/kg bodyweight/day over a 5 day period. Alternatively, a single dose of 2000 mg (40 mL)/kg body weight may be given i.v. In addition, in the case of 5 day treatment, this period may be		Normally given as human immunoglobulin G either i.v. or by direct i.v. infusion, at 200 mg (4 mL)/kg bodyweight/day over a 5 day period. Alternatively, a single dose of 2000 mg (40 mL)/kg bodyweight may be given i.v. In addition, in the case of 5 day treatment, this period may		Normally given as human immunoglobulin G either i.v. or by direct i.v. infusion, at 400 mg (8 mL)/kg bodyweight/day over a 5 day period. Alternatively, a single dose of 2000 mg (40 mL)/kg bodyweight may be given i.v. The dose may be reduced according to patient age and condition.		Normally given as human immunoglobulin G either i.v. or by direct i.v. infusion, at 200 mg (4 mL)/kg bodyweight/day, over a 5 day period. Alternatively, a single dose of 2000 mg (40 mL)/kg bodyweight may be given i.v. In addition, in the case of 5 day treatment, this period may be adjusted	

adjusted according to patient age and condition. In the case of 1-time i.v., the dose may be similarly reduced as required.	be adjusted according to patient age and condition. In the case of 1-time i.v. treatment, the dose may be similarly reduced as required.		according to patient age and condition. In the case of 1-time i.v. treatment, the dose may be similarly reduced as required.

A sudden drop in blood pressure may result if the medication is given too rapidly (special care is required when the patient's blood contains little or no endogenous γ-globulin).

Points to consider in treatment and dosing	Treatment speed:	Treatment speed:	Treatment speed:	Treatment speed:
		As there is the possibility of shock or other serious side-effects during the first hour of treatment on the first day, and also when treatment speed is increased, the patient must be carefully monitored during these times.	As there is a possibility of shock or other serious side-effects during the first hour of treatment on the first day, and also when treatment speed is increased, the patient must be carefully monitored during these times.	
	1) On the first day, the first 30 min should be at a rate of 0.01–0.02 mL/kg/min. If no side-effects or other abnormalities are observed, treatment speed may gradually be increased to 0.03–0.06 mL/kg/min.	1) On the first day, the treatment speed should be 0.01 mL/kg/min during the first hour. When the absence of side-effects and other problems has been confirmed, the speed may be gradually increased.	1) On the first day, the treatment speed should be 0.01 mL/kg/min during the first hour. When the absence of side-effects and other problems has been confirmed, the rate may gradually be increased.	1) On the first day, the drug should be delivered at a rate of 0.01–0.02 mL/kg/min during the first 30 min. If no side-effects or other abnormalities are observed, the rate may gradually be increased to 0.03–0.06 mL/kg/min. From the second day onward, the patient may be started at the highest speed tolerated on the previous day.

(continued)

Table 2 (continued)

	From the second day onward, the patient may be started at the highest rate tolerated on the previous day.	However, it should not exceed 0.03 mL/kg/min. On the second day and later, treatment may be started at the highest rate tolerated on the previous day.	However, it should not exceed 0.03 mL/kg/min. On the second day and thereafter, treatment may be started at the highest rate tolerated on the previous day.	
	2) In cases of 1-time treatment of 2000 mg (40 mL)/kg to KD patients, treatment rates in 1) above should basically be adhered to, and the i.v. infusion should given over a period of at least 12 h.	2) In the cases of 1-time treatment of 2000 mg (40 mL)/kg i.v. to KD patients, the rates in 1) should basically be adhered to, with careful attention to sudden increases in circulatory blood volume. The i.v. should be given over a period of at least 20 h.	2) In the case of 1-time treatment of 2000 mg (40 mL)/kg i.v. to KD patients, the rates in 1) should basically be adhered to, with careful attention to sudden increases in circulating blood volume. The i.v. should be given over a period of at least 20 h.	2) In the case of 1-time treatment of 2000 mg (40 mL)/kg to KD patients, the treatment rates in 1) above should basically be adhered to. The i.v. should be given over a period of at least 12 h.
Contraindications	Patients with a history of shock after receiving any component of this medication.	Patients with a history of shock after receiving any of the components of this medication	Patients with a history of shock after receiving any of the components of this medication; patients with inherited glucose intolerance	Patients with a history of shock after receiving any of the components of this medication
Important fundamental points	For KD patients who do not satisfactorily respond to initial IVIG treatment (e.g. patients with persistent fever) and whose symptoms do not improve, additional IVIG should only be given when judged necessary (the	For KD patients who do not satisfactorily respond to initial IVIG treatment (e.g. patients with persistent fever) and whose symptoms do not improve, additional IVIG should only be given when judged necessary (the	For KD patients who do not satisfactorily respond to initial IVIG (e.g. patients with persistent fever) and whose symptoms do not improve, additional IVIG should only be given when judged necessary (the data do not	For KD patients who do not satisfactorily respond to initial IVIG treatment (e.g. patients with persistent fever) and whose symptoms do not improve, additional IVIG should only be given when judged necessary (the

		data do not conclusively demonstrate the efficacy and safety of additional doses of this drug.	data do not conclusively demonstrate the efficacy and safety of additional doses of this drug).	conclusively demonstrate the efficacy and safety of additional doses of this drug). The incidence of liver dysfunction, including elevated AST and ALT, is high when this preparation is given to KD patients, especially to infants younger than 1 year. Patients should be closely monitored after treatment.	data do not conclusively demonstrate the efficacy and safety of additional doses of this drug.
Side-effects	All patients	1.24% (165/13,339)	8.8% (79/893)	11.46% (285/2486)	5.11% (269/5260)
	Acute KD	1.08% (15/1389)	5.6% (9/160)	NA	8.30% (95/1144)
Incidence of side-effects reported in KD patients		1.14% (12/1053 patients), but incidence of severe side-effects was 0% (0 events in 0 cases), including shock in 0% (0 events in 0 patient), symptoms of suspected shock (e.g. cyanosis, hypotension) in 0.28% (4 events in 3 patients)	6.62% (48/725 patients), with severe side-effects occurring in 1.93% (30 events in 14 patients), including shock in 0.14% (1 event in 1 patient), symptoms of suspected shock (e.g. cyanosis, hypotension) in 2.07% (21 events in 15 patients)	10.96% (224/2044 patients), with severe side-effects in 2.89% (84 events in 59 patients), including shock in 0.78% (18 events in 16 patients) and symptoms of suspected shock (e.g. cyanosis, hypotension) in 2.74% (67 events in 56 patients)	8.97% (78/870 patients); severe side-effects in 1.15% (11 events in 10 patients), including shock 0% (0 events in 0 patients) and symptoms of suspected shock (e.g. cyanosis, hypotension) in 0.23% (2 events in 2 patients)
Severe side-effects		Shock, anaphylactic symptoms (<0.1%)	Shock, anaphylactic symptoms (0.1% to <5%)	Shock, anaphylactic symptoms (0.1 to <5%)	Shock, anaphylactic symptoms (0.1 to <5%)
		Hepatic dysfunction, jaundice (incidence unknown)	Hepatic dysfunction, jaundice (incidence unknown)	Hepatic dysfunction (0.1 to <5%), jaundice (incidence unknown)	Hepatic dysfunction, jaundice (0.1 to <5%)
		Aseptic meningitis (incidence unknown)	Aseptic meningitis (incidence unknown)	Aseptic meningitis (0.1 to <5%)	Aseptic meningitis (incidence unknown)

(continued)

Table 2 (continued)

		Acute renal failure (incidence unknown) Thrombocytopenia (incidence unknown) Pulmonary edema (incidence unknown) Thromboembolism (incidence unknown) Heart failure (incidence unknown)	Acute renal failure (incidence unknown) Thrombocytopenia (incidence unknown) Pulmonary edema (incidence unknown) Thromboembolism (incidence unknown) Heart failure (incidence unknown)	Acute renal failure (incidence unknown) Thrombocytopenia (incidence unknown) Pulmonary edema (incidence unknown) Thromboembolism (incidence unknown) Heart failure (incidence unknown)	Acute renal failure (incidence unknown) Thrombocytopenia (incidence unknown) Thromboembolism (incidence unknown) Heart failure (incidence unknown)
Severe side-effects	Allergic reactions	Rash (0.1% to <5%), sensation of heat, urticaria, pruritus, localized edema etc. (<0.1%), redness, swelling, blistering, dyshidrosis	Rash, urticaria, pruritus, blistering, pompholyx (0.1 to <5%), facial flushing, localized edema, generalized redness, purpuric rash, eczema, papule (<0.1%)	Rash, urticaria (0.1 to <5%), facial flushing, localized edema (<0.1%), pruritus, general erythema (incidence unknown) etc.	Fever, rash (0.1 to <5%), pruritus (<0.1%)
	Psychological/ neurological		Seizure, trembling (0.1 to <5%), dizziness, numbness (less than 0.1%), impaired consciousness (incidence unknown)	Trembling, convulsions (0.1 to <5%), drowsiness (<0.1%), impaired consciousness, discomfort (incidence unknown)	
	Circulatory system	Reduced blood pressure, increased blood pressure (incidences unknown)	Abnormal facial color, cold extremities, chest tightness (0.1 to <5%), increased blood pressure, palpitations (incidence unknown)	Abnormal facial color, cold extremities (0.1 to <5%), elevated blood pressure, bradycardia (<0.1%)	
	Liver	Elevated AST, ALT etc. (0.1% to <5%)	Elevated AST, ALT, and ALP (0.1 to <5%)	Abnormal results on hepatic function tests: elevated AST, ALT, γ-GTP, ALP etc. ($\geq$5%)	

Respiratory system		Asthma symptoms, coughing (incidence unknown)	Coughing (<0.1%), asthma symptoms, hypoxemia (incidence unknown)	
Digestive organs	Nausea, vomiting, loss of appetite, abdominal pain (<0.1%)	Nausea, vomiting (0.1 to <5%), diarrhea (<0.1%), abdominal pain (incidence unknown)	Nausea, vomiting, diarrhea (0.1 to <5%), abdominal pain (<0.1%)	
Blood	Leukopenia, neutropenia, eosinophilia, hemolytic anemia, anemia (incidence unknown)	Eosinophilia, neutropenia, hemolytic anemia (<0.1%)	Neutropenia (<0.1%), leukopenia, eosinophilia, hemolytic anemia (incidence unknown)	Neutropenia, eosinophilia (0.1 to <5%), hemolytic anemia (<0.1%)
Other	Headache, fever, chills, shivering (0.1% to <5%), fatigue (<0.1%), chest pain, reduced body temperature, increased CK (CPK), asthmatic symptoms (incidence unknown)	Headache, fever, coldness, shivering, angiodynia (0.1 to <5%), fatigue (<0.1%), arthralgia, myalgia, back pain, increased CK (CPK), hot flushes, moodiness, conjunctival hyperemia, hypothermia (incidence unknown)	Headache, fever, coldness, shivering, hypothermia (0.1 to <5%), melalgia (<0.1%) fatigue, arthralgia, back pain, increased CK (CPK), hot flashes, moodiness (incidence unknown)	Headache, nausea (0.1 to <5%)
Notes on suitability for treatment	Avoid co-treatment with other medications.	Avoid co-treatment with other medications except pH-neutral infusions and fluid replacement solutions such as 5% glucose solution or biological saline solution.	Avoid co-treatment with other medications.	Avoid co-treatment with other medications.
	Do not use any preparation that is not completely dissolved.		Do not use product if it appears incompletely dissolved or there is excessive turbidity.	Do not use product if it appears incompletely dissolved or there is excessive turbidity.

(continued)

Table 2 (continued)

	Product (May 2010)	Product (April 2011)	Product (September 2011)	Product (June 2012)
	Once dissolved, the medication should be used as soon as possible.		Administer only after returning to room temperature.	Do not use the product if it has been frozen.
	Any liquid remaining after treatment should not be reused, due to the possibility of bacterial contamination.		Any liquid remaining after treatment should not be reused, due to the possibility of bacterial contamination.	Any liquid remaining after treatment should not be reused, due to the possibility of bacterial contamination.
				When administering the product i.v., ensure that none of the medication leaks out of the blood vessel (in infants, if there is leakage during i.v. treatment, the skin near the insertion point may become ulcerated; cases of skin necrosis have been reported)
Storage	Store at <30°C; do not freeze		Store at <10°C; do not freeze	Store at ≤ 10°C; do not freeze
	Information based on revised product manual (May 2010)	Information based on revised product manual (April 2011)	Information based on revised product manual (September 2011)	Information based on revised product manual (June 2012)

ALP, alkaline phosphatase; ALT, alanine aminotransferase; AST, aspartate aminotransferase; CK, creatine kinase; CPK, creatine phosphokinase; IVIG, i.v. immunoglobulin; KD, Kawasaki disease

IVIG retreatment for IVIG-resistant patients

Although IVIG is the established first-line treatment for KD, approximately 15–20 % of all KD patients (16.6 % of patients in the 21st Nationwide Survey of KD[1]) have persistent or recrudescent fever after 2 g/kg of IVIG, and there has been considerable debate regarding the optimal second-line treatment for such patients. The 21st Nationwide Survey of KD reported that additional IVIG was given to a large majority (91.5 %) of the 3231 IVIG-resistant patients reported during the survey period. Steroid was given together with IVIG in 29.0 % of patients, IFX in 4.3 %, immunosuppressants in 3.7 %, and PE in 2.2 % of patients. IVIG retreatment alone was effective in approximately half of the patients.[24]

In recent years, various scoring systems have been developed to evaluate the likelihood of IVIG resistance at the time of diagnosis. Representative scoring systems are listed in Table 3.[8-10] If such scores suggest that patients are at high risk of IVIG resistance, more aggressive primary therapy in combination with the usual first-line treatment of 2 g/kg IVIG plus aspirin can be considered. In the RAISE study, Kobayashi et al. found that IVIG plus PSL, started at 2 mg/kg per day and halved every 5 days, was effective in preventing CAL formation and initial treatment failure.[8, 13] In addition, Egami et al. and Ogata et al. as well as Sano et al. and Okada et al. reported the effectiveness of methylprednisolone (MP; 1–3 doses of 30 mg/kg of IVMP) in combination with IVIG.[9-12] As compared with

Table 3 Representative scoring systems for evaluating potential IVIG resistance

	Cut-off point	Points
Kobayashi score[8] (≥5 points; 76 % sensitivity, 80 % specificity)		
Sodium	≤133 mmol/L	2
Day of illness at initial IVIG (= KD diagnosed)	Day 4 or earlier	2
AST	≥100 IU/L	2
Neutrophil ratio	≥80 %	2
CRP	≥10 mg/dL	1
Platelet counts	≤30.0 × 10^4/mm^3	1
Age	≤12 months	1
Egami score[9] (≥3 points; 78 % sensitivity, 76 % specificity)		
ALT	≥80 IU/L	2
Day of illness at initial IVIG (= KD diagnosed)	Day 4 or earlier	1
CRP	≥8 mg/dL	1
Platelet counts	≤30.0 × 10^4/mm^3	1
Age	≤6 months	1
Sano score[10] (≥2 points; 77 % sensitivity, 86 % specificity)		
AST	≥200 IU/L	1
Total bilirubin	≥0.9 mg/dL	1
CRP	≥7 mg/dL	1

AST, aspartate aminotransferase; CRP, C-reactive protein; IVIG, i.v. immunoglobulin; KD, Kawasaki disease

patients receiving only IVIG plus aspirin, defervescence was significantly more likely, and the incidence of CAL was significantly lower, among patients receiving IVIG plus steroids. Although further research is necessary, it seems advisable to adapt this risk-stratified strategy for severe cases so as to reduce the number of IVIG-resistant patients and further lower the incidence of CAL.

Effectiveness

I.v. immunoglobulin was found to be quite safe and, at present, has the greatest effectiveness. For these reasons, its effectiveness has been widely recognized both in Japan and in other countries, and it is also included in the recommendations of many relevant textbooks.

The incidence of cardiac complications reported in the latest Nationwide KD survey decreased to approximately half that in 1997–1998, when patients only rarely received 2 g/kg IVIG. During the acute phase of the illness, that is, until approximately 1 month after disease onset, the incidence of cardiac complications was 9.3 %, including dilation, 7.26 %; valvular insufficiency, 1.19 %; coronary aneurysm, 1.04 %; giant coronary aneurysm, 0.24 %; coronary artery stenosis, 0.03 %; and myocardial infarction, 0.01 %. Even during the convalescent phase, that is, >28 days after disease onset, complications persisted in 3.0 % of patients, including dilation, 1.90 %; aneurysm, 0.78 %; valvular insufficiency, 0.29 %; giant aneurysm, 0.22 %; stenosis, 0.03 %; and myocardial infarction, 0.02 %. Furthermore, the number of deaths in Japan within 2 years of KD onset was 51 during the 10 year period 1991–2000, which decreased by more than 60 % to 19 cases with the introduction of 2 g/kg IVIG during the subsequent 10 year period, 2001–2010 (Fig. 2).[1]

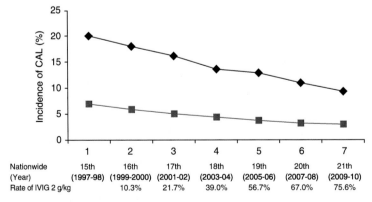

Fig. 2 Incidence of coronary artery lesions (CAL) vs rate of 2 g/kg i.v. immunoglobulin (IVIG) treatment. image, <30 days; image, ≥30 days

Side-effects

I.v. immunoglobulin is derived from human plasma and is considered to have very few adverse effects and a high level of safety (Table 4). It is necessary, however, to carefully explain the possibilities of rare side-effects to patients and/or their families and to obtain their informed consent before treatment

In Japan, there have been no reports of viral contamination of any IVIG product. Donated blood is carefully screened to confirm the absence of HBs antigens, anti-HCV antibodies, anti-HIV-1 antibodies, anti-HIV-2 antibodies, and anti-HTLV-1 antibodies and to verify normal ALT. Furthermore, when plasma is pooled, the nucleic acid amplification testing (NAT) is used to test for HIV, hepatitis B virus (HBV), hepatitis C virus (HCV), hepatitis A virus, and human parvovirus B19, and only plasma that tests negative for all these infections is used. Using present pharmaceutical production processes, the absence of viruses that are undetectable even by NAT (e.g. abnormal prion proteins and human parvovirus B19), cannot be determined with 100 % certainty, but there have been no reports of viral infection due to IVIG. Side-effects are infrequent but include post-treatment chills and shivering, shock (such as cyanosis and hypotension), anaphylactic reactions, aseptic meningitis,[25] hemolytic anemia,[26] hepatic dysfunction, jaundice, acute renal failure, thrombocytopenia, and pulmonary edema. Thus, patients should be careful monitored for these side-effects. Particularly immediately after the start of i.v. treatment and when the infusion rate is increased, the physician should monitor for coldness and shivering, altered consciousness, discomfort, trembling, cyanosis, hypotension, and shock. Finally, cardiac dysfunction or even acute heart failure

Table 4 General side-effects of immunoglobulin

	High incidence	Rare
General	Fatigue, fever, facial erythema, coldness	Anaphylaxis
Systemic side-effects	Loss of appetite, myalgia, arthralgia, swollen joints	Common cold symptoms, anaphylaxis, blepharedema
Neurological	Headache, migraine, dizziness	Aseptic meningitis, weakness, abnormal sensations
Respiratory	Shortness of breath, cough, bronchial spasms	Pleural effusion, blood transfusion-related lung disorders, pulmonary edema
Cardiovascular	Hypotension, hypertension, chest pain	Irregular pulse, myocardial infarction
Gastrointestinal	Loss of appetite, nausea, vomiting, abdominal pain, diarrhea	Taste disorder
Renal		Renal tubular disorders, renal failure
Dermatological	Urticaria, erythema, pimples, pruritus	Multiform exudative erythema
Hematological	Hemolysis	Thromboembolism, hyperviscosity syndrome, leukopenia

Table 5 Post-marketing survey of adverse effects of Ig for KD (no. treatments, 7259)

Side-effect	No. events
Hepatic dysfunction	69
Abnormal findings of liver enzyme tests	40
Pruritus, rash	78
Hypothermia	50
Hypotension	19
Aseptic meningitis	19
Pallor	15
Cyanosis	14
Heart failure	13
Shock	13
Peripheral coldness	13
Hemolytic anemia	4

KD, Kawasaki disease

may develop during acute KD, so close attention should be paid to patient vital signs, and to preventing sudden increases in circulating blood volume, throughout the duration of i.v. treatment.[27, 28]

Other considerations when using IVIG are as follows.

(1) Patients with IgA deficiency: allergic reactions may occur in response to IVIG in patients with anti-IgA antibodies.
(2) Patients with renal damage: risk of further impairment of renal function.
(3) Patients with cerebral or cardiovascular damage or a history of these conditions: blood viscosity may increase when high-dose IVIG is given rapidly, thus leading to thromboembolic events such as cerebral or myocardial infarction.
(4) Patients at risk for thromboembolism: rapid use of high-dose IVIG could increase blood viscosity and lead to thromboembolic events.
(5) Patients with hemolytic anemia, blood loss anemia, immune deficiencies, or immunosuppressive disorders: the possibility of human parvovirus B19 infection cannot be completely excluded. If such infection occurs, severe systemic effects such as fever and sudden or persistent anemia may result.
(6) Patients with reduced cardiac function: high-dose IVIG may lead to cardiac dysfunction or could worsen existing heart failure.

A post-marketing survey of IVIG for KD noted that among 7259 patients who received IVIG treatment, 484 had a total of 697 adverse events (9.6 %) and only 68 patients experienced 78 severe adverse events (1.1 %; Table 5).[29]

Evidence levels

First-line IVIG treatment: class Ia, grade A.

Additional IVIG treatment in IVIG-resistant patients: class III, grade B.

Combined therapy with IVIG and steroid as first-line treatment for suspected IVIG-resistant patients: class Ib, grade B.

Methylprednisolone pulse

Purpose

I.v. methylprednisolone pulse is usually given because of its powerful and rapid immunosuppressive effect (Table 6). Among available steroids, MP treatment is often selected for high-dose i.v. infusion because it is less likely to disrupt electrolyte balance. IVMP is widely used in treating severe pediatric illnesses such as rheumatic disease and kidney disease and is also used in treating confirmed and suspected IVIG-resistant KD.

Mechanism of action

Steroids bind with glucocorticoid receptors in cytoplasm and regulate nuclear expression of proteins such as NF-κB, which produces an anti-inflammatory effect referred to as genomic action.[30] When high-dose MP is given i.v., however, the saturation point of these glucocorticoid receptors is greatly exceeded; thus, mechanisms other than genomic action are thought to contribute to its efficacy. Such mechanisms may include acting through proteins that dissociate from complexes with cytosolic glucocorticoid receptors, membrane-bound glucocorticoid receptors, and functional modification of membrane-bound protein after interlocation of the cell membrane. These mechanisms precede genomic action.[30, 31]

When used for KD patients, the effects of IVMP are very rapid, which suggests that non-genomic mechanisms stimulate immunocytological activity and suppress inflammatory cytokines. In confirmed and suspected IVIG-resistant patients, IVMP was reported to limit production of cytokines involved in inflammation and CAL, [32] and to reduce transcription at the genetic level.[33]

Indications

Patients suspected of being IVIG resistant on the basis of clinical symptoms and laboratory findings.

Patients found to be IVIG resistant after first-line IVIG treatment.

It should be noted that IVMP treatment for KD is an off-label use.

Treatment method and dosage

In patients with kidney disease or connective-tissue disease, the standard dose of IVMP is 20–30 mg/kg IVMP, given once a day over a period of 2–3 h, for 1–3 consecutive days.[31] For KD patients, studies of IVMP in combination with first-line IVIG investigated a single dose of 30 mg/kg IVMP.[11, 12, 34] Studies of

Table 6 Treatments other than IVIG for acute KD

General name	Mode of action	Treatment route, dose, and methods	Principal side-effects	Important notices
Methylprednisolone	Suppresses transcription of inflammatory proteins arising from glucocorticoid receptors	When used in combination with first-line IVIG: 1 dose of 30 mg/kg methylprednisolone.	Sinus bradycardia (6–82 %), hypertension (10–91 %), hyperglycemia (6–55 %), hypothermia (6–9 %) etc.	Vital signs – including electrocardiogram, body temperature, and blood pressure – should be continuously monitored
	Suppresses immune cells and inflammatory cytokines arising due to non-genomic activity, such as functional changes in cell membranes etc.	When used to treat IVIG-resistant patients: 30 mg/kg methylprednisolone once a day, for 1–3 days. Some reports suggest additional prednisolone (started at 1–2 mg/kg/day and gradually tapered over a period of 1–3 weeks) after methylprednisolone.	In rare cases, patients may develop infections, gastrointestinal ulcers, mental disorders, femur head necrosis, and suppressed adrenal function.	
Prednisolone	Inhibits gene transcription of inflammatory proteins and promotes gene transcription of anti-inflammatory proteins	During fever: 2 mg/kg/day of prednisolone, i.v. in 3 divided doses	Some viral infections (a few percent), moon facies (most who receive this treatment), hypothermia immediately after defervescence (a few percent), occult blood positivity (approx. 1 %), hyperlipidemia (a large proportion), neutrophil-predominant leukocytosis (in almost all cases) etc.	
		After defervescence: Once patient is no longer febrile and general status has improved, prednisolone is given orally. When CRP normalizes, the dose of prednisolone is tapered	General side-effects of steroid treatment: infections, gastrointestinal ulcers, mental disorders, femur head necrosis, suppressed adrenal function etc.	

		over 15 days, in 5 day steps, from 2 mg/kg/day in 3 divided doses to 1 mg/kg/day in 2 divided doses to 0.5 mg/kg/day in a single dose.		
Infliximab	Neutralizes biological activity of soluble TNF-a Damages membrane-bound TNF-a-expressing cells, with complement- and antibody-dependent cell damage Dissociates TNF-a bound to TNF-a receptors	i.v. drip infusion of 5 mg/kg (may only be given once)	Of Of 708 adult cases in Japan, nasopharyngitis (19.6 %), fever, (11 %), exanthema (8.9 %), headache (5.8 %), cough (5.1 %), elevated ALT (12.6 %), elevated AST (9.9 %), elevated LDH (9.3 %) etc.	Avoid mixing with IVIG in treatment route
Ulinastatin	Inhibits elastase release from neutrophils and platelets, and rendering it inactive after release	i.v. drip of 5000 units/kg, 3–6 times a day, for 3–4 days	Anaphylaxis, hepatic dysfunction (0.5 %), leukopenia (0.2 %), allergic symptoms such as exanthema and pruritus (0.1 %), diarrhea, angiodynia (0.1 %), elevated AST, elevated ALT, eosinophilia, vascular pain at injection site etc.	
		No treatment may exceed 50 000 units.		
Cyclosporine A	Suppresses cytokine production such as IL-2 by inhibiting nuclear factor of activated T cells	Start on 2 divided oral doses (1 each before meal) of 4–5 mg/kg/day Target trough level: 60–200 ng/mL	Subclinical hyperkalemia (with lower values in plasma than in serum; no reports of adverse events such as arrhythmia etc.)	
			General adverse reactions include increased blood pressure, nausea and vomiting, shivering, hyperglycemia, hyperuricemia, hyperlipidemia (1–5%) etc.	

(continued)

Table 6 (continued)

General name	Mode of action	Treatment route, dose, and methods	Principal side-effects	Important notices
Methotrexate	Suppresses proliferation of several immunomodulatory cells by inhibiting synthesis of DNA as a folic acid antagonist	One oral dose of 10 mg/body surface area per week	Side-effects appearing at standard doses (gastrointestinal injury, hair loss, myelosuppression etc.) are not reported at lower doses	
Plasma exchange	Mechanical removal of inflammatory cytokines	Displacing solution set at 5 % albumin; 1–1.5x the patient's circulating plasma volume is exchanged Usually given for 3 continuous days (upper limit: 6 days)	Hypotension, hypovolemia, shock, anaphylactoid reactions, hypocalcemia, fever/coldness/shivering, nausea/vomiting, coagulopathies, pneumothorax at time of catheter insertion	
Aspirin	Blocks synthesis of PGE2 from arachidonic acid during PG synthesis	Febrile period: Oral dose of 30–50 mg/kg/day, in 3 divided doses	Bleeding, hepatic dysfunction, gastrointestinal ulcer, hematemesis, induction of asthmatic attacks, urticaria, exanthema (incidence unknown), loss of appetite (0.1 to < 5 %), nephropathy (<0.1 %) etc.	Special care should be taken when patient has chickenpox or influenza, as aspirin might induce Reye syndrome
		After defervescence: Single oral doses of 3–5 mg/kg/day		

ALT, alanine aminotransferase; AST, aspartate aminotransferase; CRP, C-reactive protein; IL, interleukin; IVIG, i.v. immunoglobulin; LDH, lactate dehydrogenase; PG, prostaglandin

second-line IVIG treatment in IVIG-resistant patients investigated the same IVMP dose given once a day, for 1–3 days.[32, 33, 35-39] Because the half-life of IVMP is only 3 h,[31] some studies used additional therapy with PSL started at 1–2 mg/kg per day and gradually tapered over a period of 1–3 weeks.[38, 39]

Effectiveness

First-line therapy with IVIG plus IVMP for all KD patients has not been proven to prevent CAL.[40] There is, however, no evidence that IVMP increases CAL incidence. In a double-blind randomized controlled trial comparing IVIG plus IVMP with IVIG plus placebo, no significant differences were found in factors such as duration of fever, incidence of additional treatment, incidence of CAL, and coronary artery diameter, as indicated by Z score.[34] A post-hoc analysis of patients requiring additional treatment, however, found that the incidence of CAL was significantly lower among those who had received IVIG plus IVMP, which suggests that the combined regimen had been effective among IVIG-resistant patients. Studies have also reported that suspected IVIG-resistant patients (as determined by Egami score or Sano score) who received first-line IVIG plus IVMP had earlier defervescence and a significantly lower rate of CAL than did those who had received IVIG alone.[11, 12]

For patients resistant to initial IVIG, some studies compared IVMP as a second-line treatment to additional treatment with IVIG and found that duration of fever was shorter after IVMP but that CAL incidence was similar.[32, 36-40] The researchers, however, highlighted the fact that IVMP therapy was less expensive than retreatment of IVIG.[36, 37] Nevertheless, the finding of equal efficacy for IVIG and IVMP has not been shown in non-inferiority trials and requires confirmation. One study reported that IVIG-resistant patients who did not respond to additional IVIG had a lower rate of CAL after subsequent IVMP followed by PSL treatment.[39]

Side-effects

The reported side-effects of IVMP treatment for KD patients include sinus brady-cardia (6–82 %), hypertension (10–91 %), hyperglycemia (6–55 %), and hypother-mia (6–9 %).[39, 41] Therefore, patient vital signs must be very carefully monitored during IVMP, including monitoring of electrocardiogram and blood pressure.

To avoid development of gastrointestinal ulcer, patients can be given H2 blockers and/or other antacid agents. Additional heparin can also be given as thrombosis prophylaxis.[38, 39] Nevertheless, the necessity of these medications has not been proven.

Evidence levels

Initial IVIG plus IVMP for all KD patients: class Ib, grade C.
   Initial IVIG plus IVMP for suspected IVIG-resistant patients: class Ib, grade B.
   Second-line IVMP use for IVIG-resistant patients: class IIb, grade B.

Prednisolone

Purpose

The primary purpose of PSL therapy is to take advantage of its powerful anti-inflammatory effects (Table 6). PSL may quickly resolve KD vasculitis and suppress the potential risk for remodeling of coronary arteries.

Mechanism of action

Prednisolone is the most widely used synthetic corticosteroid hormone, and its glucocorticoid action is stronger than that of cortisol. Through cytoplasmic steroid receptors, PSL inhibits gene transcription of inflammatory cytokines and promotes gene transcription of anti-inflammatory cytokines.[30] PSL also suppresses inflammation by inhibiting production of inflammatory cytokines (e.g. tumor necrosis factor-α [TNF-α], interleukin [IL]-6, IL-8), chemokines, and cell adhesion molecules. In addition, PSL stimulates production of anti-inflammatory proteins such as lipocortin, IL-1 receptor antagonists, β-2 adrenergic receptors, and IκB kinase.

Indications

Patients suspected of being IVIG resistant, based on evaluation of clinical symptoms and laboratory findings.
   Patients found to be IVIG resistant after first-line IVIG treatment.
   PSL treatment for KD is an off-label use.

Treatment method and dosage

When used in combination with initial IVIG, 2 mg/kg per day of PSL is given i.v. in three divided doses.[13] After defervescence and improvement in the patient's general condition, PSL can be given orally. After CRP normalizes, the patient is continued for 5 days on the same dosage in three divided doses of 2 mg/kg per day. Thereafter, if fever does not recur, the dosage of PSL is decreased to 1 mg/kg per day in two divided doses on the subsequent 5 days and then a single dose of 0.5 mg/

kg per day on the final 5 days. If fever recurs after dose reduction, additional treatment should be considered, including an increase in PSL dose, IVIG retreatment, or other treatments. The most common periods for relapse are 4–5 days after the start of PSL and after the dose reduction from 2 mg/kg to 1 mg/kg.

For patients resistant to initial IVIG, the regimen for second-line PSL should, in principle, involve the same dosages and timings as specified for first-line PSL therapy.

Effectiveness

Although corticosteroids are the treatment of choice for other forms of vasculitis, their use has been limited in KD. In 1975, a case–control study showed that fatal cases were more frequently treated with PSL as compared with matched non-fatal cases.[42] In addition, a retrospective study found that PSL had a detrimental effect when used as initial therapy.[14] Finally, a prospective randomized controlled trial of three groups (receiving either aspirin, flurbiprofen, or PSL plus dipyridamole) did not confirm the efficacy of PSL. These results led to PSL being contraindicated for KD in the 1980s.[43] A retrospective study, however, in the 1990s of a PSL plus aspirin regimen found this combination to be useful in preventing CAL and shortening duration of fever,[44] which led to a reconsideration of PSL therapy. In 2006, a prospective randomized controlled trial comparing initial IVIG plus PSL to initial IVIG alone reported a significantly lower incidence of CAL in the IVIG plus PSL group.[45] A subsequent retrospective study suggested that risk stratification of initial treatment might be possible using the Kobayashi score;[8, 46] therefore, a randomized controlled trial to assess immunoglobulin plus steroid efficacy for KD (RAISE study) was carried out. The RAISE Study showed that among patients with a Kobayashi score ≥ 5, initial treatment with IVIG plus PSL significantly decreased the incidence of CAL and rate of resistance to initial treatment.[13] Although its external validity remains unproven, initial therapy with IVIG plus PSL for patients at high risk of IVIG resistance could become the standard therapy for severe KD.

Reports have also shown the effectiveness of PSL as a second-line therapy for IVIG-resistant patients.[47] One study however, reported that PSL therapy might induce CAL formation in IVIG-resistant patients, given that more days have elapsed since the onset of illness.[48] No randomized controlled trials have assessed PSL therapy for IVIG-resistant patients; thus, the efficacy of PSL for this subgroup is unknown.

Side-effects

According to the product labeling, PSL may lead to side-effects such as shock (0.08 %), infection (2.54 %), Legg-Calvé-Perthes disease (0.36 %), gastrointestinal perforation (0.02 %), gastrointestinal hemorrhage (0.80 %), gastrointestinal ulcer (0.02 %), diabetes (3.95 %), posterior subcapsular cataract (0.09 %), pancreatitis

(0.03 %), congestive heart failure (0.02 %), and impaired hepatic function (1.21 %), as well as circulatory collapse, arrhythmia, secondary adrenocortical insufficiency, osteoporosis, myopathy, thrombosis, increased intracranial pressure, seizure, abnormal mental function, glaucoma, central serous chorioretinopathy, esophagitis, and jaundice (incidences unknown).

Prednisolone is contraindicated for patients with (i) infections for which there is no effective antimicrobial agent, such as systemic mycoses; (ii) severe infections accompanied by reduced renal function or chronic renal failure; or (iii) a history of acute myocardial infarction.

Evidence levels

Initial IVIG plus PSL for suspected IVIG-resistant patients: class Ib, grade B.
    Second-line treatment for IVIG-resistant patients: class IIb, grade C.

Biologics (infliximab)

Purpose

The serum concentration of TNF-α is elevated in KD patients, and several reports have shown a significant association between KD severity and incidence of CAA. IFX suppresses inflammation by blocking the action of TNF-α (Table 6).

Mechanism of action

Infliximab was originally developed in mice as a mouse antibody with human TNF-α. IFX is a chimeric monoclonal antibody and is produced by bonding 25 % V-region – a specific antibody derived from mice – with 75 % C-region of the human immunoglobulin G1 κ-chain. Because each IFX molecule contains 25 % mouse protein, anti-chimeric antibodies (neutralizing antibodies) develop in approximately 40 % of patients; thus, among patients undergoing repeated use, its efficacy decreases and allergic reactions might occur. Production of neutralizing antibodies is inhibited in patients with rheumatoid arthritis (RA) who receive IFX in combination with MTX. IFX binds specifically to TNF-α, not to TNF-β. The mechanisms of action are believed to be as follows: (i) neutralize soluble TNF-α and block binding of TNF-α to TNF receptors (p55 and p75); (ii) bind membrane-associated TNF-α expressed on the surface of TNF-α-producing cells, inducing apoptosis through complement-dependent cytotoxicity and antibody-dependent cellular cytotoxicity and inhibiting production of TNF-α; and (iii) dissociate TNF-α bound to receptors. As a result of these mechanisms, IFX suppresses activation of inflammatory cells and production of inflammatory cytokines such as IL-1 and IL-6.

Indications

IVIG-resistant patients.
   The use of IFX for treating KD is off-label.

Treatment method and dosage

In Japan, IFX is presently approved for use in adults with (i) RA; (ii) inflammatory bowel disease (IBD; Crohn's disease, ulcerative colitis); (iii) intractable uveitis accompanying Behçet disease; (iv) pruritus; and (v) ankylosing spondylitis (AS). In Europe and the USA, it has also been approved for use in treating Crohn's disease in children aged $\geq$6 years.[49]
   Children treated with IFX usually receive one dose of 5 mg/kg. In patients with Crohn's disease, however, there are reports of other dosages such as 3 mg/kg or 6 mg/kg. For adults with RA, 3–10 mg/kg IFX is given i.v. once every 8 weeks. IFX has a half-life of approximately 9.5 days and is usually given by i.v. drip infusion mixed in 200–500 mL of saline, over a period of at least 2 h. Unlike RA, KD is an acute disease, and MTX and steroids are not usually given as they would be for RA. A single-dose IFX regimen is recommended because KD is an acute disease, unlike RA, and MTX or steroids are not usually concomitantly used. Studies in the USA have not established a lower age limit for IFX use, but there is no assurance of complete safety when IFX is given to newborns and infants.

Effectiveness

The first experience of the effectiveness of IFX for treating KD was reported in 2004 by Weiss et al., who used it with positive results to treat a 3-year-old patient who had not responded to treatment with IVIG and IVMP at the 45th day of illness. [50] Later, several reports confirmed the effectiveness of IFX in suppressing inflammation among patients resistant to both IVIG and IVMP. These reports suggested that IFX is safe and effective within a relatively short time.[51-61] IFX lowered serum levels of inflammatory markers such as IL-6, CRP, and soluble TNF-α receptor 1.[52, 62] By 2009, a total of 39 cases (patient age range, 1 month–13 years; CAA development, 22 of 39) of IFX use in treating KD that did not respond to IVIG and/or IVMP had been reported.[58] In the USA, IFX was used in approximately 1 % of the 4811 IVIG-resistant cases, and its use had increased from 0 % in 2001 to 2.3 % by 2006.[63] In a recent review of additional treatment for IVIG-resistant patients, either additional IVIG, 3 days of IVMP, or IFX was recommended.[64] The effectiveness of anti-TNF-α antibody in reducing vasculitis severity was demonstrated in an animal model of KD vasculitis.[65]
   In Japan, 6 years have passed since IFX was first used as an off-label treatment for a patient who failed to respond to IVIG.[52] The Japanese Society of Kawasaki Disease surveyed the use of IFX during 2006–2011 and found a total of 192 patients

treated with IFX during that period. It was effective in around 80 % of cases but was unsuccessful in reducing fever in 10–15 % of cases. Experimental studies have not reported any severe side-effects; thus, IFX appears to be relatively safe for use in most patients. In general, the incidence of CAA is lower when IFX is used before the 10th day after onset.

Side-effects

After IFX had been approved for RA, it was given to >5000 adult patients with RA in Japan. Adverse events were reported in 28 % of these patients within 6 months of first use; 6.2 % of these were severe adverse events, including bacterial pneumonia (2.2 %, 108 patients), Pneumocystis pneumonia (0.4 %, 22 patients), sepsis (0.2 %, 10 patients), tuberculosis (0.3 %, 14 patients), and severe infusion reaction (0.5 %, 24 patients; Table 7).[66-76] As for patients with juvenile idiopathic arthritis (JIA), there is a report that adverse events were more frequent at lower doses (3 mg/kg) than at higher doses (6 mg/kg).[69] There are limited data, however, on the safety of IFX in children. Therefore, the indication of IFX for KD should be determined only after carefully assessing the risk–benefit balance on a case-by-case basis.

Table 7 Severe adverse effects and contraindications of anti-TNF-α treatment for children 66–76

Severe adverse effects
Overresponse at treatment site
Infusion reaction
Varicella infection
Latent infections (tuberculosis etc.)
Neurological demyelination diseases (multiple sclerosis etc.)
Neuropsychiatric side-effects
Fatigue, headache, vertigo, depression, anxiety
Pain amplification syndrome
Malignant tumors
Immunogenicity
Contraindications
Complete contraindications
Active infections
Recurrent infections and history of chronic infections
Existing untreated tuberculosis Multiple sclerosis, optic neuritis
Combined use with anakinra (anti-IL-1 receptor antagonist)
Active or recent (previous 10 years) malignant tumor (except skin tumors)
Relative contraindications
Pregnancy, breastfeeding
HIV, HBV, or HCV infection

IL, interleukin

Infusion-associated reaction

Because IFX is a chimeric monoclonal antibody, it might induce anaphylactic reactions. For this reason, patients receiving IFX should be carefully observed for symptoms such as fever, rash, pruritus, and headache, along with regular monitoring of vital signs. The patient should also be carefully monitored for other side-effects, such as respiratory distress, bronchial spasms, angioedema, cyanosis, hypoxia, and urticaria.[70]

Premedication with acetaminophen and/or antihistamines is considered ineffective for preventing anaphylactic symptoms.[70] As for long-term IFX treatment, in a study of 163 patients with JIA (68 receiving IFX and 95 receiving etanercept; mean age, 17 years; mean treatment period, 22.9 months), there were 71 adverse events, and 62.9 % of the events occurred in patients treated with IFX. In contrast, another report found IFX to be safe and well-tolerated, with few side-effects.[73] Among patients with JIA who had been receiving IFX for 1 year, the incidence of infusion reaction was 3.3 % among those who had been receiving a dose of 3 mg/kg and 7 % among those receiving 6 mg/kg.[74, 75] In addition, neutralizing human antichimeric antibodies (HACA) were found in many patients who developed an infusion-associated reaction. HACA was also found in 7.1–12.1 % of pediatric patients with Crohn's disease.[76]

Delayed hypersensitivity symptoms were seen ≥3 days after repeated use of IFX (24 h–3 weeks after treatment), including myalgia, rash, fever, fatigue, arthralgia, pruritus, edema of the hands and face, dysphagia, urticaria, pharyngeal pain, and headache. Table 7 lists the points of concern when giving IFX to pediatric patients. For these reasons, additional use of IFX in patients with acute KD is not recommended.

Exacerbation of heart failure

Infliximab worsened symptoms of heart failure in adults with New York Heart Association (NYHA) class III or IV disease and left ventricular ejection fraction <50 %. Even among NYHA class II patients, IFX should be used with caution because serum brain natriuretic peptide is elevated in acute KD, which suggests asymptomatic cardiac impairment, including subclinical myocarditis, cardiac hypofunction, pericardial effusion, and atrioventricular valvular regurgitation.[70]

Exacerbation of infectious diseases

The possibility of worsening of infectious disease is especially important for infants who have not yet been vaccinated against BCG. QuantiFERON (QFT-TB Gold; Japan BCG Laboratory, Tokyo, Japan) testing is not affected by BCG vaccination or mycobacterial infection, but a false-positive result may occur if a patient has a history of past infection. Although pediatric patients sometimes show false-negative results, QuantiFERON testing may nevertheless be useful. It is essential to conduct a careful diagnostic interview, including questions on infections in family members and the patient's BCG vaccination status. Findings from chest radiography or computed tomography, if required, are also important.

As for live vaccines other than BCG, such as the rotavirus vaccine, use of IFX should be postponed if the patient has had such a vaccination <2 months previously or has had vaccines for measles–rubella, mumps, or chickenpox <1 month previously. IFX is contraindicated if any active infection is present.

Unfortunately, evidence is limited regarding the interval necessary between inoculation with a live vaccine and IFX treatment. Some specialists suggest an interval of 2–3 months to ensure patient safety.

Development of malignant tumors

When etanercept was used to treat 1200 patients with JIA, five patients developed malignancies, including Hodgkin lymphoma, non-Hodgkin lymphoma, thyroid carcinoma, yolk-sac cancer, and cervical dysplasia of the uterus. All these patients, however, had also been treated with other immunosuppressants, and two had received adalimumab and IFX as well. Before IFX is given, the possible side-effects should be carefully explained to the patient and/or family, and written informed consent should be obtained.[71] The US Food and Drug Administration reported that 48 patients developed malignant carcinomas (of which half were lymphomas) after receiving anti-TNF-α agents, and 11 patients died. Among the patients, IFX was given to 31, etanercept to 15, and adalimumab to two patients; 88 % of the patients developing malignant carcinomas had also received other immunosuppressants (e.g. azathioprine and MTX).[72] The present data do not show a conclusive association between IFX and malignant disease.

Carriers of hepatitis B and C

Among adult patients with rheumatic diseases, asymptomatic carriers of HBV or chronic hepatitis may experience reactivation of HBV or de novo hepatitis.[77, 78] Thus, testing for HBs antigens and HBs and HBc antibodies is necessary before IFX treatment. Because HBV carrier status and presence of chronic viral hepatitis are associated with higher risk of activation of these viruses and exacerbation of existing hepatitis, IFX use in such patients should be avoided, as recommended by the Japan College of Rheumatology.[78]

Screening for HCV infection should be done before IFX treatment. IFX is also contraindicated for patients with active hepatitis C. Patients who are positive for HCV but do not have active hepatitis should be carefully monitored if IFX is used. Although the safety of IFX for hepatitis C patients has not been confirmed, there are no reports in Japan or other countries of IFX worsening hepatitis C. Nevertheless, consultation with a pediatric liver specialist is recommended before beginning IFX treatment.

Other

Infliximab is contraindicated in patients with demyelination disorders or allergy to IFX. For patients with KD, severe complications due to IFX are likely to be uncommon because IFX is mostly given as one dose and because KD patients usually have no other chronic active infectious disease. Many children, however, become susceptible to acute infectious disease at early infancy thus, IFX should be used only after careful examination for active infections such as pneumonia, otitis media, and urinary tract infections. In addition, long-term follow up of possible side-effects is required.

Evidence levels

When used for IVIG-resistant patients: class IIb, grade C.

Ulinastatin

Purpose

The principal action of UTI is to reduce inflammatory vascular lesions caused by proteolysis, edema, necrosis, and hemorrhage (Table 6).[79]

Mechanism of action

Ulinastatin is a human urinary trypsin inhibitor, purified from human urine. UTI is a polyvalent enzyme inhibitor – a serine protease inhibitor – with a molecular weight of 67 000 kDa and blocks various protein-degrading pancreatic enzymes, including trypsin. UTI is produced by many organs, including liver, kidney, pancreas, lungs, heart, adrenals, stomach, large intestine, brain, and testes.

Suppression of TNF-α

Ulinastatin suppresses production and secretion of inflammatory cytokines, for example TNF-α, IL-6, and IL-8 from neutrophils or TNF-α from monocytes. [80] It also inhibits expression of intercellular adhesion molecule-1 on the surface of vascular endothelial cells activated by TNF-α, thereby playing a protective role with regard to endothelial cells.

Blocking of neutrophil elastase

Ulinastatin has a dual action, first blocking elastase release, especially from neutrophils and platelets, and then deactivating elastase as it is released. UTI removes oxygen radicals and reduces the activity of cytokines and cell adhesion factors. By stabilizing lysosome membranes, UTI suppresses the release of various protein-degrading enzymes. Finally, it also blocks the release of inflammatory cytokines of myocardial inhibitory factor containing TNF-α and hypercoagulopathy.[81]

Indications

IVIG-resistant patients.
   Initial treatment in combination with IVIG.
   Its use in KD treatment is off-label.

Treatment method and dosage

Although optimal dosage has not been determined for pediatric patients, several reports show that a dose of 5000 U/kg given 3–6 times/day, not exceeding 50 000 units/dose, is suitable for KD patients. UTI has a half-life of only 40 min when given i.v. at 300 000 U/10 mL. UTI is officially approved to treat two conditions: (i) acute pancreatitis in the earlier phase (adult dosage, 25 000–50 000 units i.v. 1–3 times/day with dose tapering thereafter); and (ii) acute circulatory collapse (adult dosage, 100 000 units i.v. 1–3 times/day).

Effectiveness

Ulinastatin has been reported to inhibit mRNA transcription of prostaglandin H2 and thromboxane A2 in polynuclear leukocytes.[82] It also prevented neutrophil-induced damage to endothelial cells.[83] The first use of UTI was reported in 1993, after which several case studies were reported. These reports appeared to support the effectiveness and safety of UTI treatment under certain conditions, such as (i) when given as a single dose to patients with clinically mild disease; (ii) when it allowed a reduction in IVIG dose in the context of combination therapy; and (iii) when IVIG was ineffective due to non-response or resistance to IVIG.[84, 85] Although these studies enrolled only a small number of patients, and there have been no well-designed clinical studies of UTI, it has been recognized and used as an additional option for treating IVIG-resistant patients.[86] Recent retrospective cohort studies showed that as a first-line treatment UTI in combination with IVIG plus aspirin was less likely to require second-line treatment and had a lower risk of CAA among patients at high risk for IVIG resistance, as defined by Kobayashi score.[87]

Side-effects

The most important side-effect of UTI is anaphylactic shock. UTI should be used carefully if the patient has a history of drug allergies or allergic reactions to products containing gelatin or a past history of UTI use. Other side-effects include liver dysfunction (0.5 %), leukopenia (0.2 %), rash, pruritus (0.1 %), diarrhea (0.1 %), angialgia (0.1 %), increased AST and/or ALT, eosinophilia, and vascular pain at the injection site. Also, if UTI is given along the same route as IVIG and the medications are thus mixed, the drug will become white and turbid. To avoid this, a different i.v. route can be selected. Alternatively, IVIG may be paused and the i.v. route can be flushed with saline before and after UTI infusion, after which IVIG infusion can continue.

Evidence level

First-line treatment with IVIG plus UTI: class IIa, grade B.
   IVIG-resistant patients: class IIb, grade C.

Immunosuppressants

Cyclosporin A

Purpose

In 2008, Onouchi et al. reported a susceptibility gene of KD: inositol 1,4,5-trisphosphate 3-kinase C (ITPKC), composed of inositol triphosphate (Table 6). [88] ITPKC suppresses T-cell activity through the calcineurin/nuclear factor of activated T-cells (calcineurin/NFAT) cascade. Patients with suppressed ITPKC function may produce more cytokines, such as IL-2. For this reason, ITPKC was thought to be a critical gene contributing to IVIG resistance and development of CAA. CsA is used to block calcineurin function and suppress cytokine production.

   Several studies evaluated the efficacy of CsA in IVIG-resistant patients.[89-91] Accumulating evidence of its effectiveness spurred multicenter observational studies in Japan and other countries, and the results of these studies indicate that CsA is safe and well-tolerated.[90, 91]

Mechanism of action

Cyclosporin A binds and inhibits calcineurin, which has a major role in signal transduction that results in increased T-cell activity. By dephosphorylating NFAT, the transcription factor for IL-2 genes, the nuclear import of NFAT is blocked, and production of cytokines such as IL-2 is inhibited.[92]

Indications

IVIG-resistant patients.
   Its use in treating KD is off-label.

Treatment method and dosage

Usually, 4 mg/kg per day of Neoral® (Novartis Pharmaceuticals UK, Surrey, UK) is given orally in two divided doses before meals.[90] The required dose is drawn into a 1 mL syringe and can be given to infants. Outside Japan, some researchers believe that the absorption of CsA is reduced during acute KD. Thus, they start patients on i.v. 3–5 mg/kg per day. After resolution of fever, 10 mg/kg per day of Neoral is given orally in two divided doses of 5 mg/kg.[91] In principle, before the fifth dose on the third day, the trough level of CsA should be monitored to confirm that it is within the therapeutic range (60–200 ng/mL). If it is not within the therapeutic range and fever remains, the dose may be increased by 5–8 mg/kg per day.[90] There is no established duration of treatment, but CsA is usually given until CRP again normalizes, or for a period of 10–14 days. This period may be extended if the dose is tapered.[91] Therapeutic doses of aspirin 30–50 mg/kg per day should be given in combination with CsA until defervescence is confirmed.

Effectiveness

Cyclosporin A has not been evaluated in prospective randomized trials, but observational studies of its use as a third-line treatment in IVIG-resistant patients showed that fever was reduced within 72 h in most patients receiving CsA, and CRP returned to normal.[90, 91] Additional IVIG, however, was occasionally required for cases in which CsA was ineffective.[90] It should be noted that there are no reports of its use in infants younger than 4 months.[90, 91]

Side-effects

There have been no reports of severe side-effects in treating KD. In approximately 40 % of patients, asymptomatic hyperkalemia was observed in serum samples 3–7 days after treatment. Because plasma samples did not show evidence of hyperkalemia, these may have been cases of pseudohyperkalemia.[90] There have also been reports of hypomagnesemia,[91] but no reports have noted arrhythmias due to electrolyte imbalances. Other side-effects reported in patients receiving long-term CsA include hirsutism and hypertension in a few patients.

Evidence level

Class III, grade C.

Methotrexate

Purpose

In 2008, Lee et al. reported that MTX reduced fever and suppressed inflammation in IVIG-resistant patients.[93]

Mechanism of action

Methotrexate (4-amino-N10-methylpteroyl glutamic acid) is a folic acid antagonist. Pharmacologically, MTX (i) inhibits synthesis of purine bodies; (ii) increases adenosine release; (iii) inhibits production of inflammatory cytokines; (iv) suppresses lymphoproliferation; and (v) suppresses migration and adhering of neutrophils; and (vi) suppresses serum immunoglobulin. The mechanism by which low-dose MTX suppresses inflammation, however, has not been confirmed.

Indications

IVIG-resistant patients.
    Use of MTX in treating KD is off-label.
    Treatment method and dosage
    Dosage: 10 mg/m2, given orally once a week. Do not provide folic acid supplements. MTX is given until defervescence. In the report by Lee et al. describing the use of MTX, the median total dosage was 20 mg/m2 (range, 10–50) given in two divided doses.[93]

Effectiveness

Although there have been no prospective randomized trials of MTX, in a case series describing 17 IVIG-resistant patients who received MTX, fever recurred 7 days after the start of MTX in three patients and 14 days after the start of MTX in one patient. Fever resolved, however, in all four of these patients after they received their second or third dose of MTX. Finally, there was no fever recurrence after MTX was discontinued.

Side-effects

The side-effects of MTX at standard doses include gastrointestinal disturbances, hair loss, and myelosuppression, but these side-effects were not seen at low doses. [93] In general, side-effects could include shock or anaphylaxis, myelosuppression, infection, hepatic dysfunction, and acute renal failure.

Evidence levels

Class III, Grade C.

Plasma exchange

Purpose

Plasma exchange directly removes cytokines and chemokines from blood and induces quick recovery from cytokine storm (Table 6).

Mechanism of action

Cytokine storm is thought to be a major contributor to KD pathology. PE might reduce this inflammatory reaction by removing soluble cytokines, even in IVIG-resistant patients. After PE, the serum level of cytokines and chemokines, especially IL-6 and soluble TNF receptor, is markedly reduced.

Indications

IVIG-resistant patients.

Treatment method and dosage

The replacement solution is 5 % albumin, and the total volume to be exchanged is approximately 1–1.5-fold the circulating plasma volume (mL), calculated as follows: [bodyweight (kg)/13 × (1–Hct/100) × 1000] (Hct, hematocrit [%]).

Treatment is via the femoral vein, subclavian vein, or internal or external jugular veins, using a 6–7 Fr pediatric dialysis double-lumen catheter. During treatment, heparin 15–30 U/kg, first as a bolus i.v. infusion and 15–30 U/kg per h thereafter, may also be given for its anticoagulant effect, with the activated clotting time adjusted to 180–250 s. It is also necessary to keep the patient sedated.

Effectiveness

There have been no prospective randomized trials of PE for treatment of pediatric diseases, including KD. Two retrospective studies assessed the effectiveness of PE. [94, 95] One compared PE with IVIG given to 20 patients within 15 days of KD onset.[96] Although the findings were not statistically significant, no patients developed CAL, and there were no adverse effects.

In studies of the safety and efficacy of PE, multivariate analysis comparing PE with additional IVIG yielded an odds ratio of 0.052 and showed a significant reduction in CAL incidence among PE patients.[97, 98] Among PE-resistant patients, some already had CAL. Thus, to ensure optimal outcome PE should probably be started before development of CAL.[99]

Side-effects

In general, the side-effects of PE include hypotension, hypovolemia, and shock. In addition, the replacement solution (in the case of fresh frozen plasma) might induce urticaria, allergic reactions, anaphylactic reactions, and hypocalcemia, as well as fever, chills, shivering, nausea, vomiting, and coagulopathies.[100]

Because the volume of extracorporeal circulation will exceed circulating blood volume in pediatric patients, it may be necessary to reduce the volume to lower the risk of hypotension.

Evidence level

Class III, grade C.

Antiplatelets/anticoagulants

Aspirin

Purpose

Because the mechanism of action of aspirin differs by dosage, medium–high doses are usually given to treat KD in the febrile phase, due to decreased absorption and hypoalbuminemia, to obtain the expected anti-inflammatory benefits (Tables 6, 8). Low doses, however, are usually given to inhibit platelet aggregation after the febrile phase, when the risk of CAA is much lower.

Mechanism of action

Aspirin irreversibly inhibits platelet aggregation to block synthesis of thromboxane A2 by cyclooxygenase-1 activity. It also exerts an anti-inflammatory effect by blocking synthesis of prostaglandin E2 from arachidonic acid during prostaglandin synthesis.

Indications

Approved for all patients.

Treatment method and dosage

Aspirin is given orally. In the USA, high-dose aspirin 80–100 mg/kg per day is usually given in combination with IVIG as an initial treatment.[101] In Japan, a moderate dose of 30–50 mg/kg per day is usually given in three divided doses per day, together with IVIG. Thereafter, 48–72 h after defervescence, dosage can be reduced to one dose of 3–5 mg/kg per day. Even among patients without CAA, aspirin is typically continued for 6–8 weeks after onset of symptoms.

Effectiveness

Two meta-analyses in the late 1990s showed that CAA incidence was not associated with aspirin dose, although it was associated with IVIG dose and IVIG effectiveness.[102, 103]

Table 8 Antiplatelet, anticoagulant, and thrombolytic drugs

Name of medication (trade name)	Mechanism of action	Dose and method of treatment	Side-effects (%)	Important considerations
Flurbiprofen	Anti-inflammatory effect by inhibiting cyclooxygenase	3–5 mg/kg, in 3 divided doses	Gastric discomfort (1.56 %), loss of appetite (1.03 %), rash (0.24 %), rare cases of thrombopenia etc.	
Dipyridamole	Inhibits phosphodiesterase	2–5 mg/kg, in 3 divided doses	Headache (0.91–4.37 %), palpitations (0.43–0.56 %); severe side-effects: worsening of angina symptoms ($<$0.1 %), tendency to bleed (incidence unknown) etc.	
Ticlopidine	Suppresses antiplatelet coagulation; reinforces activity of platelet adenylate cyclase	2–5 mg/kg, in 3 divided doses	TTP, agranulocytosis, severe liver damage (incidence unknown) etc.	Indications for treatment should be carefully examined. Blood tests required every 2 weeks during initial treatment.
Unfractionated heparin	Displays anticoagulant activity by binding AT-III, a factor in physiological inhibition of coagulation factors II, VII, IX, X, XI, XII	Start patient on slow i.v. 50 units/kg (duration of treatment: $\geq$10 min), then continuous i.v. infusion with 20–25 units/kg/h	Hemorrhage is the principal side-effect (incidence unknown) HIT (incidence unknown), impaired hepatic function (0.1 to $<$5 %), rash (incidence unknown), hair loss/vitiligo (incidence unknown) etc.	APTT should be controlled within 60–85 s (1.5–2.5X that of controls)

(continued)

Table 8 (continued)

Name of medication (trade name)	Mechanism of action	Dose and method of treatment	Side-effects (%)	Important considerations
LMWH	Displays anticoagulant effect through AT-III indirectly	Infants <12 months	Lower incidence of hemorrhage than unfractionated heparin	APTT should be controlled within 60–85 s (1.5–2.5X that of controls)
		Treatment: 300 units/kg/day in 2 divided doses (every 12 h)	Subcutaneous bleeding (3.8 %), HIT (0.4 %), headache/vertigo (1 to <10 %), constipation/ diarrhea (1 to <10 %), abnormal hepatic functioning (1 to <10 %) etc.	
		Prevention: 150 units/kg/day in 2 divided doses (every 12 h)		
		Children/ adolescents		
		Treatment: 200 units/kg/day in 2 divided doses (every 12 h)		
		Prevention: 100 units/kg/day in 2 divided doses (every 12 h)		
		Subcutaneous injection		
Warfarin	Achieves anticoagulant effect by inhibiting biosynthesis of vitamin K-dependent coagulation factors II, VII, IX, and X	0.05-0.12 mg/kg, in a single dose Orally	Hemorrhage (incidence unknown), allergic reactions (incidence unknown), impaired hepatic function/jaundice (incidence unknown) etc.	PT-INR should be adjusted to 1.6–2.5 and thrombotest to 10–25 %
				Because warfarin is passed through the placenta, it is contraindicated for pregnant women in their first trimester

(continued)

Table 8 (continued)

Name of medication (trade name)	Mechanism of action	Dose and method of treatment	Side-effects (%)	Important considerations
Urokinase	Degrades fibrin and encourages activation of plasmin	Systemic treatment 10 000–16 000 units kg (maximum 960 000 units), given in an i.v. drip over 30–60 min	Hemorrhagic cerebral infarction (0.1 to <0.5 %), cerebral hemorrhage (<0.1 %), gastrointestinal hemorrhage (<0.1 %), impaired liver function (<0.1 %), rash and other allergic reactions (<0.1 %) etc.	Additive effect with heparin, warfarin, aspirin, dipyridamole, ticlopidine hydrochloride, and other t-PA medications, leading to increased risk of hemorrhage
		Intracoronary thrombolysis 4000 units/kg over 10 min, maximum 4 times		When given with aprotinin medications, urokinase may have weakened capacity for fibrinolysis
Alteplase	Degrades fibrin and enhances activation of plasmin	290 000–435 000 units/kg; first administer 10 % of total volume of medication i.v. for 1–2 min, and the remaining volume by i.v. drip over 60 min	Tendency to bleed, including cerebral hemorrhage (0.4 %), gastrointestinal hemorrhage (0.6 %), pulmonary hemorrhage (0.08 %).	Increased risk of hemorrhage when given with other thrombolytics, anticoagulants, antiplatelet medications etc.
			After reperfusion, arrhythmias such as premature ventricular contraction, ventricular tachycardia, and ventricular fibrillation (incidence unknown), shock/anaphylactic symptoms (0.1 %), abnormal hepatic function (0.1 to <0.5 %) etc.	

(continued)

Table 8 (continued)

Name of medication (trade name)	Mechanism of action	Dose and method of treatment	Side-effects (%)	Important considerations
Monteplase	Its half-life, affinity for fibrin, and plasminogen activator activity are greater than those of alteplase	27 500 units/kg, i.v. over 2–3 min	Cerebral and gastrointestinal hemorrhage (0.1 to <5 %), tendency to bleed including pulmonary hemorrhage (incidence unknown), cardiac rupture/perforation of intraventricular septum (0.1 to <5 %). After reperfusion, arrhythmias such as premature ventricular contraction, ventricular tachycardia, and ventricular fibrillation (incidence unknown), shock/anaphylactic symptoms (0.1 %), abnormal hepatic function (0.1 to <0.5 %) etc.	Same as above
Pamiteplase	Same as above	65 000 units/kg, i.v. over 1 min	Severe bleeding, including cerebral hemorrhage, retroperitoneal hemorrhage, gastrointestinal hemorrhage etc. (0.1 to <5 %), cardiac rupture/ cardiac tamponade (0.1 to <5 %), ventricular tachycardia/ventricular fibrillation (0.1 to <5 %), shock (<0.1 %).	Same as above

APTT, activated partial thromboplastin time; AT-III, anti-thrombin III; HIT, heparin-induced thrombocytopenia; IVIG, i.v. immunoglobulin; LMWH, low-molecular-weight heparin; PT-INR, prothrombin time international normalized ratio; TTP, thrombotic thrombocytopenic purpura

Side-effects

High-dose aspirin is associated with hemorrhage, asthma attacks, impaired liver function, and gastrointestinal ulcers (incidence rates unknown). Other side-effects include hematemesis, urticarial, rash (incidence rates unknown), loss of appetite (0.1 to <5 %), and renal impairment (<0.1 %). Hepatic dysfunction is common, so routine testing of liver enzymes is necessary. If abnormalities are found, it is necessary to reduce the dose or temporarily cease treatment. In children with chickenpox or influenza, it is important to be aware of the possible development of Reye syndrome. Current evidence does not indicate an increased risk of Reye syndrome among children receiving long-term low-dose aspirin after acute KD, but these patients should receive influenza vaccinations to ensure safety.

Evidence level

Initial therapy with IVIG plus aspirin: class Ia, grade A.

Other antiplatelet medications

Flurbiprofen (Froben®)

A total of 3–5 mg/kg per day, in three divided doses.

Flurbiprofen is sometimes given instead of aspirin for patients with severely impaired hepatic function, but there is insufficient evidence of its effectiveness. Furthermore, in patients with hepatic dysfunction related to onset of acute KD, such dysfunction often resolves after IVIG treatment.

Side-effects include epigastric discomfort (1.56 %), loss of appetite (1.03 %), rash (0.24 %), and, rarely, thrombopenia.

Dipyridamole (Persantin® tablets, Anginal®)

A total of 2–5 mg/kg per day, in three divided doses.

Dipyridamole is sometimes given in combination with aspirin for patients with CAA. Its adverse events include headache (0.91–4.37 %) and tachycardia (0.43–0.56 %); more severe side-effects include worsening of angina symptoms (<0.1 %) and hemorrhage (incidence unknown).

Ticlopidine (Panaldine®)

A total of 2–5 mg/kg, in three divided doses.

Ticlopidine is sometimes used to treat patients with CAA. The incidence of side-effects is unknown, but reported adverse events include thrombotic thrombocytopenic purpura and agranulocytosis, and severe liver damage may develop up to 2 months after treatment and is sometimes fatal. Therefore, indications should be carefully examined before use. During treatment, patients should undergo blood testing at least every 2 weeks.

Clopidogrel (Plavix®)

A total of 1.0 mg/kg per day, as a single dose (for patients aged 0–24 months, 0.2 mg/kg per day).

Clopidogrel is sometimes used in treating patients with CAA. The mechanism of action is similar to that of ticlopidine, although the incidence of liver damage is lower for clopidogrel. Sufficient antiplatelet action is achieved at a dose of only 0.2 mg/kg per day in patients aged 0–24 months.[104] Unfortunately, there are no data for patients aged ≥25 months; some centers use a dose of 1.0 mg/kg per day for these patients.

Use of the antiplatelet medications flurbiprofen, dipyridamole, ticlopidine and clopidogrel for treating KD is off-label.

Other cardiovascular agents

Anticoagulants

The coagulation/fibrinolytic systems are activated during the acute phase of KD. Therefore, patients with CAA require some form of anticoagulant to counteract this, although patients without CAL usually do not require anticoagulant treatment in the convalescent phase. Warfarin is widely used as an oral anticoagulant but, among patients requiring urgent treatment, i.v. unfractionated heparin (UFH) later switched to warfarin is the treatment of choice.

Warfarin

Warfarin prevents formation of intra-aneurysmal thrombi caused by increased activity in the coagulation/fibrinolytic system.

Mechanism of action

Warfarin blocks synthesis of vitamin K-dependent blood coagulation factors II, VII, IX, and X in liver.

Recent comprehensive genetic studies of the warfarin metabolic enzyme found that stable dosing of warfarin is related to genetic polymorphisms, including 30 different alleles, such as CYP2C9. Of these, the genotypes of CYP2C9*2 and *3 seem to be most affected by warfarin. CYP2C9*3, a poor metabolizer genotype, is prevalent among Japanese people; thus, warfarin dosage may need to be reduced in Japanese patients.[105]

Indications

Patients with medium–giant CAA.
   Patients with a history of acute myocardial infarction.
   Patients with a history of thrombogenesis in a CAA.

Treatment method and dosage

To achieve stable dosing, the patient can be started on 0.05–0.12 mg/kg per day o. d., which is increased to the optimal dosage in 4–5 days. Prothrombin time (PT) and the international normalized ratio (PT-INR) screens for coagulant factors II, V, VII, and X are useful for estimating the optimal dose of warfarin. In patients with KD, warfarin dosage should be adjusted so that the PT-INR is 1.6–2.5 (Thrombotest values: 10–25 %).[106] In addition, the American Heart Association (AHA) KD Guidelines recommend a dose of 0.05–0.34 mg/kg warfarin, which is then adjusted to maintain PT-INR between 2.0 and 2.5.[101]

Usefulness

There have been no large-scale studies of the efficacy of warfarin. In CAA, and particularly in giant CAA, thrombi frequently form because of reduced shear stress, due to impaired vascular endothelial function and increased platelet count and aggregation.[107] In such cases, oral warfarin treatment is sometimes impossible because the patient's general status is unfavorable. These patients may require continuous infusion of UFH. After the anticoagulant effect induced by UFH has been confirmed, patients can be switched to oral warfarin. Natto (Japanese fermented soybeans), chlorella, and green and yellow vegetables contain significant amounts of vitamin K and may decrease the effectiveness of warfarin, as may commercial infant formula fortified with vitamin K. Breast-fed infants require special attention because of overdosing. Other medications may also influence the effectiveness of warfarin. Trimethoprim–sulfamethoxazole combinations, acetaminophen, antimicrobials such as erythromycin, antifungals such as fluconazole, anabolic steroids, amiodarone, and statins enhance the effect of warfarin. In contrast, the effects of warfarin may be reduced in patients taking phenobarbital, carbamazepine, or rifampicin.

Side-effects

The major side-effect of warfarin is hemorrhage. Epistaxis and gingival hemorrhage are common. The patient should also be carefully monitored for intracranial and intraperitoneal hemorrhage. Warfarin, which passes through placenta, is contraindicated for use in pregnant women due to the possibility of embryopathies such as dysostosis/dyschondroplasia, central nervous system disorders, and microcephaly. The incidence of embryopathies is reported to be around 5 %, and the risk is even lower at a dose of ≤ 5 mg/day.[108]

Evidence level

Class IIb, grade C.

Unfractionated heparin

Unfractionated heparin is obtained from the intestinal mucosa, liver, and lungs of healthy animals. It achieves its anticoagulant effect by binding to anti-thrombin III (AT-III), a physiological inhibitor of many clotting factors (II, VII, IX, X, XI, XII). The effective half-life of UFH is 1–2 h. An initial dose of 50 U/kg should be given i.v. over a period of 10 min or longer, which may be followed by a dose of 20–25 U/kg per h, to maintain an activated partial thromboplastin time (APTT) of 60–85 s (1.5–2.5-fold the APTT in controls). Infants may need proportionately larger doses than older children or adults.

There is insufficient evidence of the effectiveness of UFH when given to patients with acute KD. For patients with CAA at very high risk of thrombus formation, however, UFH should first be given as a continuous i.v. infusion, after which it may be switched to oral warfarin after the anticoagulant effect induced by UFH has been confirmed. The most significant side-effect is hemorrhage; other side-effects include heparin-induced thrombocytopenia (HIT), hepatic dysfunction, rash, diarrhea, and hair loss. Long-term UFH may cause osteoporosis.

Evidence level

Class III, grade C.

Low-molecular-weight heparin

Low-molecular-weight heparin (LMWH) achieves its anticoagulant effect along the same pathway as UFH. As compared with UFH, its inhibition of thrombin is weaker. In addition, the incidences of side-effects such as HIT and osteoporosis are lower. Enoxaparin, an LMWH, was found to be safe and effective for coronary intervention/thrombolytic therapy in adult patients with acute coronary syndrome. [109]

Evidence level

Class III, grade C.

Thrombolytics

Purpose

Patients with large CAA have a higher risk of acute coronary syndrome. Most KD-related acute myocardial infarctions occur within 2 years of KD onset, and most of these events result from the formation of new thrombi.

Thrombolytic therapy is indicated when a thrombus is detected in a CAA or when thrombotic occlusion and myocardial infarction develop. In adults with acute myocardial infarction, the treatment of choice is almost always percutaneous coronary intervention. At present, thrombolytics have an important role in clinical practice, and earlier treatment is associated with better results. American College of Cardiology/AHA guidelines state that it is best to start the patient on thrombolytic therapy within 12 h of thrombotic events.[110]

Mechanism of action

Thrombolytics are proteins belonging to the plasminogen activators (PA), enzymes that stimulate the activity of the fibrinolytic system. Activation of the fibrinolytic system is started by conversion of plasminogen to plasmin. Increased plasmin enzyme activity leads to catabolization of fibrin (a component of thrombi) and thrombolysis. Plasmin also catabolizes fibrinogen (the precursor of fibrin), which can induce hemorrhaging. The thrombolytics are classed as follows.

(1) First-generation thrombolytic: urokinase.
(2) Second-generation thrombolytics: tisokinase and its genetically modified analog alteplase are tissue plasminogen activators (tPA). They have a stronger affinity than first-generation thrombolytics for fibrin (a component of thrombi) and an enhanced thrombolytic effect. This category also includes nasaruplase, the precursor of the fibrinolytic agent urokinase.
(3) Third-generation thrombolytic: the further refined tPA monteplase has a longer half-life and even greater affinity for fibrin and results in greater plasminogen activation.

Thrombolytics are currently given systemically or for intracoronary thrombolysis (ICT). The research committee recommends systemic treatment with thrombolytics, which may be followed by ICT if necessary.

Indications

Patients with acute myocardial infarction or intra-aneurysm thrombi.
Patients with sudden enlargement of thrombi in a coronary artery.
Their use in KD patients is off-label.

Treatment method and dosage

The safety of thrombolytics has not been established in pediatric patients. Furthermore, because there is insufficient clinical evidence to recommend suitable standards, dosages, and treatment methods for pediatric patients, the following reference values for adult patients are included.

Urokinase

Covered by the Japanese health insurance system when given to adults as thrombolytic therapy for coronary thrombosis in cases of acute myocardial infarction. Although urokinase is the only thrombolytic also covered for use in ICT cases, however, it is almost never used in such cases.

Systemic i.v. treatment: 10 000–16 000 units/kg urokinase; upper limit, 96 000 units i.v. over a period of 30–60 min.

ICT: 4000 units/kg urokinase, injected over a period of 10 min. Maximum of four doses.

Alteplase (Activacin®, Grtpa®)

Systemic i.v. treatment: 290 000–435 000 units/kg, 10 % of which should be first given i.v. over a period of 1–2 min, after which the remaining dose may be given by i.v. infusion over a 60 min period.

Monteplase (Cleactor®)

Systemic i.v. treatment: 27 500 units/kg, i.v. over 2–3 min.

Effectiveness

Evidence of effectiveness is insufficient because no large-scale study has evaluated thrombolytic therapy in KD patients. Theoretically, as in adult patients, thrombolytic therapy should be used as an acute-phase therapy when required, to hasten reperfusion.[111-113] After systemic use of thrombolytics, recanalization occurs in 70–80 % of patients. When ICT is added, these rates improve by approximately 10 %.[106]

Side-effects

When reperfusion is achieved in cases of acute myocardial infarction, reported side-effects include arrhythmias such as paroxysmal ventricular contraction, ventricular tachycardia, and ventricular fibrillation, and even cardiac rupture. There is a tendency toward bleeding, including hemorrhage from the catheter insertion point, hematuria, and gingival hemorrhage. Digestive symptoms such as nausea and vomiting have also been reported. Furthermore, gelatin is used as a stabilizer in the formulation of urokinase; therefore, shock or anaphylactic symptoms may occur (including during tPA treatment). Before using these drugs, the patient's history should be carefully investigated, and his/her progress carefully monitored after treatment has begun.

When anticoagulants such as heparin and warfarin are given in combination with antiplatelets such as aspirin, dipyridamole, ticlopidine hydrochloride, or other tPA medications, an additive effect may increase bleeding tendency. Thus, in cases of combined use, coagulation tests (clotting time, PT) should be performed regularly and all clinical data carefully monitored. Conversely, co-treatment with aprotinin and urokinase could inhibit the fibrinolytic capacity of the latter.

Evidence level

Class IIb, grade C.

Anti-anginals and coronary vasodilators

Angina symptoms are extremely rare during the acute phase of KD, and patients with such symptoms are typically aged 1–2 years and thus cannot easily explain their symptoms to caregivers. In adult patients, the characteristics of angina symptoms may allow classification of angina as stable or unstable.

The principal therapeutic goal for angina is to reduce heart rate (thereby reducing cardiac workload), decrease preload and afterload, and increase coronary artery flow. For these reasons, beta-blockers, calcium antagonists and nitrovasodilators may be useful.

(1) Beta-blockers are the first choice for stable effort angina. To avoid side-effects in other body organs, beta-blockers that selectively block β-1 are recommended. As well as reducing myocardial workload and suppressing oxygen consumption, beta-blockers increase coronary blood flow accompanying bradydiastole, thereby preventing development of myocardial ischemia. Although atenolol, bisoprolol, and metoprolol have all been found to be effective,[114] beta-blockers may worsen prognosis in patients with coronary vasospasm, because upregulated α-receptor function may induce exacerbation of coronary tonus and symptoms of coronary spastic angina.[115] Carvedilol is a non-selective beta-blocker that also blocks α-1, and it increases coronary flow by lowering peripheral resistance in coronary arteries.[116]

(2) Calcium antagonists suppress the flow of Ca2+ into vascular smooth muscle cells. They are therefore extremely useful in preventing coronary vasospasm and are the first choice in treating coronary spastic angina.[117] KD-related myocardial infarction often occurs during sleep and may be induced by coronary spasms.[118] The ability of calcium antagonists to protect cardiovascular function seems to be due to stimulation of NO production. Because diltiazem blocks the L-type Ca2+ channel in cardiac myocytes, however, it is contraindicated for use in newborns up to early infancy.

(3) Nitrates exert their effect by dilating coronary arteries and reducing preload. Nitrates increase coronary blood flow and reduce both preload and afterload, which reduces the workload of the left ventricle, thereby relieving myocardial ischemia. Acute KD, however, is characterized by persistent damage to endothelial cells. Therefore, nitrates may not be effective in dilating impaired coronary arteries. A sublingual tablet of nitroglycerine or an oral spray of nitroglycerine or isosorbide dinitrate may alleviate angina symptoms. Nitrovasodilators are contraindicated in patients with glaucoma, in those taking phosphodiesterase inhibitors, and in those with cardiogenic shock, severe hypotension, or severe anemia.

(4) Nicorandil is a hybrid medication (a nitrovasodilator that opens the ATP-sensitive potassium channel) and can selectively dilate coronary arteries and inhibit coronary vasospasm.[119] It is therefore useful in preventing angina. Nicorandil also affects mitochondria, resulting in pharmacological preconditioning that protects against myocardial ischemia.

Evidence level

Class IIb, grade C.

Indication

The use of the aforementioned medications, both in cases of KD and in pediatric patients in general, is off-label.

This article is based on a study first reported in *Pediatric Cardiology and Cardiac Surgery*, 2012; 28 (Suppl. 3): 1–s28.[120]

References

1. Nakamura Y, Yashiro M, Uehara R et al. Epidemiologic features of Kawasaki disease in Japan: Results of the 2009–2010 nationwide survey. J. Epidemiol. 2012; 22: 216–221.
2. Ayusawa M, Sonobe T, Uemura S et al. Revision of diagnostic guidelines for Kawasaki disease (the 5th revised edition). Pediatr. Int. 2005; 47: 232–234.
3. Jennette JC, Falk RJ, Bacon PA et al. 2012 revised International Chapel Hill Consensus Conference Nomenclature of Vasculitides. Arthritis Rheum. 2013; 65: 1–11.
4. Naoe S, Takahashi K, Masuda H et al. Kawasaki disease. With particular emphasis on arterial lesions. Acta Pathol. Jpn 1991; 41: 785–797.
5. Asai T. Diagnosis and prognosis of coronary artery lesions in Kawasaki disease. Coronary angiography and the conditions for its application (a score chart). Nihon Rinsho. 1983; 41: 2080–2085 (in Japanese).
6. Iwasa M, Sugiyama K, Ando T, Nomura H, Katoh T, Wada Y. Selection of high-risk children for immunoglobulin therapy in Kawasaki disease. Prog. Clin. Biol. Res. 1987; 250: 543–544.
7. Harada K. Intravenous gamma-globulin treatment in Kawasaki disease. Acta Paediatr Jpn. 1991; 33: 805–810.
8. Kobayashi T, Inoue Y, Takeuchi K et al. Prediction of intravenous immuno-globulin unresponsiveness in patients with Kawasaki disease. Circulation 2006; 113: 2606–2612.
9. Egami K, Muta H, Ishii M et al. Prediction of resistance to intravenous immunoglobulin treatment in patients with Kawasaki disease. J. Pediatr. 2006; 149: 237–240.
10. Sano T, Kurotobi S, Matsuzaki K et al. Prediction of nonresponsiveness to standard high-dose gamma-globulin therapy in patients with acute Kawasaki disease before starting initial treatment. Eur. J. Pediatr. 2007; 166: 131–137.
11. Okada K, Hara J, Maki I et al. Pulse methylprednisolone with gammaglobulin as an initial treatment for acute Kawasaki disease. Eur. J. Pediatr. 2009; 168: 181–185.
12. Ogata S, Ogihara Y, Honda T et al. Corticosteroid pulse combination therapy for refractory Kawasaki disease: A randomized trial. Pediatrics 2012; 129: e17–23.
13. Kobayashi T, Saji T, Otani T et al. Efficacy of immunoglobulin plus prednis-olone for prevention of coronary artery abnormalities in severe Kawasaki disease: A prospective, randomised, open, blinded-endpoint trial. Lancet 2012; 379: 1613–1620.
14. Kato H, Koike S, Yokoyama T. Kawasaki disease: Effect of treatment on coronary artery involvement. Pediatrics 1979; 63: 175–179.

15. Furusho K, Kamiya T, Nakano H et al. High-dose intravenous gammaglobulin for Kawasaki disease. Lancet 1984; 2: 1055–1058.
16. Newburger JW, Takahashi M, Burns JC et al. The treatment of Kawasaki syndrome with intravenous gamma globulin. N. Engl. J. Med. 1986; 315: 341–347.
17. Newburger JW, Takahashi M, Beiser AS et al. A single intravenous infusion of gamma globulin as compared with four infusions in the treatment of acute Kawasaki syndrome. N. Engl. J. Med. 1991; 324: 1633–1639.
18. Oates-Whitehead RM, Baumer JH, Haines L et al. Intravenous immunoglobulin for the treatment of Kawasaki disease in children. Cochrane Database Syst. Rev. 2003; (4): CD004000.
19. Leung DY, Cotran RS, Kurt-Jones E et al. Endothelial cell activation and high interleukin-1 secretion in the pathogenesis of acute Kawasaki disease. Lancet 1989; 2: 1298–1302.
20. Abe J, Jibiki T, Noma S et al. Gene expression profiling of the effect of high-dose intravenous Ig in patients with Kawasaki disease. J. Immunol. 2005; 174: 5837–5845.
21. Terai M, Jibiki T, Harada A et al. Dramatic decrease of circulating levels of monocyte chemoattractant protein-1 in Kawasaki disease after gamma globulin treatment. J. Leukoc. Biol. 1999; 65: 566–572.
22. Bayary J, Dasgupta S, Misra N et al. Intravenous immunoglobulin in autoimmune disorders; an insight into the immunoregulatory mechanisms. Int. Immunopharmacol. 2006; 6: 528–534.
23. Tse SM, Silverman ED, McCrindle BW et al. Early treatment with intravenous immunoglobulin in patients with Kawasaki disease. J. Pediatr. 2002; 140: 450–455.
24. Uehara R, Yashiro M, Oki I et al. Re-treatment regimens for acute stage of Kawasaki disease patients who failed to respond to initial intravenous immunoglobulin therapy: Analysis from the 17th nationwide survey. Pediatr. Int. 2007; 49: 427–430.
25. Boyce TG, Spearman P. Acute aseptic meningitis secondary to intravenous immunoglobulin in a patient with Kawasaki syndrome. Pediatr. Infect. Dis. J. 1998; 17: 1054–1056.
26. Nakagawa M, Watanabe N, Okuno M et al. Severe hemolytic anemia following high-dose intravenous immunoglobulin administration in a patient with Kawasaki disease. Am. J. Hematol. 2000; 63: 160–161.
27. Bonilla FA. Intravenous immunoglobulin: Adverse reactions and management. J. Allergy Clin. Immunol. 2008; 122: 1238–1239.
28. Nimmerjahan F, Ravetch J. Anti-inflammatory actions of intravenous immunoglobulin. Annu. Rev. Immunol. 2008; 26: 513–533.
29. Saji T, Sonobe T, Hamaoka K et al. Safety and effectiveness of intravenous immunoglobulin preparations for the treatment of Kawasaki disease. Prog. Med. 2012; 32: 1369–1375.
30. Stahn C, Buttgereit F. Genomic and nongenomic effects of glucocorticoids. Nat. Clin. Pract. Rheumatol. 2008; 4: 525–533.

31. Sinha A, Bagga A. Pulse steroid therapy. Indian J. Pediatr. 2008; 75: 1057–1066.
32. Miura M, Kohno K, Ohki H et al. Effects of methylprednisolone pulse on cytokine levels in Kawasaki disease patients unresponsive to intravenous immunoglobulin. Eur. J. Pediatr. 2008; 167: 1119–1123.
33. Ogata S, Ogihara Y, Nomoto K et al. Clinical score and transcript abundance patterns identify Kawasaki disease patients who may benefit from addition of methylprednisolone. Pediatr. Res. 2009; 66: 577–584.
34. Newburger JW, Sleeper LA, McCrindle BW et al. Randomized trial of pulsed corticosteroid therapy for primary treatment of Kawasaki disease. N. Engl. J. Med. 2007; 356: 663–675.
35. Wright DA, Newburger JW, Baker A et al. Treatment of immune globulin-resistant Kawasaki disease with pulsed dose of corticosteroids. J. Pediatr. 1996; 128: 146–149.
36. Hashino K, Ishii M, Iemura M et al. Re-treatment for immune globulin-resistant Kawasaki disease: A comparative study of additional immune globulin and steroid pulse therapy. Pediatr. Int. 2001; 43: 211–217.
37. Ogata S, Bando Y, Kimura S et al. The strategy of immune globulin resistant Kawasaki disease: A comparative study of additional immune globulin and steroid pulse therapy. J. Cardiol. 2009; 53: 15–19.
38. Furukawa T, Kishiro M, Akimoto K et al. Effects of steroid pulse therapy on immunoglobulin-resistant Kawasaki disease. Arch. Dis. Child. 2008; 93: 142–146.
39. Miura M, Tamame T, Naganuma T et al. Steroid pulse therapy for Kawasaki disease unresponsive to additional immunoglobulin therapy. Paediatr Child Health. 2011; 16: 479–484.
40. Zhu BH, Lv HT, Sun L et al. A meta-analysis on the effect of corticosteroid therapy in Kawasaki disease. Eur. J. Pediatr. 2012; 171: 571–578.
41. Miura M, Ohki H, Yoshiba S et al. Adverse effects of methylprednisolone pulse therapy in refractory Kawasaki disease. Arch. Dis. Child. 2005; 90: 1096–1097.
42. Okawa S, Kawasaki T, Kosaki A et al. Study of deaths from acute mucocutaneous lymph node syndrome (MCLS). Syonika Shinryo 1975; 38: 608–614 (in Japanese).
43. Kusakawa S, Tatara K. Research on treatment of acute-stage Kawasaki disease (third report): A prospective study of three treatment options: Aspirin, flurbiprofen, prednisolone + dipyridamole. Nihon Shonika Gakkai Zasshi 1986; 90: 1844–1849 (in Japanese).
44. Shinohara M, Sone K, Tomomasa T, Morikawa A. Corticosteroids in the treatment of the acute phase of Kawasaki disease. J. Pediatr. 1999; 135: 465–469.
45. Inoue Y, Okada Y, Shinohara M et al. A multicenter prospective randomized trial of corticosteroids in primary therapy for Kawasaki disease: Clinical course and coronary artery outcome. J. Pediatr. 2006; 149: 336–341.

46. Kobayashi T, Inoue Y, Otani T et al. Risk stratification in the decision to include prednisolone with intravenous immunoglobulin in primary therapy of Kawasaki disease. Pediatr. Infect. Dis. J. 2009; 28: 498–502.
47. Hibino K, Ashida M, Iwashima S et al. A cooperative, multicenter study of treatments for Kawasaki disease. Nihon Shonika Gakkai Zasshi 2008; 112: 1227–1232 (in Japanese).
48. Millar K, Manlhiot C, Yeung RS, Somji Z, McCrindle BW. Corticosteroid administration for patients with coronary artery aneurysms after Kawasaki disease may be associated with impaired regression. Int. J. Cardiol. 2012; 154: 9–13.
49. Breda L, Del Torto M, De Sanctis S et al. Biologics in children's autoimmune disorders: Efficacy and safety. Eur. J. Pediatr. 2010; 170: 157–167.
50. Weiss JE, Eberhard A, Chowdhury D et al. Infliximab as a novel therapy for refractory Kawasaki disease. J. Rheumatol. 2004; 31: 808–810.
51. Burns JC, Mason WH, Hauger SB et al. Infliximab treatment for refractory Kawasaki syndrome. J. Pediatr. 2005; 146: 662–667.
52. Saji T, Kemmotsu Y. Infliximab for Kawasaki syndrome. J. Pediatr. 2006; 149: 426.
53. Stenbog EV, Windelborg B, Horlyck A et al. The effect of TNFalpha blockade in complicated, refractory Kawasaki disease. Scand. J. Rheumatol. 2006; 35: 318–321.
54. O'Connor MJ, Saulsbury FT. Incomplete and atypical Kawasaki disease in a young infant: Severe, recalcitrant disease responsive to infliximab. Clin Pediatr 2007; 46: 345–348.
55. Oishi T, Fujieda M, Shiraishi T et al. Infliximab treatment for refractory Kawasaki disease with coronary artery aneurysm. Circ. J. 2008; 72: 850–852.
56. Girish M, Subramaniam G. Infliximab treatment in refractory Kawasaki syndrome. Indian J. Pediatr. 2008; 75: 521–522.
57. Burns JC, Best BM, Mas PD et al. Infliximab treatment of intravenous immunoglobulin-resistant Kawasaki disease. J. Pediatr. 2008; 153: 833–838.
58. Brogan RJ, Eleftheriou D, Gnanapragasam J et al. Infliximab for the treatment of intravenous immunoglobulin resistant Kawasaki disease complicated by coronary artery aneurysms: A case report. Pediatr. Rheumatol. 2009; 7: 1–5.
59. Saji T, Nakagawa N, Ogawa S et al. Committee Report: Nationwide survey report on the use of the biopharmaceutical biologics infliximab (Remicade) in treating IVIG resistant cases of acute Kawasaki disease: Safety and usefulness. J. Jpn. Soc. Pediatr. Cardiol. Cardiac Surg. 2009; 25: 268–269 (in Japanese).
60. Mori M, Imagawa T, Hara R et al. Efficacy and limitation of infliximab treatment for children with Kawasaki disease intractable to intravenous immunoglobulin therapy: Report of an open-label case series. J. Rheumatol. 2012; 39: 864–867.
61. Shirley DA, Stephens I. Primary treatment of incomplete Kawasaki disease with infliximab and methylpredonisolone in a patient with a contraindication to intravenous immune globulin. Pediatr. Infect. Dis. J. 2010; 29: 978–979.

62. Hirono K, Kemmotsu Y, Wittkowski H et al. Infliximab reduces the cytokine-mediated inflammation but does not suppress cellular infiltration of the vessel wall in refractory Kawasaki disease. Pediatr. Res. 2009; 65: 696–701.
63. Son MB, Gauvreau K, Ma L et al. Treatment of Kawasaki disease: Analysis of 27 US pediatric hospitals from 2001 to 2006. Pediatrics 2009; 124: 1–8.
64. Rowley AH, Shulman ST. Pathogenesis and management of Kawasaki disease. Expert Rev. Anti Infect. Ther. 2010; 8: 197–203.
65. Hii-Yuen JS, Duong TT, Yeung RSM. TNF-α is necessary for induction of coronary artery inflammation and aneurysm formation in an animal model of Kawasaki disease. J. Immunol. 2006; 176: 6294–6301.
66. Carter JD, Ladhani A, Ricca LR et al. A safety assessment of tumor necrosis factor antagonists during pregnancy: A review of the Food and Drug Administration database. J. Rheumatol. 2009; 36: 635–641.
67. Molloy ES, Langford CA, Clark TM et al. Anti-tumor necrosis factor therapy in patients with refractory Takayasu arteritis: Long-term follow-up. Ann. Rheum. Dis. 2008; 67: 1567–1569.
68. Koh MJ, Tay YK. An update on Stevens-Johnson syndrome and toxic epidermal necrolysis in children. Curr. Opin. Pediatr. 2009; 21: 505–510.
69. Ruperto N, Lovell DJ, Cuttica R et al. Pediatric Rheumatology International Trials Organization; Pediatric Rheumatology Collaborative Study Group. A randomized, placebo-controlled trial of infliximab plus methotrexate for the treatment of polyarticular-course juvenile rheumatoid arthritis. Arthritis Rheum. 2007; 56: 3096–3106.
70. Saag KG, Teng GG, Patkar M et al. American College of Rheumatology 2008 recommendations for the use of nonbiologic and biologic disease-modifying antirheumatic drugs in rheumatoid arthritis. Arthritis Rheum. 2008; 59: 762–784.
71. Horneff G. Malignancy and tumor necrosis factor inhibitors in juvenile idiopathic arthritis. J. Rheumatol. 2010; 69: 516–526.
72. Diak P, Siegel J, Grenade L, Choi L, Lemery S, McMahon A. Malignancy in children and tumor necrosis factor-alpha blockers: Forty-eight cases reported to the Food and Drug Administration. Arthritis Rheum. 2010; 62: 2517–2524.
73. Lahdenne P, Wikstrom AM, Aalto K et al. Prevention of acute adverse events related to infliximab infusions in pediatric patients. Arthritis Care Res. (Hoboken) 2010; 62: 785–790.
74. Gerloni V, Pontikaki I, Gattinnara M et al. Focus on adverse events of tumour necrosis factor alpha blockade in juvenile idiopathic arthritis in an open monocentric long-term prospective study of 163 patients. Am. Rheum. Dis. 2008; 67: 1145–1152.
75. Ruperto N, Lovell DJ, Cuttica R et al. Long-term efficacy and safety of infliximab plus methotrexate for the treatment of polyarticular course juvenile rheumatoid arthritis: Findings from an open-label treatment extension. Ann. Rheum. Dis. 2010; 69: 718–722.

76. de Rodder L, Rings EH, Damen GM et al. Infliximab dependency in pediatric Crohn's disease. Long-term follow-up of an unselected cohort. Inflamm. Bowel Dis. 2008; 14: 353–356.

77. Singh JA, Furst DE, Bharat A et al. 2012 update of the 2008 American College of Rheumatology: Recommendations for the use of disease-modifying anti-rheumatic drugs and biologic agents in the treatment of rheumatoid arthritis. Arthritis Care Res. (Hoboken) 2012; 64: 625–639.

78. Harigai M, Mochida S, Koike T et al. A proposal for management of rheumatic disease patients with hepatitis B virus infection receiving immunosppressive therapy. Mod. Rheumatol. 2014; 24: 1–7.

79. Saji T. Therapy with the protein-degradation enzyme blocker Ulinastatin. Shonika Shinryo 2008; 66: 343–348 (in Japanese).

80. Aosasa S, Ono S, Mochizuki H et al. Mechanism of the inhibitory protease inhibitor on tumor necrosis factor alpha production of monocytes. Shock 2001; 15: 101–105.

81. Aosasa S, Ono S, Seki S et al. Inhibitory effect of protease inhibitor on endothelial cell activation. J. Surg. Res. 1998; 80: 182–187.

82. Zaitsu M, Hamasaki Y, Tashiro K et al. Ulinastatin, an elastase inhibitor, inhibits the increased mRNA expression of prostaglandin H2 synthase-type 2 in Kawasaki disease. J. Infect. Dis. 2000; 181: 1101–1109.

83. Nakatani K, Takeshita S, Tsujimoto H et al. Inhibitory effect of serine protease inhibitors on neutrophil-mediated endothelial cell injury. J. Leukoc. Biol. 2001; 69: 241–247.

84. Okada M, Nakai S, Ookado K et al. The results of ulinastatin and antithrombin III medications administered to severe Kawasaki disease patients displaying shock symptoms. Nihon Shonika Gakkai Zasshi. 1993; 97: 43–48 (in Japanese).

85. Saji T, Ozawa Y, Takeuchi M et al. Treating Kawasaki disease with ulinastatin. Syonika 1999; 40: 1049–1054 (in Japanese).

86. Nakatani K, Takeshita S, Kawamura Y. Please tell me the mechanism of action of ulinastatin during acute-stage Kawasaki disease and the clinical results obtained with it. Syouni Naika 2003; 9: 1578–1581 (in Japanese).

87. Kanai T, Ishiwata T, Kobayashi T et al. Ulinastatin, a urinary trypsin inhibitor, for the initial treatment of patients with Kawasaki disease: As retrospective study. Circulation 2011; 124: 2822–2828.

88. Onouchi Y, Gunji T, Burns JC et al. ITPKC functional polymorphism associated with Kawasaki disease susceptibility and formation of coronary artery aneurysms. Nat. Genet. 2008; 40: 35–42.

89. Raman V, Kim J, Sharkey A et al. Response of refractory Kawasaki disease to pulse-steroid and cyclosporine A therapy. Pediatr. Infect. Dis. J. 2001; 20: 635–637.

90. Suzuki H, Terai M, Hamada H et al. Cyclosporin A treatment for Kawasaki disease refractory to initial and additional intravenous immunoglobulin. Pediatr. Infect. Dis. J. 2011; 30: 871–876.

91. Tremolet AH, Pancoast P, Franco A et al. Calcineurin inhibitor treatment of IVIG-resistant Kawasaki disease. J. Pediatr. 2012; 161: 506–512.
92. Amazaki Y. The calcineurin and NFAT system and its inhibition. Jpn J. Clin. Immunol. 2010; 33: 249–261.
93. Lee TJ, Kim KH, Chun JK, Kim DS. Low-dose methotrexate therapy for intravenous immunoglobulin-resistant Kawasaki disease. Yonsei Med. J. 2008; 49: 714–718.
94. Joh K. Effects of plasma exchange in Kawasaki disease. In: Oda T (ed). Therapeutic Plasmapheresis (IV). Schattauer, New York, 1985; 519–524.
95. Takagi N, Kihara M, Yamaguchi S et al. Plasma exchange in Kawasaki disease. Lancet 1995; 346: 1307.
96. Villain E, Kachaner J, Sidi D et al. Trial of prevention of coronary aneurysm in Kawasaki's disease using plasma exchange or infusion of immunoglobulins. Arch. Fr. Pediatr. 1987; 44: 79–83 (in French).
97. Imagawa T, Mori M, Miyamae T et al. Plasma exchange for refractory Kawasaki disease. Eur. J. Pediatr. 2004; 163: 263–264.
98. Mori M, Imagawa T, Katakura S et al. Efficacy of plasma exchange therapy for Kawasaki disease intractable to intravenous gamma-globulin. Mod. Rheumatol. 2004; 14: 43–47.
99. Hokosaki T, Mori M, Nishizawa T et al. Long-term efficacy of plasma exchange treatment for refractory Kawasaki disease. Pediatr. Int. 2012; 54: 99–103.
100. Japan Apheresis Society Scientific Committee. The present state of apheresis (results of the 2002 survey). Japan Apher. Soc. 2005; 54: 99–103.
101. Newburger JW, Takahashi M, Gerber MA et al. Diagnosis, treatment, and long-term management of Kawasaki disease. A Statement for Health Professionals From the Committee on Rheumatic Fever, Endocarditis and Kawasaki Disease, Council on Cardiovascular Disease in the Young, American Heart Association. Circulation 2004; 110: 2747–2771.
102. Durongpisitkul K, Gururaj VJ, Park JM et al. The prevention of coronary artery aneurysm in Kawasaki disease: A meta-analysis on the efficacy of aspirin and immunoglobulin treatment. Pediatrics 1995; 96: 1057–1061.
103. Terai M, Shulman ST. Prevalence of coronary artery abnormalities in Kawasaki disease is highly dependent on gamma globulin dose but independent of salicylate dose. J. Pediatr. 1997; 131: 888–893.
104. Li JS, Yow E, Berezny KY et al. Dosing of clopidogrel for platelet inhibition in infants and young children. Primary results of the platelet inhibition in children on Clopidogrel (PICOLO) trial. Circulation 2008; 117: 553–559.
105. Takahashi H, Wilkinson GR, Nutescu EA et al. Different contributions of polymorphisms in VKORC1 and CYP2C9 to intra- and inter-population differences in maintenance dose of warfarin in Japanese, Caucasians and African-Americans. Pharmacogenet. Genomics 2006; 16: 101–110.
106. JCS Joint Working Group. Guidelines for diagnosis and management of cardiovascular sequelae in Kawasaki disease (JCS 2008) – digest version. Circ. J. 2010; 74: 1989–2020.

107. Ohkubo T, Fukazawa R, Ikegami E et al. Reduced shear stress and disturbed flow may lead to coronary aneurysm and thrombus formations. Pediatr. Int. 2007; 49: 1–7.

108. Hanania G. Management of anticoagulants during pregnancy. Heart 2001; 86: 125–126.

109. Petersen JL, Mahaffey KW, Hasselblad V et al. Efficacy and bleeding complications among patients randomized to enoxaparin or unfractionated heparin for antithrombin therapy in non-ST-Segment elevation acute coronary syndromes: A systematic overview. JAMA 2004; 292: 89–96.

110. Smith SC Jr, Allen J, Blair SN et al. AHA/ACC guidelines for secondary prevention for patients with coronary and other atherosclerotic vascular disease: 2006 update: endorsed by the National Heart, Lung, and Blood Institute. Circulation 2006; 113: 2363–2372.

111. Shiraishi J, Sawada T, Tatsumi T et al. Acute myocardial infarction due to a regressed giant coronary aneurysm as possible sequela of Kawasaki disease. J. Invasive Cardiol. 2001; 13: 569–572.

112. Kato H, Inoue O, Ichinose E et al. Intracoronary urokinase in Kawasaki disease: Treatment and prevention of myocardial infarction. Acta Paediatr. Jpn. 1991; 33: 27–35.

113. Tsubata S, Ichida F, Hamamichi Y, Miyazaki A, Hashimoto I, Okada T. Successful thrombolytic therapy using tissue-type plasminogen activator in Kawasaki disease. Pediatr. Cardiol. 1995; 16: 186–189.

114. Onouchi Z, Hamaoka K, Sakata K et al. Long-term changes in coronary artery aneurysms in patients with Kawasaki disease: Comparison of therapeutic regimens. Circ. J. 2005; 69: 265–272.

115. Ito A, Fukumoto Y, Shimokawa H. Changing characteristics of patients with vasospastic angina in the era of new calcium channel blockers. J. Cardiovasc. Pharmacol. 2004; 44: 480–485.

116. Bruns LA, Chrisant MK, Lamour JM et al. Carvedilol as therapy in pediatric heart failure: An initial multicenter experience. J. Pediatr. 2001; 138: 505–511.

117. Kimura E, Kishida H. Treatment of variant angina with drugs: A survey of 11 cardiology institutes in Japan. Circulation 1981; 63: 844–848.

118. Tsuda E, Yasuda T, Naito H. Vasospastic angina in Kawasaki disease. J. Cardiol. 2008; 51: 65–69.

119. Aizawa T, Ogasawara K, Kato K. Effects of nicorandil on coronary circulation in patients with ischemic heart disease: Comparison with nitroglycerin. J. Cardiovasc. Pharmacol. 1987; 10: S123–129.

120. Saji T, Ayusawa M, Miura M et al. Guidelines for medical treatment of acute Kawasaki disease: Report of the Research Committee of the Japanese Society of pediatric cardiology and cardiac surgery (2012 revised version). Jpn. Soc. Pediatr. Cardiol. Cardiac Surg. 2012; 28 (Suppl. 3): 1–s28.

Reference

1. Research Committee of the Japanese Society of Pediatric Cardiology, Cardiac Surgery Committee for Development of Guidelines for Medical Treatment of Acute Kawasaki Disease. Guidelines for medical treatment of acute Kawasaki disease: report of the Research Committee of the Japanese Society of Pediatric Cardiology and Cardiac Surgery. Pediatr Int. 2014 Apr (2012 revised version);56(2):135–58.

Tumor Necrosis Factor-α Blockade for Treatment of Acute Kawasaki Disease

Adriana H. Tremoulet

Abstract Tumor necrosis factor (TNF)-α has a key role in the development of coronary artery aneurysms in acute KD. Blockade of the TNF-α inflammatory cascade is thus a logical therapeutic aim. Infliximab, a chimeric monoclonal antibody that specifically binds TNF-α, and etanercept, a TNF-α receptor blocker, have both been used as rescue therapy for treatment-resistant KD. A prospective trial of intensification of primary therapy with infliximab in acute KD demonstrated that infliximab was safe and reduced inflammation, days of fever, and left anterior descending coronary artery diameter more rapidly than IVIG alone. A trial of etanercept as adjunctive therapy in acute KD is currently in progress.

Keywords Tumor necrosis factor-α • Monoclonal antibody • Infliximab • Etanercept

Introduction

Levels of TNF-α and TNF-α soluble receptors (sTNFR) I and II are elevated in acute KD and are highest in children who subsequently develop coronary artery aneurysms [1, 2]. In addition, approximately 10–20 % of Kawasaki disease (KD) patients develop persistent or recrudescent fever after standard therapy with a single infusion of intravenous immunoglobulin (IVIG) and aspirin [3, 4]. This subset of IVIG-resistant patients is at highest risk for developing coronary artery aneurysms and requires additional therapy to interrupt the inflammatory process. Given the importance of TNF-α in the formation and maintenance of inflammation in KD [5], primary treatment of KD patients, or treatment of highly resistant KD patients, with a TNF-α antagonist is a logical therapeutic intervention.

A.H. Tremoulet, M.D., MAS (✉)
Pediatrics, University of California San Diego, La Jolla, CA, USA, 9500 Gilman Drive Mail Code 0641, CA 92093

Rady Children's Hospital San Diego, San Diego, CA, USA, 3020 Children's Way, CA 92123
e-mail: atremoulet@ucsd.edu

© Springer Japan 2017
B.T. Saji et al. (eds.), *Kawasaki Disease*, DOI 10.1007/978-4-431-56039-5_17

Current Understanding

The two TNF-α inhibitors that have been most widely used in treating children with KD are infliximab, a chimeric monoclonal antibody that specifically binds TNF-α, and etanercept, a TNF-α receptor blocker.

Infliximab

The first reported use of infliximab in acute KD was in 2004 in a 3-year-old boy with giant coronary artery aneurysms. He was unresponsive to multiple doses of IVIG and methylprednisolone but defervesced and had improvement in laboratory measures after a single dose of infliximab (Weiss JE, Gottlieb) [6]. This was soon followed by a report of 16 KD patients (age, 0.12–13 years) treated with infliximab for treatment-resistant KD or persistent fever and arthritis, 13 of whom responded with cessation of fever [7]. Since then infliximab has been used in refractory cases of acute KD [8–12]. In 2008 a phase I, randomized, multicenter clinical trial in KD children with persistent or recrudescent fever after standard therapy found no infusion reactions or serious adverse events attributable to a single infusion of 5 mg/kg of infliximab [13]. In a subsequent two-center retrospective study of IVIG-resistant KD, patients treated with infliximab had faster resolution of fever and fewer days of hospitalization than did those treated with a second dose of IVIG [9]. Given the importance of the expansion of regulatory T cells in controlling inflammation during acute KD, the effect of infliximab was evaluated in seven patients treated initially with IVIG and infliximab [14]. As compared with those treated with IVIG alone, there was no inhibition of the generation of tolerogenic myeloid dendritic cells, regulatory T cells, or memory T cells. Most recently, a two-center, phase III, randomized, double-blind, placebo-controlled trial of infliximab plus IVIG for initial treatment of KD patients was completed [15]. Although the addition of infliximab to primary treatment did not reduce treatment resistance, infliximab was determined to be safe and well-tolerated and reduced fever, markers of inflammation, left anterior descending coronary artery Z score, and intravenous immunoglobulin reaction rates (Table 1 and Fig. 1).

Etanercept

Two studies demonstrated that etanercept reduced vasculitis in a mouse model of arteritis induced by *Candida albicans* cell wall extract. One group showed that etanercept was more effective than IVIG, cyclosporine, or methylprednisolone [5, 16]. Etanercept has been used in ill infants with refractory KD and resulted in improvement of inflammatory marker and resolution of fever [17, 18]. An open-

Table 1 Comparison of outcome measures by treatment arm for infliximab randomized trial

	Infliximab	Placebo	P value
Treatment resistance, N (%)	11 (11.2)	11 (11.3)	0.81
IVIG infusion reaction, N (%)	0 (0)	13 (13.4)	<0.0001
Days of fever, median (range)[a]	1 (0–4)	2 (0–6)	<0.0001
Change from baseline in absolute neutrophil count, $\times 10^9$/L (CI)			
24 h	−6.18 (−6.892 to −5.468)	−5.019 (−5.735 to −4.303)	0.024
Week 2	−6.522 (−6.91 to −6.135)	−7.053 (−7.444 to −6.661)	0.06
Change from baseline in CRP, mg/dl (CI)			
24 h	−6.6 (−7.7 to −5.4)	−3.6 (−4.8 to −2.5)	<0.001
Week 2	−10.628 (−11.0 to −10.2)	−10.38 (−10.7 to −10.1)	0.37
Change from baseline in ESR, mm/hr (CI)			
Week 2	−23 (−27 to −18)	−14 (−18 to −9)	0.009

Abbreviations: *CI* confidence interval, *CRP* C-reactive protein, *ESR* erythrocyte sedimentation rate, *IVIG* intravenous immunoglobulin

[a]Days of fever = number of calendar days from the day of enrollment with any temperature ≥38 °C

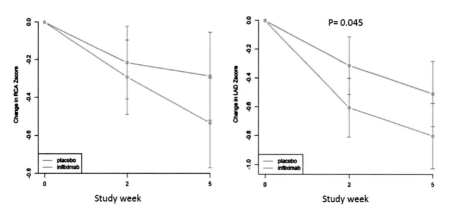

Fig. 1 Change in Z score of the right coronary artery (RCA) and left anterior descending coronary artery (LAD) from baseline to 2 and 5 weeks after randomization to receive IVIG plus placebo (*blue circles*) or IVIG plus infliximab (*red circles*), estimated from a mixed effects model for repeated measures. Change in the Z score of LAD from baseline to 2 weeks is significantly different between the two study arms

label trial of etanercept in 15 children (age, 6 months to 5 years) with KD demonstrated that etanercept (0.4–0.8 mg/kg subcutaneously weekly for 3 doses) added to primary treatment of IVIG and aspirin was safe, well-tolerated, and not associated with recrudescence of fever [19]. A randomized, placebo-controlled trial to assess etanercept (0.8 mg/kg subcutaneously weekly for 3 doses) as adjunctive therapy to standard treatment with IVIG is currently in progress.

Safety of TNF-α Inhibitors

Despite concerns of immune suppression with blockade of TNF-α, use of infliximab and etanercept during acute KD has not raised any major safety concerns. In the phase III trial of infliximab 11 infants aged 2–11 months were treated with infliximab, and none had any significant adverse events from a single dose of this medication. Although there is concern regarding activation of latent tuberculosis infection, this has not been observed in any KD patient receiving infliximab as adjunctive therapy. In Japan, use of infliximab in infants has been limited due to theoretical concerns of disseminated infection after BCG vaccination.

In summary, there is evidence to support the use of 5 mg/kg of infliximab as adjunctive therapy in KD patients with severe inflammation. Recommendations regarding the use of etanercept must await the results of the clinical trial currently in progress. Future studies could focus on dose-finding, as a higher dose of infliximab might benefit patients with severe inflammation, and randomized trials should investigate infliximab as the first rescue therapy for patients with IVIG resistance.

References

1. Furukawa S, Matsubara T, Jujoh K, Yone K, Sugawara T, Sasai K, et al. Peripheral blood monocyte/macrophages and serum tumor necrosis factor in Kawasaki disease. Clin Immunol Immunopathol. 1988;48(2):247–51. http://dx.doi.org/10.1016/0090-1229(88)90088-8 PMID:3390972.
2. Matsubara T. Serum gamma interferon levels in relation to tumor necrosis factor and interleukin 2 receptor in patients with Kawasaki disease involving coronary-artery lesions. Arerugi. 1990;39(2 Pt 1):118–23. PMID:2112909.
3. Burns JC, Capparelli EV, Brown JA, Newburger JW. Glode MP; US/Canadian Kawasaki Syndrome Study Group. Intravenous gamma-globulin treatment and retreatment in Kawasaki disease. Pediatr Infect Dis J. 1998;17(12):1144–8. http://dx.doi.org/10.1097/00006454-199812000-00009 PMID:9877364.
4. Tremoulet AH, Best BM, Song S, Wang S, Corinaldesi E, Eichenfield JR, et al. Resistance to intravenous immunoglobulin in children with Kawasaki disease. J Pediatr. 2008;153 (1):117–21. http://dx.doi.org/10.1016/j.jpeds.2007.12.021 PMID:18571548.
5. Oharaseki T, Yokouchi Y, Yamada H, Mamada H, Muto S, Sadamoto K, et al. The role of TNF-alpha in a murine model of Kawasaki disease arteritis induced with a Candida albicans cell wall polysaccharide. Mod Rheumatol. 2014;24(1):120–8. http://dx.doi.org/10.3109/14397595.2013.854061.

6. Weiss JE, Eberhard BA, Chowdhury D, Gottlieb BS. Infliximab as a novel therapy for refractory Kawasaki disease. J Rheumatol. 2004;31(4):808–10. PMID:15088313.

7. Burns JC, Mason WH, Hauger SB, Janai H, Bastian JF, Wohrley JD, et al. Infliximab treatment for refractory Kawasaki syndrome. J Pediatr. 2005;146(5):662–7. http://dx.doi.org/10.1016/j.jpeds.2004.12.022 PMID:15870671.

8. Saji T, Kemmotsu Y. Infliximab for Kawasaki syndrome. J Pediatr. 2006;149(3):426. http://dx.doi.org/10.1016/j.jpeds.2005.07.039 PMID:16939768.

9. Son MB, Gauvreau K, Burns JC, Corinaldesi E, Tremoulet AH, Watson VE, et al. Infliximab for intravenous immunoglobulin resistance in Kawasaki disease: a retrospective study. J Pediatr. 2011;158(4):644–9 e1. http://dx.doi.org/10.1016/j.jpeds.2010.10.012.

10. Son MB, Gauvreau K, Ma L, Baker AL, Sundel RP, Fulton DR, et al. Treatment of Kawasaki disease: analysis of 27 US pediatric hospitals from 2001 to 2006. Pediatrics. 2009;124(1):1–8. http://dx.doi.org/10.1542/peds.2008-0730 PMID:19564276.

11. Mori M, Imagawa T, Hara R, Kikuchi M, Hara T, Nozawa T, et al. Efficacy and limitation of infliximab treatment for children with Kawasaki disease intractable to intravenous immunoglobulin therapy: report of an open-label case series. J Rheumatol. 2012;39(4):864–7. http://dx.doi.org/10.3899/jrheum.110877 PMID:22337241.

12. Jimenez-Fernandez SG, Tremoulet AH. Infliximab treatment of pancreatitis complicating acute Kawasaki disease. Pediatr Infect Dis J. 2012;31(10):1087–9. PMID:22653489.

13. Burns JC, Best BM, Mejias A, Mahony L, Fixler DE, Jafri HS, et al. Infliximab treatment of intravenous immunoglobulin-resistant Kawasaki disease. J Pediatr. 2008;153(6):833–8. http://dx.doi.org/10.1016/j.jpeds.2008.06.011 PMID:18672254.

14. Burns JC, Song Y, Bujold M, Shimizu C, Kanegaye JT, Tremoulet AH, et al. Immune-monitoring in Kawasaki disease patients treated with infliximab and intravenous immunoglobulin. Clin Exp Immunol. 2013;174(3):337–44. http://dx.doi.org/10.1111/cei.12182 PMID:23901839.

15. Tremoulet AH, Jain S, Jaggi P, Jimenez-Fernandez S, Pancheri JM, Sun X, et al. Infliximab for intensification of primary therapy for Kawasaki disease: a phase 3 randomised, double-blind, placebo-controlled trial. Lancet. 2014;383(9930):1731–8. http://dx.doi.org/10.1016/S0140-6736(13)62298-9 PMID:24572997.

16. Ohashi R, Fukazawa R, Watanabe M, Tajima H, Nagi-Miura N, Ohno N, et al. Etanercept suppresses arteritis in a murine model of kawasaki disease: a comparative study involving different biological agents. Int J Vasc Med. 2013;2013:543141. http://dx.doi.org/10.1155/2013/543141.

17. Peyre M, Laroche C, Etchecopar C, Brosset P. The role of immunosuppressive agents in Kawasaki disease: a discussion of two cases. Arch Pediatr. 2013;20(7):748–53. http://dx.doi.org/10.1016/j.arcped.2013.04.002 PMID:23693156.

18. de Magalhaes CM, Alves NR, de Melo AV, Junior CA, Nomicronbrega YK, Gandolfi L, et al. Catastrophic Kawasaki disease unresponsive to IVIG in a 3-month-old infant: a diagnostic and therapeutic challenge. Pediatr Rheumatol Online J. 2012;10(1):28. http://dx.doi.org/10.1186/1546-0096-10-28 PMID:22929725.

19. Choueiter NF, Olson AK, Shen DD, Portman MA. Prospective open-label trial of etanercept as adjunctive therapy for kawasaki disease. J Pediatr. 2010;157(6):960–6 e1. http://dx.doi.org/10.1016/j.jpeds.2010.06.014.

Methylprednisolone Pulse Therapy for Nonresponders to Immunoglobulin Therapy

Masaru Miura

Abstract Intravenous methylprednisolone pulse (IVMP) therapy is administered to children with severe illnesses, such as Kawasaki disease (KD), collagen disease, and kidney disease, because of its powerful, rapid, and probably nongenomic immunosuppressive action. In a randomized controlled trial, IVMP plus initial intravenous immunoglobulin (IVIG) therapy did not decrease the incidence of coronary artery lesions (CAL) in KD patients as compared with IVIG plus placebo. Predicted nonresponders to IVIG treated with initial IVIG plus IVMP had earlier defervescence and lower incidence of CAL than did those treated with IVIG alone. Some studies showed that IVMP was effective for fast defervescence and prevention of CAL in nonresponders to initial or additional IVIG. The adverse effects of IVMP for KD patients include sinus bradycardia, hypertension, hyperglycemia, and hypothermia, but these effects were usually transient and not serious. Present evidence indicates that IVMP should be given as initial therapy for predicted IVIG nonresponders and as rescue therapy for confirmed nonresponders to initial or additional IVIG.

Keywords Coronary artery lesions • Nonresponders to immune globulin therapy • Intravenous methylprednisolone pulse

Introduction

Steroid pulse therapy involves intravenous infusion of high-dose glucocorticoids such as methylprednisolone, which is often selected because it is less likely to disrupt electrolyte balance. Because of its powerful and rapid immunosuppressive effect, intravenous methylprednisolone pulse (IVMP) therapy is widely used to treat children with severe or refractory illnesses such as collagen disease and kidney disease. IVMP is also used to treat severe or refractory cases of Kawasaki disease, especially nonresponders to standard intravenous immunoglobulin (IVIG) therapy.

M. Miura (✉)
Division of Cardiology, Tokyo Metropolitan Children's Medical Center, 2-8-29, Musashidai, Fuchu, Tokyo 183-8561, Japan
e-mail: masaru_miura@tmhp.jp

© Springer Japan 2017

175

B.T. Saji et al. (eds.), *Kawasaki Disease*, DOI 10.1007/978-4-431-56039-5_18

History

Kijima et al. [1] were the first to report initial treatment with IVMP for KD patients in 1982. IVMP then fell out of favor, probably because of the establishment of IVIG therapy and criticisms of steroid therapy, which were subsequently disproven. A worldwide re-evaluation of IVMP was triggered by a report on the effectiveness of IVMP in IVIG nonresponders by Wright et al. [2] in 1996. Subsequent studies of IVIG nonresponders during 2001–2009 [3–6] showed that IVMP decreased the incidence of coronary artery lesions (CAL) to the same extent as additional IVIG. In 2007 Newburger et al. [7] conducted a double-blind, randomized, controlled trial comparing initial treatment with IVMP plus IVIG to IVIG alone for KD patients and did not demonstrate superior efficacy for the IVMP plus IVIG regimen. Thus, IVMP is now indicated only for confirmed [3–6] or predicted [8, 9] nonresponders to IVIG therapy.

Current Understanding and Recognition [10–12]

Among nonresponders to IVIG, studies comparing IVMP as rescue therapy to additional IVIG showed that duration of fever was shorter after IVMP and that incidence of CAL was similar [3–6]. Nevertheless, equal efficacy has not been demonstrated in noninferiority analyses and requires confirmation. The cost of IVMP was less than that of additional IVIG in some studies [4, 6] but similar in another recent study [13]. In many institutions, IVMP seems to be given to non-responders to additional IVIG, in accordance with American Heart Association guidelines [11]. One study [14] reported that the incidence of CAL was low, 0.7–1.9 % overall, when nonresponders to additional IVIG were treated with IVMP followed by oral prednisolone.

Initial therapy with IVIG plus IVMP for all KD patients has not been proven to prevent CAL. A double-blind, randomized, controlled study [7] found no significant difference between this regimen and conventional primary therapy in duration of fever, incidence of additional treatment, incidence of CAL, or coronary artery diameters. However, a post-hoc analysis of patients requiring additional treatment showed that the incidence of CAL was significantly lower among those receiving IVIG plus IVMP. In studies of initial therapy for predicted nonresponders to IVIG [8, 9], IVIG plus IVMP significantly decreased the incidence of CAL in comparison with IVIG alone.

The dosage and method of IVMP administration are shown in Table 1. Studies of IVMP in combination with initial IVIG investigated the use of a single dose of 30 mg/kg of IVMP [7–9]. Studies of nonresponders to initial or additional IVIG used the same IVMP dose given once a day, for 1–3 days [3–6, 13, 14]. Because the half-life of IVMP is only 3 h [15], some studies [3, 14] administered prednisolone 1–2 mg/kg/day initially and gradually tapered the dose for 1–3 weeks after IVMP.

Table 1 Dosage and method of administering intravenous methylprednisolone pulse (IVMP) therapy

Dosage	30 mg/kg/dose
Administration method	Drip infusion over 2–3 h, once a day, for 1–3 days
Combination therapy[a]	Oral prednisolone, started at 1–2 mg/kg/day, followed by tapering over 1–3 weeks after IVMP
	Continuous infusion of heparin, 15–20 units/kg/h
	Anti-ulcer drug such as oral famotidine, 0.5 mg/kg/day
Adverse effects	Relatively common: sinus bradycardia, hypertension, hyperglycemia hypothermia
	Rare: infections, gastrointestinal ulcers, mental disorders, severe arrhythmias, femur head necrosis, suppressed adrenal function

[a]These therapies are combined with IVMP at some centers [3, 5, 14], but the necessity of such combination therapies is unclear

The reported adverse effects of IVMP for KD patients [3, 14] include sinus bradycardia, hypertension, hyperglycemia, and hypothermia; hence, vital signs must be carefully monitored during IVMP administration. These symptoms are usually transient and do not require treatment. Although anti-ulcer drugs (such as H_2 blockers) are used to avoid gastrointestinal bleeding, and continuous infusion of heparin is used to prevent thrombosis in some institutions [3, 5, 14], the necessity of such treatments has not been proven (Table 1).

Glucocorticoids bind to cytoplasmic receptors and regulate nuclear expression of inflammatory proteins, thereby producing a genomic anti-inflammatory effect [15]. Because a high dose of IVMP is administered, the saturation point of glucocorticoid receptors is greatly exceeded. Thus, mechanisms other than genomic alteration are likely responsible for the observed effects. Possible nongenomic effects include action through proteins that dissociate from complexes with cytosolic glucocorticoid receptors, glucocorticoid receptors located on the cell membrane, and functional modification of membrane-binding protein after penetration into the cell membrane. These mechanisms precede genomic effects [15, 16] (Fig. 1 [17]). When used in KD patients, IVMP acts rapidly, which suggests the presence of nongenomic suppression of immune cell and inflammatory cytokine activity. In confirmed and predicted nonresponders to IVIG, IVMP limited production of cytokines involved in inflammation and CAL [18] and reduced transcription at the genetic level [19].

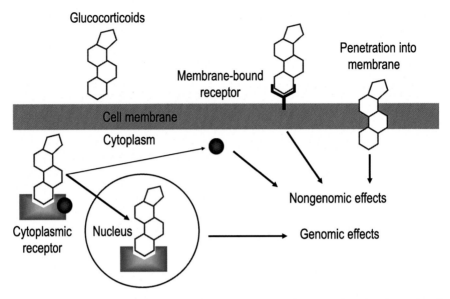

Fig. 1 Mechanisms of intravenous methylprednisolone pulse therapy (Adapted and reproduced with permission from M. Miura [17])

Assigned Evidence Class and Recommendation [10–12]

Initial therapy with IVIG plus IVMP should not be given to all KD patients but is indicated for patients with clinical symptoms and laboratory findings that indicate IVIG nonresponder is likely. Rescue therapy with IVMP is recommended for nonresponders to initial or additional IVIG.

References

1. Kijima Y, Kamiya T, Suzuki A, Hirose O, Manabe H. A trial procedure to prevent aneurysm formation of the coronary arteries by steroid pulse therapy in Kawasaki disease. Jpn Circ J. 1982;46(11):1239–42. http://dx.doi.org/10.1253/jcj.46.1239 PMID:7131714.
2. Wright DA, Newburger JW, Baker A, Sundel RP. Treatment of immune globulin-resistant Kawasaki disease with pulsed doses of corticosteroids. J Pediatr. 1996;128(1):146–9. http://dx.doi.org/10.1016/S0022-3476(96)70447-X PMID:8551407.
3. Furukawa T, Kishiro M, Akimoto K, Nagata S, Shimizu T, Yamashiro Y. Effects of steroid pulse therapy on immunoglobulin-resistant Kawasaki disease. Arch Dis Child. 2008;93 (2):142–6. http://dx.doi.org/10.1136/adc.2007.126144 PMID:17962370.
4. Hashino K, Ishii M, Iemura M, Akagi T, Kato H. Re-treatment for immune globulin-resistant Kawasaki disease: a comparative study of additional immune globulin and steroid pulse therapy. Pediatr Int. 2001;43(3):211–7. http://dx.doi.org/10.1046/j.1442-200x.2001.01373.x.
5. Miura M, Ohki H, Yoshiba S, Ueda H, Sugaya A, Satoh M, et al. Adverse effects of methylprednisolone pulse therapy in refractory Kawasaki disease. Arch Dis Child. 2005;90 (10):1096–7. http://dx.doi.org/10.1136/adc.2004.062299 PMID:16177169.

6. Ogata S, Bando Y, Kimura S, Ando H, Nakahata Y, Ogihara Y, et al. The strategy of immune globulin resistant Kawasaki disease: a comparative study of additional immune globulin and steroid pulse therapy. J Cardiol. 2009;53(1):15–9. http://dx.doi.org/10.1016/j.jjcc.2008.08.002 PMID:19167633.

7. Newburger JW, Sleeper LA, McCrindle BW, Minich LL, Gersony W, Vetter VL, et al. Pediatric Heart Network Investigators. Randomized trial of pulsed corticosteroid therapy for primary treatment of Kawasaki disease. N Engl J Med. 2007;356(7):663–75. http://dx.doi.org/10.1056/NEJMoa061235 PMID:17301297.

8. Ogata S, Ogihara Y, Honda T, Kon S, Akiyama K, Ishii M. Corticosteroid pulse combination therapy for refractory Kawasaki disease: a randomized trial. Pediatrics. 2012;129(1):e17–23. http://dx.doi.org/10.1542/peds.2011-0148 PMID:22144699.

9. Okada K, Hara J, Maki I, Miki K, Matsuzaki K, Matsuoka T, et al. Osaka Kawasaki Disease Study Group. Pulse methylprednisolone with gammaglobulin as an initial treatment for acute Kawasaki disease. Eur J Pediatr. 2009;168(2):181–5. http://dx.doi.org/10.1007/s00431-008-0727-9 PMID:18446365.

10. Eleftheriou D, Levin M, Shingadia D, Tulloh R, Klein NJ, Brogan PA. Management of Kawasaki disease. Arch Dis Child. 2014;99(1):74–83. http://dx.doi.org/10.1136/archdischild-2012-302841 PMID:24162006.

11. Newburger JW, Takahashi M, Gerber MA, Gewitz MH, Tani LY, Burns JC, et al. American Academy of Pediatrics. Diagnosis, treatment, and long-term management of Kawasaki disease: a statement for health professionals from the Committee on Rheumatic Fever, Endocarditis and Kawasaki Disease, Council on Cardiovascular Disease in the Young, American Heart Association. Circulation. 2004;110(17):2747–71. http://dx.doi.org/10.1161/01.cir.0000145143.19711.78 PMID:15505111.

12. Saji T, Ayusawa M, Miura M, Kobayashi T, Suzuki H, Mori M, et al. Guidelines for medical treatment of acute Kawasaki disease: report of the Research Committee of the Japanese Society of Pediatric Cardiology and Cardiac Surgery (2012 revised version); Research Committee of the Japanese Society of Pediatric Cardiology and Cardiac Surgery, Committee for Development of Guidelines for Medical Treatment of Acute Kawasaki Disease. Pediatr Int. 2014;56:135–58.

13. Teraguchi M, Ogino H, Yoshimura K, Taniuchi S, Kino M, Okazaki H, et al. Steroid pulse therapy for children with intravenous immunoglobulin therapy-resistant Kawasaki disease: a prospective study. Pediatr Cardiol. 2013;34(4):959–63. http://dx.doi.org/10.1007/s00246-012-0589-9 PMID:23184018.

14. Miura M, Tamame T, Naganuma T, Chinen S, Matsuoka M, Ohki H. Steroid pulse therapy for Kawasaki disease unresponsive to additional immunoglobulin therapy. Paediatr Child Health. 2011;16(8):479–84. PMID:23024586.

15. Stahn C, Buttgereit F. Genomic and nongenomic effects of glucocorticoids. Nat Clin Pract Rheumatol. 2008;4(10):525–33. http://dx.doi.org/10.1038/ncprheum0898 PMID:18762788.

16. Sinha A, Bagga A. Pulse steroid therapy. Indian J Pediatr. 2008;75(10):1057–66. http://dx.doi.org/10.1007/s12098-008-0210-7 PMID:19023530.

17. Miura M. Steroid pulse [in Japanese]. J Pediatr Practice. 2011;74:1189–94.

18. Miura M, Kohno K, Ohki H, Yoshiba S, Sugaya A, Satoh M. Effects of methylprednisolone pulse on cytokine levels in Kawasaki disease patients unresponsive to intravenous immunoglobulin. Eur J Pediatr. 2008;167(10):1119–23. http://dx.doi.org/10.1007/s00431-007-0642-5 PMID:18175148.

19. Ogata S, Ogihara Y, Nomoto K, Akiyama K, Nakahata Y, Sato K, et al. Clinical score and transcript abundance patterns identify Kawasaki disease patients who may benefit from addition of methylprednisolone. Pediatr Res. 2009;66(5):577–84. http://dx.doi.org/10.1203/PDR.0b013e3181baa3c2 PMID:19680167.

Prednisolone

Tohru Kobayashi

Abstract There are no specific therapies for Kawasaki disease patients, because the causes of the disease have not been identified. Currently, treatment with intravenous immunoglobulin (2 g/kg single infusion) plus aspirin (30 mg/kg/day) is considered the standard therapy. However, 20 % of patients do not become afebrile despite completion of intravenous immunoglobulin therapy. These intravenous immunoglobulin nonresponders are considered to be at high risk for coronary artery lesions. Recent clinical trials indicate a combined regimen of prednisolone and intravenous immunoglobulin is effective, especially for patients at high risk for nonresponse to initial intravenous immunoglobulin treatment. Although reproducibility and generalizability have been confirmed, prednisolone therapy should be an option for Kawasaki disease patients.

Keywords Prednisolone • Intravenous immunoglobulin • Risk stratification

Introduction

Although prednisolone (PSL) is an important treatment for several forms of vasculitis, such as Takayasu vasculitis and antineutrophil cytoplasmic antibody–associated vasculitis, its use is limited in children with Kawasaki disease (KD). However, recent clinical studies indicate that PSL plus intravenous immunoglobulin (IVIG) is effective in reducing the proportion of patients with initial or rescue treatment failure and might prevent coronary artery abnormalities (CAAs). This chapter reviews evidence regarding PSL therapy for KD patients.

T. Kobayashi, M.D., Ph.D. (✉)
Division of Clinical Research Planning, Department of Development Strategy, Center for Clinical Research and Development, National Center for Child Health and Development, 2-10-1, Okura, Setagaya-ku, Tokyo 157-8535, Japan
e-mail: torukoba@nifty.com

© Springer Japan 2017
B.T. Saji et al. (eds.), *Kawasaki Disease*, DOI 10.1007/978-4-431-56039-5_19

History

PSL was the initial therapy for KD, long before the first report of IVIG efficacy, by Furusho et al., in 1984 [1]. In Kawasaki's original report [2], 22 of 50 KD patients (44 %) were treated with combinations of intravenous, intramuscular, and oral corticosteroid, including PSL. He concluded that it was "very difficult to evaluate the efficacy of this therapeutic modality." In 1975, a case–control study [3] showed that fatal cases were more frequently treated with PSL as compared with matched non-fatal cases, although the causal relationship was unproven. In 1979, a retro-spective study by Kato et al. [4] reported that PSL as initial therapy might have adverse effects on CAA development. In 1983, a prospective randomized con-trolled trial [5] of three treatment groups (receiving either aspirin, flurbiprofen, or PSL plus dipyridamole) did not confirm the efficacy of PSL. The findings of these clinical studies led to contraindication of PSL for KD, in the 1980s.

In 1999, Shinohara et al. [6] reported that a PSL plus aspirin regimen might be useful in preventing CAAs and shortening duration of fever, which led to a reconsideration of PSL therapy. In 2006, a prospective randomized controlled trial [7] comparing initial IVIG plus PSL to initial IVIG alone reported a signifi-cantly lower incidence of CAAs in the IVIG plus PSL group. That study enrolled 178 patients, who were allocated randomly to either an IVIG group (n = 88) or an IVIG + PSL group (n = 90). The incidence of CAAs during the first month was 11.4 % in the IVIG group and 2.2 % in the IVIG + PSL group (P = 0.017). Similarly, the incidence of CAAs at 1 month was 3.4 % in the IVIG group and 0 % in the IVIG + PSL group (P = 0.12). No giant coronary aneurysms (internal diameter >8 mm) were observed in the trial. Nonresponse to initial treatment was less frequent in the IVIG + PSL group than in the IVIG group (5.6 % vs 18.2 %, P = 0.010). No serious adverse events were observed in either treatment group. Although the results were highly promising, the randomized trial had several methodologic flaws, including lack of adequate statistical power (only half the projected sample number was enrolled in the study) and the method of IVIG administration (1 g/kg/day for two consecutive days). Therefore, initial treatment with IVIG + PSL did not become a standard therapy for KD patients. A subsequent retrospective study [8] suggested that risk stratification of initial treatment, using the Kobayashi score [9], might be a more promising therapeutic strategy for improving clinical and coronary outcomes. Therefore, a new randomized controlled trial was designed in order to confirm the efficacy of intensified initial therapy with PSL in KD patients at high risk for IVIG nonresponse.

Current Understanding and Recognition

In 2012, the RAISE Study Group conducted a multicenter, prospective, random-ized, open-label, blinded-endpoints trial to assess the efficacy of IVIG (2 g/kg for a day) and aspirin (30 mg/kg/day) plus intravenous PSL (2 mg/kg/day) for 5 days, followed by an oral taper for 2–3 weeks [10]. Table 1 shows the coronary and clinical outcomes in the RAISE Study. The incidence of CAAs during the study period was significantly lower in the IVIG + PSL group than in the IVIG group (3 % vs 23 %, P < 0.001). Similarly, the incidence of CAAs at week 4 after enrollment was significantly lower in the IVIG + PSL group than in the IVIG group (3 % vs 13 %, P = 0.014). Patients in the IVIG + PSL group had more rapid fever resolution than did those in the IVIG group (P < 0.001). The incidence of additional rescue therapies was lower in the IVIG + PSL group than in the IVIG group (13 % vs 40 %, P < 0.001). A recent meta-analysis [11], using different steroid regimens and different prediction scores, found that a combination of corticosteroid with the standard dose of IVIG as initial treatment reduced the rate of coronary abnormal-ities. Thus, addition of corticosteroid therapy to IVIG and aspirin in primary therapy for KD lowers the prevalence of CAAs, duration of fever, and inflammation among Japanese children with the highest risk for IVIG resistance. However, the Japanese scoring systems for IVIG resistance and aneurysms have low sensitivity in North American [12] and Chinese populations [13]. Therefore, further research is needed in order to develop predictive instruments or scores for reliable identifica-tion of high-risk children outside Japan and to test the efficacy of the RAISE steroid regimen in non-Japanese populations. It should also be noted that reproducibility of the RAISE Study results has not yet been demonstrated, even in Japan.

As an additional rescue therapy for patients who fail to respond to initial IVIG treatment, Kobayashi et al. [14] assessed the efficacy of intravenous PSL (2 mg/kg/

Table 1 Coronary and clinical outcomes for two initial treatments

	IVIG + PSL group	IVIG group	
	(n = 121)	(n = 121)	P-value
Coronary artery abnormalities during study period	4/121 (3)	28/121 (23)	<0.001
Coronary artery abnormality at week 4	4/120 (3)	15/120 (13)	0.014
Maximum Z score, by coronary artery (n = 242)			
Proximal right coronary artery	1.92 (1.28-2.53)	2.32 (1.58-3.36)	0.001
Left main coronary artery	1.91 (1.48-2.24)	2.27 (1.83-2.83)	<0.001
Proximal left anterior descending artery	1.98 (1.45-2.50)	2.26 (1.79-2.91)	0.001
Duration of fever after enrollment (days)	1 (1–1)	2 (1–4)	<0.001
Additional therapy required, n (%)	16/121 (13)	48/121 (40)	<0.001
Nonresponse to primary therapy	6/121 (5)	36/121 (30)	<0.001
Relapse	13/121 (11)	15/121 (12)	0.84

Table 2 Clinical and coronary outcomes for three first-line additional rescue treatments

	IVIG (n = 136)	PSL (n = 72)	IVIG + PSL (n = 151)	P value
Univariate analysis				
Nonresponse to first-line rescue therapy, n (%)	51 (37.5)*	23 (31.9)*	18 (11.9)	<0.001
Coronary artery lesion within 1 mo, n (%)	39 (28.7)†	22 (30.6)†	24 (15.9)	0.010
Coronary artery lesion at 1 mo, n (%)	21 (15.4)	12 (16.7)	10 (6.6)	0.023

Chi-square analysis with post-hoc Holm's test
*P < 0.001, IVIG + PSL vs IVIG, PSL; †P < 0.05, IVIG + PSL vs IVIG, PSL

day tapered over 2 weeks after normalization of C-reactive protein) followed by an oral taper in a retrospective study of a database of 359 consecutive IVIG-resistant patients. Subjects treated with IVIG plus PSL had significantly lower rates of persistent or recrudescent fever and CAAs as compared with patients receiving IVIG monotherapy (Table 2). Because of the lack of adequately powered, randomized, controlled trials, steroid therapy for nonresponders to initial IVIG remains controversial.

Assigned Evidence Class and Recommendation

The research committee of the Japanese Society of Pediatric Cardiology and Cardiac Surgery revised their guideline for medical treatment of acute KD in 2012. [14] According to the guideline, evidence for initial IVIG plus PSL for suspected IVIG-resistant patients was classified as class Ib, grade B (recommended based on randomized controlled trials), and additional rescue treatment for nonresponders to initial IVIG treatment was classified as class IIb grade C (recommended based on observational trials, but evidence is uncertain). In North America and other regions, scoring systems are used to predict IVIG nonresponse. Therefore, administration of a longer course of corticosteroids, together with IVIG 2 g/kg and aspirin, may be considered for treatment of high-risk patients with acute KD, when such risk is identified before initiation of treatment.

References

1. Furusho K, Kamiya T, Nakano H, Kiyosawa N, Shinomiya K, Hayashidera T, et al. High-dose intravenous gammaglobulin for Kawasaki disease. Lancet. 1984;2(8411):1055–8. http://dx.doi.org/10.1016/S0140-6736(84)91504-6 PMID:6209513.
2. Kawasaki T, Kosaki F, Okawa S, Shigematsu I, Yanagawa H. A new infantile acute febrile mucocutaneous lymph node syndrome (MLNS) prevailing in Japan. Pediatrics. 1974;54 (3):271–6. PMID:4153258.

3. Okawa S, Kawasaki T, Kosaki A, et al. Fetal cases of mucocutaneous lymph node syndrome (MCLS) [in Japanese]. J Pediatr Prac. 1975;38:608–14.

4. Kato H, Koike S, Yokoyama T. Kawasaki disease: effect of treatment on coronary artery involvement. Pediatrics. 1979;63(2):175–9. PMID:440805.

5. Kusakawa S, Tatara K, Kawasaki T, et al. A randomized controlled study of three different therapies for patients having Kawasaki disease [in Japanese]. J Jpn Pediatr Soc. 1986;90:1844–9.

6. Shinohara M, Sone K, Tomomasa T, Morikawa A. Corticosteroids in the treatment of the acute phase of Kawasaki disease. J Pediatr. 1999;135(4):465–9. http://dx.doi.org/10.1016/S0022-3476(99)70169-1 PMID:10518080.

7. Inoue Y, Okada Y, Shinohara M, Kobayashi T, Kobayashi T, Tomomasa T, et al. A multi-center prospective randomized trial of corticosteroids in primary therapy for Kawasaki disease: clinical course and coronary artery outcome. J Pediatr. 2006;149(3):336–41. http://dx.doi.org/10.1016/j.jpeds.2006.05.025 PMID:16939743.

8. Kobayashi T, Inoue Y, Otani T, Morikawa A, Kobayashi T, Takeuchi K, et al. Risk stratification in the decision to include prednisolone with intravenous immunoglobulin in primary therapy of Kawasaki disease. Pediatr Infect Dis J. 2009;28(6):498–502. http://dx.doi.org/10.1097/INF.0b013e3181950b64 PMID:19504733.

9. Kobayashi T, Inoue Y, Takeuchi K, Okada Y, Tamura K, Tomomasa T, et al. Prediction of intravenous immunoglobulin unresponsiveness in patients with Kawasaki disease. Circulation. 2006;113(22):2606–12. http://dx.doi.org/10.1161/CIRCULATIONAHA.105.592865 PMID:16735679.

10. Kobayashi T, Saji T, Otani T, Takeuchi K, Nakamura T, Arakawa H, et al. RAISE study group investigators. Efficacy of immunoglobulin plus prednisolone for prevention of coronary artery abnormalities in severe Kawasaki disease (RAISE study): a randomised, open-label, blinded-endpoints trial. Lancet. 2012;379(9826):1613–20. http://dx.doi.org/10.1016/S0140-6736(11)61930-2 PMID:22405251.

11. Chen S, Dong Y, Yin Y, Krucoff MW. Intravenous immunoglobulin plus corticosteroid to prevent coronary artery abnormalities in Kawasaki disease: a meta-analysis. Heart. 2013;99 (2):76–82. http://dx.doi.org/10.1136/heartjnl-2012-302126 PMID:22869678.

12. Sleeper LA, Minich LL, McCrindle BM, et al. Evaluation of Kawasaki disease risk-scoring systems for intravenous immunoglobulin resistance. Pediatr Infect Dis J. 2011;158:831–5 e3. http://dx.doi.org/10.1016/j.jpeds.2010.10.031.

13. Fu PP, Du ZD, Pan YS. Novel predictors of intravenous immunoglobulin resistance in Chinese children with Kawasaki disease. Pediatr Infect Dis J. 2013;32(8):e319–23. PMID:23446442.

14. Kobayashi T, Kobayashi T, Morikawa A, Ikeda K, Seki M, Shimoyama S, et al. Efficacy of intravenous immunoglobulin combined with prednisolone following resistance to initial intravenous immunoglobulin treatment of acute Kawasaki disease. J Pediatr. 2013;163(2):521–6. http://dx.doi.org/10.1016/j.jpeds.2013.01.022 PMID:23485027.

Cyclosporin A for IVIG Nonresponders

Hiroyuki Suzuki

Abstract The 2012 treatment guideline for Kawasaki disease (KD) proposes several second- and third-line therapies for patients unresponsive to intravenous immunoglobulin (IVIG). However, there are still no definite treatment recommendations for refractory KD. In 2005 we used cyclosporin A (CsA) to treat a case of refractory KD, and in 2008 it was reported that functional polymorphism of inositol 1,4,5-trisphosphate 3-kinase-C *(ITPKC)* is associated with susceptibility to KD and the risk of developing coronary arterial lesions. Because ITPKC acts as a negative regulator of T-cell activation through the NFAT pathway, activated T cells may be important in KD. CsA suppresses the activity of T cells through the same pathway and might therefore be a promising candidate for treatment of refractory KD. Here, we summarize the results of our clinical trials of CsA for refractory KD and propose a new CsA treatment option for KD.

Keywords Kawasaki disease • IVIG nonresponder • Cyclosporin A • T-cell activation

Introduction

Although the incidence of coronary arterial lesions (CAL) has been reduced to around 3 % by standard therapy with intravenous immunoglobulin (IVIG) and aspirin [1], prevalence is high among the 10–20 % of KD patients who do not respond to IVIG. In 2012 the Scientific Committee of the Japanese Society of Pediatric Cardiology and Cardiac Surgery published clinical guidelines for medical treatment of acute KD [2]. Several options, including steroid [3], steroid pulse [4], ulinastatin [5], infliximab [6], plasma exchange [7], and immunosuppressants, were proposed as second- and third-line therapies for patients resistant to IVIG. The goal of treatment for KD is total prevention of CAL. Currently, however, there are still no definite treatment options for refractory KD. This chapter describes a clinical

H. Suzuki, M.D., Ph.D. (✉)
Department of Pediatrics, Wakayama Medical University, 811-1 Kimiidera, Wakayama 641-8509, Japan
e-mail: hsuzuki@wakayama-med.ac.jp

© Springer Japan 2017   187
B.T. Saji et al. (eds.), *Kawasaki Disease*, DOI 10.1007/978-4-431-56039-5_20

trial of cyclosporin A (CsA) for refractory KD and proposes a future direction for treatment of acute KD using CsA.

Historical Overview

The first report of CsA treatment for refractory KD was published by Raman et al. [8] in 2001. They demonstrated that potent immunosuppressive treatment using a combination of high-dose steroid and CsA might be effective against refractory KD.

In 2005, we treated a case of refractory KD with CsA (Fig. 1). The patient had not responded to initial or second treatment with IVIG (1 g/kg/day). Although she responded to intravenous methylprednisolone, her high fever relapsed, and she developed CAL and arthritis of the hip joint, with severe pain. We administered oral CsA, and the effects were dramatic: the high fever, inflammatory response, and severe pain disappeared within 2 days. This experience suggested that CsA might be an excellent option for KD patients unresponsive to IVIG.

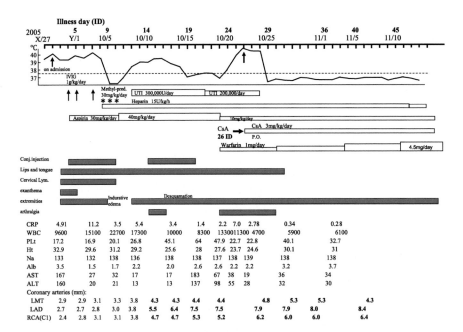

Fig. 1 Clinical course of our initial case. *UTI* urinary trypsin inhibitor, *Methyl-pred.* methylprednisolone, *CsA* cyclosporin A, *CRP* C-reactive protein, *WBC* white blood cell, *PLt* platelets, *Ht* hematocrit, *AST* alanine aminotransferase, *ALT* alanine transamirase, *LMT* left main coronary artery, *LAD* left anterior descending artery, *RCA* right coronary artery

Current Understanding and Recognition

Onouchi et al. reported that functional polymorphisms of inositol 1,4,5-trisphosphate 3-kinase C *(ITPKC)* and caspase-3 *(CASP3)* are associated with susceptibility to KD and risk of CAL [9–11]. Because *ITPKC* and *CASP3* act as negative regulators of T-cell activation via the Ca^{2+}/NAFT pathway, CsA—which potently suppresses the activity of T cells by the same pathway—may be a promising candidate for treatment of acute KD, especially refractory KD. Therefore, we carried out a pilot study to evaluate the effectiveness of CsA for refractory KD [12].

Pilot Study [12]

Patients

Between January 2008 and June 2010, study subjects were enrolled from among 329 Japanese patients who met the diagnostic criteria for KD [13].

Protocol

All patients received initial IVIG infusion (2 g/kg for 24 h) and aspirin (30–50 mg/kg/day) within 7 days after the onset of KD (Fig. 2). Patients resistant to initial and additional IVIG were treated with oral CsA (Neoral, oral solution, Novartis Pharma Co. Ltd., Tokyo, Japan). The initial dose of CsA was 4 mg/kg/day, and patients received oral CsA divided into two equal daily doses every 12 h. CsA dose was adjusted to between 4 and 8 mg/kg/day to maintain a trough level of 60–200 ng/ml by reference to clinical and laboratory data such as body temperature and C-reactive protein level. If patients remained febrile more than 5 days after the start of CsA treatment, or if fever returned after an afebrile period within 5 days after the start of CsA treatment, CsA treatment was judged to be ineffective, and patients were then given a third course of IVIG. Patients younger than 4 months who were resistant to initial and additional IVIG were given a third course of IVIG.

Results and Discussion of the Pilot Study

Of the 329 patients with KD, 245 (74.5 %) became afebrile within 24 h after completion of initial IVIG therapy, and 84 (25.5 %) continued to be febrile (Fig. 3). The latter 84 patients received additional IVIG, and 54 became afebrile

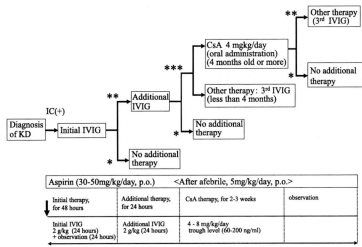

Aspirin (30-50mg/kg/day, p.o.)   <After afebrile, 5mg/kg/day, p.o.>

Initial therapy, for 48 hours	Additional therapy, for 24 hours	CsA therapy, for 2-3 weeks	observation
Initial IVIG 2 g/kg (24 hours) + observation (24 hours)	Additional IVIG 2 g/kg (24 hours)	4 - 8 mg/kg/day trough level (60-200 ng/ml)	

Total periods: 4 weeks after initial IVIG therapy

Fig. 2 Protocol. *KD* Kawasaki disease, *IVIG* intravenous immunoglobulin, *CsA* cyclosporin A, *IC* informed consent. * Responders to each treatment; ** Patients resistant to initial IVIG or CsA; *** Patients resistant to additional IVIG. All patients with KD received initial IVIG infusion (2 g/kg) and aspirin (30–50 mg/kg/day). Patients resistant to initial IVIG received additional IVIG (2 g/kg). In addition, patients at least 4 months of age who were resistant to additional IVIG were treated with CsA. Patients younger than 4 months who were resistant to additional IVIG were treated with a third course of IVIG

before completion of the additional IVIG course. The other 30 failed to become afebrile, and 28 of them who were older than 4 months were treated with CsA. The remaining two patients, who were younger than 4 months, received a third course of IVIG (2 g/kg) and subsequently became afebrile (Fig. 3). Although four patients developed CAL, coronary arteries were already dilated before CsA treatment in two of them.

Third IVIG as an Effective Option for CsA-Resistant Patients

In this pilot study, CsA appeared to exert antifebrile and anti-inflammatory effects in patients with refractory KD (Fig. 4) [14, 15]. The effect of CsA was particularly clear in 18 of the 28 resistant patients, as they became afebrile within 3 days after the start of CsA treatment. Although it took 4–5 days for four of the 28 patients to become afebrile, their body temperature decreased to a level close to the definition of "afebrile" within 2 days after the start of CsA treatment. In contrast, six of the 28 patients failed to become afebrile within 5 days after the start of CsA and/or high fever returned within 5 days after an afebrile period, despite having an adequate trough level of CsA. Four of these six patients received a third course of IVIG, after which they rapidly became afebrile. These findings suggest that certain subgroups

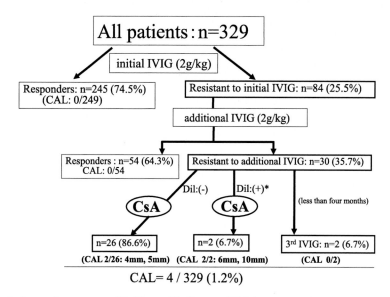

Fig. 3 Protocol outcomes. *KD* Kawasaki disease, *IVIG* intravenous immunoglobulin, *CsA* cyclosporin A, *CAL* coronary arterial lesions. Of 329 patients with KD, 245 (74.5%) became afebrile after initial IVIG. A total of 84 patients resistant to initial IVIG received additional IVIG, of whom 30 failed to become afebrile within the treatment completion time. Among these 30 patients, 28 who were at least 4 months old were treated with CsA; the other two patients were younger than 4 months and received a third course of IVIG (2 g/kg). * CAL developed in these two patients before CsA treatment (during additional IVIG)

of patients with refractory KD may be resistant to CsA. It may be that CsA treatment was started too late or that the suppressive effect of CsA on the calcineurin or NFAT pathway was insufficient to control severe vasculitis. Future studies might be able to clarify these issues.

Prevention of CAL Development by CsA

It is difficult to determine whether CsA inhibits development of CAL. Our pilot study was not a randomized controlled trial. Four of the 30 patients resistant to both initial and additional IVIG developed CAL. Thus, four (1.2%) of 329 patients developed CAL. All four of those patients were resistant to initial and additional IVIG treatment and received CsA. However, coronary arterial dilatation occurred during additional IVIG (i.e., before CsA treatment) in two of the four patients, and CsA did not inhibit progression of CAL in these patients. In the other two patients, CAL developed after the start of CsA treatment.

Summary of patients treated with CsA

```
┌─────────────────────────────────────────────┐
│        Patients treated with CsA : n=28      │
└─────────────────────────────────────────────┘
          ↙                             ↘
┌─────────────────────────┐   ┌──────────────────────────────┐
│  Responders to CsA:      │   │  Resistant to CsA:            │
│     n=22 (78.6%)         │   │             n=6 (21.4%)       │
└─────────────────────────┘   └──────────────────────────────┘
          ↓                                  ↓
┌─────────────────────────┐   ┌──────────────────────────────────────┐
│ 1. Additional IVIG(-)    │   │ 1. 3rd-IVIG : Effective (4 patients)   │
│ 2. CAL (+) : 3/22        │   │ 2. CAL(+) : 1/6                        │
│       (4, 6*, 10*mm)     │   │           (5**mm)                      │
└─────────────────────────┘   └──────────────────────────────────────┘
```

Fig. 4 Summary of patients treated with CsA. Twenty-two (78.6 %) of the 28 patients became afebrile within 5 days after the start of CsA treatment. Although three of these 28 patients developed CAL, coronary arterial dilatation occurred during IVIG (before CsA treatment) in two* of three patients who developed CAL (6 mm, 10 mm). Six (21.4 %) of the 28 patients failed to become afebrile within 5 days after the start of CsA and/or high fever returned within 5 days after an afebrile period. Four of these six patients received a third course of IVIG, after which they rapidly became afebrile. One** of these six patients developed CAL (5 mm) after the start of CsA treatment

Adverse Events

Hyperkalemia developed after the start of CsA treatment. Although serum potassium levels increased after CsA treatment, plasma potassium levels did not increase, and serum creatinine and estimated glomerular filtration rate did not change significantly. In addition, there were no serious adverse effects such as ventricular arrhythmia. These findings suggest that the hyperkalemia was actually pseudohyperkalemia, although the precise mechanism remains unclear. As for electrolyte disorders, a previous study reported that hypomagnesemia developed in two of ten patients [16]. No clinical problems have been reported in relation to either pseudohyperkalemia or hypomagnesemia.

Trough CsA Levels

We examined the time course of serum trough levels of CsA, which ranged between 60 and 200 ng/mL and were regarded as optimal. Examination of trough values showed that oral administration of CsA was satisfactory for obtaining sufficiently high serum concentrations (60–200 ng/mL). Further analyses of trough values in more patients with refractory KD will be needed in order to determine the optimal therapeutic levels of CsA. In this study, we did not examine C2 levels of CsA, which, as compared with trough level, might better correlate with the area under the concentration–time curve from 0 to 4 h (AUC0–4). Future studies should examine C0 and C2 levels of CsA.

Route of CsA Administration

We had no information on whether oral administration or intravenous infusion of CsA would be more effective. We selected oral administration because it is easier and more tolerable for young children and infants, who need to be treated for 2–3 weeks. The volume of CsA was small, and the patients were therefore able to ingest the medication without major problems.

Summary and Future Direction

In summary, CsA treatment is a promising, well tolerated, and safe option for patients with refractory KD. Oral administration of CsA offers good treatment compliance and has both antifebrile and anti-inflammatory effects in KD patients who are resistant to IVIG. In addition, a third course of IVIG is an effective option for patients resistant to CsA. To further decrease the incidence of CAL, a new strategy that rapidly decreases severe inflammatory responses is needed. In May 2014 we started a prospective, randomized clinical trial (the KAICA trial) of intensified initial treatment comprising IVIG plus CsA in patients predicted to be IVIG-resistant based on the Gunma score. Future studies should investigate dosing, safety, optimal timing, and duration of CsA treatment.

References

1. Nakamura Y, Yashiro M, Uehara R, Sadakane A, Tsuboi S, Aoyama Y, et al. Epidemiologic features of Kawasaki disease in Japan: results of the 2009–2010 nationwide survey. J Epidemiol. 2012;22(3):216–21. http://dx.doi.org/10.2188/jea.JE20110126 PMID:22447211.
2. The Clinical Guideline for Medical Treatment of Acute Stage Kawasaki Disease from the Scientific Committee. Pediatr Cardiol Card Surg. 2012;28 Suppl 3:s1–28.
3. Lang BA, Yeung RS, Oen KG, Malleson PN, Huber AM, Riley M, et al. Corticosteroid treatment of refractory Kawasaki disease. J Rheumatol. 2006;33(4):803–9. PMID:16583481.
4. Hashino K, Ishii M, Iemura M, Akagi T, Kato H. Re-treatment for immune globulin-resistant Kawasaki disease: a comparative study of additional immune globulin and steroid pulse therapy. Pediatr Int. 2001;43(3):211–17. http://dx.doi.org/10.1046/j.1442-200x.2001.01373.x PMID:11380911.

5. Kanai T, Ishiwata T, Kobayashi T, Sato H, Takizawa M, Kawamura Y, et al. Ulinastatin, a urinary trypsin inhibitor, for the initial treatment of patients with Kawasaki disease: a retrospective study. Circulation. 2011;124(25):2822–8. http://dx.doi.org/10.1161/CIRCULATIONAHA.111.028423 PMID:22104548.

6. Burns JC, Best BM, Mejias A, Mahony L, Fixler DE, Jafri HS, et al. Infliximab treatment of intravenous immunoglobulin-resistant Kawasaki disease. J Pediatr. 2008;153(6):833–8. http://dx.doi.org/10.1016/j.jpeds.2008.06.011 PMID:18672254.

7. Mori M, Imagawa T, Katakura S, Miyamae T, Okuyama K, Ito S, et al. Efficacy of plasma exchange therapy for Kawasaki disease intractable to intravenous gamma-globulin. Mod Rheumatol. 2004;14(1):43–7. http://dx.doi.org/10.3109/s10165-003-0264-3 PMID:17028804.

8. Raman V, Kim J, Sharkey A, Chatila T. Response of refractory Kawasaki disease to pulse steroid and cyclosporin a therapy. Pediatr Infect Dis J. 2001;20(6):635–7. http://dx.doi.org/10.1097/00006454-200106000-00022 PMID:11419513.

9. Onouchi Y, Gunji T, Burns JC, Shimizu C, Newburger JW, Yashiro M, et al. ITPKC functional polymorphism associated with Kawasaki disease susceptibility and formation of coronary artery aneurysms. Nat Genet. 2008;40(1):35–42. PMID:18084290.

10. Onouchi Y, Ozaki K, Buns JC, Shimizu C, Hamada H, Honda T, et al. Common variants in CASP3 confer susceptibility to Kawasaki disease. Hum Mol Genet. 2010;19(14):2898–906. http://dx.doi.org/10.1093/hmg/ddq176 PMID:20423928.

11. Onouchi Y, Suzuki Y, Suzuki H, Terai M, Yasukawa K, Hamada H, et al. ITPKC and CASP3 polymorphisms and risks for IVIG unresponsiveness and coronary artery lesion formation in Kawasaki disease. Pharmacogenomics J. 2013;13(1):52–9. http://dx.doi.org/10.1038/tpj.2011.45 PMID:21987091.

12. Suzuki H, Terai M, Hamada H, Honda T, Suenaga T, Takeuchi T, et al. Cyclosporin a treatment for Kawasaki disease refractory to initial and additional intravenous immunoglobulin. Pediatr Infect Dis J. 2011;30(10):871–6. http://dx.doi.org/10.1097/INF.0b013e318220c3cf PMID:21587094.

13. Japanese Kawasaki disease Research Committee. Diagnostic guidelines of Kawasaki disease (in Japanese). 5th ed. Tokyo: Japanese Kawasaki disease Research Committee; 2002.

14. Suzuki H, Suenaga T, Takeuchi T, Shibuta S, Yoshikawa N. Marker of T-cell activation is elevated in refractory Kawasaki disease. Pediatr Int. 2010;52(5):785–9. http://dx.doi.org/10.1111/j.1442-200X.2010.03163.x PMID:20487370.

15. Hamada H, Suzuki H, Abe J, Suzuki Y, Suenaga T, Takeuchi T, et al. Inflammatory cytokine profiles during cyclosporin treatment for immunoglobulin-resistant Kawasaki disease. Cytokine. 2012;60(3):681–5. http://dx.doi.org/10.1016/j.cyto.2012.08.006 PMID:22944461.

16. Tremoulet AH, Pancoast P, Franco A, Bujold M, Shimizu C, Onouchi Y, et al. Calcineurin inhibitor treatment of intravenous immunoglobulin-resistant Kawasaki disease. J Pediatr. 2012;161(3):506–12.e1.. http://dx.doi.org/10.1016/j.jpeds.2012.02.048 PMID:22484354.

Other Challenging Therapies

Tohru Kobayashi

Abstract Previous chapters described initial and rescue treatment for patients with Kawasaki disease. Other immunosuppressive agents, such as biological agents, methotrexate, cyclophosphamide, and plasma exchange, may also be effective for patients with Kawasaki disease. However, most of these agents have not been carefully evaluated for their efficacy in suppressing inflammation due to Kawasaki disease and preventing formation of coronary artery lesions, and most of the present evidence is from case reports or case series. Further research is needed before recommendations can be developed for these agents.

Keywords Methotrexate • Etanercept • Cytotoxic agents • Plasma exchange

Introduction

Immunosuppressive agents, such as biological agents, methotrexate, cyclophosphamide, and plasma exchange (PE), are sometimes used to treat patients with Kawasaki disease (KD) who do not respond to intravenous immunoglobulin (IVIG), steroids, anti-tumor necrosis factor (TNF) α antibody, cyclosporine, and/or ulinastatin. Although no confirmatory trials have been completed, there is considerable accumulating evidence regarding these immunosuppressive agents and PE. This chapter focuses on the potential efficacy and safety of these therapies.

T. Kobayashi, M.D., Ph.D. (✉)
Division of Clinical Research Planning, Department of Development Strategy, Center for Clinical Research and Development, National Center for Child Health and Development, 2-10-1, Okura, Setagaya-ku, Tokyo 157-8535, Japan
e-mail: torukoba@nifty.com

© Springer Japan 2017   195
B.T. Saji et al. (eds.), *Kawasaki Disease*, DOI 10.1007/978-4-431-56039-5_21

Biological Agents

Infliximab has been used as an adjunctive primary treatment or additional rescue treatment for IVIG nonresponders. Etanercept is a soluble TNF receptor that functions as a TNF antagonist and has a mechanism believed to be similar to that of infliximab. In 2010, Choueiter et al. [1] reported the results of a phase II trial of etanercept for intensification of initial therapy. In this prospective, open-label trial, 15 patients were given subcutaneous etanercept (0.4 mg/kg for four patients and 0.8 mg/kg for 11 patients) immediately after IVIG infusion; the patients were followed-up at 1 and 2 weeks. The pharmacokinetic profile was similar to that reported in older children, and there were no adverse reactions related to etanercept. None of the patients treated in this study required retreatment, and no patient had an increase in coronary artery diameter or cardiac dysfunction. On the basis of preliminary data, researchers designed a multicenter, double-blind, randomized, placebo-controlled trial of the efficacy of etanercept in addition to IVIG plus aspirin as initial therapy to reduce the incidence of initial treatment failure (ClinicalTrials. gov identifier NCT00841789).

Anakinra blocks interleukin-1, high levels of which lead to inflammation during acute KD. Anakinra has been shown in a KD mouse model to prevent development of coronary artery damage [2]. Cohen et al. [3] reported that a boy with severe KD was successfully treated with anakinra for 7 days after nonresponse to IVIG and intravenous methylprednisolone and for a period of 6 weeks after he developed recurrent KD. Currently, a phase I dose escalation trial has been launched in the United States to assess the safety of anakinra for KD patients with CAL (ClinicalTrials.gov identifier NCT02179853).

A marked increase in circulating B cells and production of cytotoxic immuno-globulins directed against endothelial cells has been documented in patients with KD. Thus, B-cell suppression seems to be a potential treatment option. A case report described the successful use of rituximab, a chimeric monoclonal antibody against the protein CD20, for treatment of highly refractory KD [4]. Rapid clinical, biological, and cardiac improvement was observed in the patient.

These biological agents seems to be well-tolerated and effective for refractory KD patients. However, current evidence is insufficient to develop recommendations regarding administration. These biological agents should be considered only for the most severe cases, i.e., patients resistant to other agents, or for patients who are enrolled in a well-designed clinical study.

Cytotoxic Agents

Evidence from a case report and a case series of four KD patients from Korea suggests that methotrexate might be an effective treatment [5, 6]. A subsequent trial by Lee et al. [7] reported the results of low-dose methotrexate (10 mg/m^2, once weekly until normalization of C-reactive protein levels) treatment for 17 patients with refractory KD. Methotrexate resulted in defervescence and improvement in inflammatory markers such as C-reactive protein level and erythrocyte sedimentation rate. No patient developed recurrent fever after discontinuation of methotrexate. However, the small sample size of this single-center study yielded insufficient statistical power to assess the efficacy and safety of methotrexate. Cyclophosphamide has also been used to treat refractory KD [8], but the evidence remains limited.

Plasma Exchange

Increases in inflammatory cytokines and chemokines such as interleukin (IL)-1, IL-6, IL-8, and TNF-α are thought to be major contributors to KD vasculitis. In theory, PE directly removes these cytokines and chemokines from blood and ameliorates clinical symptoms and inflammation.

In 1995, Takagi et al. [9] reported refractory KD patients who were successfully treated with PE. Imagawa et al. [10] reported a single-center retrospective trial that included 27 refractory KD patients treated with PE over three consecutive days after a second course of IVIG. Of the 27 patients treated with PE, 24 did not develop CAL during the acute phase, in contrast to the 23 of 48 children who did not undergo PE after the second IVIG but developed CAL during the acute phase.

Later, Hokosaki et al. [11] reported long-term follow-up data from the same center, in 2012. A total of 125 KD patients refractory to IVIG were treated with PE. The incidences of CAL before PE (i.e., during the acute period) and during the late period were examined retrospectively. During the acute period, within 1 month of onset, 41 of 125 patients had CAL. One year after onset, six patients developed CAL requiring systemic drug treatment (including five with giant aneurysms exceeding 8 mm). Fujimaru et al. [12] reported serial changes in 13 cytokines in nine children with IVIG-resistant KD before and after PE. Among those cytokines, interleukin-6, TNF-α, TNF receptor 1, TNF receptor 2, granulocyte colony-stimulating factor, and IL-17 were significantly lower after, as compared with before, PE, which reflects the potential central efficacy of PE.

The Research Committee of the Japanese Society of Pediatric Cardiology and Cardiovascular Surgery published a guideline for medical treatment of acute KD, in 2012 [13], which specified the method to be used for PE. In that guideline, the replacement solution is 5 % albumin, and the total volume to be exchanged is approximately 1- to 1.5-fold the circulating plasma volume (mL), calculated as follows: [bodyweight (kg)/13 × (1−Hematocrit (%)/100) × 1000]. Treatment is via the femoral vein, subclavian vein, or internal or external jugular veins, using a 6- or 7-Fr pediatric dialysis double-lumen catheter. During treatment, heparin 15–30 U/kg, first as a bolus intravenous infusion and 15–30 U/kg/h thereafter, may also be given for its anticoagulant effect, with the activated clotting time adjusted to 180–250 s. It is also necessary to keep the patient sedated. In general, the side effects of PE include hypotension, hypovolemia, and shock. Because the volume of extracorporeal circulation will exceed circulating blood volume in pediatric patients, it may be necessary to reduce the volume to lower the risk of hypotension. Because of its potential risks, PE should be reserved for KD patients in whom reasonable medical therapies have failed to improve clinical symptoms and laboratory findings. PE is not the first choice for patients with refractory KD.

References

1. Choueiter NF, Olson AK, Shen DD, Portman MA. Prospective open-label trial of etanercept as adjunctive therapy for Kawasaki disease. J Pediatr. 2010;157(6):960–6. http://dx.doi.org/10. 1016/j.jpeds.2010.06.014 PMID:20667551.
2. Chen S, Lee Y, Crother TR, Fishbein M, Zhang W, Yilmaz A, et al. Marked acceleration of atherosclerosis after Lactobacillus casei-induced coronary arteritis in a mouse model of Kawasaki disease. Arterioscler Thromb Vasc Biol. 2012;32(8):e60–71. http://dx.doi.org/10. 1161/ATVBAHA.112.249417 PMID:22628430.
3. Cohen S, Tacke CE, Straver B, Meijer N, Kuipers IM, Kuijpers TW. A child with severe relapsing Kawasaki disease rescued by IL-1 receptor blockade and extracorporeal membrane oxygenation. Ann Rheum Dis. 2012;71(12):2059–61. http://dx.doi.org/10.1136/annrheumdis-2012-201658 PMID:22689319.
4. Sauvaget E, Bonello B, David M, Chabrol B, Dubus JC, Bosdure E. Resistant Kawasaki disease treated with anti-CD20. J Pediatr. 2012;160(5):875–6. http://dx.doi.org/10.1016/j. jpeds.2012.01.018 PMID:22341587.
5. Lee MS, An SY, Jang GC, Kim DS. A case of intravenous immunoglobulin-resistant Kawasaki disease treated with methotrexate. Yonsei Med J. 2002;43(4):527–32. http://dx.doi.org/10. 3349/ymj.2002.43.4.527 PMID:12205742.
6. Ahn SY, Kim DS. Treatment of intravenous immunoglobulin-resistant Kawasaki disease with methotrexate. Scand J Rheumatol. 2005;34(2):136–9. PMID:16095010.
7. Lee TJ, Kim KH, Chun JK, Kim DS. Low-dose methotrexate therapy for intravenous immunoglobulin-resistant Kawasaki disease. Yonsei Med J. 2008;49(5):714–18. http://dx. doi.org/10.3349/ymj.2008.49.5.714 PMID:18972590.
8. Wallace CA, French JW, Kahn SJ, Sherry DD. Initial intravenous gammaglobulin treatment failure in Kawasaki disease. Pediatrics. 2000;105(6):E78. http://dx.doi.org/10.1542/peds.105. 6.e78 PMID:10835091.
9. Takagi N, Kihara M, Yamaguchi S, Tamura K, Yabana M, Tokita Y, et al. Plasma exchange in Kawasaki disease. Lancet. 1995;346(8985):1307. http://dx.doi.org/10.1016/S0140-6736(95) 91916-3 PMID:7475760.
10. Imagawa T, Mori M, Miyamae T, Ito S, Nakamura T, Yasui K, et al. Plasma exchange for refractory Kawasaki disease. Eur J Pediatr. 2004;163(4–5):263–4. http://dx.doi.org/10.1007/ s00431-003-1267-y PMID:14986117.
11. Hokosaki T, Mori M, Nishizawa T, Nakamura T, Imagawa T, Iwamoto M, et al. Long-term efficacy of plasma exchange treatment for refractory Kawasaki disease. Pediatr Int. 2012;54 (1):99–103. http://dx.doi.org/10.1111/j.1442-200X.2011.03487.x PMID:22004042.
12. Fujimaru T, Ito S, Masuda H, Oana S, Kamei K, Ishiguro A, et al. Decreased levels of inflammatory cytokines in immunoglobulin-resistant Kawasaki disease after plasma exchange. Cytokine. 2014;70(2):156–60. http://dx.doi.org/10.1016/j.cyto.2014.07.003 PMID:25082649.
13. Research Committee of the Japanese Society of Pediatric CardiologyCardiac Surgery Committee for Development of Guidelines for Medical Treatment of Acute Kawasaki Disease. Guidelines for medical treatment of acute Kawasaki disease: report of the Research Committee of the Japanese Society of Pediatric Cardiology and Cardiac Surgery (2012 revised version). Pediatr Int. 2014;56(2):135–58. http://dx.doi.org/10.1111/ped.12317 PMID:24730626.

Antiplatelet and Antithrombotic Therapy for Giant Coronary Aneurysm

Kenji Suda

Abstract After treatment of acute Kawasaki disease, 0.2–0.3 % of patients have giant coronary aneurysms (≥8 mm in diameter). These aneurysms are less likely to regress and may result in stenosis leading to coronary thrombosis and myocardial infarction. Although there has been no randomized controlled trial of treatments to prevent thrombosis of giant coronary aneurysms, several case-control studies have compared warfarin plus aspirin with antiplatelet medications given without warfarin. In addition, a recent meta-analysis confirmed the efficacy of warfarin plus aspirin in decreasing the incidence of coronary artery occlusion, myocardial infarction, and cardiac death. Anticoagulant therapy must be carefully monitored because warfarin can cause serious hemorrhagic complications. The efficacy of new drug regimens, including double antiplatelet treatment and factor Xa inhibitors, should be investigated.

Keywords Aspirin • Warfarin • Myocardial infarction

Introduction

Coronary artery aneurysms are classified on the basis of internal diameter as small, medium, and giant (≥8 mm) [1]. In recent years, the proportion of patients with Kawasaki disease (KD) who have coronary artery dilation or aneurysms after treatment for acute disease has decreased to 3 % [2]. However, 0.2–0.3 % of patients have giant coronary aneurysms (GA) at 1 month after KD onset. GA are less likely to regress and may persist or develop into stenosis. Hence, patients with GA have the highest risk of cardiac events, such as acute myocardial infarction, and death [3, 4].

K. Suda, M.D., Ph.D. (✉)
Department of Pediatrics and Child Health, Kurume University School of Medicine,
67 Asahi-machi, Kurume-shi, Fukuoka-ken 830-0011, Japan
e-mail: suda_kenji@med.kurume-u.ac.jp

© Springer Japan 2017   199
B.T. Saji et al. (eds.), *Kawasaki Disease*, DOI 10.1007/978-4-431-56039-5_22

Historical Overview

The first Japanese nationwide survey of KD, in 1970, showed that 1.7 % of patients
with KD died from acute myocardial infarction, and the four autopsies conducted
showed thrombotic occlusion of coronary aneurysms. A report describing multiple
coronary artery aneurysms in 12 of 20 patients with KD was the first recognition of
KD as a systemic vasculitis syndrome [3]. Follow-up of these patients for a period
of 10–21 years showed that about half of the aneurysms regressed within 2 years
after onset, whereas obstructive lesion developed gradually with time [4]. In particular, GA were less likely to regress and had a high probability of developing into
ischemic heart disease and myocardial infarction [4–6]. In an analysis of
195 patients with myocardial infarction in a nationwide survey of KD, 22 % died
at the first attack, and 57 % of survivors of the first and subsequent attacks had
cardiac dysfunction [7].

Current Understanding and Recognition

Studies using the Doppler flow guidewire and pressure monitoring wire showed that
average peak velocity index and shear stress index significantly decreased as
aneurysm size increased [8, 9]. Decreased shear stress and stagnant flow increase
platelet aggregation and coagulation activity but reduce fibrinolysis, thus leading to
thrombus formation [10]. Flow stagnation and reduction of shear stress in GA were
associated with mural thrombus formation [8]. In addition, fractional flow reserve
in patients with GA and no stenosis was significantly lower than in those without
GA. Multiple coronary aneurysms or GA with mild stenosis could easily trigger
coronary thrombosis [11]. Therefore, antiplatelet and anticoagulant therapy is
important to prevent thrombosis of GA.

Assigned Evidence Class and Recommendations

Although thrombosis of GA can cause acute myocardial infarction leading to poor
outcomes, there has been no randomized controlled trial comparing treatment
options. Two case-control studies found that treatment with aspirin plus warfarin
was more effective than other regimens [12, 13]. Onouchi et al. followed patients
with coronary aneurysms for a mean period of 9 years [12] and found that the
incidence of coronary occlusion was significantly lower in those receiving warfarin
plus aspirin than in those receiving warfarin alone or no medication ($p < 0.01$).
Incidence in the warfarin plus aspirin group was also lower than that for aspirin
alone but not significantly so ($p < 0.10$) (Fig. 1). In a study of patients with GA,
Sugawara et al. [13] reported that the incidence of myocardial infarction was

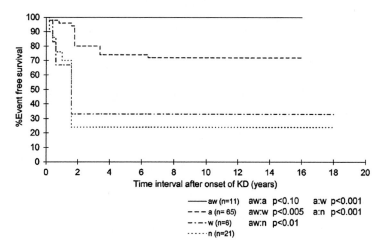

Fig. 1 Kaplan–Meier curves for rate of freedom from occlusion/recanalization of giant aneurysms Prophylactic therapy after acute Kawasaki disease (a: aspirin, w: warfarin, aw: aspirin plus warfarin, n: none). The rates of Event free survival at the last observation were 72 %, 33 %, 100 %, and 24 % for treatments {a}, {w}, {aw}, and {n}, respectively. No occlusion/recanalization was noted for {aw}, and this rate significantly differed from the rates for {w} and {n}. Furthermore, {aw} had a tendency toward lower incidence of occlusion/recanalization as compared with {a} (Adapted from Onouchi et al. [12] with permission)

significantly lower in patients receiving warfarin plus aspirin than in those receiving antiplatelet medications without warfarin (5.2 % vs. 32.7 %, p < 0.05). The rate of freedom from myocardial infarction was 95 % after a mean follow-up period of 7.7 years in patients assigned to the combined regimen (Fig. 2). There were no deaths among patients treated with warfarin plus aspirin; however, seven of the 49 patients who did not receive warfarin died (p = 0.18). Additionally, a multicenter case study of 87 patients treated with warfarin plus aspirin showed that 91 % were free from cardiac events at 10 years [14] (Fig. 3). A meta-analysis of several descriptive observational studies [15, 16] showed that warfarin plus aspirin reduced the incidence of coronary artery occlusion (odds ratio [OR], 0.08; 95 % CI, 0.02–0.29; p < 0.0001), myocardial infarction (OR, 0.27; 95 % CI, 0.11–0.63; p = 0.003), and death (OR, 0.18; 95 % CI, 0.04–0.88; p = 0.03) [16]. On the basis of this evidence, warfarin and antiplatelet therapy is classified as a class 1 treatment for GA with or without coronary stenosis [1, 17]. Other antiplatelet medications, such as dipyridamole, flurbiprofen, and ticlopidine (Table 1) [1], have been given alone or in combination with aspirin or warfarin. However, evidence regarding the effectiveness of these drugs is limited.

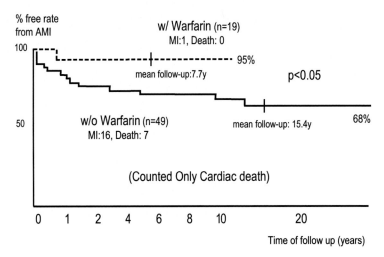

Fig. 2 Kaplan–Meier curves for rate of freedom from acute myocardial infarction: warfarin plus aspirin vs. aspirin alone The incidence of acute myocardial infarction was significantly lower in patients given warfarin plus aspirin (*dotted line*) than in those given aspirin alone (*solid line*). *AMI* acute myocardial infarction, *MI* myocardial infarction (Adapted from Sugahara et al. [13] with permission)

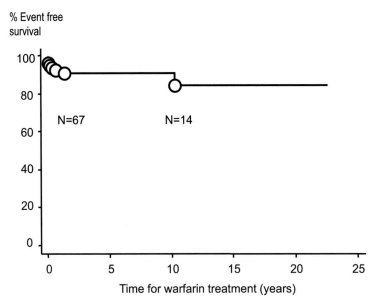

Fig. 3 Kaplan–Meier curve for rate of freedom from cardiac events in patients receiving warfarin plus aspirin A multicenter case study of 87 patients receiving warfarin plus aspirin showed that 91 % were free from cardiac events at 10 years. (Adapted from Suda et al. [14] with permission)

Table 1 Antiplatelet and anticoagulant drugs used in the treatment of Kawasaki disease

Drugs	Dosage
Aspirin	3–5 mg/kg, qd
	3–5 mg/kg, tid
Dipyridamole	2–5 mg/kg, tid
Ticlopidine	5–7 mg/kg, bid
Clopidogrel	1 mg/kg, qd
Unfractionated heparin	Loading 50 U/kg + maintenance 20 U/kg
	Target APTT 60–85 s
	(1.5–2.5 times the reference)
Low molecular heparin	ex) enoxaparin
Infants (<12 months)	1.5 mg/kg/day, bid
Children	1 mg/kg/day, bid
Warfarin	0.05–0.12 mg/kg, qd
	Target INR 2.0–2.5

Abbreviations: *APTT* activated partial-thromboplastin time, *INR* international normalized ratio

The former treatment guideline of the Japanese Circulation Society established a target international normalized ratio of 1.6–2.5 for antithrombotic treatment using warfarin [1]. This was later changed to 2.0–2.5, to match the recommendations of the American Heart Association [17]. In a multicenter case study, hemorrhagic complications occurred eight times in five patients, a frequency of 1.7 % per patient-year, at a target international normalized ratio of 1.5–2.5 or higher [14].

Recent Advances and Future Directions

A recent computational simulation model of coronary artery aneurysms provided strong evidence that thrombotic risk is more accurately predicted by hemodynamic parameters than by aneurysm diameter alone [18]. Therefore, hemodynamic factors [8] should be incorporated in the selection of patients for anticoagulation therapy. In addition, studies should investigate new drugs, such as factor Xa inhibitor [19], that may be better at producing stable anticoagulant activity and minimizing the risk of bleeding complications, especially for small infants with KD who are at high risk for developing GA.

References

1. JCS Joint Working Group. Guidelines for diagnosis and management of cardiovascular sequelae in Kawasaki disease (JCS 2008). Circ J. 2010;74(9):1989–2020. http://www.j-circ. or.jp/guideline/pdf/JCS2008_ogawasy_d.pdf. Accessed August 26, 2014.

2. Nakamura Y, Yashiro M, Uehara R, Sadakane A, Tsuboi S, Aoyama Y, et al. Epidemiologic features of Kawasaki disease in Japan: results of the 2009–2010 nationwide survey. J Epidemiol. 2012;22(3):216–21. http://dx.doi.org/10.2188/jea.JE20110126 PMID:22447211.

3. Kato H, Koike S, Yamamoto M, Ito Y, Yano E. Coronary aneurysms in infants and young children with acute febrile mucocutaneous lymph node syndrome. J Pediatr. 1975;86 (6):892–8. http://dx.doi.org/10.1016/S0022-3476(75)80220-4 PMID:236368.

4. Kato H, Sugimura T, Akagi T, Sato N, Hashino K, Maeno Y, et al. Long-term consequences of Kawasaki disease. A 10- to 21-year follow-up study of 594 patients. Circulation. 1996;94 (6):1379–85. http://dx.doi.org/10.1161/01.CIR.94.6.1379 PMID:8822996.

5. Takahashi K, Oharaseki T, Yokouchi Y, Naoe S, Saji T. Kawasaki disease: basic and pathological findings. Clin Exp Nephrol. 2013;17(5):690–3. http://dx.doi.org/10.1007/ s10157-012-0734-z PMID:23188196.

6. Suda K, Iemura M, Nishiono H, Teramachi Y, Koteda Y, Kishimoto S, et al. Long-term prognosis of patients with Kawasaki disease complicated by giant coronary aneurysms: a single-institution experience. Circulation. 2011;123(17):1836–42. http://dx.doi.org/10.1161/ CIRCULATIONAHA.110.978213 PMID:21502578.

7. Kato H, Ichinose E, Kawasaki T. Myocardial infarction in Kawasaki disease: clinical analyses in 195 cases. J Pediatr. 1986;108(6):923–7. http://dx.doi.org/10.1016/S0022-3476(86)80928-3 PMID:3712157.

8. Kuramochi Y, Ohkubo T, Takechi N, Fukumi D, Uchikoba Y, Ogawa S. Hemodynamic factors of thrombus formation in coronary aneurysms associated with Kawasaki disease. Pediatr Int. 2000;42(5):470–5. http://dx.doi.org/10.1046/j.1442-200x.2000.01270.x PMID:11059533.

9. Ohkubo T, Fukazawa R, Ikegami E, Ogawa S. Reduced shear stress and disturbed flow may lead to coronary aneurysm and thrombus formations. Pediatr Int. 2007;49(1):1–7. http://dx.doi. org/10.1111/j.1442-200X.2007.02312.x PMID:17250496.

10. Wolberg AS, Aleman MM, Leiderman K, Machlus KR. Procoagulant activity in hemostasis and thrombosis: Virchow's triad revisited. Anesth Analg. 2012;114(2):275–85. http://dx.doi. org/10.1213/ANE.0b013e31823a088c PMID:22104070.

11. Murakami T, Tanaka N. The physiological significance of coronary aneurysms in Kawasaki disease. EuroIntervention. 2011;7(8):944–7. http://dx.doi.org/10.4244/EIJV7I8A149 PMID:22157479.

12. Onouchi Z, Hamaoka K, Sakata K, Ozawa S, Shiraishi I, Itoi T, et al. Long-term changes in coronary artery aneurysms in patients with Kawasaki disease: comparison of therapeutic regimens. Circ J. 2005;69(3):265–72. http://dx.doi.org/10.1253/circj.69.265 PMID:15731529.

13. Sugahara Y, Ishii M, Muta H, Iemura M, Matsuishi T, Kato H. Warfarin therapy for giant aneurysm prevents myocardial infarction in Kawasaki disease. Pediatr Cardiol. 2008;29 (2):398–401. http://dx.doi.org/10.1007/s00246-007-9132-9 PMID:18027010.

14. Suda K, Kudo Y, Higaki T, Nomura Y, Miura M, Matsumura M, et al. Multicenter and retrospective case study of warfarin and aspirin combination therapy in patients with giant coronary aneurysms caused by Kawasaki disease. Circ J. 2009;73(7):1319–23. http://dx.doi. org/10.1253/circj.CJ-08-0931 PMID:19436123.

15. Levy DM, Silverman ED, Massicotte MP, McCrindle BW, Yeung RS. Longterm outcomes in patients with giant aneurysms secondary to Kawasaki disease. J Rheumatol. 2005;32 (5):928–34. PMID:15868632.

16. Su D, Wang K, Qin S, Pang Y. Safety and efficacy of warfarin plus aspirin combination therapy for giant coronary artery aneurysm secondary to Kawasaki disease: a meta-analysis [Epub ahead of print]. Cardiology. 2014;129(1):55–64. http://dx.doi.org/10.1159/000363732 PMID:25116427.

17. Newburger JW, Takahashi M, Gerber MA, Gewitz MH, Tani LY, Burns JC, et al. American academy of pediatrics. Diagnosis, treatment, and long-term management of Kawasaki disease: a statement for health professionals from the Committee on Rheumatic Fever, Endocarditis and Kawasaki Disease, Council on Cardiovascular Disease in the Young, American Heart Association. Circulation. 2004;110(17):2747–71. http://dx.doi.org/10.1161/01.CIR. 0000145143.19711.78 PMID:15505111.

18. Sengupta D, Kahn AM, Kung E, Esmaily Moghadam M, Shirinsky O, Lyskina GA, et al. Thrombotic risk stratification using computational modeling in patients with coronary artery aneurysms following Kawasaki disease [Epub ahead of print]. Biomech Model Mechanobiol.   2014;13(6):1261–76.   http://dx.doi.org/10.1007/s10237-014-0570-z PMID:24722951.

19. Granger CB, Alexander JH, McMurray JJ, Lopes RD, Hylek EM, Hanna M, et al. ARISTOTLE Committees and Investigators. Apixaban versus warfarin in patients with atrial fibrillation. N Engl J Med. 2011;365(11):981–92. http://dx.doi.org/10.1056/NEJMoa1107039 PMID:21870978.

Characteristics of Sudden Cardiac Death Late After Acute Kawasaki Disease

Etsuko Tsuda

Abstract When present, giant aneurysms typically occlude coronary arteries within the first year after onset of Kawasaki disease (KD) and can cause acute myocardial infarction. Bilateral giant aneurysm is major risk factor for sudden death after KD and leads to myocardial infarction, decreased left ventricular ejection fraction, multifocal premature ventricular contractions, and asymptomatic nonsustained ventricular tachycardia. Prevention of myocardial infarction and left ventricular (LV) dysfunction depends on careful follow-up, anticoagulation therapy, and coronary revascularization. LV dysfunction predisposes patients to arrhythmic sudden death; however, angiotensin-converting enzyme inhibitors and beta-blockers improve prognosis for patients with LV dysfunction. Such patients may also benefit from antiarrhythmic treatment with amiodarone or sotalol. If critical ventricular tachycardia is detected, catheter ablation or an implantable cardioverter–defibrillator should be considered. Sudden death can occur more than 20 years after acute KD in patients with LV dysfunction (left ventricular ejection fraction <40 %). Multifocal premature ventricular contractions and nonsustained ventricular tachycardia are probable risk factors in such patients.

Keywords Giant aneurysm • Acute myocardial infarction • Sudden death • Left ventricular dysfunction • Nonsustained ventricular tachycardia

Introduction

Although mortality from Kawasaki disease (KD) and its cardiac sequelae has decreased recently [1], lifetime prognosis is unclear. Death in this population is either sudden or from heart failure. Coronary artery lesions after KD are rarely symptomatic, and there is often no evidence of ischemia until actual infarction or sudden death occurs. Therefore, an important challenge is preventing late sudden death in patients with coronary artery lesions resulting from KD. The author and

E. Tsuda, M.D. (✉)
Department of Pediatric Cardiology, National Cerebral and Cardiovascular Center,
5-7-1 Fujishirodai, Suita-shi, Osaka 565-8565, Japan
e-mail: etsuda@hsp.ncvc.go.jp

© Springer Japan 2017
B.T. Saji et al. (eds.), *Kawasaki Disease*, DOI 10.1007/978-4-431-56039-5_23

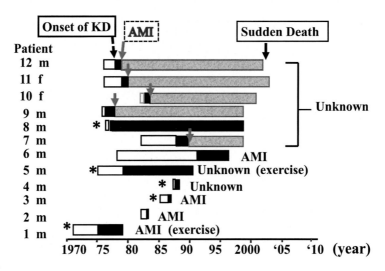

Fig. 1 Interval from onset of Kawasaki disease to sudden death, and cause of death in 12 patients with KD. *KD* Kawasaki disease, *AMI* acute myocardial infarction. * Patient had asymptomatic coronary occlusion of more than one major branch. During the 1980s, three infants with bilateral giant aneurysms were included, two of whom had acute myocardial infarction. In the late 1990s and the 2000s, there were five cases of sudden death in patients with left ventricular dysfunction (ejection fraction <40 %), more than 20 years after acute KD. The causes of death were unknown

colleagues analyzed clinical course and cause of death in 12 cases of sudden death in KD patients, to identify risk factors for sudden death and determine if cause of death changed over the last three decades, a period which saw improvements in medical and surgical treatments for KD [2] (Fig. 1).

History

The first national survey of KD in Japan, in 1970, reported 10 deaths (1 %) out of 1100 patients with KD. Seven of the decedents were male and three were female. Age at death ranged from 3 month to 2 years 7 months, and the interval from KD onset to death was 10–60 days. Eight of the 10 deaths were classified as sudden death. Four patients were autopsied, and the findings revealed thrombotic occlusion of a coronary aneurysm due to vasculitis, resulting in acute myocardial infarction (MI). Records in Japan show that 272,749 patients had acute KD and 436 died, as of 2010. Although the mortality rate for KD in Japan was 0.4 % in the 1970s and 1980s, it decreased to <0.1 % during the 1990s [1]. National surveys of KD in Japan have been performed every 2 years since 1976. Recent surveys show an incidence of about 10,000 KD cases per year. At 1 month after onset, giant (>8 mm) coronary aneurysms (GA), the cause of cardiac sequelae leading to sudden death, are present in about 0.2 % of KD patients. The male: female ratio for incidence of death after KD is about 3:1, as is the male:female ratio in the prevalence of GAs as cardiac sequelae.

The principal causes of sudden death after KD onset differ by decade (Fig. 1) [2]. In the 1970s, most exercise-related sudden deaths occurred in patients with occult coronary artery disease resulting from KD. Unfortunately, these cases were not identified until after sudden death. Appropriate treatments for acute KD and precise diagnostic techniques for cardiac sequelae had not yet been established in the 1970s and 1980s. Until the early 1980s most sudden deaths were caused by acute MI within several years of the acute episode. In addition to missed diagnoses, the contemporaneous anticoagulation regimen for KD coronary artery lesions was insufficient for preventing MI. In the late 1990s and early 2000s several sudden deaths occurred in patients with left ventricular dysfunction and nonsustained ventricular tachycardia (NSVT). The patients were born in the 1970s and 1980s and developed MI soon after acute KD. They had no history of cardiac events in the many years before their deaths. Fatal ventricular arrhythmia was the most likely cause of death. There are probably many such at-risk patients, now adults. Thus, determining the cause of sudden death and preventing such deaths in this population are important concerns.

Current Understanding

Acute sudden death from aneurysms is usually caused by aneurysm rupture. Such ruptures are rare in aneurysms with a diameter <10 mm. In autopsy reports by the Japan Pathologic Society, rupture was found in 20 (10 %) of 204 KD patients [3]. The interval from KD onset to rupture of a giant aneurysm was 10–28 days, and the rate was higher for aneurysms in the left coronary artery than for those in the right coronary artery. The pathologists noted that the coronary walls were thin and that the internal and external elastic lamina were destroyed. Continuous steroid therapy should be avoided in patients with aneurysms when aneurysm diameter is progressively increasing during acute KD.

GA are likely to occlude with thrombosis, especially during the first year. Thrombosis often results in acute MI [4], which occasionally causes sudden death or impaired left ventricular function, a major determinant of outcome in this population (Table 1). In most patients acute MI after KD is caused by sudden coronary occlusion due to a thrombus in the GA. These thrombi are triggered by three factors, as described by Virchow, namely, endothelial dysfunction in the injured coronary arterial wall due to severe acute vasculitis, turbulence or stasis within the giant aneurysm, and hypercoagulability caused by acceleration of coagulant and thrombolytic systems in the first year after KD. Antithrombotic therapy for GA patients is also beneficial during the first year after acute KD [5]. More effective anticoagulation, including the use of coumadin, has likely decreased the prevalence of acute MI. GA due to KD can cause acute coronary syndromes in adults, and age at onset in patients with such syndromes is younger than in the

Table 1 Risk factors of sudden death late after Kawasaki disease

Bilateral giant aneurysm (multivessel disease)
Occlusion of one or more coronary arteries
Previous myocardial infarction
Nonviable infarct area
Low left ventricular ejection fraction ($<40\%$)
Nonsustained ventricular tachycardia

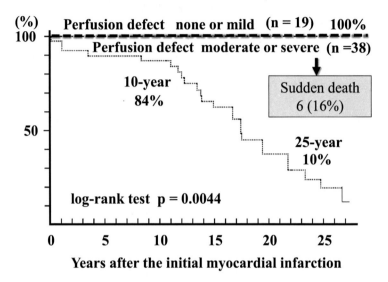

Fig. 2 Kaplan–Meier curves of freedom from nonsustained ventricular tachycardia after initial myocardial infarction, as determined by presence of abnormalities in ^{99m}-Tc myocardial perfusion imaging

general population. Even when aneurysms regress during adulthood, a few patients develop AMI [6]. Smoking is clearly contraindicated in at-risk individuals.

Successful revascularization for AMI also increases survival after AMI. However, more information on precise diagnosis and optimal treatment of AMI is critically needed. Most late deaths after AMI were due to heart failure or were sudden. Recurrent MI and fatal ventricular arrhythmia were also noted. Nonsustained ventricular tachycardia (NSVT) and ventricular tachycardia (VT) can develop more than 10 years after initial MI, mostly in patients with nonviable myocardium secondary to MI (Fig 2) [5]. Development of NSVT and VT in patients with low left ventricular ejection fraction (LVEF) adversely influenced outcomes.

The incidence of stenotic lesions in GA progressively increases, and the degree of stenosis worsens with aging [7]. Stenotic lesions were found in most working GA branches after 20 years, although the incidence of stenosis was very low in vessels without GA. Patients with bilateral GA had a higher incidence of stenosis and a low cardiac event-free rate. The hazard ratio for the risk of death and cardiac events associated with bilateral GA was about four times that associated with unilateral GA. Prognosis was significantly poorer for patients with bilateral GA than for those with unilateral GA. Multivessel disease and previous infarction are risk factors for sudden death (Table 1). Therefore, coronary bypass grafting (CABG) as a means of coronary revascularization is more effective in multivessel disease. Patients with bilateral GA require at least one good revascularization in the long-term period after KD, as it increases survival [8].

Evidence Quality and Recommendations

Coronary artery lesions caused by KD require medical and possibly surgical management. Intracoronary thrombolysis using tissue plasminogen activator and percutaneous coronary intervention (PCI) is indicated for acute MI. After infarction, medical treatment for heart failure and arrhythmia may be necessary.

Late localized stenosis due to intimal thickening may eventually completely occlude one or more coronary arteries, causing severe myocardial ischemia. Coronary artery revascularization aims to improve myocardial ischemia from impaired flow secondary to stenosis and is achieved either surgically by CABG or by one or more PCI procedures [9]. CABG using the internal thoracic artery (ITA) has been successfully performed since the middle of the 1980s and has been widely accepted as the most reliable means of ensuring myocardial revascularization [10]. Experience with PCI during the late period after KD suggests it can be effective, although information on PCI in children is limited. A combination of procedures is often needed in patients with multivessel disease, to optimize the possibility of long-term survival.

Selection of the best approach for revascularization is critical and involves determining whether CABG, PCI, or both is better for a given patient. Large body size and the presence of multivessel disease favor surgery. One must decide if the affected vessels are appropriate for PCI. In some cases delayed intervention might result in a better long-term outcome. In some respects, CABG is a better approach than PCI for coronary revascularization. Although PCI may improve myocardial ischemia for localized stenosis with GAs, the risk of MI from thrombotic occlusion remains. In contrast, if good flow is present in an ITA graft 1 year after surgery, long-term patency is virtually assured [9]. It improves patient quality of life, and the risk of restenosis of target vessels is low. Complete recovery of coronary blood flow by CABG might permit discontinuation of long-term anticoagulant therapy in patients without persistent GAs or coronary artery lesions in other vessels. However, coronary revascularization in children does not always have to be complete, because the interval to development of stenotic lesions varies in each patient. CABG should be performed only when native flow is severely impaired.

Electrophysiological studies may be needed in order to detect potentially fatal arrhythmias in such patients. Sudden deaths in patients with left ventricular dysfunction due to KD can occur more than 20 years after previous MI. Amiodarone or sotalol can prevent fatal ventricular arrhythmia, a late complication of MI. The ACC/AHA/HRS 2008 Guidelines for Device-Based Therapy of Cardiac Rhythm Abnormalities state that implantable cardioverter–defibrillator (ICD) therapy is indicated in patients who are at least 40 days post-MI and have LV dysfunction due to prior MI, an LVEF <30 %, and NYHA functional class I disease (Level of Evidence: A). Furthermore, ICD therapy is indicated in patients with NSVT caused by prior MI, an LVEF less than 40 %, and inducible ventricular fibrillation or sustained VT in an electrophysiological study (Level of Evidence: B) These groups were included in class I. Some patients with low LVEF and nonviability after KD may be suitable for inclusion in these groups.

Recent Advances

Research on myocardial disease is continuing to explore the possibility of transplanting cells that regenerate and are well-tolerated. Ongoing trials are investigating the feasibility of cell therapies, including the evaluation of cell types and injection methods.

References

1. Nakamura Y, Yashiro M, Uehara R, Sadakane A, Chihara I, Aoyama Y, et al. Epidemiologic features of Kawasaki disease in Japan: results of the 2007–2008 nationwide survey. J Epidemiol. 2010;20(4):302–7. http://dx.doi.org/10.2188/jea.JE20090180 PMID:20530917.
2. Tsuda E, Arakaki Y, Shimizu T, Sakaguchi H, Yoshimura S, Yazaki S, et al. Changes in causes of sudden deaths by decade in patients with coronary arterial lesions due to Kawasaki disease. Cardiol Young. 2005;15(5):481–8. http://dx.doi.org/10.1017/S1047951105001344 PMID:16164786.
3. Imai Y, Sunagawa K, Ayusawa M, Miyashita M, Abe O, Suzuki J, et al. A fatal case of ruptured giant coronary artery aneurysm. Eur J Pediatr. 2006;165(2):130–3. http://dx.doi.org/10.1007/s00431-005-0016-9 PMID:16215725.
4. Tsuda E, Hirata T, Matsuo O, Abe T, Sugiyama H, Yamada O. The 30-year outcome for patients after myocardial infarction due to coronary artery lesions caused by Kawasaki disease. Pediatr Cardiol. 2011;32(2):176–82. http://dx.doi.org/10.1007/s00246-010-9838-y PMID:21120463.
5. Tsuda E, Abe T, Tamaki W. Acute coronary syndrome in adult patients with coronary artery lesions caused by Kawasaki disease: review of case reports. Cardiol Young. 2011;21(1):74–82. http://dx.doi.org/10.1017/S1047951110001502 PMID:21070690.
6. Tsuda E, Hamaoka K, Suzuki H, Sakazaki H, Murakami Y, Nakagawa M, et al. A survey of the 3-decade outcome for patients with giant aneurysms caused by Kawasaki disease. Am Heart J. 2014;167(2):249–58. http://dx.doi.org/10.1016/j.ahj.2013.10.025 PMID:24439987.
7. Tsuda E, Kamiya T, Ono Y, Kimura K, Kurosaki K, Echigo S. Incidence of stenotic lesions predicted by acute phase changes in coronary arterial diameter during Kawasaki disease. Pediatr Cardiol. 2005;26(1):73–9. http://dx.doi.org/10.1007/s00246-004-0698-1 PMID:15136903.

8. Tsuda E, Kitamura S, Kimura K, Kobayashi J, Miyazaki S, Echigo S, et al. Long-term patency of internal thoracic artery grafts for coronary artery stenosis due to Kawasaki disease: comparison of early with recent results in small children. Am Heart J. 2007;153 (6):995–1000. http://dx.doi.org/10.1016/j.ahj.2007.03.034 PMID:17540201.

9. Muta H, Ishii M. Percutaneous coronary intervention versus coronary artery bypass grafting for stenotic lesions after Kawasaki disease. J Pediatr. 2010;157(1):120–6. http://dx.doi.org/10.1016/j.jpeds.2010.01.032 PMID:20304414.

10. Kitamura S, Tsuda E, Kobayashi J, Nakajima H, Yoshikawa Y, Yagihara T, et al. Twenty-five-year outcome of pediatric coronary artery bypass surgery for Kawasaki disease. Circulation. 2009;120 (1):60–8. http://dx.doi.org/10.1161/CIRCULATIONAHA.108.840603 PMID:19546384.

Kawasaki Disease Diagnosis and Complication Rates in the United States and Japan

Shohei Ogata

Abstract Clear diagnostic criteria and definitions of coronary artery lesions (CALs) were established in Japan by the Japanese Ministry of Health Research Committee (Fifth Revised Edition, February 2002) and the Japanese Circulation Society (JCS), and in the United States by the American Heart Association (AHA) and American Academy of Pediatrics (AAP), in 2004. Definitions and criteria for Kawasaki disease diagnosis slightly differ between the AHA/AAP and Japanese guidelines. The diagnostic criteria for classical Kawasaki disease in AHA/AAP guidelines include fever persisting at least 5 days and at least four of five other criteria. The criteria in the Japanese guidelines include fever as a sixth, equally important criterion, and patients must meet five of six criteria for diagnosis, including fever that subsides within 5 days in response to therapy. It is difficult to compare CAL rates in these countries because the definitions of CALs are completely different in the respective guidelines. The Japanese JCS guidelines for CALs use the diameter of each segment of coronary arteries. However, in the AHA/APP guidelines aneurysms are classified using z-scores. Previously reported differences in CAL rates between the United States and Japan likely resulted from use of different definitions and nomenclature. Development of standard criteria for CALs in both countries would allow meaningful comparisons between countries and facilitate collaborative international clinical trials.

Keywords Kawasaki disease • Epidemiology • Diagnosis • Complication • Guidelines

S. Ogata (✉)
Department of Pediatrics, Kitasato University School of Medicine, 1-15-1 Kitazato, Minami-ku, Sagamihara, Kanagawa 252-0375, Japan
e-mail: shogata@kitasato-u.ac.jp

© Springer Japan 2017   215
B.T. Saji et al. (eds.), *Kawasaki Disease*, DOI 10.1007/978-4-431-56039-5_24

Guidelines for Kawasaki Disease in the United States and Japan

Children with Kawasaki disease (KD) are febrile and extremely irritable, much more so than children with other febrile illnesses. No specific and sensitive diagnostic test for KD is available. Current diagnostic criteria and definitions of coronary artery lesions (CALs) were established in Japan by the Japanese Ministry of Health Research Committee (Fifth Revised Edition, February 2002) and the Japanese Circulation Society (JCS), and in United States by the American Heart Association (AHA) and American Academy of Pediatrics (AAP) [1–4].

AHA/AAP published the first US KD guidelines in 2004, and they have been widely used in that country and elsewhere. The guidelines from the Japanese Ministry of Health Research Committee have been used for KD diagnosis in Japan since 1984, and the Scientific Committee of the JCS published guideline criteria for CALs in 2005, which have been used for CAL diagnosis in Japan. Although the criteria for KD diagnosis are described in the JCS guidelines, the diagnostic criteria in both guidelines are very similar in content because the JCS guidelines were designed based on the guidelines from the Japan Ministry of Health Research Committee.

The definitions and criteria for KD diagnosis slightly differ between the AHA/AAP and Japanese guidelines. It is difficult to compare rates of CALs between countries because the definitions for CALs are completely different. In addition, KD complication rates differ between the United States and Japan. This chapter describes the characteristics and diagnostic findings for KD and CALs in these guidelines and complication rates in the United States and Japan.

Diagnosis

Complete KD

The diagnostic criteria for classical KD in the AHA/AAP guidelines are a fever persisting at least 5 days accompanied by at least four of five other criteria, which are largely mucocutaneous (i.e., nonexudative bilateral conjunctival injection, changes in lips and oral cavity, polymorphous eruption, changes in distal extremities, and acute nonpurulent cervical lymphadenopathy). Patients with a fever persisting at least 5 days and fewer than four principal features receive a diagnosis of KD when coronary artery disease is detected by 2-D echocardiography or coronary angiography. In the presence of the principal criteria, a KD diagnosis can be made on day 4 of illness.

The Japanese criteria include fever as a sixth, equally important criterion, and patients must meet five of six criteria for diagnosis, including fever that subsides before the fifth day in response to therapy (Table 1). Other common clinical

Table 1 Diagnostic criteria for Kawasaki disease in the AHA/AAP and Japanese Ministry of Health Research Committee guidelines

AHA/AAP guidelines
Patients with fever persisting at least 5 days and <4 of the principal criteria receive a Kawasaki disease diagnosis when coronary artery abnormalities are detected by 2-D echocardiography or angiography.
1. Fever persisting at least 5 days*
Presence of at least four principal features:
2. Change in extremities
Acute: Erythema of palms, soles; edema of hands, feet
Subacute: Periungual peeling of fingers, toes in weeks 2 and 3
3. Polymorphous exanthema
4. Bilateral bulbar conjunctiva injection without exudate
5. Changes in lips and oral cavity: erythema, lips cracking, strawberry tongue, diffuse injection of oral and pharyngeal mucosae
6. Cervical lymphadenopathy (>1.5 cm diameter), usually unilateral
The Japanese Ministry of Health Research Committee guidelines
At least five of items 1–6 should be satisfied for a diagnosis of Kawasaki disease. However, Kawasaki disease can be diagnosed when patients with four of the principal symptoms have coronary aneurysm or dilatation, as confirmed by 2-D echocardiography or angiography.
1. Fever persisting at least 5 days (including patients in whom fever has subsided before day 5 in response to therapy)
2. Bilateral conjunctival congestion
3. Changes in lips and oral cavity: erythema of lips, strawberry tongue, diffuse injection of oral and pharyngeal mucosa
4. Polymorphous exanthema
5. Changes in peripheral extremities
Acute phase: Erythema of palms and soles; indurative edema
Convalescent phase: Membranous desquamation from fingertips
6. Acute nonpurulent cervical lymphadenopathy

When ≥4 of the principal criteria are present, a diagnosis of Kawasaki disease can be made on day 4 of illness. Experienced clinicians who have treated many Kawasaki disease patients may establish a diagnosis before day 4
* The diagnostic criteria for classical Kawasaki disease in AHA/AAP guidelines include fever persisting at least 5 days and at least four of five other criteria. On the other hand, the criteria in the Japanese guidelines include fever as one of sixth symptoms

findings are not required for diagnosis in either the US or Japanese guidelines. KD may also be diagnosed when only four of the aforementioned symptoms are present if, during the period of illness, either 2-D echocardiography or coronary angiography shows coronary artery aneurysms (CAAs), including coronary artery dilation, and all other causes of CAAs can be excluded.

Although fever occurs in 80–90 % of patients with KD, the diagnostic criteria defined by the AHA are comparable to the Japanese diagnostic guidelines because 99 % of KD patients who receive a diagnosis based on the Japanese diagnostic guidelines also satisfy the fever criterion [5, 6].

Incomplete KD

The definitions for a diagnosis of incomplete or atypical KD are similar in the United States and Japan. The Japanese guidelines state that a KD diagnosis is possible even when five or more of the principal symptoms are absent, if other conditions can be excluded and KD is suspected, a condition known as incomplete KD. Indeed, approximately 15–20 % of KD patients have incomplete KD in Japan [7]. However, even if a patient has four or fewer principal symptoms, the illness should not be regarded as less severe, because cardiovascular abnormalities are not rare in patients with incomplete KD [8]. In Japan, redness and crusting at a bacille Calmette-Guérin (BCG) inoculation site in infants younger than 1 year is an important finding, and erythema or crusting at a BCG site is one of the other significant symptoms or findings in the Japanese guidelines. This finding is not included in the AHA/AAP guidelines because BCG vaccination is uncommon in the United States.

The AHA/AAP guidelines include an algorithm for evaluation and treatment of suspected patients with incomplete or atypical KD (Fig. 1). The algorithm indicates that incomplete KD should be diagnosed in a patient with a fever persisting at least 5 days, two or three additional clinical diagnostic criteria, and abnormal laboratory values typical of KD. The incidence rate of incomplete KD in the United States is reported to be approximately 20–27 % [9]. The AHA/AAP specifies that the term "atypical" should be used to describe patients who have a sign or symptom not typically seen in KD, such as renal impairment [3].

Complication: Coronary Artery Aneurysms

Coronary artery aneurysms develop as a sequela of vasculitis in 20–25 % of untreated children. Currently, studies report an aneurysm rate of approximately 4.0–5.0 %, while the rate in Japan is reported to be about 1.0 % for patients receiving treatment for KD [7, 10]. However, it has been difficult to compare coronary artery outcomes between the two countries because of different definitions for CALs [11].

Validation methods for CALs are very similar between countries. On echocardiography, CALs are observed during acute KD as increased echo intensity of the coronary artery wall, and coronary aneurysms or "regression" of coronary aneurysms is observed on coronary angiography within 1–2 years after onset, typically in patients with small or medium aneurysms, in both countries. However, the criteria for CALs differ between the United States and Japan.

The JCS guidelines classify coronary arteries as small aneurysms or dilatation if the internal lumen diameter is ≤4 mm in children <5 years or the internal diameter of a segment measures <1.5 times that of an adjacent segment in children ≥5 years; as medium aneurysms if the internal lumen diameter is >4 to ≤8 mm in children

Evaluation of Suspected Incomplete Kawasaki Disease (KD)[1]

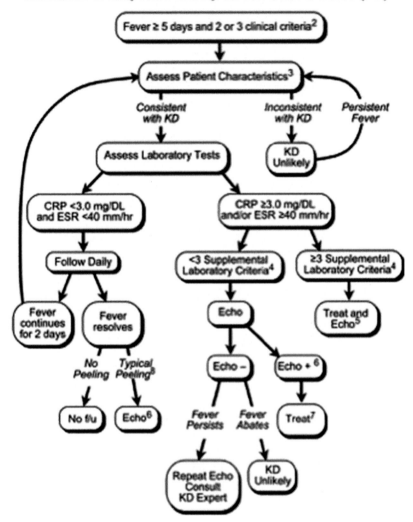

Jane W. Newburger et al. Circulation. 2004;110:2747-2771

Fig. 1 Evaluation of Suspected Incomplete Kawasaki disease. Evaluation of suspected incomplete Kawasaki disease. (1) In the absence of a gold standard for diagnosis, this algorithm cannot be evidence-based but rather represents the informed opinion of an expert committee. Consultation with an expert should be sought anytime assistance is needed. (2) Infants aged ≤6 months with fever persisting at least 7 days, in the absence of another explanation, should undergo laboratory testing. If evidence of systemic inflammation is found, echocardiography should be performed even if the patient has no other clinical symptoms. (3) Patient characteristics suggesting Kawasaki disease are listed in Table 1. Characteristics suggesting diseases other than Kawasaki disease include exudative conjunctivitis, exudative pharyngitis, discrete intraoral lesions, bullous or vesicular rash, and generalized adenopathy. Consider alternative diagnoses (see Table 2). (4) Supplemental laboratory criteria include albumin ≤3.0 g/dL, anemia for age, elevation of alanine aminotransferase, platelets after 7 days ≥450 000/mm³, white blood cell count ≥15 000/mm³, and

Table 2 Criteria for coronary artery abnormalities in the AHA/AAP and JCS guidelines

AHA/AAP guidelines	
Normal	Z-score, <2.5
Small aneurysms	Internal diameter, <5 mm
Medium aneurysms	Internal diameter, 5–8 mm
Giant aneurysms	Internal diameter, >8 mm
The Japanese Ministry of Health Research Committee guidelines	
Dilatation or small aneurysms	Localized dilatation ≤4 mm in internal diameter
	In children ≥5 years, internal diameter of a segment measures 1.5 times that of an adjacent segment
Medium aneurysms	Aneurysms with an internal diameter of >4 mm to ≤8 mm
	In children ≥5 years, the internal diameter of a segment measures 1.5–4 times that of an adjacent segment
Giant aneurysms	Aneurysms with an internal diameter of >8 mm
	In children ≥5 years, the internal diameter of a segment measures >4 times that of an adjacent segment
Transient coronary dilatation	Patients with transient coronary dilatation that typically subsides within 30 days after onset

<5 years or the internal diameter of a segment measures 1.5–4 times that of an adjacent segment in children ≥5 years; and as giant aneurysms if the internal lumen diameter is ≥8 mm in children <5 years or the internal diameter of a segment measures >4 times that of an adjacent segment in children ≥5 years (Table 2) [2]. In addition, slight, transient coronary dilations that typically subside within 30 days after onset are defined in the Japanese guidelines as transient coronary dilatations but are not described in the AHA/AAP guidelines. The Japanese guidelines recommend echocardiographic assessment for persistent aneurysms during early KD, about 30 days after onset [2].

In the AHA/APP guidelines, aneurysms are classified as small (internal diameter of vessel wall <5 mm), medium (diameter from 5–8 mm), and giant (diameter >8 mm). Although the criteria for CALs in the JCS guidelines are not based on patient body size, the US guidelines use z-scores to classify CALs because coronary artery dimensions in children without KD were shown to increase with indices of body size, such as body surface area or body length (Table 2) [3]. In the AHA/AAP

Fig. 1 (continued) urine with ≥10 white blood cells/high-power field. (5) Patients can receive treatment before echocardiography. (6) An echocardiogram is considered positive for purposes of this algorithm if any of three conditions are met: if the z-score for the LAD or RCA is ≥2.5, if coronary arteries satisfy Japanese Ministry of Health criteria for aneurysms, or if ≥3 other suggestive features exist, including perivascular brightness, lack of tapering, decreased LV function, mitral regurgitation, pericardial effusion, or LAD or RCA z scores of 2–2.5. (7) If the echocardiogram is positive, treatment should be given to children within 10 days of fever onset and to those with clinical and laboratory signs (CRP, ESR) of ongoing inflammation later than 10 days after fever onset. (8) Typical peeling begins under the nail beds, first in the fingers and then in the toes (Newburger et al. [3])

guidelines, normal coronary arteries have a z-score of <2.5. New z-score formulas for CAL evaluation have been developed (12–14). A clear advantage of using z-scores for evaluating coronary artery dimensions in pediatric populations is normalization for body surface area and the use of specific criteria for right and left coronary arteries [11]. Infants (age <1 year), older children (age 9–17 years), males, Asians, Pacific Islanders, and Hispanics have a higher risk of developing CAAs [15]. Specifically, the rate for Asians and Pacific Islanders in the United States was higher than that for whites but similar to those reported in Japan, Korea, and China [6, 11].

Use of immunoglobulin therapy as standard therapy for KD has dramatically reduced the rate of CAAs in both countries. Thus, delayed diagnosis and treatment might increase the rate of CAAs. Up to 20 % of KD patients do not respond to immunoglobulin therapy [10]. These patients are at a higher risk of developing cardiac complications and should be promptly retreated with additional therapies to reduce the occurrence of cardiac complications.

Previously reported differences in CAA rates in the United States and Japan likely resulted from the use of different definitions and nomenclature. Establishment of standard criteria for CAAs in both countries would allow for meaningful comparisons between the countries and would facilitate collaborative international clinical trials.

References

1. Ayusawa M, Sonobe T, Uemura S, Ogawa S, Nakamura Y, Kiyosawa N, et al. Revision of diagnostic guidelines for Kawasaki disease (the 5th revised edition). Pediatr Int. 2005;47(2):232–4.
2. Japanese Circulation Society Joint Research Group. Guidelines for diagnosis and management of cardiovascular sequelae in Kawasaki disease. Pediatr Int. 2005;47(6):711–32. http://dx.doi.org/10.1111/j.1442-200x.2005.02149.x PMID:16354233.
3. Newburger JW, Takahashi M, Gerber MA, Gewitz MH, Tani LY, Burns JC, et al. Committee on rheumatic fever, endocarditis and Kawasaki disease; Council on Cardiovascular Disease in the Young; American Heart Association; American Academy of Pediatrics. Diagnosis, treatment, and long-term management of Kawasaki disease: a statement for health professionals from the Committee on Rheumatic Fever, Endocarditis and Kawasaki Disease, Council on Cardiovascular Disease in the Young, American Heart Association. Circulation. 2004;110(17):2747–71. http://dx.doi.org/10.1161/01.CIR.0000145143.19711.78 PMID:15505111.
4. Newburger JW, Takahashi M, Gerber MA, Gewitz MH, Tani LY, Burns JC, et al. Committee on Rheumatic Fever, Endocarditis, and Kawasaki Disease, Council on Cardiovascular Disease in the Young, American Heart Association. Diagnosis, treatment, and long-term management of Kawasaki disease: a statement for health professionals from the Committee on Rheumatic Fever, Endocarditis, and Kawasaki Disease, Council on Cardiovascular Disease in the Young, American Heart Association. Pediatrics. 2004;114(6):1708–33. http://dx.doi.org/10.1542/peds.2004-2182 PMID:15574639.
5. Bayers S, Shulman ST, Paller AS. Kawasaki disease: Part I. Diagnosis, clinical features, and pathogenesis. J Am Acad Dermatol. 2013;69(4):501 e1–11; quiz 11–2.
6. Uehara R, Belay ED. Epidemiology of Kawasaki disease in Asia, Europe, and the United States. J Epidemiol. 2012;22(2):79–85.

7. Makino N, Nakamura Y, Yashiro M, Ae R, Tsuboi S, Aoyama Y, et al. Descriptive epidemiology of Kawasaki disease in Japan, 2011–2012: from the results of the 22nd nationwide
   survey. J Epidemiol. 2015;25(3):239–45.
8. Sonobe T, Kiyosawa N, Tsuchiya K, Aso S, Imada Y, Imai Y, et al. Prevalence of coronary
   artery abnormality in incomplete Kawasaki disease. Pediatr Int. 2007;49(4):421–6. http://dx.
   doi.org/10.1111/j.1442-200X.2007.02396.x.
9. Yellen ES, Gauvreau K, Takahashi M, Burns JC, Shulman S, Baker AL, et al. Performance of
   2004 American Heart Association recommendations for treatment of Kawasaki disease.
   Pediatrics. 2010;125(2):e234–41. http://dx.doi.org/10.1542/peds.2009-0606 PMID:20100771.
10. Tremoulet AH, Best BM, Song S, Wang S, Corinaldesi E, Eichenfield JR, et al. Resistance to
    intravenous immunoglobulin in children with Kawasaki disease. J Pediatr. 2008;153
    (1):117–21. http://dx.doi.org/10.1016/j.jpeds.2007.12.021 PMID:18571548.
11. Ogata S, Tremoulet AH, Sato Y, Ueda K, Shimizu C, Sun X, et al. Coronary artery outcomes
    among children with Kawasaki disease in the United States and Japan. Int J Cardiol. 2013;168
    (4):3825–8. http://dx.doi.org/10.1016/j.ijcard.2013.06.027 PMID:23849968.
12. Dallaire F, Dahdah N. New equations and a critical appraisal of coronary artery Z scores in
    healthy children. J Am Soc Echocardiogr. 2011;24(1):60–74. http://dx.doi.org/10.1016/j.echo.
    2010.10.004 PMID:21074965.
13. Manlhiot C, Millar K, Golding F, McCrindle BW. Improved classification of coronary artery
    abnormalities based only on coronary artery z-scores after Kawasaki disease. Pediatr Cardiol.
    2010;31(2):242–9. http://dx.doi.org/10.1007/s00246-009-9599-7 PMID:20024653.
14. de Zorzi A, Colan SD, Gauvreau K, Baker AL, Sundel RP, Newburger JW. Coronary artery
    dimensions may be misclassified as normal in Kawasaki disease. J Pediatr. 1998;133(2):254–8.
    http://dx.doi.org/10.1016/S0022-3476(98)70229-X PMID:9709715.
15. Belay ED, Maddox RA, Holman RC, Curns AT, Ballah K, Schonberger LB. Kawasaki
    syndrome and risk factors for coronary artery abnormalities: United States, 1994–2003. Pediatr
    Infect Dis J. 2006;25(3):245–9. http://dx.doi.org/10.1097/01.inf.0000202068.30956.16
    PMID:16511388.

Mechanism of Action of Immunoglobulin: Sialylated IgG

Toshiyuki Takai

Abstract Glycosylation of IgG, including sialylation of the Fc region, influences binding of IgG to receptors. In addition to the classical Fc receptor members, we now know of several sugar-binding lectins that recognize sialylated oligosaccharides of IgG. These lectins, particularly human dendritic cell-specific intercellular adhesion molecule-3-grabbing non-integrin (DC-SIGN), may regulate immune reactions and are thus candidate molecules in the initiation of the sequence of IVIG-mediated anti-inflammatory events. This chapter reviews the emerging role of sialylated IgG Fc in the IVIG-mediated therapeutic effect, in particular the importance of DC-SIGN-initiated events.

Keywords DC-SIGN • Lectin • Fc receptor • Dendritic cell • Oligosaccharide

Introduction

The mechanisms underlying the action of IVIG involve blocking or neutralizing the effects of IgG Fc receptors (FcγRs), complements, pathogenic antibodies, superantigens, and cytokines. The effects of receptors and complements are attributed to the Fc region of IgG, and the effects of pathogenic antibodies, superantigens, and cytokines are ascribed to the Fab region and induction of regulatory cells including regulatory T (Treg) cells. The pluripotential nature of IgG and related molecules with which IgG molecules interact (Fig. 1) suggests the presence of multiple mechanisms by which IVIG alleviates disease. A recent series of studies by Ravetch and colleagues showed that IVIG mechanisms involve recognition of sialylated IgG Fc by a carbohydrate receptor on sensor macrophages and dendritic cells (DCs), namely DC-specific intercellular adhesion molecule-3-grabbing non-integrin (DC-SIGN or CD209), which indirectly leads to upregulation of a unique inhibitory FcγR, FcγRIIB, on effector macrophages [1].

T. Takai (✉)
Department of Experimental Immunology, Institute of Development, Aging and Cancer,
Tohoku University, Seiryo-machi 4-1, Aoba-ku, Sendai 980-8575, Japan
e-mail: toshiyuki.takai.b8@tohoku.ac.jp

© Springer Japan 2017 223
B.T. Saji et al. (eds.), *Kawasaki Disease*, DOI 10.1007/978-4-431-56039-5_25

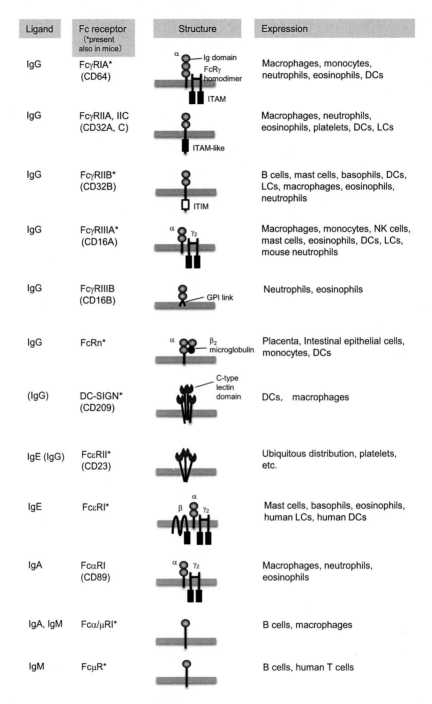

Ligand	Fc receptor (*present also in mice)	Structure	Expression
IgG	FcγRIA* (CD64)		Macrophages, monocytes, neutrophils, eosinophils, DCs
IgG	FcγRIIA, IIC (CD32A, C)		Macrophages, neutrophils, eosinophils, platelets, DCs, LCs
IgG	FcγRIIB* (CD32B)		B cells, mast cells, basophils, DCs, LCs, macrophages, eosinophils, neutrophils
IgG	FcγRIIIA* (CD16A)		Macrophages, monocytes, NK cells, mast cells, eosinophils, DCs, LCs, mouse neutrophils
IgG	FcγRIIIB (CD16B)		Neutrophils, eosinophils
IgG	FcRn*		Placenta, Intestinal epithelial cells, monocytes, DCs
(IgG)	DC-SIGN* (CD209)		DCs, macrophages
IgE (IgG)	FcεRII* (CD23)		Ubiquitous distribution, platelets, etc.
IgE	FcεRI*		Mast cells, basophils, eosinophils, human LCs, human DCs
IgA	FcαRI (CD89)		Macrophages, neutrophils, eosinophils
IgA, IgM	Fcα/µRI*		B cells, macrophages
IgM	FcµR*		B cells, human T cells

Fig. 1 Schematic view of Ig Fc-binding receptors

The schematic structures of human IgG Fc receptor proteins are shown with ligands and expression profiles. The structures of IgE-, IgA-, and IgM-binding Fc receptors are also shown. In the classical IgG Fc receptors FcγRI, RII, and RIII (and RIV in mice), FcγRI is a high-affinity receptor that

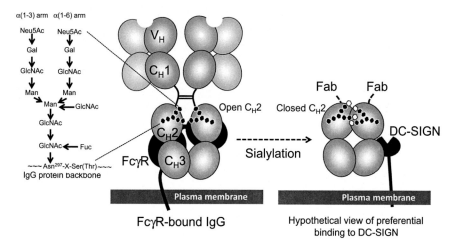

FcγR-bound IgG   Hypothetical view of preferential
                                  binding to DC-SIGN

Fig. 2 Binding of glycosylated IgG to a canonical Fcγ receptor
A schematic view of an IgG molecule bound to a classical FcγR. Note that low-affinity FcγR receptors bind IgG molecules as multivalent immune complexes (not shown in figure). The N-linked oligosaccharides (*black hexagons*) are located in the Fc portions, as biantennary chains bound to Asn297 of C_H2 domains (for composition of the residues, *left*) [2], and in variable regions of the L and H chains (not shown), depending on the N-glycosylation consensus sequence, Asn–X–Ser/Thr. It has been proposed that sialylation (*white hexagons*) at the termini of oligosaccharides induces conformational change of the Fc C_H2-C_H3 domains, from "open" to "closed", and reduces IgG binding to the Fc receptor [3], although this has not been verified by X-ray crystallography [4]. Man, mannose; GlcNAc, N-acetylglucosamine; Gal, galactose; Fuc, fucose; Neu5Ac, N-acetylneuraminic acid (sialic acid)

Glycosylated IgG

N-linked oligosaccharides of human serum IgG are present in the Fc portion (Fig. 2) and sometimes in the V_H and V_L regions, depending on the consensus sequence, Asn–X–Ser/Thr. Sialyl residues may be located at the termini of biantennary carbohydrate chains. Studies of the relation of IgG glycosylation to physiology and pathology began over 50 years ago [5]. An analysis of the composition of carbohydrate residues in glycosylated IgG [6] suggested the presence of one sialic acid residue per IgG molecule on average. It was also shown that the carbohydrates

<hr/>

Fig. 1 (continued) binds monomeric IgG. FcγRII and RIII (and RIV) show low affinities to IgG, so they bind IgG as immune complexes. FcγRI and RIIIA associate with a homodimeric Fc receptor common γ chain harboring an immunoreceptor tyrosine-based activation motif (ITAM), and FcγRIIA harbors an endogenous ITAM-like motif. Upon ligand binding, these receptors deliver activating signaling within cells. FcγRIIB has an immunoreceptor tyrosine-based inhibitory motif (ITIM) and delivers inhibitory signals upon ligand binding. DC-SIGN (CD209) and FcγRII (CD23) are C-type lectin family members and are proposed sialyl Fc IgG receptors. LCs, Langerhans cells

of IgG Fc determine the half-life of IgG in plasma and its deposition in tissues [7]. The serum level of IgG with no terminal galactose residues is associated with the rheumatoid arthritis (RA) pathology, eg, in the production of IgG rheumatoid factor (RF) [8]. This suggests that *N*-glycosylation of Fc may be linked to immune response and disease states in general. Fucose residues in oligosaccharides of IgG may also modulate immune responses, because fucosylation of IgG reduces binding to FcγRs, and a fucose-less anti-CD20 monoclonal antibody, rituximab, exhibits more active antibody-dependent cell-mediated cytotoxicity toward Raji human B cells of human NK cells *in vitro* [9].

Sialylation of IgG Fc

Findings from earlier studies suggest that terminal sialylation of Fc is important in IgG turnover [5, 6]. In addition, the sialic acid content of RF isolated from an RA patient was lower than that of normal IgG [7], suggesting that sialylation is related to disease. However, the potential significance of sialyl IgG in health and disease was not well recognized until recent studies by Ravetch and colleagues, which highlighted sialyl IgG Fc and its relation to immune regulation. Their research suggests that FcγRIIB has a role in feedback regulation of B cells and in inflammatory responses by effector cells, a notion already widely accepted. Several lines of evidence indicate that the therapeutic activity of IVIG is mediated through its Fc portion and FcγRIIB in mouse models of immune thrombocytic purpura (ITP), RA, and nephrotoxic nephritis [10], and it was associated with upregulated expression of FcγRIIB on splenic macrophages in an ITP model.

Kaneko et al. [11] demonstrated the significance of sialyl Fc in the anti-inflammatory action of IVIG. Measurement of the affinities of the sialyl and non-sialyl forms of IgG to FcγRs indicated that sialylation reduces binding affinities by five- to ten-fold. In addition, sialyl Fc, but not non-sialyl IVIG, mediated anti-inflammatory activity in an arthritis model, suggesting that the sialic acids of Fc are responsible for the effect. They also found that the sialic acid content of IgG was reduced upon induction of an antigen-specific immune response, which suggests that differential sialylation constitutes a switch from steady-state anti-inflammatory activity to pro-inflammatory effects upon antigenic challenge (Fig. 3).

Anthony et al. [12] developed a fully recombinant sialyl IgG1 Fc fragment with greatly enhanced potency, as compared with IVIG, in arthritis and ITP models. A specific receptor for sialyl Fc was believed to be involved in this pathway. This receptor was later identified as a C-type lectin, SIGNR1 (specific ICAM-3-grabbing non-integrin-related 1), which is expressed in the splenic marginal zone in mice [13]. Genetic deletion of SIGNR1 in mice abrogated the anti-inflammatory activity of IVIG and sialylated Fc. The study authors also suggested that human DC-SIGN, a homolog of murine SIGNR1, could be a receptor for sialyl Fc and a mediator of anti-inflammation because of the similarity to SIGNR1 in its binding to sialyl Fc *in vitro*.

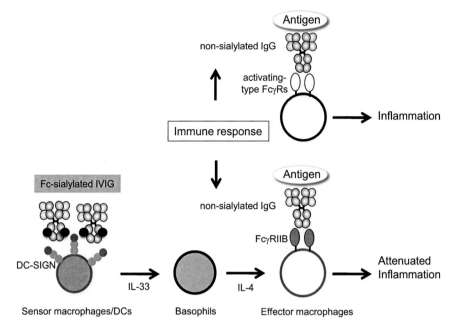

Fig. 3 Proposed mechanism of sialylated IgG Fc–DC-SIGN–FcγRIIB-mediated anti-inflammation
On the basis of data from animal models, a model for DC-SIGN-mediated anti-inflammation has been proposed in which sialylated Fc binds to DC-SIGN on sensor macrophages and DCs, thereby inducing production of IL-33, which then induces basophils to produce IL-4. These basophils then promote increased expression of FcγRIIB on effector macrophages [1]

General Characteristics of DC-SIGN

DC-SIGN is preferentially expressed on human peripheral and lymph node DCs and some macrophages [14] (Fig. 1) and was initially characterized as a receptor for the HIV envelope glycoprotein gp120. *In vitro* analyses of DC-SIGN have revealed that this receptor recognizes a broad range of pathogen-derived ligands and self-glycoproteins as a pattern recognition receptor and is capable of mediating different aspects of DC biology, including intercellular communication, migration, pathogen recognition, signaling, and antigen presentation [14]. However, the *in vivo* function of DC-SIGN is difficult to ascertain, in part because there are multiple genetic homologs (SIGNR1–8) in mice with no clear DC-SIGN ortholog. While human DC-SIGN is expressed on DCs and some macrophages, mouse SIGNR1 is expressed exclusively on marginal zone macrophages, not on DCs. SIGNR1 and SIGNR3 knockout and human DC-SIGN transgenic mouse models have failed to reproduce the predicted *in vitro* physiological functions of DC-SIGN. Thus, available mouse models may be limited in their capacity to reveal the physiological role of DC-SIGN in *in vivo* models [14].

The Potential DC-SIGN-Mediated IVIG Mechanism

Anthony et al. [1] proposed a cascade by which sialylated IVIG Fc and DC-SIGN induce anti-inflammatory activity in an arthritis model expressing human DC-SIGN as a transgene. They found that IVIG action was attained by transfer of macrophages or DCs treated with sialylated Fc into naïve recipient mice. Sialylated Fc administration to mice induced a T helper (Th)2 cytokine, IL-33, which then induced basophils to produce another Th2 cytokine, IL-4. These basophils ultimately increased expression of FcγRIIB on inflammatory effector macrophages (Fig. 3). To better understand the structural basis of sialylated Fc binding to DC-SIGN, Sondermann et al. [3] used circular dichroism spectrometry to examine alterations in Fc structure and found that sialylation induced significant structural alterations, from an "open" to "closed" state in the C_H2 domain of Fc (Fig. 2). CD23, a low-affinity receptor for IgE (Fig. 1), bound IgG upon Fc sialylation in a cell-based binding assay. On the basis of these results, they hypothesized that Fc domains undergo a shift between an "open" activating conformation and a "closed" anti-inflammatory state, thereby regulating Fc binding to FcγRs or DC-SIGN, which could be a general immunoregulatory mechanism for maintaining homeostasis. Crispin et al. [4] tested this hypothesis by means of X-ray crystallography but observed no conformational changes upon sialylation of Fc, whose structure was strikingly similar to that of a previously reported IgG-bearing nonsialylated Fc. Thus, the mechanism by which sialyl IgG Fc mediates anti-inflammatory activity remains unclear.

Massoud et al. [15] observed that DC immunoreceptor, or DCIR, which is also a C-type lectin on DCs, mediates the effect of sialylated IVIG. In this case, the anti-inflammatory effect was associated with induction of Treg cells in an airway hyperresponsiveness model. This suggests that sialyl IgG can also be bound by DCIR, which induces inhibitory signaling and makes the DC tolerogenic. This mechanism differs from that of the DC-SIGN–FcγRIIB. Käsermann et al. [16] found that the action of IVIG on human monocytes *in vitro* depends on sialylated Fab rather than on the Fc portion. Additionally, a mechanism in human DCs for IVIG-mediated reciprocal regulation of Th17 and Th1 cells, and Treg cell induction is Fab-dependent [17], and DC-SIGN on DCs directly interacts with Fab of IVIG, thus inducing expansion of Treg cells [18].

Taken together, these observations caution against oversimplification of the IVIG action of DC-SIGN and sialyl Fc and against overestimation of the sialyl Fc–DC-SIGN–FcγRIIB axis in different mouse disease models and its extrapolation to IVIG therapy in humans [19]. The mechanisms of action of IVIG involve a wide spectrum of Fab-mediated and, probably, distinct Fc-mediated mechanisms, which may or may not depend on IVIG sialylation. For example, upregulation of FcγRIIB expression by IVIG could not be confirmed by gene expression profiling, even in Kawasaki disease [20]. von Gunten et al. [19] stressed that many of the disease-specific mechanisms of IVIG observed in mouse models must be validated in humans, as animal models offer only limited insight into human disease and might be biased due to the xenogeneic or species-specific properties of IVIG.

Conclusion

DC-SIGN expressed on macrophages and DCs may be responsible for initiating IVIG Fc-mediated anti-inflammatory events leading to upregulation of FcγRIIB on effector macrophages. Because IVIG is a pluripotent drug, its mode of action allows for multiple scenarios, potentially including the sialyl Fc–DC-SIGN–FcγRIIB cascade.

Acknowledgements The author thanks Nicholas Halewood for editorial assistance. This work is supported in part by a Grant-in-Aid from the Ministry of Education, Culture, Sports, Science and Technology of Japan (to TT).

References

1. Anthony RM, Kobayashi T, Wermeling F, Ravetch JV. Intravenous gammaglobulin suppresses inflammation through a novel T_H2 pathway. Nature. 2011;475(7354):110–3. http://dx.doi.org/10.1038/nature10134 PMID:21685887.
2. Dwek RA, Lellouch AC, Wormald MR. Glycobiology: 'the function of sugar in the IgG molecule'. J Anat. 1995;187(Pt 2):279–92. PMID:7591992.
3. Sondermann P, Pincetic A, Maamary J, Lammens K, Ravetch JV. General mechanism for modulating immunoglobulin effector function. Proc Natl Acad Sci U S A. 2013;110 (24):9868–72. http://dx.doi.org/10.1073/pnas.1307864110 PMID:23697368.
4. Crispin M, Yu X, Bowden TA. Crystal structure of sialylated IgG Fc: implications for the mechanism of intravenous immunoglobulin therapy. Proc Natl Acad Sci U S A. 2013;110(38): E3544–6. http://dx.doi.org/10.1073/pnas.1310657110 PMID:23929778.
5. Rosevear JW, Smith EL. Glycopeptides. I. Isolation and properties of glycopeptides from a fraction of human gamma-globulin. J Biol Chem. 1961;236:425–35. PMID:13743526.
6. Clamp JR, Putnam FW. The carbohydrate prosthetic group of human γ-globulin. J Biol Chem. 1964;239:3233–40. PMID:14245367.
7. Dodon MD, Quash GA. The antigenicity of asialylated IgG: its relationship to rheumatoid factor. Immunology. 1981;42(3):401–8. PMID:6162783.
8. Parekh RB, Roitt IM, Isenberg DA, Dwek RA, Ansell BM, Rademacher TW. Galactosylation of IgG associated oligosaccharides: reduction in patients with adult and juvenile onset rheumatoid arthritis and relation to disease activity. Lancet. 1988;1(8592):966–9. http://dx.doi.org/10.1016/S0140-6736(88)91781-3 PMID:2896829.
9. Shinkawa T, Nakamura K, Yamane N, Shoji-Hosaka E, Kanda Y, Sakurada M, et al. The absence of fucose but not the presence of galactose or bisecting N-acetylglucosamine of human IgG1 complex-type oligosaccharides shows the critical role of enhancing antibody-dependent cellular cytotoxicity. J Biol Chem. 2003;278(5):3466–73. http://dx.doi.org/10.1074/jbc.M210665200 PMID:12427744.
10. Samuelsson A, Towers TL, Ravetch JV. Anti-inflammatory activity of IVIG mediated through the inhibitory Fc receptor. Science. 2001;291(5503):484–6. http://dx.doi.org/10.1126/science.291.5503.484 PMID:11161202.
11. Kaneko Y, Nimmerjahn F, Ravetch JV. Anti-inflammatory activity of immunoglobulin G resulting from Fc sialylation. Science. 2006;313(5787):670–3. http://dx.doi.org/10.1126/science.1129594 PMID:16888140.

12. Anthony RM, Nimmerjahn F, Ashline DJ, Reinhold VN, Paulson JC, Ravetch JV. Recapitulation of IVIG anti-inflammatory activity with a recombinant IgG Fc. Science. 2008;320(5874):373–6. http://dx.doi.org/10.1126/science.1154315 PMID:18420934.
13. Anthony RM, Wermeling F, Karlsson MC, Ravetch JV. Identification of a receptor required for the anti-inflammatory activity of IVIG. Proc Natl Acad Sci U S A. 2008;105(50):19571–8. http://dx.doi.org/10.1073/pnas.0810163105 PMID:19036920.
14. Garcia-Vallejo JJ, van Kooyk Y. The physiological role of DC-SIGN: a tale of mice and men. Trends Immunol. 2013;34(10):482–6. http://dx.doi.org/10.1016/j.it.2013.03.001 PMID:23608151.
15. Massoud AH, Yona M, Xue D, Chouiali F, Alturaihi H, Ablona A, et al. Dendritic cell immunoreceptor: a novel receptor for intravenous immunoglobulin mediates induction of regulatory T cells. J Allergy Clin Immunol. 2014;133(3):853–63.e5. http://dx.doi.org/10.1016/j.jaci.2013.09.029 PMID:24210883.
16. Käsermann F, Boerema DJ, Rüegsegger M, Hofmann A, Wymann S, Zuercher AW, et al. Analysis and functional consequences of increased Fab-sialylation of intravenous immunoglobulin (IVIG) after lectin fractionation. PLoS ONE. 2012;7(6):e37243. http://dx.doi.org/10.1371/journal.pone.0037243 PMID:22675478.
17. Maddur MS, Sharma M, Hegde P, Lacroix-Desmazes S, Kaveri SV, Bayry J. Inhibitory effect of IVIG on IL-17 production by Th17 cells is independent of anti-IL-17 antibodies in the immunoglobulin preparations. J Clin Immunol. 2013;33(S1 Suppl 1):S62–6. http://dx.doi.org/10.1007/s10875-012-9752-6 PMID:22864643.
18. Trinath J, Hegde P, Sharma M, Maddur MS, Rabin M, Vallat JM, et al. Intravenous immunoglobulin expands regulatory T cells via induction of cyclooxygenase-2-dependent prostaglandin E2 in human dendritic cells. Blood. 2013;122(8):1419–27. http://dx.doi.org/10.1182/blood-2012-11-468264 PMID:23847198.
19. von Gunten S, Shoenfeld Y, Blank M, Branch DR, Vassilev T, Käsermann F, et al. IVIG pluripotency and the concept of Fc-sialylation: challenges to the scientist. Nat Rev Immunol. 2014;14(5):349. http://dx.doi.org/10.1038/nri3401-c1 PMID:24762829.
20. Abe J, Jibiki T, Noma S, Nakajima T, Saito H, Terai M. Gene expression profiling of the effect of high-dose intravenous Ig in patients with Kawasaki disease. J Immunol. 2005;174(9):5837–45. http://dx.doi.org/10.4049/jimmunol.174.9.5837 PMID:15843588.

Treatment Options for Refractory Kawasaki Disease: Alternative Treatments for Infliximab Nonresponders

Shinichi Takatsuki, Kazuyoshi Saito, Fukiko Ichida, and Tsutomu Saji

Abstract In a recent study, infliximab (IFX) therapy resulted in dramatic improvement in 85–90 % of children with Kawasaki disease who did not respond to repeated intravenous immunoglobulin (IVIG) infusion or steroid therapy as second-line treatment. Although studies have confirmed the clinical efficacy and safety of IFX therapy in children with refractory Kawasaki disease, there is no consensus regarding treatment of IFX nonresponse, which is defined as the presence of persistent fever (>37 °C) despite optimal treatment. In a treatment algorithm from two Japanese institutions, IFX was given to children who did not respond to second IVIG or methylprednisolone pulse (IMP) therapy. Overall, 10–26 % were IFX nonresponders, and treatments for this group included IVIG, methylprednisolone pulse, and cyclosporin A. Persistent fever resolved in IFX nonresponders after these additional treatments, although some patients developed coronary artery abnormalities. There has been no evidence-based study of optimal treatment for IFX nonresponders. If fever or elevation of C-reactive protein does not resolve after IFX therapy, therapies other than IFX, such as re-IVIG, re-IMP, and other immunosuppressive agents, should be started.

Keywords Infliximab • Intravenous immunoglobulin • Refractory Kawasaki disease • Methylprednisolone pulse

Introduction

Approximately 20 % of children with Kawasaki disease (KD) have persistent or recurrent fever at or later than 36 h after initial intravenous immunoglobulin (IVIG) administration [1]. Nonresponders to initial IVIG have a higher risk of developing coronary artery abnormalities (CAAs). A second dose of IVIG and steroid pulse therapy are used as second-line treatment strategies. However, a small subset of patients will remain febrile after such therapies. There are no guidelines for

S. Takatsuki, M.D. (✉) • K. Saito, M.D. • F. Ichida, M.D. • T. Saji, M.D.
Department of Pediatrics, Toho University Omori Medical Center, 6-11-1 Omori-nishi Ota-ku, Tokyo 143-8541, Japan
e-mail: s-taka@med.toho-u.ac.jp

© Springer Japan 2017   231
B.T. Saji et al. (eds.), *Kawasaki Disease*, DOI 10.1007/978-4-431-56039-5_26

management of these children, who have persistent inflammation and are at high risk for CAAs. Reported third-line therapies for refractory KD include infliximab (IFX).

IFX is a humanized mouse monoclonal antibody that binds to tumor necrosis factor-α (TNF-α), a pro-inflammatory cytokine that has an important role in rheumatoid arthritis and other vasculitis syndromes. TNF-α levels are elevated in patients with acute KD [2], and the highest serum levels were observed in patients with CAAs [3]. Clinical studies have investigated the effectiveness of IFX therapy for IVIG-resistant KD. Although several found that IFX had potential benefits for this population [4–6], a recent study reported that the incidence of IFX nonresponse was 11.2 % [4]. Unfortunately, there have been no large studies of treatment strategies for this population. This chapter describes recent findings from patients with rheumatic disease and KD that did not respond to treatment with IFX.

IFX Nonresponders

IFX Therapy in KD

In a recent study of IFX therapy for children with KD who did not respond to repeated IVIG infusion or steroid therapy, IFX resulted in dramatic improvements in 85–90 % of children, without treatment-related serious adverse events. In Japan, IFX therapy has been used since 2006 for cases of refractory KD. As was noted in previous US reports, Japanese patients with KD markedly improved, with no IFX-related adverse events [7–10]. These findings suggest that IFX therapy reduces the risk of subsequent CAAs in patients who have an unsatisfactory therapeutic response to conventional treatments. Numerous studies have confirmed the clinical efficacy and safety profile of IFX therapy in children with refractory KD. However, no treatment strategies for IFX nonresponders are available.

IFX Nonresponse in Inflammatory Disease

In pediatric populations, IFX has been approved for treatment of immune-modulated inflammatory disorders such as Crohn's disease. Although data on IFX therapy in KD are limited, previous studies have investigated pediatric IFX non-responders with inflammatory bowel disease. In studies of children with Crohn's disease, clinical improvement was observed in children treated with 5 mg/kg IFX. Additionally, disease activity frequently relapsed after discontinuation of IFX treatment. A previous study found that 29 % of children with Crohn's disease were unresponsive to IFX, whereas 29 % had a prolonged response after discontinuation of IFX and 42 % were dependent on IFX therapy [11]. Similarly, several studies investigated clinical response to IFX therapy in children with ulcerative colitis. Clinical improvement was not seen in approximately 25–35 % of these patients [12, 13].

Definition and Incidence of IFX Nonresponse in KD

IFX nonresponse is defined as persistence of fever (>37 °C) despite optimal treatment for refractory KD, ie, IVIG or steroid. In a nonrandomized, open-label, single-center trial of 76 Japanese children unresponsive to additional IVIG therapy [5], 70 responded to IFX therapy. The remaining six children (8 %), who were nonresponsive to IFX, were treated with plasma exchange. However, 12 of the 76 patients (16 %) developed coronary artery dilatation and three had CAAs, whereas five had coronary dilatation and one had a CAA before IFX administration. All CAAs resolved during follow-up.

A phase III, randomized, double-blind, placebo-controlled trial of the clinical effect of IFX plus IVIG treatment on adverse outcomes in patients with refractory KD [4] showed no significant difference in the rate of treatment resistance (11.2 % for IFX vs 11.3 % for placebo) or CAA incidence between the two groups at 5 weeks, although the IFX group had faster resolution of fever and fewer days of hospitalization as compared with the placebo group. None of the patients who received IFX therapy developed serious adverse events. Children resistant to IFX received a second infusion of IVIG, but responsiveness was not described. The authors concluded that addition of IFX to IVIG as a first-line therapy did not reduce treatment resistance.

Treatment of IFX Nonresponders

In a treatment algorithm from two Japanese institutions, IFX was given to nonresponders to second IVIG or methylprednisolone pulse (IMP) therapy (Fig. 1). Overall, 26 % of children were IFX nonresponders, and treatments for this group included IVIG (1 or 2 g/kg), IMP (15–30 mg/kg), and cyclosporin A (5 mg/kg/day, po). After these additional treatments, clinical improvements were noted in all nonresponders. There has been no evidence-based study of optimal treatment for children with KD who do not respond to IFX. Table 1 shows our proposed treatment for this population. Treatment options are based on those commonly used for other inflammatory diseases such as rheumatoid arthritis and Crohn's disease. In a study of the rate and reasons for discontinuation of IFX therapy in adults with active rheumatoid arthritis during a 10-year follow-up period [14], 34 of 144 patients (24 %) discontinued IFX therapy because of loss of effectiveness. Methotrexate and tacrolimus resulted in satisfactory clinical improvement in the treatment of rheumatoid arthritis in IFX nonresponders [15].

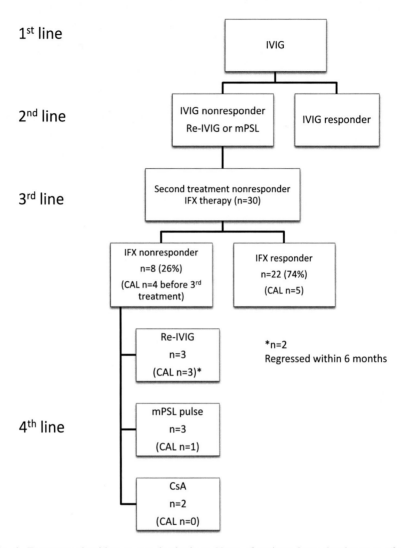

Fig. 1 Treatment algorithm at two institutions. None of patients have development of new coronary artery abnormalities after IFX therapies. The 32nd annual meeting of the Japanese Society of Kawasaki Disease (unpublished data). *CsA* cyclosporin A, *IFX* infliximab, *IVIG* intravenous immunoglobulin, *mPSL* methylprednisolone

Table 1 Proposed treatment plan for infliximab nonresponders	
	1. Re-IVIG treatment
	2. Steroid: prednisolone or methylprednisolone pulse
	3. Immunosuppressive agents
	(a) Other anti–TNF-α agent: etanercept, adalimumab
	(b) Cyclosporin A
	4. Plasma exchange

Transition to other TNF-α agents, such as etanercept and adalimumab, may also be effective for IFX nonresponders. Like IFX, etanercept is a TNF-α inhibitor and has been used as additional therapy for patients with refractory KD. Etanercept is approved by the US Food and Drug Administration for children older than 2 years with juvenile idiopathic arthritis. In an experimental study, etanercept significantly reduced arteritis severity as compared with IVIG, methylprednisolone, and cyclosporin A [16]. A mouse model of KD was induced by injecting *Candida albicans* water-soluble fractions. In a study of four agents, the severity of experimental vasculitis at 2 weeks was reduced by etanercept. Although IVIG and cyclosporin A attenuated inflammation, only etanercept significantly improved vasculitis. A prospective, open-label trial evaluated the clinical efficacy and safety profile in children with KD treated with etanercept [17]. The children, aged 6 months to 5 years, were all IVIG-resistant. Three doses of etanercept (0.8 mg/kg/dose) were given subcutaneously within 2 weeks after IVIG and resulted in resolution of prolonged fever, without serious adverse events. No CAAs developed after etanercept infusion. These findings suggest that etanercept is a satisfactory alternative immunosuppressive treatment for IVIG-resistant KD, although there are no data on etanercept treatment for KD patients who did not respond to IFX.

Adalimumab is another anti–TNF-α agent and has been approved for adults with rheumatoid disease. It improved inflammatory markers in patients who did not respond to IFX or etanercept, without serious adverse events [18].

Although transition to other immunosuppressive treatment is effective for IFX nonresponders, uptitration of IFX is another method for treating unresolved clinical symptoms. In a randomized, double-blind study of the efficacy and safety of 10 mg/kg and 3 mg/kg infliximab treatment for methotrexate-refractory rheumatoid arthritis [19], the higher dosage was beneficial for patients who had not responded to three infusions of 3 mg/kg. Incidence of adverse events did not differ between groups.

Conclusion

IFX nonresponse is defined as persistent fever despite optimal treatment. Approximately 10–26 % of children with KD are IFX nonresponders. However, there has been no evidence-based study of optimal treatments for this population. Treatments for IFX nonresponders include IVIG, methylprednisolone pulse, and cyclosporin A.

References

1. Burns JC, Capparelli EV, Brown JA, Newburger JW, Glode MP. US/Canadian Kawasaki Syndrome Study Group. Intravenous gamma-globulin treatment and retreatment in Kawasaki

disease. Pediatr Infect Dis J. 1998;17(12):1144–8. http://dx.doi.org/10.1097/00006454-199812000-00009 PMID:9877364.

2. Oharaseki T, Yokouchi Y, Yamada H, Mamada H, Muto S, Sadamoto K, et al. The role of TNF-α in a murine model of Kawasaki disease arteritis induced with a Candida albicans cell wall polysaccharide. Mod Rheumatol. 2014;24(1):120–8. http://dx.doi.org/10.3109/14397595.2013.854061 PMID:24261768.

3. Matsubara T, Furukawa S, Yabuta K. Serum levels of tumor necrosis factor, interleukin 2 receptor, and interferon-gamma in Kawasaki disease involved coronary-artery lesions. Clin Immunol Immunopathol. 1990;56(1):29–36. http://dx.doi.org/10.1016/0090-1229(90)90166-N PMID:2113446.

4. Tremoulet AH, Jain S, Jaggi P, Jimenez-Fernandez S, Pancheri JM, Sun X, et al. Infliximab for intensification of primary therapy for Kawasaki disease: a phase 3 randomised, double-blind, placebo-controlled trial. Lancet. 2014;383(9930):1731–8. http://dx.doi.org/10.1016/S0140-6736(13)62298-9 PMID:24572997.

5. Sonoda K, Mori M, Hokosaki T, Yokota S. Infliximab plus plasma exchange rescue therapy in Kawasaki disease. J Pediatr. 2014;164(5):1128–32.e1. http://dx.doi.org/10.1016/j.jpeds.2014.01.020 PMID:24560183.

6. Son MB, Gauvreau K, Burns JC, Corinaldesi E, Tremoulet AH, Watson VE, et al. Infliximab for intravenous immunoglobulin resistance in Kawasaki disease: a retrospective study. J Pediatr. 2011;158(4):644–9.e1. http://dx.doi.org/10.1016/j.jpeds.2010.10.012 PMID:21129756.

7. Saji T, Kemmotsu Y. Infliximab for Kawasaki syndrome. J Pediatr. 2006;149(3):426. http://dx.doi.org/10.1016/j.jpeds.2005.07.039 PMID:16939768.

8. Oishi T, Fujieda M, Shiraishi T, Ono M, Inoue K, Takahashi A, et al. Infliximab treatment for refractory Kawasaki disease with coronary artery aneurysm. Circ J. 2008;72(5):850–2. http://dx.doi.org/10.1253/circj.72.850 PMID:18441471.

9. Hirono K, Kemmotsu Y, Wittkowski H, Foell D, Saito K, Ibuki K, et al. Infliximab reduces the cytokine-mediated inflammation but does not suppress cellular infiltration of the vessel wall in refractory Kawasaki disease. Pediatr Res. 2009;65(6):696–701. http://dx.doi.org/10.1203/PDR.0b013e31819ed68d PMID:19430379.

10. Mori M, Imagawa T, Hara R, Kikuchi M, Hara T, Nozawa T, et al. Efficacy and limitation of infliximab treatment for children with Kawasaki disease intractable to intravenous immuno-globulin therapy: report of an open-label case series. J Rheumatol. 2012;39(4):864–7. http://dx.doi.org/10.3899/jrheum.110877 PMID:22337241.

11. Wewer V, Riis L, Vind I, Husby S, Munkholm P, Paerregaard A. Infliximab dependency in a national cohort of children with Crohn's disease. J Pediatr Gastroenterol Nutr. 2006;42 (1):40–5. http://dx.doi.org/10.1097/01.mpg.0000189137.06151.33 PMID:16385252.

12. Mamula P, Markowitz JE, Cohen LJ, von Allmen D, Baldassano RN. Infliximab in pediatric ulcerative colitis: two-year follow-up. J Pediatr Gastroenterol Nutr. 2004;38(3):298–301. http://dx.doi.org/10.1097/00005176-200403000-00013 PMID:15076630.

13. Russell GH, Katz AJ. Infliximab is effective in acute but not chronic childhood ulcerative colitis. J Pediatr Gastroenterol Nutr. 2004;39(2):166–70. http://dx.doi.org/10.1097/00005176-200408000-00008.

14. De Keyser F, De Kock J, Leroi H, Durez P, Westhovens R, Ackerman C, et al. Infliximab EAP Study Group. Ten-year followup of infliximab therapy in rheumatoid arthritis patients with severe, longstanding refractory disease: a cohort study. J Rheumatol. 2014;41(7):1276–81. http://dx.doi.org/10.3899/jrheum.131270 PMID:24882838.

15. Bao J, Yue T, Li T, et al. Good response to infliximab in rheumatoid arthritis following failure of interleukin-1 receptor antagonist. Int J Rheum Dis. 2014.[Epub ahead of print]. http://dx.doi.org/10.1111/1756-185X.12387.

16. Ohashi R, Fukazawa R, Watanabe M, Tajima H, Nagi-Miura N, Ohno N, Tsuchiya S, Fukuda Y, Ogawa S, Itoh Y. Etanercept suppresses arteritis in a murine model of Kawasaki disease: a comparative study involving different biological agents. Int J Vasc Med. 2013;2013:543141. http://dx.doi.org/10.1155/2013/543141.

17. Choueiter NF, Olson AK, Shen DD, Portman MA. Prospective open-label trial of etanercept as adjunctive therapy for Kawasaki disease. J Pediatr. 2010;157(6):960–6.e1. http://dx.doi.org/ 10.1016/j.jpeds.2010.06.014 PMID:20667551.
18. Burmester GR, Mariette X, Montecucco C, Monteagudo-Sáez I, Malaise M, Tzioufas AG, et al. Adalimumab alone and in combination with disease-modifying antirheumatic drugs for the treatment of rheumatoid arthritis in clinical practice: the Research in Active Rheumatoid Arthritis (ReAct) trial. Ann Rheum Dis. 2007;66(6):732–9. http://dx.doi.org/10.1136/ard. 2006.066761 PMID:17329305.
19. Takeuchi T, Miyasaka N, Inoue K, Abe T, Koike T. RISING study. Impact of trough serum level on radiographic and clinical response to infliximab plus methotrexate in patients with rheumatoid arthritis: results from the RISING study. Mod Rheumatol. 2009;19(5):478–87. http://dx.doi.org/10.3109/s10165-009-0195-8 PMID:19626391.

Ulinastatin

Seiichiro Takeshita, Takashi Kanai, and Yoichi Kawamura

Abstract In acute Kawasaki disease (KD), circulating neutrophils proliferate and are functionally activated as levels of reactive oxygen species and elastase increase. This suggests that neutrophil-mediated injury of endothelial cells is involved in the pathogenesis of KD vasculitis. Ulinastatin (urinary trypsin inhibitor; UTI) is a serine protease inhibitor and inhibits neutrophil-mediated injury of endothelial cells *in vitro*, mainly by inactivating neutrophil elastase. UTI has been used in Japan as an additional therapeutic option for KD patients resistant to initial treatment with high-dose intravenous immunoglobulin (IVIG). In a recent study, the percentage of KD patients requiring additional rescue treatment and incidence of coronary artery lesions were lower after initial UTI therapy combined with IVIG than after IVIG alone. UTI, in combination with IVIG, may thus be a candidate for initial treatment of KD.

Keywords Ulinastatin • Neutrophil • Endothelial cell

Introduction

Human polymorphonuclear neutrophils ingest and destroy infectious agents and are thus important in host defense. Neutrophils contain a number of proteases in their granules, and these proteases are involved in the physiological processes of matrix proteolysis such as intercellular migration and tissue remodeling and repair [1, 2]. However, if the activity of proteases secreted from neutrophils is uncontrolled or excessive, as in severe inflammatory disease, the extracellular matrix may be degraded, thereby leading to tissue self-destruction. The strongest serine protease, elastase, is stored in its active form in azurophilic granules and is

S. Takeshita (✉)
Division of Nursing, School of Medicine, National Defense Medical College, 3-2 Namiki, Tokorozawa, Saitama 359-8513, Japan
e-mail: takeshit@ndmc.ac.jp

T. Kanai • Y. Kawamura
Department of Pediatrics, National Defense Medical College, 3-2 Namiki, Tokorozawa, Saitama 359-8513, Japan

© Springer Japan 2017
B.T. Saji et al. (eds.), *Kawasaki Disease*, DOI 10.1007/978-4-431-56039-5_27

reported to be the primary agent of neutrophil-mediated injury of endothelial cells (ECs) [1]. EC injury mediated by activated neutrophils is seen in systemic inflammatory response syndrome, adult respiratory distress syndrome, and multiple organ failure [3]. Ulinastatin (urinary trypsin inhibitor; UTI) is a glycoprotein derived from human urine and has a molecular weight of 67,000 Da. It is a serine protease inhibitor (SPI) and inhibits neutrophil elastase activity [4] and trypsin activity [5]. UTI has clinical applications in the treatment of inflammatory disorders such as pancreatitis, circulatory shock, septic shock, adult respiratory distress syndrome, and disseminated intravascular coagulation [6].

Historical Overview

Toxic neutrophils proliferate during acute Kawasaki disease (KD). These are morphologically characterized by cytotoxic vacuolization, swelling, and toxic granulation, with or without Döhle bodies, in conjunction with leukocytosis and leftward shift [7] (Fig. 1). Neutrophil apoptosis is inhibited during acute KD, and delayed neutrophil apoptosis may be related to proliferation of peripheral neutrophils [8]. The function of neutrophils in early KD is enhanced, and there is a marked increase in oxygen intermediate production [9]. Plasma neutrophil elastase and myeloperoxidase increase during acute KD [10]. A histopathological study found that numerous neutrophils (anti–elastase-positive neutrophils) infiltrate coronary arterial lesions (CAL) of KD patients at 7–9 days after onset, which suggests that neutrophils are involved in damage to coronary arteries [11]. Therefore, activated neutrophil-mediated EC injury may be involved in the pathogenesis of KD vasculitis. If so, neutrophils are potential therapeutic targets in KD.

Fig. 1 A toxic neutrophil collected from a patient with acute KD

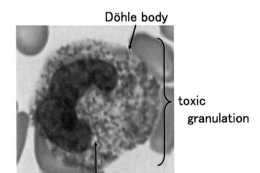

Current Understanding

The several types of therapeutic SPIs have distinct functions. UTI and sivelestat sodium hydrate (SSH) inactivate neutrophil elastase, while other SPIs (gabexate mesilate, nafamostat mesilate, aprotinin, and argatroban) do not. In an *in vitro* study, UTI and SSH inhibited neutrophil-mediated EC injury, whereas other SPIs did not [12]. Furthermore, UTI and SSH inactivated extracellular elastase secreted by neutrophils and directly suppressed production of intracellular elastase in neutrophils. Therefore, by protecting ECs against neutrophil-mediated injury, these drugs may be clinically beneficial in treating inflammatory diseases characterized by the presence of activated neutrophils.

The therapeutic mechanisms of UTI vary (Fig 2) and include (1) activity inhibition of elastase and other proteases secreted from neutrophils, (2) suppression of protease secretion from neutrophils via stabilization of the lysosomal membrane, (3) suppression of extracellular release of reactive oxygen species from neutrophils, (4) inhibition of adhesion molecule expression on ECs, and (5) inhibition of neutrophil–EC adhesion and transendothelial migration of neutrophils [12–15]. In addition, UTI may inhibit the inflammatory response by reducing release of proinflammatory cytokines (TNF-α, IL-6, and IL-8) [16].

Assigned Evidence Class and Recommendation

Although high-dose intravenous immunoglobulin (IVIG) is the established initial treatment for acute KD, 15–20 % of KD patients are resistant to this therapy. CAL, including transient dilation on echocardiography during acute KD, develop in

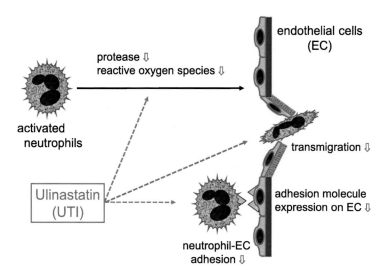

Fig. 2 Inhibitory effect of ulinastatin (UTI) on neutrophil-mediated endothelial cell injury

appropriately 10 % of KD patients receiving IVIG therapy. The limited efficacy of IVIG therapy has led to research on other drugs for treatment of KD. Zaitsu et al. reported that UTI inhibits increased mRNA expression of prostaglandin H_2 synthase-type 2 in KD, which suggests that it may be a useful additional therapeutic approach for KD [17]. UTI has been used in Japan as an additional option for KD patients who do not respond to initial IVIG treatment, but there have been no well-designed clinical studies of additional UTI therapy as a second-line treatment for KD. The level of evidence for additional UTI therapy for KD patients resistant to initial IVIG is Class IIb (other quasi-experimental studies) and Grade C (recommended, but evidence is uncertain), according to the Clinical Guideline for Medical Treatment of Acute Stage Kawasaki Disease from the Scientific Committee, the Japanese Society of Pediatric Cardiology and Cardiac Surgery [18].

UTI is usually administered by intravenous infusion, and a dose of 5,000 U/kg given 3–6 times/day (not to exceed 100,000 U/dose or 300,000 U/day) is suitable for KD patients. Although the possible side effects of UTI include anaphylaxis, liver dysfunction, leukopenia, rash, pruritus, and diarrhea, they are rare. No adverse events associated with UTI were observed in KD patients [19, 20]; thus, the drug is considered relatively safe.

Recent Advances

As mentioned above, neutrophils infiltrate CAL early in the course of KD [11] and produce elastase, various inflammatory cytokines, and superoxide anions, which may contribute to CAL formation [9, 10, 21]. Thus, UTI may be more clinically beneficial during initial treatment rather than as additional rescue (second-line) treatment. Iwashima et al. reported that initial therapy with UTI combined with IVIG had a better antipyretic effect than IVIG alone, and that use of UTI for initial treatment of KD may reduce the medical cost of IVIG therapy [19].

Recently, Kanai et al. reported that initial combined therapy with UTI and IVIG increased the success rate of initial IVIG treatment and thus reduced the proportion of KD patients that required additional rescue treatment [20]. Furthermore, as shown in Table 1, the incidence of CAL in the UTI group (UTI plus IVIG) was significantly lower than in the control group (IVIG alone), particularly among patients with a Gunma score (a predictor of IVIG unresponsiveness) of 7–11 points (ie, those at high risk of CAL, with extremely high specificity) [20]. Therefore, UTI may be effective for initial treatment of KD in combination with IVIG. The level of evidence for initial UTI therapy combined with IVIG is classified as Class IIa (nonrandomized controlled trials) and Grade B (recommended) for initial treatment in the Clinical Guideline for Medical Treatment of Acute Stage Kawasaki Disease from the Scientific Committee, the Japanese Society of Pediatric Cardiology and Cardiac Surgery.

Table 1 Development of coronary artery lesions [20]

Gunma score	Control group	UTI group	Crude OR (95 % CI)	P	Adjusted OR (95 % CI)[a]	P
0–6	41/1034	7/300	0.58	0.19	0.48	0.08
	(4)	(2)	(0.26–1.31)		(0.21–1.09)	
7–11	39/141	5/69	0.20	0.002	0.21	0.002
	(28)	(7)	(0.08–0.55)		(0.08–0.57)	
All patients	80/1178	12/369	0.46	0.01	0.32	<0.001
	(7)	(3)	(0.25–0.86)		(0.17–0.60)	

Data are proportions of patients with coronary artery lesions (CAL) in each category (%)
OR odds ratio, *CI* confidence interval
[a]Adjusted OR for CAL in the UTI group was obtained using multiple logistic regression analysis adjusted for sex, Gunma score, and dosage of initial intravenous immunoglobulin (IVIG) (1 or 2 g/kg)

References

1. Smedly LA, Tonnesen MG, Sandhaus RA, Haslett C, Guthrie LA, Johnston RB, et al. Neutrophil-mediated injury to endothelial cells. Enhancement by endotoxin and essential role of neutrophil elastase. J Clin Invest. 1986;77(4):1233–43. http://dx.doi.org/10.1172/JCI112426 PMID:3485659.
2. Owen CA, Campbell EJ. The cell biology of leukocyte-mediated proteolysis. J Leukoc Biol. 1999;65(2):137–50. PMID:10088596.
3. Chen X, Christou NV. Relative contribution of endothelial cell and polymorphonuclear neutrophil activation in their interactions in systemic inflammatory response syndrome. Arch Surg. 1996;131(11):1148–53. http://dx.doi.org/10.1001/archsurg.1996.01430230030006 PMID:8911254.
4. Ogawa M, Nishibe S, Mori T, Neumann S. Effect of human urinary trypsin inhibitor on granulocyte elastase activity. Res Commun Chem Pathol Pharmacol. 1987;55(2):271–4. PMID:3644371.
5. Ohwada M, Watanabe N, Maeda M, Gotoh M, Teramoto J, Moriya H, et al. New endoscopic treatment for chronic pancreatitis, using contrast media containing ulinastatin and prednisolone. J Gastroenterol. 1997;32(2):216–21. http://dx.doi.org/10.1007/BF02936371 PMID:9085171.
6. Inoue K, Takano H. Urinary trypsin inhibitor as a therapeutic option for endotoxin-related inflammatory disorders. Expert Opin Investig Drugs. 2010;19(4):513–20. http://dx.doi.org/10.1517/13543781003649533 PMID:20367192.
7. Takeshita S, Sekine I, Fujisawa T, Yoshioka S. Studies of peripheral blood toxic neutrophils as a predictor of coronary risk in Kawasaki disease – The pathogenetic role of hematopoietic colony-stimulating factors (GM-CSF, G-CSF). Acta Paediatr Jpn. 1990;32(5):508–14. http://dx.doi.org/10.1111/j.1442-200X.1990.tb00871.x PMID:1704677.
8. Tsujimoto H, Takeshita S, Nakatani K, Kawamura Y, Tokutomi T, Sekine I. Delayed apoptosis of circulating neutrophils in Kawasaki disease. Clin Exp Immunol. 2001;126(2):355–64. http://dx.doi.org/10.1046/j.1365-2249.2001.01675.x PMID:11703382.
9. Niwa Y, Sohmiya K. Enhanced neutrophilic functions in mucocutaneous lymph node syndrome, with special reference to the possible role of increased oxygen intermediate generation in the pathogenesis of coronary thromboarteritis. J Pediatr. 1984;104(1):56–60. http://dx.doi.org/10.1016/S0022-3476(84)80589-2 PMID:6690675.
10. Takeshita S, Nakatani K, Kawase H, Seki S, Yamamoto M, Sekine I, et al. The role of bacterial lipopolysaccharide-bound neutrophils in the pathogenesis of Kawasaki disease. J Infect Dis. 1999;179(2):508–12. http://dx.doi.org/10.1086/314600 PMID:9878040.

11. Takahashi K, Oharaseki T, Naoe S, Wakayama M, Yokouchi Y. Neutrophilic involvement in the damage to coronary arteries in acute stage of Kawasaki disease. Pediatr Int. 2005;47 (3):305–10. http://dx.doi.org/10.1111/j.1442-200x.2005.02049.x PMID:15910456.

12. Nakatani K, Takeshita S, Tsujimoto H, Kawamura Y, Sekine I. Inhibitory effect of serine protease inhibitors on neutrophil-mediated endothelial cell injury. J Leukoc Biol. 2001;69 (2):241–7. PMID:11272274.

13. Nishijima J, Hiraoka N, Murata A, Oka Y, Kitagawa K, Tanaka N, et al. Protease inhibitors (gebexate mesylate and ulinastatin) stimulate intracellular chemiluminescence in human neutrophils. J Leukoc Biol. 1992;52(3):262–8. PMID:1326018.

14. Aosasa S, Ono S, Seki S, Takayama E, Tadakuma T, Hiraide H, et al. Inhibitory effect of protease inhibitor on endothelial cell activation. J Surg Res. 1998;80(2):182–7. http://dx.doi.org/10.1006/jsre.1998.5474 PMID:9878311.

15. Okumura Y, Inoue H, Fujiyama Y, Bamba T. Effects of serine protease inhibitors on accumulation of polymorphonuclear leukocytes in the lung induced by acute pancreatitis in rats. J Gastroenterol. 1995;30(3):379–86. http://dx.doi.org/10.1007/BF02347515 PMID:7647905.

16. Bingyang J, Jinping L, Mingzheng L, Guyan W, Zhengyi F. Effects of urinary protease inhibitor on inflammatory response during on-pump coronary revascularisation. Effect of ulinastatin on inflammatory response. J Cardiovasc Surg (Torino). 2007;48(4):497–503. PMID:17653011.

17. Zaitsu M, Hamasaki Y, Tashiro K, Matsuo M, Ichimaru T, Fujita I, et al. Ulinastatin, an elastase inhibitor, inhibits the increased mRNA expression of prostaglandin H2 synthase-type 2 in Kawasaki disease. J Infect Dis. 2000;181(3):1101–9. http://dx.doi.org/10.1086/315332 PMID:10720537.

18. The Clinical Guideline for Medical Treatment of Acute Stage Kawasaki Disease from the Scientific Committee (in Japanese). Pediatric Cardiology and Cardiac Surgery. 2012;28(Supplement 3):s1–28.

19. Iwashima S, Seguchi M, Matubayashi T, Ohzeki T. Ulinastatin therapy in kawasaki disease. Clin Drug Investig. 2007;27(10):691–6. http://dx.doi.org/10.2165/00044011-200727100-00004 PMID:17803344.

20. Kanai T, Ishiwata T, Kobayashi T, Sato H, Takizawa M, Kawamura Y, et al. Ulinastatin, a urinary trypsin inhibitor, for the initial treatment of patients with Kawasaki disease: a retrospective study. Circulation. 2011;124(25):2822–8. http://dx.doi.org/10.1161/CIRCULATIONAHA.111.028423 PMID:22104548.

21. Hamamichi Y, Ichida F, Yu X, Hirono KI, Uese KI, Hashimoto I, et al. Neutrophils and mononuclear cells express vascular endothelial growth factor in acute Kawasaki disease: its possible role in progression of coronary artery lesions. Pediatr Res. 2001;49(1):74–80. http://dx.doi.org/10.1203/00006450-200101000-00017.

Part IV
Diagnosis and Examinations

Diagnosis and Management of Cardiovascular Risk Factors

Brian W. McCrindle

Abstract Given that Kawasaki disease is a systemic vasculitis causing arterial dysfunction and injury, there is concern that this may contribute to atherosclerosis. While the vascular pathology differs from atherosclerosis, it is unclear whether traditional cardiovascular risk factors produce further injury or superimpose atherosclerotic changes. Most studies show that patients with a history of Kawasaki disease do not have a predisposition to cardiovascular risk factors, although those with ongoing coronary artery involvement may have chronic inflammation. Nonetheless, all patients should undergo assessment and management of cardiovascular risk factors to maintain optimal cardiovascular health across the lifespan. Lifestyle counselling for healthy behaviors is recommended as the cornerstone of management, and motivational interviewing is advocated as a more effective counselling technique. Specific attention should be focused on counselling for physical activity participation, particularly if a precaution is indicated.

Keywords Atherosclerosis • Cardiovascular risk factors • Lifestyle management • Dyslipidemia • Inflammation

Introduction

While data suggest that, in the long-term, patients who have had Kawasaki disease (KD) without cardiac sequelae have mortality rates equivalent to that of the general population[1], questions remain as to whether these patients are at increased risk for premature or accelerated atherosclerosis and cardiovascular (CV) disease. This controversy is driven by sometimes conflicting reports regarding the presence of traditional and nontraditional CV risk factors, the nature of the chronic vascular process in coronary arteries, and the extent and nature of abnormalities in unaffected coronary artery segments or other systemic arteries. Using

B.W. McCrindle, M.D. MPH (✉)
Division of Cardiology, Department of Pediatrics, University of Toronto, Labatt Family Heart Centre, The Hospital for Sick Children, 555 University Avenue, Toronto, ON M5G 1X8, Canada
e-mail: brian.mccrindle@sickkids.ca

© Springer Japan 2017   247
B.T. Saji et al. (eds.), *Kawasaki Disease*, DOI 10.1007/978-4-431-56039-5_28

pathology specimens obtained at various intervals during and after the acute episode from 41 patients who had severe coronary artery involvement, Orenstein et al. characterized both a chronic vasculitis and a process of luminal myofibroblastic proliferation, which were also noted in some patients in non-coronary arteries and veins [2]. Often superimposed on this pathology was the presence of organizing and/or organized thrombus. Imaging studies have variously documented and characterized coronary artery lesions, which were interpreted as atherosclerosis. Atherosclerosis is a nonspecific vascular response to injury from cardiovascular risk factors, often mediated by endothelial damage and dysfunction, some features of which may overlap with the vascular processes of KD. The degree to which the vascular processes of KD interact with CV risk factors and atherosclerotic processes is not known. Nonetheless, it seems prudent that patients who have had KD be screened and managed for CV risk factors [3].

Cardiovascular Risk Factors and Vascular Disease

KD patients and normal control subjects have been reported to differ in CV risk factors. Regarding lipids, KD patients may have lower levels of high-density lipoprotein cholesterol (HDL-C), lower levels of apolipoproteins AI and AII, and higher levels of triglycerides. These differences in lipid levels are more prominent during and soon after the acute illness but may persist over the long term in some patients [4, 5]. The structure and function of HDL particles are adversely affected by inflammation, and correlations of HDL changes in KD patients with acute and chronic markers of inflammation and severe coronary artery involvement have been reported [6]. Ongoing abnormalities in other lipid levels, as compared with normal controls, have not been noted [7]. with the exception of a single study, which reported that higher total cholesterol and low-density lipoprotein cholesterol (LDL-C) levels were associated with increased arterial stiffness [8]. The impact of observed HDL changes on CV risk in KD patients is not known. Likewise, KD patients do not appear to have abnormal blood pressure or blood pressure regulation, although one study noted reduced night-time dipping on ambulatory blood pressure monitoring [9]. KD patients do not appear to have abnormal glucose homeostasis, although one case-control study did note higher levels of glycosylated hemoglobin [9]. A higher prevalence of obesity has not been reported, although one study reported lower levels of physical activity [10]. It would appear that KD patients do not have important differences in their profile of traditional CV risk factors.

There is some evidence that KD may be associated with a chronic inflammatory state, particularly in patients with important and ongoing coronary artery aneurysms. Examination of pathology specimens showed evidence of chronic inflammatory vasculitis in some patients who died with severe coronary artery involvement [2]. Clinical studies have noted higher levels of inflammation biomarkers in KD patients and a variable relationship to coronary artery complications.

There is evidence that inflammation promotes atherosclerosis, both directly and as a mediator of the effects of traditional CV risk factors [11].

Several studies have suggested that KD patients may have systemic arterial abnormalities indicative of a chronic vascular process or early atherosclerosis. Case-control studies using noninvasive vascular measures have variably shown increases in arterial stiffness, intima-media thickness, and endothelial dysfunction, and a varying relationship to the degree of coronary artery involvement. It is not yet known whether these systemic arterial abnormalities are of clinical importance or, importantly, if they are indicative of a predisposition to accelerated atherosclerosis. Regardless, HMG CoA-reductase inhibitors, or statins, have been used in a few small studies, primarily to target potentially beneficial pleiotropic effects, with some evidence that these agents improve endothelial function, reduce arterial stiffness, reduce oxidative stress, and reduce inflammation in KD patients [12, 13].

Assessment

In 2006, a scientific statement from the American Heart Association identified pediatric populations at risk for premature CV disease [3]. KD patients with current coronary artery aneurysms were defined as high-risk based on clinical evidence of manifest coronary artery disease before age 30 years. KD patients with regressed aneurysms were defined as moderate-risk based on pathophysiological evidence of accelerated atherosclerosis. KD patients without coronary artery involvement were defined as at-risk based on presumed epidemiological evidence of a high-risk setting for accelerated atherosclerosis. However, the evidence base for this classification is not robust. Nonetheless, it was recommended that all KD patients undergo careful assessment of CV risk factors and behaviors. This recommendation has been incorporated into KD management guidelines in North America [14] and Japan [15]. The assessment can be included as part of cardiology care or primary health care for these patients. The need for more in-depth assessment depends on the presence of detected abnormalities, but patients with ongoing coronary artery abnormalities may require periodic routine assessment.

Recommendations for assessment are outlined in Table 1 [16]. Assessment should include a detailed medical history of associated conditions that increase CV risk, such as diabetes. A detailed family history of premature CV disease and CV risk factors should be obtained. Lifestyle behavior assessment should evaluate diet, activity and sedentary pursuits, smoking, and sleep. Physical examination should include assessment of blood pressure and anthropometric measures. Fasting blood work should be obtained to assess lipids and glucose homeostasis. Characterization of abnormalities should be based on defined cutpoints derived from population-based data, which are available in the Expert Panel integrated CV risk guidelines [17]. Additionally, actionable cutpoints for KD patients may be lowered depending on the extent of coronary artery abnormalities, as well as the presence of multiple CV risk factors [3].

Table 1 Assessment for cardiovascular risk factors

Family history	Early cardiovascular disease, defined as angina, myocardial infarction, sudden cardiac death, stroke, and coronary artery interventions in a parent, grandparent, aunt, or uncle, occurring in males $\leq$55 years or females $\leq$65 years of age
	Dyslipidemia, hypertension, smoking, obesity, or diabetes in first-degree relatives
Dyslipidemia	Fasting lipid profile
Hypertension	Measure on three separate occasions; determine percentile for systolic and diastolic blood pressure, based on age, gender, and height percentile
Dysglycemia	Medical history for type 1 or 2 diabetes
	Fasting glucose, hemoglobin A1c
Overweight/ obesity	Measure height and weight; calculate and plot body mass index
	Measure waist circumference; plot or calculate waist/height ratio
Lifestyle behaviors	Eating behaviors and dietary quality
	Type, frequency, duration, and intensity of physical activity
	Type and time spent in sedentary pursuits
	Tobacco use and smoke exposure
	Sleep habits: duration and quality

Management

KD patients with CV risk factors require treatment similar to that recommended for the general population. In general, the cornerstone of management is adoption of healthy lifestyle behaviors, although selected patients may require drug therapy for specific risk factors that fail to respond to lifestyle management and exceed cutpoints indicating high risk. Overweight/obesity is likely to be the predominant risk factor and may further compound overall risk by its association with other risk factors, particularly dyslipidemia, hypertension, and type 2 diabetes. The presence of multiple risk factors exponentially accelerates atherosclerosis; hence, patients with KD should be assessed and counseled with a view to prevent CV risk factors and facilitate early and effective intervention. It is not known if treatment of CV risk factors alters the KD vascular processes or outcomes.

Lifestyle Management

All KD patients should be counseled to adopt healthy lifestyle behaviors (Table 2) [16]. This can be done by the cardiologist or primary care provider and may involve ancillary personnel such as nurses, dieticians, and activity counselors. Overweight and obese patients may require more intensive support, including referral to weight management programs and assessment for additional comorbidities. Counseling regarding physical activity for the KD patient needs to be calibrated to additional

Table 2 Targets of lifestyle management

Diet	Avoid skipping meals
	Increase daily intake and variety of fruits and vegetables
	Reduce consumption of refined starches
	Reduce consumption of protein sources (primarily meats) high in saturated fat/cholesterol; more fish
	Change food preparation to reduce frying and added fat and salt
	Change fat consumption from saturated fats to mono-/polyunsaturated fats
	Eliminate consumption of foods with trans fats
	Increase intake of dietary fiber
	Increase intake of dietary calcium (eg, fat-free or fat-reduced dairy products)
	Reduce intake of junk food snacks and highly processed foods
	Eliminate sugar-sweetened beverages
	Reduce restaurant/fast-food meals/snacks
	Assess and counsel regarding appropriate meal portion sizes
Physical activity	Increase daily time spent in moderate to vigorous physical activity
	Accumulate 1 h of moderate to vigorous physical activity every day
	Participate in vigorous physical activity at least 3 days per week
	Counsel regarding precautions related to KD (eg, anticoagulation, ischemia)
	Give clear and written instructions
	Counsel with a goal to promote physical activity
Sedentary pursuits	Limit overall leisure screen time (television, video games, computer, phone/devices) to no more than 1–2 h per day
Sleep	Avoid caffeinated beverages and other stimulants
	Improve sleep environment
	Remove media from sleeping room
	Improve sleep habits
	Regular and reasonable bedtime; relaxing bedtime routine
Smoking	Eliminate passive smoke exposure
	Counsel smoking prevention
	Counsel smoking cessation; provide support and resources

factors, such as cautioning about contact/trauma for those on anticoagulation therapy and restrictions on extreme exertion for those at risk for cardiac ischemia and those with arrhythmia. All patients, regardless of precautions, should be counseled to participate, and the emphasis should be on promoting physical activity [17]. It is important to ask families if they have any questions or concerns about physical activity.

Lifestyle counseling should be supportive and nonjudgmental. Motivational interviewing has emerged as an effective counseling technique that guides patients to find their own intrinsic motivation and strategies for achieving behavior change. The patient sets the agenda and the counselor elicits and supports arguments for change in an empathetic manner that respects patient autonomy [17].

Drug Therapy

Selected patients with high levels of risk factors may additionally require drug therapy, although this would be expected to be a small proportion of patients. Antihypertensive drug therapy is recommended for patients with Stage 2 hypertension (blood pressure >99th percentile + 5 mmHg, based on age and sex and height percentile), Stage 1 hypertension (blood pressure ≥95th percentile), or secondary hypertension that has not responded to lifestyle management, and those with symptoms, target organ damage (increased left ventricular mass), or associated diabetes [16, 18, 19]. Patients considered for drug therapy should be assessed for left ventricular hypertrophy, and 24-h ambulatory blood pressure monitoring may useful in defining blood pressure burden and response to therapy [20]. There is insufficient evidence to recommend a specific initial agent.

Statin therapy may be indicated for high LDL-C levels [16]. A statin is recommended for patients older than 10 years with an LDL-C ≥190 mg/dL (4.90 mmol/L), who are likely to have an underlying familial dyslipidemia. If LDL-C is <190 mg/dL but ≥160 mmol/L (4.10 mmol/L), a statin is indicated if the patient has a positive family history of premature CV disease or if other risk factors are present, which may include KD with regressed or current coronary artery aneurysms. Statins may be recommended for selected patients with an LDL-C ≥130 mg/dL (3.35 mmol/L), but a greater number of risk factors must be present. It has been estimated that about 0.85 % of the pediatric population will meet the criteria for statin therapy [21]. KD patients rarely require a statin for treatment of dyslipidemia, although, as mentioned previously, an argument for empiric statin therapy has been suggested. For patients with isolated low HDL-C, treatment is usually focused on lifestyle management and optimizing LDL-C levels. For patients with significant hypertriglyceridemia, lifestyle management is recommended, particularly decreased sugar intake and increased intake of dietary fiber and omega-3 fatty acid (fish, fish oil). Rarely patients will require drug therapy and should be referred to a lipid specialist.

Summary

After KD, patients should be assessed for CV risk factors and counselled regarding healthy lifestyle behaviors; a select few may require drug therapy for management of dyslipidemia or hypertension. Obesity prevention and management are important goals. Counselling should address anxieties and concerns regarding physical activity, particularly if precautions are indicated, and all should be allowed to participate. Patients with regressed or ongoing coronary complications require continuing monitoring for CV risk factors and may merit lower thresholds for initiating specific therapies. The aim should be to promote and protect overall CV health across the lifespan for these at-risk patients.

References

1. Nakamura Y, Aso E, Yashiro M, Tsuboi S, Kojo T, Aoyama Y, et al. Mortality among Japanese with a history of Kawasaki disease: results at the end of 2009. J Epidemiol. 2013;23(6):429–34. http://dx.doi.org/10.2188/jea.JE20130048 PMID:24042393.

2. Orenstein JM, Shulman ST, Fox LM, Baker SC, Takahashi M, Bhatti TR, et al. Three linked vasculopathic processes characterize Kawasaki disease: a light and transmission electron microscopic study. PLoS One. 2012;7(6), e38998. http://dx.doi.org/10.1371/journal.pone.0038998 PMID:22723916.

3. Kavey RE, Allada V, Daniels SR, Hayman LL, McCrindle BW, Newburger JW, et al. American Heart Association Expert Panel on Population and Prevention Science; American Heart Association Council on Cardiovascular Disease in the Young; American Heart Association Council on Epidemiology and Prevention; American Heart Association Council on Nutrition, Physical Activity and Metabolism; American Heart Association Council on High Blood Pressure Research; American Heart Association Council on Cardiovascular Nursing; American Heart Association Council on the Kidney in Heart Disease; Interdisciplinary Working Group on Quality of Care and Outcomes Research. Cardiovascular risk reduction in high-risk pediatric patients: a scientific statement from the American Heart Association Expert Panel on Population and Prevention Science; the Councils on Cardiovascular Disease in the Young, Epidemiology and Prevention, Nutrition, Physical Activity and Metabolism, High Blood Pressure Research, Cardiovascular Nursing, and the Kidney in Heart Disease; and the Interdisciplinary Working Group on Quality of Care and Outcomes Research: endorsed by the American Academy of Pediatrics. Circulation. 2006;114(24):2710–38. http://dx.doi.org/10.1161/CIRCULATIONAHA.106.179568 PMID:17130340.

4. Okada T, Harada K, Okuni M. Serum HDL-cholesterol and lipoprotein fraction in Kawasaki disease (acute mucocutaneous lymph node syndrome). Jpn Circ J. 1982;46(10):1039–44. http://dx.doi.org/10.1253/jcj.46.1039 PMID:6956753.

5. Newburger JW, Burns JC, Beiser AS, Loscalzo J. Altered lipid profile after Kawasaki syndrome. Circulation. 1991;84(2):625–31. http://dx.doi.org/10.1161/01.CIR.84.2.625 PMID:1860206.

6. Ou CY, Tseng YF, Lee CL, Chiou YH, Hsieh KS. Significant relationship between serum high-sensitivity C-reactive protein, high-density lipoprotein cholesterol levels and children with Kawasaki disease and coronary artery lesions. J Formos Med Assoc. 2009;108 (9):719–24. http://dx.doi.org/10.1016/S0929-6646(09)60395-8 PMID:19773210.

7. Lin J, Jain S, Sun X, Liu V, Sato YZ, Jimenez-Fernandez S, et al. Lipoprotein particle concentrations in children and adults following Kawasaki disease. J Pediatr. 2014;165 (4):727–31. http://dx.doi.org/10.1016/j.jpeds.2014.06.017 PMID:25039043.

8. Cho HJ, Yang SI, Kim KH, Kim JN, Kil HR. Cardiovascular risk factors of early atherosclerosis in school-aged children after Kawasaki disease. Korean J Pediatr. 2014;57(5):217–21. http://dx.doi.org/10.3345/kjp.2014.57.5.217 PMID:25045363.

9. McCrindle BW, McIntyre S, Kim C, Lin T, Adeli K. Are patients after Kawasaki disease at increased risk for accelerated atherosclerosis? J Pediatr. 2007;151:244–8, 8 e1. http://dx.doi.org/10.1016/j.jpeds.2007.03.056 PMID:17719931.

10. Banks L, Lin YT, Chahal N, Manlhiot C, Yeung RS, McCrindle BW. Factors associated with low moderate-to-vigorous physical activity levels in pediatric patients with Kawasaki disease. Clin Pediatr (Phila). 2012;51(9):828–34. http://dx.doi.org/10.1177/0009922812441664 PMID:22523278.

11. Libby P. Inflammation in atherosclerosis. Arterioscler Thromb Vasc Biol. 2012;32 (9):2045–51. http://dx.doi.org/10.1161/ATVBAHA.108.179705 PMID:22895665.

12. Hamaoka A, Hamaoka K, Yahata T, Fujii M, Ozawa S, Toiyama K, et al. Effects of HMG-CoA reductase inhibitors on continuous post-inflammatory vascular remodeling late after Kawasaki disease. J Cardiol. 2010;56(2):245–53. http://dx.doi.org/10.1016/j.jjcc.2010.06.006 PMID:20678900.

13. Duan C, Du ZD, Wang Y, Jia LQ. Effect of pravastatin on endothelial dysfunction in children with medium to giant coronary aneurysms due to Kawasaki disease. World J Pediatr. 2014;10 (3):232–7. http://dx.doi.org/10.1007/s12519-014-0498-5 PMID:25124974.

14. Newburger JW, Takahashi M, Gerber MA, Gewitz MH, Tani LY, Burns JC, et al. American Academy of Pediatrics. Diagnosis, treatment, and long-term management of Kawasaki disease: a statement for health professionals from the Committee on Rheumatic Fever, Endocarditis and Kawasaki Disease, Council on Cardiovascular Disease in the Young, American Heart Association. Circulation. 2004;110(17):2747–71. http://dx.doi.org/10.1161/01.CIR.0000145143. 19711.78 PMID:15505111.

15. JCS Joint Working Group. Guidelines for diagnosis and management of cardiovascular sequelae in Kawasaki disease (JCS 2008) – digest version. Circ J. 2010;74(9):1989–2020. http://dx.doi.org/10.1253/circj.CJ-10-74-0903 PMID:20724794.

16. Expert Panel on Integrated Guidelines for Cardiovascular Health and Risk Reduction in Children and Adolescents. National Heart, Lung, and Blood Institute. Expert panel on integrated guidelines for cardiovascular health and risk reduction in children and adolescents: summary report. Pediatrics. 2011;128(Suppl 5):S213–56. http://dx.doi.org/10.1542/peds. 2009-2107C PMID:22084329.

17. Longmuir PE, Brothers JA, de Ferranti SD, Hayman LL, Van Hare GF, Matherne GP, et al. American Heart Association Atherosclerosis, Hypertension and Obesity in Youth Committee of the Council on Cardiovascular Disease in the Young. Promotion of physical activity for children and adults with congenital heart disease: a scientific statement from the American Heart Association. Circulation. 2013;127(21):2147–59. http://dx.doi.org/10.1161/ CIR.0b013e318293688f PMID:23630128.

18. National High Blood Pressure Education Program Working Group on High Blood Pressure in Children and Adolescents. The fourth report on the diagnosis, evaluation, and treatment of high blood pressure in children and adolescents. Pediatrics. 2004;114(2 Suppl 4th Report):555–76. http://dx.doi.org/10.1542/peds.114.2.S2.555 PMID:15286277.

19. McCrindle BW. Assessment and management of hypertension in children and adolescents. Nat Rev Cardiol. 2010;7(3):155–63. http://dx.doi.org/10.1038/nrcardio.2009.231 PMID:20065950.

20. Flynn JT, Daniels SR, Hayman LL, Maahs DM, McCrindle BW, Mitsnefes M, et al. American Heart Association Atherosclerosis, Hypertension and Obesity in Youth Committee of the Council on Cardiovascular Disease in the Young. Update: ambulatory blood pressure monitoring in children and adolescents: a scientific statement from the American Heart Association. Hypertension. 2014;63(5):1116–35. http://dx.doi.org/10.1161/ HYP.0000000000000007 PMID:24591341.

21. McCrindle BW, Tyrrell PN, Kavey RE. Will obesity increase the proportion of children and adolescents recommended for a statin? Circulation. 2013;128(19):2162–5. http://dx.doi.org/ 10.1161/CIRCULATIONAHA.113.002411 PMID:24190936.

Diagnosis and Characteristics of Typical and Incomplete Kawasaki Disease

Mamoru Ayusawa and Keiji Tsuchiya

Abstract Kawasaki disease (KD) is diagnosed on the basis of six characteristic symptoms, and several reference findings are used to confirm the diagnosis. Most patients are younger than 5 years. Fever is the first sign of KD in most patients, and although Japanese guidelines give equal weight to fever and the other five symptoms, the American Heart Association guidelines regard fever as indispensable to a KD diagnosis. The other principal signs are bilateral bulbar conjunctival injection, changes in the lips and oral cavity, polymorphous exanthema, changes in the extremities (including membranous desquamation from the fingertips), and cervical lymphadenopathy, which is less frequent than the other five symptoms. If KD is suspected in a patient with four or fewer principal symptoms, incomplete KD is diagnosed. Careful differential diagnosis is necessary in such cases because patients with incomplete KD can develop coronary artery aneurysms.

Keywords Diagnostic criteria • Principal symptoms • Conjunctival injection • Strawberry tongue • Desquamation • Cervical lymphadenopathy • Bacille Calmette–Guérin (BCG) inoculation site

Introduction

Kawasaki disease (KD) is diagnosed on the basis of its characteristic symptoms. Although Kawasaki first described KD approximately 50 years ago [1], the cause has not been determined. Diagnosis is based on the presence of six characteristic symptoms. Reference findings are used to confirm the diagnosis. The Fifth Edition of the Japan Diagnostic Guideline (Table 1) was published in 2003 by the

M. Ayusawa (✉)
Department of Pediatrics and Child Health, Nihon University School of Medicine, 30-1, Oyaguchi Kami-cho, Itabashi-ku, Tokyo 173-8610, Japan
e-mail: ayusawa.mamoru@nihon-u.ac.jp

K. Tsuchiya
Department of Pediatrics, Japan Red Cross Medical Center, Tokyo, Japan
e-mail: jrcped3@k4.dion.ne.jp

© Springer Japan 2017
B.T. Saji et al. (eds.), *Kawasaki Disease*, DOI 10.1007/978-4-431-56039-5_29

Table 1 Diagnostic guidelines for Kawasaki disease

This is a disease of unknown cause that most frequently affects infants and children younger than 5 years. The symptoms can be classified as principal symptoms and other significant symptoms or findings

Principal symptoms

1.	Fever persisting 5 days or longer (inclusive of cases in whom fever has subsided before the fifth day in response to therapy)
2.	Bilateral conjunctival congestion
3.	Changes of lips and oral cavity: reddening of lips, strawberry tongue, diffuse injection of oral and pharyngeal mucosa
4.	Polymorphous exanthema
5.	Changes in peripheral extremities. *Initial stage*: reddening of palms and soles, indurative edema; *Convalescent stage*: membranous desquamation from fingertips
6.	Acute non-purulent cervical lymphadenopathy

At least five of these items must be satisfied for a diagnosis of Kawasaki Disease. However, patients with four of the principal symptoms can be diagnosed with Kawasaki Disease when coronary aneurysm or dilatation is confirmed by 2-D echocardiography or coronary angiography.

Other significant symptoms or findings

The following symptoms and findings should be considered in the clinical evaluation of suspected patients:

1.	Cardiovascular: auscultation (heart murmur, gallop rhythm, distant heart sounds), electrocardiogram changes (prolonged PR/QT intervals, abnormal Q wave, low-voltage QRS complexes, ST-T changes, arrhythmias), chest X-ray findings (cardiomegaly), 2-D echo findings (pericardial effusion, coronary aneurysms), aneurysm of peripheral arteries other than the coronary artery (axillary etc.), angina pectoris or myocardial infarction
2.	Gastrointestinal tract: diarrhea, vomiting, abdominal pain, hydrops of gall bladder, paralytic ileus, mild jaundice, slight elevation in serum transaminase
3.	Blood: leukocytosis with leftward shift, thrombocytosis, increased erythrocyte sedimentation ratio, positive C-reactive peptide, hypoalbuminemia, increased $\alpha 2$-globulin, slight decrease in erythrocyte and hemoglobin levels
4.	Urine: proteinuria, increase in leukocytes in urine sediment
5.	Skin: redness and crust at site of Bacille Calmette–Guèrin inoculation, small pustules, transverse furrows of the fingernails
6.	Respiratory: cough, rhinorrhea, abdominal shadow on chest X-ray
7.	Joint: pain, swelling
8.	Neurological: cerebrospinal fluid pleocytosis, convulsion, unconsciousness, facial palsy, paralysis in extremities

Remarks

1.	For item 5 under principal symptoms, the convalescent stage is considered important.
2.	During the acute phase, non-purulent cervical lymphadenopathy is less frequent (approximately 65 %) than the other principal symptoms.
3.	Male:female ratio, 1.3–1.5:1; patients younger than 5 years, 80–85 %; mortality rate, 0.1 %.
4.	Recurrence rate, 2–3 %; proportion of siblings cases, 1–2 %.
5.	Other diseases can be excluded and KD is suspected in approximately 10 % of all patients with fewer than five of the six principal symptoms. Coronary artery aneurysms (including so-called coronary artery ectasia) have been confirmed in some of these patients.

MCLS: Infantile Acute Febrile Mucocutaneous Lymph Node Syndrome, The 5th Revised Edition, February 2002 [3]

Committee for the Diagnostic Guideline of KD, which was supported by the Japan Ministry of Health, Labour and Welfare [2].

Patient Characteristics

Age

The diagnostic guideline indicates that KD is more common in infants younger than 5 years. In the 21st Nationwide Survey of Japan (NSJ) [3], which analyzed cases during 2009–2011, 88 % of all registered patients were in this age group. In an analysis of 6-month age groups, the largest proportion of cases was among children aged 6–11 months (16 % of all cases), followed by those aged 12–17 months (13 % of cases). Although KD has been reported in newborns, school-age children, and even adults, incidence is low in these groups.

Sex

The male:female ratio for KD incidence is approximately 1.5:1. In the NSJ for 2009–2010, incidence was 247.5 per 100,000 males and 196.9 per 100,000 females. Coronary artery lesions (CALs) were more prevalent in males than in females; however, the number and severity of symptoms during acute KD did not differ by sex [3].

Symptoms and Diagnostic Criteria

Principal Symptoms (Table 1)

The characteristics of the six principal symptoms used to diagnose KD are described below.

Fever

Fever is the first sign of KD in most patients. However, the definition of fever is somewhat confusing. The Japanese Society of Kawasaki Disease (JSKD) defines a significant fever as an axillary body temperature of 37.5 °C or higher or an oral or rectal temperature of 38.0 °C or higher. Typically, an axillary temperature of greater than 38.0 °C to 40.0 °C is the first symptom of KD, regardless of the

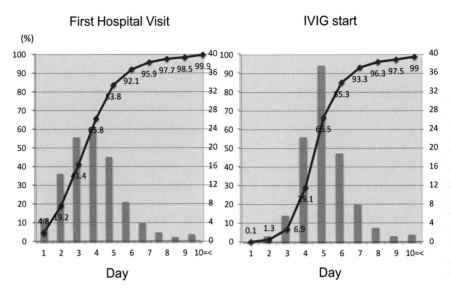

Fig. 1 Distribution of patients (2009–2010 Nationwide Survey in Japan). The right-hand axis shows the percentage totaled up on and before each day of illness (for the line graph); the left-hand axis shows the percentage for each day (for the bar graph)

presence of the other principal KD symptoms. The previous Japanese diagnostic guideline (Fourth Edition) stated that fever resistant to antibiotic treatment was a definitive characteristic of KD; however, this was removed from the Fifth Edition of the guideline, as it was felt that antibiotic use should not be necessary to confirm a KD diagnosis. Recent NSJ data show that 41.4 % of KD patients present for treatment by the third day from onset, and 65.8 % do so by the fourth day. As a result, approximately 30 % of patients were treated with intravenous γ-globulin (IVIG) before the fourth day from onset (Fig. 1). Therefore, the present diagnostic guideline also includes "patients in whom fever has subsided before the fifth day in response to therapy". The Diagnostic Guidelines of the American Heart Association (AHA) [4] indicate that in a patient with more than four of the principal criteria, a KD diagnosis can be made on day 4 of illness. Experienced clinicians who have treated many KD patients may be able to establish a diagnosis before day 4.

The AHA guidelines regard fever as an indispensable symptom in KD diagnosis, and it is therefore described separately from the other five symptoms. In the Japanese literature, there have been reports of patients without fever who presented with the other five symptoms, were diagnosed as having KD, and ultimately developed coronary artery aneurysms [5]. Therefore, the Japanese guidelines give equal weight to fever and the other five symptoms. According to the 17th NSJ, for 2001–2002, the rate (frequency) of fever was 99.3 % (23 of 16,952 cases were afebrile) [3].

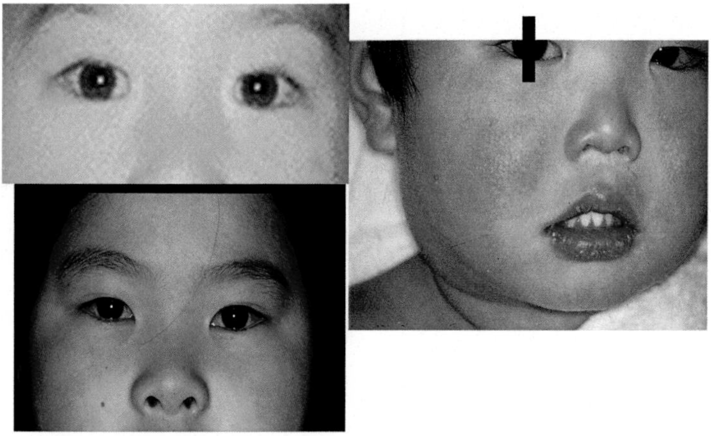

Fig. 2 Bilateral conjunctival injection

Bilateral Bulbar Conjunctival Injection (Fig. 2)

Conjunctiva bulbi is bilateral diffuse redness of the conjunctiva. This condition is not a result of conjunctival infection; thus, there is little eye discharge, and pain and photophobia are infrequent. Small vessels on the conjunctiva expand and fill with blood, and the eyes exhibit a similar degree of redness. This frequency of this symptom is close to that of fever: 92.6 % in the 17th NSJ. Iritis is another infrequent ocular manifestation of KD and is described under the category "other significant symptoms or findings".

Changes in the Lips and Oral Cavity (Fig. 3)

Reddening of the lips, strawberry tongue, and diffuse injection of oral and pharyngeal mucosae of various degrees may develop. Mild bleeding of the lips has been reported. The greatest difference with Stevens–Johnson syndrome is that patients with KD never develop oral erosions or ulcers. There is no pus or white coating of the tonsils. The frequency of oral symptoms was 89.3 % in the 17th NSJ.

Polymorphous Exanthema (Fig. 4)

The typical skin manifestation of KD resembles polymorphous exudative exanthema or urticaria with fever. A macular spotty rash may also develop, although vesicles are rare. Skin manifestations are not always diffusely distributed and frequently appear on the mucocutaneous borders, eg, around the umbilicus or genital mucosa in infants and young children. These manifestations sometimes

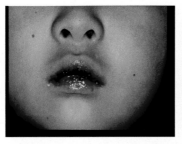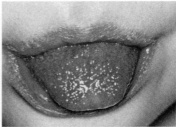

Fig. 3 Reddened lips and strawberry-like tongue

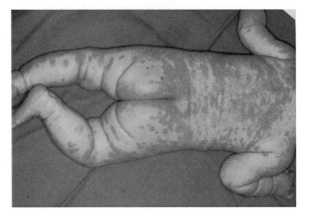

Fig. 4 Exanthema

resolve within several hours or half a day and may thus be missed. The frequency of these symptoms was 88.4 % in the 17th NSJ.

Changes in Extremities (Fig. 5)

Erythema of the palms and soles, called indurative edema, may develop during acute KD. Typically, the hands and feet are edematous and have a shiny appearance. Marked swelling may be present, without pitting edema. When these areas are touched during physical examinations, patients easily cry and complain of pain. Edematous swelling may complicate the identification of veins for injection. Membranous desquamation from the fingertips may develop during recovery. This usually begins after defervescence, when blood inflammatory markers are improving. This condition does not cause pain or discomfort. The overall frequency of changes in the extremities was 81.9 % in the 17th NSJ. At one of the present author's centers, the frequency of indurative edema was 73 % during acute KD, and desquamation was noted in 14 % of cases during the convalescent stage. However,

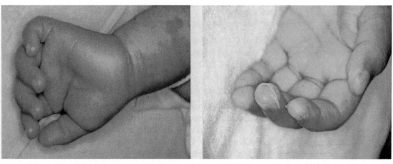

Acute phase   recovery phase

(adute phase) indurative edema of hands and paws, or erythema of palms and soles
(recovery phase) membranous desquamation from fingertip

Fig. 5 Change of hands and feet

these frequencies appear to be decreasing, probably because treatment now tends to be started during the acute stage, before peak symptom severity.

Acute Nonpurulent Cervical Lymphadenopathy (Fig 6)

Typical cervical lymphadenopathy usually presents as swelling that resembles a bowl being placed upside-down on one side of the neck. Erythema is present in some patients. The condition is usually very painful, and patients typically refuse to be touched around the affected side of the neck. When it is possible, palpation reveals no fluctuation. Cervical lymphadenopathy is one of the principal KD symptoms, and experienced pediatricians have proposed that a finding of swollen nodes with a diameter of 15 mm or larger is consistent with a KD diagnosis. These nodes resemble acute purulent lymphadenopathy. Before 1980, when KD was sometimes treated by physicians in specialties other than pediatrics, swollen lymph nodes were sometimes punctured and aspirated but failed to yield fluid or pus. This procedure is unnecessary if other KD symptoms are present.

Ultrasonographic assessment of lymph nodes may provide important information. Tashiro et al [7] noted that, in most patients with KD, ultrasonographic assessment of cervical lymphadenopathy shows multiple enlarged lymph nodes measuring 5–10 mm in diameter. This finding resembles lymphadenopathy observed in Epstein–Barr virus infection but differs from bacterial lymphadenopathy, which is usually a well-defined single mass with a large, central hypoechoic component.

The frequency of lymphadenopathy in KD differs by age (Fig. 7). It was 60.4 % among 11,357 patients 2 years or younger and 85.3 % among 5595 patients 3 years or older. The overall frequency of cervical lymphadenopathy was 68.6 % in the 17th NSJ [6]. In patients older than 3 years, fever and large, painful cervical

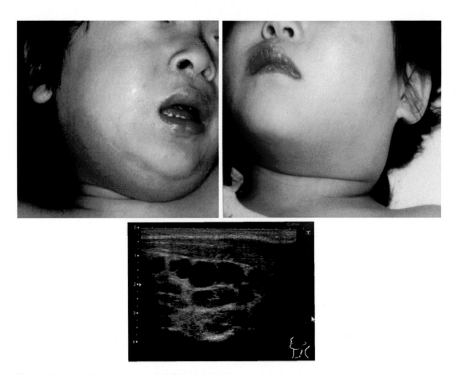

Fig. 6 Cervical lymphadenopathy (non-purulent)

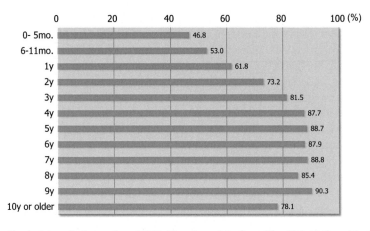

Fig. 7 Cervical lymphadenopathy of KD (Based on data from The 17th Nationwide Survey in Japan)

lymphadenopathy are often the only two initial symptoms that persist for several days. As it is difficult to distinguish KD from purulent lymphadenitis, cultures, puncture biopsy specimens, and aspirate of the lymph node are often examined and antibiotics given, but with negative results. Other KD symptoms appear within 7–10 days from the onset of these initial two signs. This course occurs in about 30 % of older KD patients.

Some patients rotate their neck to the "cock-robin position" of atlantoaxial subluxation, a condition known as Grisel syndrome [8, 9]. This occurs when patients attempt to avoid pain and their neck remains fixed even after all KD symptoms have disappeared and the patient has been discharged. Recovery usually requires 2–3 months of treatment with a brace, physiotherapy, or psychological therapy.

Definition of Final Diagnosis

KD is diagnosed when five or six principal symptoms are present, or when four symptoms are present and coronary artery aneurysm or dilatation is observed on 2-D echocardiography or coronary angiography. In the JNS, the former is categorized as "definitive KD (A)" and the latter as "definitive KD (B)". According to data from 2011 to 2012, definitive KD (A) accounted for 78.4 % of all registered patients and definitive KD (B) accounted for 1.8 % of patients. Because the prevalence of coronary artery complications has dramatically decreased, definitive KD (B) now accounts for a much smaller proportion of KD cases.

The remaining 19.8 % of cases present with four principal symptoms and no coronary artery complications or three or fewer symptoms, ie, incomplete KD (iKD). Careful differential diagnosis is necessary in such cases. Although the frequency of iKD was approximately 10 %, according to the Remarks section in the Fifth Edition of the Japanese diagnostic guideline, issued in 2003, it has been increasing recently, and the process of diagnosing iKD is now a topic of considerable interest.

One report found that patients with definitive KD (A), ie, those with six principal symptoms, were more likely to have CALs than those with five symptoms [10].

The diagnostic guidelines include other significant symptoms and findings that assist in KD diagnosis. Some of these representative findings must be confirmed for every suspected case.

Other Significant Symptoms or Findings

Gastrointestinal Tract

Gall Bladder Swelling

Most cases are accompanied by liver dysfunction and sometimes right upper abdominal pain. Ultrasonography shows a swollen gall bladder and edematous gall bladder wall. The condition improves gradually without treatment.

Liver Dysfunction

Serum alanine aminotransferase (ALT) and asparagine aminotransferase (AST) increase to about 50–500 IU/L in approximately 30 % of cases. This usually occurs during the early acute phase. Most patients improve without treatment, but bile congestion and jaundice develop rarely.

Paralytic Ileus

Paralytic ileus may develop during the early acute phase of severe KD. Typical complaints are abdominal pain and vomiting. Hypoalbuminemia is worsened by fasting.

Urine Analysis

Increased leukocyte sedimentation (>10 per high-power field) is an important finding in diagnosing KD, especially in infants younger than 6 months.

Erythema or Induration at the BCG Inoculation Site: (See Principal Symptom 4, Fig. 8)

Erythema or induration develops at the BCG inoculation site within 1 year in 80–90 % of patients. The specificity of this symptom for a KD diagnosis is very high because it is rare in other diseases. In countries that offer BCG inoculation,

Fig. 8 BCG (Bacille Calmette-Guérin) scar inoculation

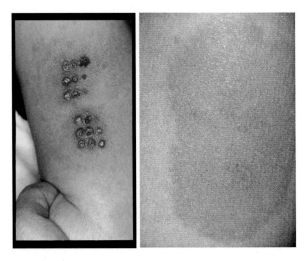

including France, South Korea, Russia, and Japan, erythema or induration at the inoculation site is a characteristic and quite specific finding for KD. However, it is not included as a principal symptom because it is limited to children younger than 2 years (ie, within approximately 1 year after BCG injection).

Cardiovascular Symptoms

During early acute KD, echocardiography may show pericarditis with pericardial effusion and carditis or myocarditis with left ventricular (LV) dysfunction. Myocardial enzymes are not always elevated in patients with LV dysfunction. Careful auscultation can reveal pericardial friction rub, distant heart sound, and gallop rhythm. Carditis/myocarditis often complicates left-side valve insufficiency. Mitral regurgitation is a frequent finding during early acute KD and improves without treatment, although treatment with IVIG and aspirin may be helpful. Aortic regurgitation is rare but sometimes develops during or after convalescence and may gradually worsen [11].

Approximately 20 % of KD patients develop coronary artery dilatation or aneurysm, including transient caliber change, usually after the seventh day from onset. However, incidence has decreased due to improvements in treatment.

Details of cardiac involvement are described in other chapters.

Other Symptoms

Facial nerve palsy is a rare complication during the acute stage and may persist for several months. However, incidence seems to be decreasing due to improvements in KD treatment. In rare severe cases, loss of consciousness due to encephalitis or encephalopathy, and death, have been reported.

During convalescence, some patients have wheezy cough or rhinorrhea.

Incomplete KD

As mentioned above, greater attention is being paid to iKD. Some reports indicate that iKD cases are increasing among children aged 10 years or older and in infants younger than 6 months.

In 2010, the JSKD indicated that the term "atypical KD" is inadequate for describing iKD. This term had previously been used for KD cases with an unusual clinical course. The 17th NSJ summarized the patient distribution with respect to the number of the six principal symptoms that were observed (Fig. 9). Patients with five or six principal symptoms accounted for 83.8 % of the total. Although patients

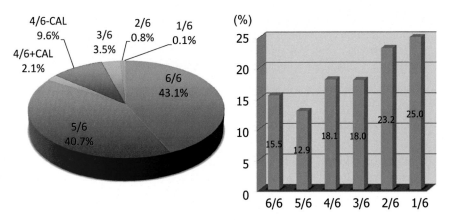

Fig. 9 Patients distribution (*left circle*) and Incidence of CAL (*right bar*) by number of KD principle symptoms (Data from the 17th NSJ: 2001–2002)

with four symptoms accounted for 11.7 % of cases, 18.1 % of these patients (2.1 % of all patients) had detectable CALs (4/6+CAL in Fig. 9). Therefore, the 9.6 % of patients with four of the principal symptoms but no CALs (4/6–CAL in Fig. 9), the 3.5 % with three symptoms, the 0.8 % with two symptoms, and the 0.1 % with one symptom were classified as iKD cases (overall frequency, 14.0 %) [12].

The incidence of coronary artery complications with respect to number of confirmed principal symptoms is shown in Figure 9 (bar graphs). Patients with fewer symptoms (iKD) were more likely to have CALs. However, it may be that some iKD cases were diagnosed because CALs were detected despite the limited number of principal symptoms (≤3). To diagnose iKD, it is essential to differentiate it from the conditions listed in Table 2.

Although we cannot conclusively determine whether all iKD is the same disease as typical KD, it is clear that some iKD patients have a high risk of CALs. Even when KD cannot be diagnosed according to standard criteria by the seventh day from onset, in the absence of an alternate diagnosis, treatment for iKD (usually IVIG) should be considered because of the imminent possibility of changes in the coronary artery wall.

In patients with four or fewer principal symptoms, laboratory data are helpful in diagnosing KD. Although inflammatory markers such as WBC and C-reactive protein may not be markedly elevated, liver enzymes (AST, ALT) and leukocyte sedimentation in urine should be carefully monitored. Brain natriuretic peptide (BNP) and N-terminal pro BNP may also reflect iKD vasculitis [13, 14], unless cardiac dysfunction is detected by echocardiography. An AHA statement [3] proposed additional items in the diagnosis of iKD, including fever of unknown origin persisting longer than 7 days in an infant younger than 6 months, serum albumin of 3.5 g/dl, anemia, elevated ALT, platelets >450,000/mm^3, WBC >15,000, or urine WBC >10/high-power field. Additional findings of interest are brightness of the coronary artery wall on imaging, lack of tapering, decreased left

Table 2 Differential diagnosis of Kawasaki disease: diseases and disorders with similar clinical findings

Infections	Viral infections (eg, measles, adenovirus, enterovirus, Epstein–Barr virus, influenza virus)
	Bacterial cervical lymphadenitis
	Yersinia pseudotuberculosis infection
	Streptococcal infection: scarlet fever, cellulitis
	Staphylococcal scalded skin syndrome
	Chlamydia pneumoniae
	Candida albicans
	Mycoplasma pneumoniae
	Rickettsia orientalis
	Rocky Mountain spotted fever
	Leptospirosis
Immunological reaction/ disorder	Toxic shock syndrome
	Drug hypersensitivity reactions, Stevens–Johnson syndrome
	Vaccinations (vaccines for measles, smallpox, DPT)
	After burns
	Insect bite (bee)
	Stevens–Johnson syndrome
	Hemophagocytic syndrome
	Mercury hypersensitivity reaction (acrodynia)
	Juvenile rheumatoid arthritis

Table 3 Harada score [15]: Indications for IVIG therapy (compiled using data from 865 cases from 18 centers)

1.	Male sex
2.	Age <12 months
3.	WBC $\geq$12,000/mm^3
4.	Platelets <350,000/mm^3
5.	CRP $\geq$4.0 mg/dl (3+)
6.	Hct <35 %
7.	Serum albumin <3.5 g/dl
	Data should be collected before the ninth day from onset
	IVIG is indicated when four or more criteria are satisfied
	In the calculation, the lowest values for platelets, Hct, and serum albumin and the highest values for WBC and CRP should be used

ventricle function, mitral regurgitation, pericardial effusion, and enlargement of the coronary artery on echocardiography.

If iKD is suspected, the Harada score (Table 3) may be helpful in determining if IVIG is indicated. This scoring system has very high specificity; thus, patients for which IVIG is determined to be unnecessary seldom develop CALs [15, 16].

Summary

When KD is suspected, the number of confirmed principal symptoms should be assessed daily. The patient's clothing should be removed before physical examination to allow for careful observation of mucocutaneous areas such as the umbilicus and genitals. BCG scars should also be carefully examined.

References

1. Kawasaki T. Infantile acute febrile mucocutaneous lymph node syndrome with specific desquamation of the fingers and toes. Clinical observation of 50 cases [Japanese]. Arerugi. 1967;16:178–222. PMID:6062087.
2. Ayusawa M, Sonobe T, Uemura S, Ogawa S, Nakamura Y, Kiyosawa N, et al. Revision of diagnostic guidelines for Kawasaki disease (the 5th revised edition). Pediatr Int. 2005;47:232–4.
3. Nakamura Y, Yashiro M, Uehara R, Sadakane A, Tsuboi S, Aoyama Y, et al. Epidemiologic features of Kawasaki disease in Japan: results of the 2009-2010 nationwide survey. J Epidemiol. 2012;22(3):216–21. http://dx.doi.org/10.2188/jea.JE20110126 PMID:22447211.
4. Newburger JW, Takahashi M, Gerber MA, Gewitz MH, Tani LY, Burns JC, et al. Committee on Rheumatic Fever, Endocarditis and Kawasaki Disease; Council on Cardiovascular Disease in the Young; American Heart Association; American Academy of Pediatrics. Diagnosis, treatment, and long-term management of Kawasaki disease: a statement for health professionals from the Committee on Rheumatic Fever, Endocarditis and Kawasaki Disease, Council on Cardiovascular Disease in the Young, American Heart Association. Circulation. 2004;110 (17):2747–71. http://dx.doi.org/10.1161/01.CIR.0000145143.19711.78 PMID:15505111.
5. Tohda Y, Yoshimura K, Tanabe Y, Kimata T, Uchiyama T, Noda Y, et al. A case of Kawasaki disease without fever complicated by significant coronary arterial lesions [Abstract]. Prog Med. 2012;32(7):1407–11.
6. Yanagawa H, Nakamura Y, Yashiro M, Uehara R, Oki I, Kayaba K. Incidence of Kawasaki disease in Japan: the nationwide surveys of 1999-2002. Pediatr Int. 2006;48(4):356–61. http://dx.doi.org/10.1111/j.1442-200X.2006.02221.x PMID:16911079.
7. Tashiro N, Matsubara T, Uchida M, Katayama K, Ichiyama T, Furukawa S. Ultrasonographic evaluation of cervical lymph nodes in Kawasaki disease. Pediatrics. 2002;109(5):E77–E7. http://dx.doi.org/10.1542/peds.109.5.e77 PMID:11986483.
8. Nozaki F, Kusunoki T, Tomoda Y, Hiejima I, Hayashi A, Kumada T, et al. Grisel syndrome as a complication of Kawasaki disease: a case report and review of the literature. Eur J Pediatr. 2013;172(1):119–21. http://dx.doi.org/10.1007/s00431-012-1858-6 PMID:23064729.
9. Wood AJ, Singh-Grewal D, De S, Gunasekera H. Kawasaki disease complicated by subluxation of cervical vertebrae (Grisel syndrome). Med J Aust. 2013;199(7):494–6. http://dx.doi.org/10.5694/mja12.11794 PMID:24099212.
10. Nakamura Y, Yashiro M, Sadakane A, Aoyama Y, Oki I, Uehara R, et al. Six principal symptoms and coronary artery sequelae in Kawasaki disease. Pediatr Int. 2009;51(5):705–8. http://dx.doi.org/10.1111/j.1442-200X.2009.02841.x PMID:19419505.
11. Akagi T, Kato H, Inoue O, Sato N, Imamura K. Valvular heart disease in Kawasaki syndrome: incidence and natural history. Am Heart J. 1990;120(2):366–72. http://dx.doi.org/10.1016/0002-8703(90)90081-8 PMID:2382613.
12. Sonobe T, Kiyosawa N, Tsuchiya K, Aso S, Imada Y, Imai Y, et al. Prevalence of coronary artery abnormality in incomplete Kawasaki disease. Pediatr Int. 2007;49(4):421–6. http://dx.doi.org/10.1111/j.1442-200X.2007.02396.x PMID:17587261.

13. Dahdah N, Siles A, Fournier A, Cousineau J, Delvin E, Saint-Cyr C, et al. Natriuretic peptide as an adjunctive diagnostic test in the acute phase of Kawasaki disease. Pediatr Cardiol. 2009;30(6):810–17. http://dx.doi.org/10.1007/s00246-009-9441-2 PMID:19365652.
14. No SJ, Kim DO, Choi KM, Eun LY. Do predictors of incomplete Kawasaki disease exist for infants? Pediatr Cardiol. 2013;34(2):286–90. http://dx.doi.org/10.1007/s00246-012-0440-3 PMID:23001516.
15. Harada K. Intravenous gamma-globulin treatment in Kawasaki disease. Acta Paediatr Jpn. 1991;33(6):805–10. http://dx.doi.org/10.1111/j.1442-200X.1991.tb02612.x PMID:1801561.
16. Tewelde H, Yoon J, Van Ittersum W, Worley S, Preminger T, Goldfarb J. The Harada score in the US population of children with Kawasaki disease. Hosp Pediatr. 2014;4(4):233–8. http://dx.doi.org/10.1542/hpeds.2014-0008 PMID:24986993.

Scoring Systems to Predict Coronary Artery Lesions and Nonresponse to Initial Intravenous Immunoglobulin Therapy

Tohru Kobayashi

Abstract Several scoring systems have been developed to predict formation of coronary artery lesions in patients with Kawasaki disease. The initial objective of such scoring systems was to identify indications for cardiac catheterization and intravenous immunoglobulin treatment. Currently, the objective is to predict response to initial intravenous immunoglobulin treatment. In Japan, three scoring system have been developed and are being used clinically.

Keywords Risk score • Coronary artery lesion • IVIG non-response

Introduction

On the basis of clinical experience treating Kawasaki disease (KD) patients, several researchers developed risk scoring systems to stratify KD patients according to the risk of coronary artery abnormalities (CAAs) or nonresponse to intravenous immunoglobulin (IVIG). Such stratification allows individualized medical treatment and/or diagnostic testing. The present chapter reviews the history of the development of scoring systems and discusses potential improvements.

History of Scoring Systems

In the 1970s until the 1980s, ie, before 2-dimensional echocardiography was widely used for routine monitoring of all KD patients, physicians focused on determining the optimal indications for cardiac catheterization and coronary angiography, because invasive procedures were the only means to identify coronary artery lesions. In 1983, Asai [1] proposed the first scoring system to determine indications

T. Kobayashi, M.D., Ph.D. (✉)
Division of Clinical Research Planning, Department of Development Strategy, Center for Clinical Research and Development, National Center for Child Health and Development, 2-10-1, Okura, Setagaya-ku, Tokyo 157-8535, Japan
e-mail: torukoba@nifty.com

© Springer Japan 2017   271
B.T. Saji et al. (eds.), *Kawasaki Disease*, DOI 10.1007/978-4-431-56039-5_30

for cardiac catheterization. It comprised 15 variables, including duration of fever, clinical symptoms, demographic characteristics, clinical data, and laboratory, electrocardiographic, and radiographic findings. This Asai and Kusakawa score (Table 1a) was confirmed to be a powerful predictor of coronary artery aneurysms in a number of studies. However, after 2-dimensional echocardiography became widely used in clinical settings in the late 1980s, the utility of this system waned. At around the same time, the efficacy of intravenous immunoglobulin (IVIG) therapy was being reported in Japan and the United States. [2,3] Although the mechanisms responsible have not been identified, IVIG therapy is clearly effective in preventing CAA formation. However, at that time, many physicians in Japan were concerned about the potential adverse effects of IVIG and sought to limit IVIG administration to patients at high risk for CAA formation. Several scoring systems [4–6] were developed to determine indications for IVIG treatment (Tables 1b, 1c and 1d). Among them, the Harada score was used by many Japanese physicians to determine whether IVIG therapy was indicated. However, their subsequent experience indicated that IVIG was safe for KD patients. When IVIG became the primary treatment for KD, the Harada score, like the Asai and Kusakawa score, was no longer necessary.

In the United States, Beiser et al. [7] developed an instrument to predict CAAs. The assessment included baseline neutrophil and band counts, hemoglobin concentration, platelet count, and temperature on the day after IVIG infusion (Fig. 1). This instrument was able to identify low-risk children for whom extensive and frequent echocardiography within 1 day of treatment would be unnecessary. However, the positive predictive value was less than satisfactory; therefore, the American Heart Association recommended that all KD patients should be treated with IVIG [8].

Table 1a Scoring systems for predicting risk of coronary artery lesions. Asai and Kusakawa score (Low risk, ≤ 5 points; moderate risk, 6–8 points; high risk, ≥ 9 points)

Variable	2 points	1 point	0 points
Sex		Male	Female
Age at onset (years)		<1	≥ 1
Duration of fever (day)	≥ 16	14–15	≤ 13
Double-peaked fever	Observed		Not observed
Double-peaked skin eruption		Observed	Not observed
Hemoglobin (g/dL)		<10	≥ 10
White blood cell count (/mm$^{3)}$)	$\geq 30,000$	26,000–29,999	$\leq 26,000$
ESR (mm/hr)	>100	60–100	<60
Days of illness until normalization of CRP or ESR	≥ 30		<30
Double-peaked CRP or ESR	Observed		Not observed
Cardiomegaly		Observed	Not observed
Arrhythmia		Observed	Not observed
Q/R ratio increase in leads II, II, and aVF	Observed		Not observed
Myocardial infarction attack symptom	Observed		Not observed
Recurrent case		Observed	Not observed

Table 1b Scoring systems for predicting risk of coronary artery lesions. Nakano Score (high risk, <0 points; low risk, ≥0 points)

Variable	Category	Points
Age at onset, y	<1	−1
	1–2	0
	≥3	+1
CRP	0 to 1+	+2
	2+ to 4+	+1
	5+	0
	6+	−3
Platelet count	$<30 \times 10^4/mm^3$	−1
	$>30 \times 10^4/mm^3$	+1

Table 1c Scoring systems for predicting risk of coronary artery lesions. Iwasa Score (high risk, ≥0 points; low risk, <0 points)

Scoring	
	$-0.01557 \times$ age in months
	$+1.004 \times$ gender (male 1, female 0)
	$-0.01501 \times$ red blood cell count $(10^4/mm^3)$
	$+0.1129 \times$ hematocrit (%)
	$-1.965 \times$ albumin (g/dL)
	$+8.462$

Table 1d Scoring systems for predicting risk of coronary artery lesions. Harada Score (high risk, ≥4 points; low risk, ≤3 points)

Variable	Cut-off	Points
White blood cell count	$\geq 12,000/m^3$	1
Platelet count	$<350,000/m^3$	1
CRP	≥3+	1
Hematocrit	<35 %	1
Albumin	<3.5 g/dL	1
Age in months	≤12	1
Gender	Male	1

Scoring System to Predict Nonresponse to Initial IVIG

Approximately 10–20 % of patients with KD have persistent or recurrent fever after primary therapy with IVIG. Many studies have shown that nonresponders to initial IVIG are at increased risk of developing CAAs, ie, nonresponse to initial IVIG is a surrogate endpoint for CAA formation. Thus, new scoring systems were developed in order to identify patients likely to be resistant to IVIG and who thus might benefit from more aggressive initial therapy. In 2000, Fukunishi et al. [9] reported that KD patients with a C-reactive protein concentration (CRP) ≥10 g/dL, lactate dehydrogenase ≥590 IU/L, and/or hemoglobin ≤10 g/dL before initial treatment (Table 1e) were likely to be nonresponders to divided dosing of initial IVIG (300 or 400 mg/kg/dose for 3–5 days). Although the predictive values were encouraging (>80 % sensitivity and specificity), the scoring system was not validated and not frequently used by physicians.

Fig. 1 Sequential
classification scheme
(Beiser et al. [7])

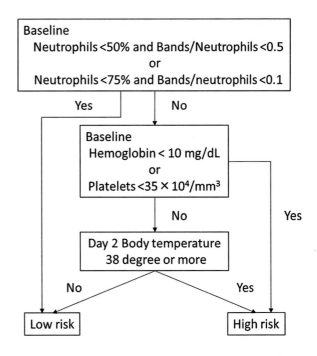

Table 1e Scoring systems for predicting risk of coronary artery lesions. Fukunishi Score (high risk>=1 point; low risk, 0 points)

Variable	Cut-off	Points
Hemoglobin	10 g/dL	1
LDH	>590 IU/L	1
CRP	>10 mg/dL	1

ESR erythrocyte sedation rate, *CRP* C-reactive protein, *AST* aspartate aminotransferase, *LDH* lactate dehydrogenase

In 2006, three Japanese groups reported new scoring systems to predict nonresponse to initial high-dose IVIG. The Kobayashi score (Table 2a) [10] was based on a multiple logistic regression analysis of 750 consecutive patients given IVIG (1 g/kg for 2 consecutive days) plus aspirin (30 mg/kg/day). In this scoring system, if a laboratory test is performed twice or more before initial therapy, the highest value is chosen for aspartate aminotransferase, %neutrophils, and CRP, while the lowest value is chosen for sodium and platelet count. Patients with KD are defined as high-risk if they have a total score of 5 points or higher. Sensitivity and specificity for predicting nonresponse to initial IVIG were 76 % and 80 %, respectively (area under the receiver-operating-characteristic curve, 0.83). The Kobayashi score was validated in a Japanese cohort treated with a single dose of IVIG 2 g/kg plus aspirin. [11] The Egami score (Table 2b) [12] was based on a multiple logistic regression analysis of 320 patients treated with IVIG (2 g/kg as a single dose) plus aspirin (30 mg/kg/day) within 9 days of fever onset. This scoring system used

Table 2a Recent scoring systems to predict nonresponse to initial intravenous immunoglobulin therapy. Kobayashi score (high risk, ≥5 points; low risk, ≤4 points)

Variable	Cut-off	Points
Sodium	≤133 mmol/L	2
Day of illness at initial IVIG (= KD diagnosed)	Day 4 or earlier	2
AST	≥100 IU/L	2
Neutrophil ratio	≥80%	2
CRP	≥10 mg/dL	1
Platelet counts	≤30.0 × 10^4/mm^3	1
Age, months	≤12	1

Table 2b Recent scoring systems to predict nonresponse to initial intravenous immunoglobulin therapy. Egami score (high risk, ≥3; low risk ≤2 points)

Variable	Cut-off	Points
ALT	≥80 IU/L	2
Day of illness at initial IVIG (= KD diagnosed)	Day 4 or earlier	1
CRP	≥8 mg/dL	1
Platelet counts	≤30.0 × 10^4/mm^3	1
Age, months	≤6	1

Table 2c Recent scoring systems to predict nonresponse to initial intravenous immunoglobulin therapy. Sano score (high risk, 2 points; low risk, 0–1 points)

Variable	Cut-off	Points
AST	≥200 IU/l	1
Total bilirubin	≥0.9 mg/dl	1
CRP	≥7 mg/dl	1

laboratory data obtained at the time of a KD diagnosis. With a cut-off of 3 or more, the sensitivity was 78% and the specificity was 76% (area under the receiver-operating-characteristic curve, 0.79). The Sano score (Table 2c) [13] was also developed using a multiple logistic regression analysis of 112 patients given IVIG (1 g/kg for 2 consecutive days). When the cut-off was set to ≥2, the sensitivity and specificity for predicting resistance to IVIG were 77 and 86%, respectively.

These three scoring systems were developed using similar methods, and the variables included in the systems are quite similar. This suggests that the three scoring system have mutually confirmed reproducibility. In addition, the three research groups used their respective scoring systems to stratify KD severity for intensification of initial therapy [14–16]. The promising results are encouraging for further development of better scoring systems and therapeutic strategies.

In the United States, Tremoulet et al. (Table 2d) [17] developed a scoring system to predict nonresponse to initial IVIG, using a database of 362 patients who received IVIG (2 g/kg for a day). With a cut-off of 2 or more, the Tremoulet

Table 2d Recent scoring systems to predict nonresponse to initial intravenous immunoglobulin therapy. Tremoulet score

Variable	Cut-off	Points
% Bands	≥ 20	2
Day of illness at initial IVIG (= KD diagnosed)	Day 4 or earlier	1
γ-GTP	≥ 60 IU/L	1
Hemoglobin z score	≤ -2	1

score had a sensitivity of 73 % and a specificity of 62 % and low predictive value as compared with the Japanese scoring systems. They also assessed the reproducibility of the Egami score in their San Diego cohort: the Egami score had insufficient sensitivity (38.3 %) but adequate specificity (83.8 %). Sleeper et al. [18] and Fu et al. [19] also applied three Japanese scoring systems to a multi-ethnic US population and a Han Chinese population in China; however, the predictive values for the scoring systems differed. Better predictive models, perhaps incorporating other biomarkers or genetic markers, are needed for countries other than Japan.

References

1. Asai T. Evaluation method for the degree of seriousness in Kawasaki disease. Acta Paediatr Jpn. 1983;25(2):170–5. http://dx.doi.org/10.1111/j.1442-200X.1983.tb01683.x.
2. Furusho K, Kamiya T, Nakano H, Kiyosawa N, Shinomiya K, Hayashidera T, et al. High-dose intravenous gammaglobulin for Kawasaki disease. Lancet. 1984;2(8411):1055–8. http://dx.doi.org/10.1016/S0140-6736(84)91504-6 PMID:6209513.
3. Newburger JW, Takahashi M, Burns JC, Beiser AS, Chung KJ, Duffy CE, et al. The treatment of Kawasaki syndrome with intravenous gamma globulin. N Engl J Med. 1986;315(6):341–7. http://dx.doi.org/10.1056/NEJM198608073150601 PMID:2426590.
4. Nakano H, Ueda K, Saito A, Tsuchitani Y, Kawamori J, Miyake T, et al. Scoring method for identifying patients with Kawasaki disease at high risk of coronary artery aneurysms. Am J Cardiol. 1986;58(9):739–42. http://dx.doi.org/10.1016/0002-9149(86)90348-6 PMID:3766414.
5. Iwasa M, Sugiyama K, Ando T, Nomura H, Katoh T, Wada Y. Selection of high-risk children for immunoglobulin therapy in Kawasaki disease. Prog Clin Biol Res. 1987;250:543–4. PMID:34230686.
6. Harada K. Intravenous gamma-globulin treatment in Kawasaki disease. Acta Paediatr Jpn. 1991;33(6):805–10. http://dx.doi.org/10.1111/j.1442-200X.1991.tb02612.x PMID:1801561.
7. Beiser AS, Takahashi M, Baker AL, Sundel RP, Newburger JW. Predictive instrument for coronary artery aneurysms in Kawasaki disease. US Multicenter Kawasaki Disease Study Group. Am J Cardiol. 1998;81(9):1116–20.
8. Newburger JW, Takahashi M, Gerber MA, Gewitz MH, Tani LY, Burns JC, et al. Committee on Rheumatic Fever, Endocarditis and Kawasaki Disease; Council on Cardiovascular Disease in the Young; American Heart Association; American Academy of Pediatrics. Diagnosis, treatment, and long-term management of Kawasaki disease: a statement for health professionals from the Committee on Rheumatic Fever, Endocarditis and Kawasaki Disease, Council on Cardiovascular Disease in the Young, American Heart Association. Circulation. 2004;110 (17):2747–71. http://dx.doi.org/10.1161/01.CIR.0000145143.19711.78 PMID:15505111.

9. Fukunishi M, Kikkawa M, Hamana K, Onodera T, Matsuzaki K, Matsumoto Y, et al. Prediction of non-responsiveness to intravenous high-dose gamma-globulin therapy in patients with Kawasaki disease at onset. J Pediatr. 2000;137(2):172–6. http://dx.doi.org/10. 1067/mpd.2000.104815 PMID:10931407.

10. Kobayashi T, Inoue Y, Takeuchi K, Okada Y, Tamura K, Tomomasa T, et al. Prediction of intravenous immunoglobulin unresponsiveness in patients with Kawasaki disease. Circulation. 2006;113(22):2606–12. http://dx.doi.org/10.1161/CIRCULATIONAHA.105.592865 PMID: 16735679.

11. Seki M, Kobayashi T, Kobayashi T, Morikawa A, Otani T, Takeuchi K, et al. External validation of a risk score to predict intravenous immunoglobulin resistance in patients with kawasaki disease. Pediatr Infect Dis J. 2011;30(2):145–7. http://dx.doi.org/10.1097/INF. 0b013e3181f386db PMID:20802375.

12. Egami K, Muta H, Ishii M, Suda K, Sugahara Y, Iemura M, et al. Prediction of resistance to intravenous immunoglobulin treatment in patients with Kawasaki disease. J Pediatr. 2006;149 (2):237–40. http://dx.doi.org/10.1016/j.jpeds.2006.03.050 PMID:16887442.

13. Sano T, Kurotobi S, Matsuzaki K, Yamamoto T, Maki I, Miki K, et al. Prediction of non-responsiveness to standard high-dose gamma-globulin therapy in patients with acute Kawasaki disease before starting initial treatment. Eur J Pediatr. 2007;166(2):131–7. http:// dx.doi.org/10.1007/s00431-006-0223-z PMID:16896641.

14. Kobayashi T, Saji T, Otani T, Takeuchi K, Nakamura T, Arakawa H, et al. RAISE study group investigators. Efficacy of immunoglobulin plus prednisolone for prevention of coronary artery abnormalities in severe Kawasaki disease (RAISE study): a randomised, open-label, blinded-endpoints trial. Lancet. 2012;379(9826):1613–20. http://dx.doi.org/10.1016/S0140-6736(11) 61930-2 PMID:22405251.

15. Ogata S, Ogihara Y, Honda T, Kon S, Akiyama K, Ishii M. Corticosteroid pulse combination therapy for refractory Kawasaki disease: a randomized trial. Pediatrics. 2012;129(1):e17–23. http://dx.doi.org/10.1542/peds.2011-0148 PMID:22144699.

16. Okada K, Hara J, Maki I, Miki K, Matsuzaki K, Matsuoka T, et al. Osaka Kawasaki Disease Study Group. Pulse methylprednisolone with gammaglobulin as an initial treatment for acute Kawasaki disease. Eur J Pediatr. 2009;168(2):181–5. http://dx.doi.org/10.1007/s00431-008-0727-9 PMID:18446365.

17. Tremoulet AH, Best BM, Song S, Wang S, Corinaldesi E, Eichenfield JR, et al. Resistance to intravenous immunoglobulin in children with Kawasaki disease. J Pediatr. 2008;153 (1):117–21. http://dx.doi.org/10.1016/j.jpeds.2007.12.021 PMID:18571548.

18. Sleeper LA, Minich LL, McCrindle BM, et al. Evaluation of Kawasaki disease risk-scoring systems for intravenous immunoglobulin resistance. J Pediatr. 2011;158:831–5 e3. http://dx. doi.org/10.1016/j.jpeds.2010.10.031.

19. Fu PP, Du ZD, Pan YS. Novel predictors of intravenous immunoglobulin resistance in Chinese children with Kawasaki disease. Pediatr Infect Dis J. 2013;32(8):e319–23. PMID:23446442.

Use of Magnetic Resonance Angiography for Assessment of Coronary Artery Lesions Caused by Kawasaki Disease

Atsuko Suzuki, Yoshiaki Hayashi, Toshitake Iiyama, Sadataka Hara, Hideo Ono, Hidekazu Ichida, and Motoyuki Yamashita

Abstract Coronary artery aneurysms caused by Kawasaki disease (KD) often progress to obstructive arterial lesions. Patients are therefore followed up throughout their lives by X-ray coronary angiography (CAG). However, CAG is invasive, hazardous, and expensive. Noninvasive magnetic resonance coronary angiography (MRCA) has remarkably improved. Since 1999, we have used MRCA to evaluate more than 1200 patients with KD, 262 of whom also underwent follow up with MRCA. We found that MRCA was useful in evaluating all types of coronary artery lesions during all stages of KD [1, 2]. In addition, when black-blood imaging sequences were used, MRCA clearly detected artery walls and thrombi in aneurysms [1, 2]. These imaging techniques are recommended to minimize use of CAG. Magnetic resonance myocardial imaging is likely to replace radioactive-isotope myocardial imaging.

Keywords Coronary aneurysms • Intimal thickening • Thrombus • Recanalized vessels

Introduction

Coronary artery lesions (CAL) due to KD are monitored by X-ray coronary angiography (CAG) throughout the patient's life. Infants with severe CAL need to be examined frequently, and children with CAL experience considerable psychological and physical stress at CAG examinations. Therefore, many adolescent

A. Suzuki, M.D. (✉)
Tokyo Teishin Hospital, 2-14-23 Fujimi, Chiyoda-ku, Tokyo 102-8798, Japan

Yaesu Clinic, 2-1-18 Nihonbashi, Chuo-ku, Tokyo 103-0027, Japan
e-mail: a.suzuki@prox.ne.jp

Y. Hayashi, RT • T. Iiyama, RT • S. Hara, RT • H. Ono, RT
Yaesu Clinic, 2-1-18 Nihonbashi, Chuo-ku, Tokyo 103-0027, Japan

H. Ichida, RT • M. Yamashita, RT
Tokyo Teishin Hospital, 2-14-23 Fujimi, Chiyoda-ku, Tokyo 102-8798, Japan

© Springer Japan 2017   279
B.T. Saji et al. (eds.), *Kawasaki Disease*, DOI 10.1007/978-4-431-56039-5_31

and adult patients neglect or refuse follow-up for severe CAL. Magnetic resonance coronary angiography (MRCA) has remarkably improved and can detect all forms of CAL caused by KD (which can be detected by CAG), as well as artery walls and thrombi in aneurysms [2] (which cannot be detected by CAG). Multidetector-row computed tomography (MDCT) is also efficient in detecting CALs but requires breath-holding and bradycardia, which are impossible for young children. Exposure to radiation and use of contrast medium are other important limitations of this technique, especially for children who need frequent MDCT.

Procedure

We used a 1.5-T Gyroscan Master gradient system with release 9 software from 1999 until 2010. An Achieva 1.5-T device with release 3.2 software was used from 2010 to 2013, and an Ingenia 1.5-T device with release 4.1 software has been used since 2013 (Philips Electronics System Co). These devices yield clearer images with shorter examination times and permit us to use various sequences during examination.

MRCA was performed using the steady-state free precession (SSFP) sequence [3]. "Bright-blood imaging" was used for whole-heart image scanning (slice thickness, 0.7–0.8 mm), followed by proton density–weighted black-blood imaging ("black-blood imaging"), such as 2-D black-blood spiral k-space order TFE (spiral BB) [4] for manual target short-axis scanning (slice thickness, 2–3 mm) and volume isotropic TSE Acquisition (VISTA-BB) [5] for whole-heart image scanning (slice thickness, 0.7–0.8 mm). Black-blood imaging was able to detect thrombi in aneurysms and coronary artery walls.

The procedure was performed without sedation, and with free breathing, in patients 8 years or older. Children younger than 8 years were given sleeping medication: those younger than 3 years were given sodium trichloroethyl phosphate syrup 1.0 mL/kg, and those aged 3–7 years were given thiopental sodium 2–4 mg/kg by intravenous infusion. A percutaneous oxygen monitor was attached and observed by a pediatrician during the examination.

MRCA: Indications in Patients with KD

More than 1200 KD patients underwent MRCA assessment, including:
(1) patients with severe CAL requiring intensive coronary angiographic monitoring, (2) patients with aneurysm or slight transient dilatation during acute KD on 2-D echocardiography (MRCA was performed in the convalescent phase, to confirm CAL and arterial wall thickness), (3) patients undergoing aortocoronary bypass surgery, who were evaluated before and after surgery, (4) patients who declined CAG and withdrew from follow-up of CAL but returned for MRCA assessment,

(5) patients with no CAL who developed new chest pain or arrhythmia, and (6) young woman with CAL who desired to have children.

MRCA is noninvasive and convenient and requires about 1–1.5 h at an outpatient clinic. Therefore, it is useful for frequent follow-up of severe CAL, occasional follow-up of less severe CAL, and for confirming the absence of CAL.

Advantages of MRCA

MRCA is advantageous for children because it does not require radiation exposure, contrast medium, breath-holding, or a decrease in heart rate. The only challenge is that patients must remain still for 1 h or longer during the examination, but this limitation is easily addressed by the safe use of sleeping medication.

CAG cannot display the ridges of large aneurysms, because the contrast medium does not satisfactorily fill the huge aneurysmal lumen (Fig. 1). Injection of a large amount of contrast medium over an extended time period can result in dangerous

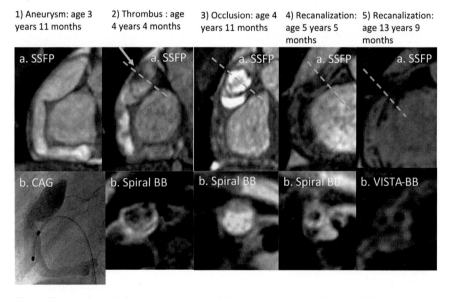

Fig. 1 Progression of giant aneurysm on right coronary artery. Onset of KD (age 3 years 8 months). CAG and MRCA were performed at age 3 years 11 months. CAG could not clearly detect the ridge of the giant aneurysm. Age 4 years 4 months. A thrombus in the aneurysm appears as a dark shadow on SSFP (*arrow*). On Spiral-BB, a grey circle surrounds the black-blood flow at the cross-section of the aneurysm (*dotted line* shows the cross-section). Age 4 years 11 months. The aneurysm is occluded by the thrombus (high-signal mass). Ages 5 years 5 months and 13 years 9 months. Right coronary artery is recanalized. Neovascularization, with a few tiny lumens and rings ("lotus root" appearance), can be seen in cross-sections of Spiral-BB and VISTA-BB images. *SSFP: steady-state free precession, CAG: coronary angiography, Spiral BB: spiral k-space order TFE black blood, VISTA BB: volume isotropic TSE Acquisition black blood*

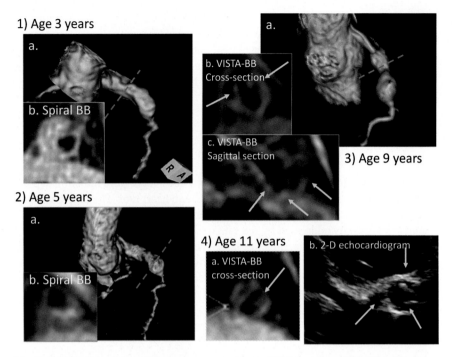

Fig. 2 Progression of thrombus in aneurysm. Onset of KD (age 4 months). Thrombus in an aneurysm on the left coronary artery appears as a white mass on Spiral BB at age 3 years. The thrombus had changed shape and location at age 5 years. At age 9 years, the mass of the thrombus had disappeared, and thin membranes and tiny polyps were seen in the aneurysm lumen. These aneurysm structures were detected by 2-D echocardiography for the first time at age 11 years (from an abstract for the 11th International Kawasaki Disease Symposium)

ventricular flutter or cardiac arrest. MRCA can detect aneurysms of any size (Fig. 1), including those with very large lumens. It can also be used to assess thrombi in aneurysms, thickened artery walls, and even developed vasa vasorum in thickened aneurysm walls. Fresh thrombi cannot be detected by 2-D echocardiography [6] but appear on MRCA at a very early phase, probably at the time of blood flow delay. Occluded aneurysms (Fig. 1) are not detectable by CAG or MDCT, but are detectable on MRCA.

Turbulent aneurysm flow can develop into a large thrombi. Such thrombi often have a small number of tiny lumens and rings (the so-called "lotus root" appearance) [7] (Fig. 1). This finding suggests neovascularity in thrombi (Fig. 1). Thrombi often change shape, location in aneurysms (Fig 2), and size. Some disappear and some develop into recanalized vessels [7].

We have recently begun to use the VISTA BB sequence routinely, and thin membranes in the aneurysm lumen (probably a fibrin net) and tiny polyps on the intima were often detected in images (Fig. 3) [8], which suggests that VISTA-BB slice thickness is thin enough to detect fine structures. In contrast, the thick slices

1) Age 1 year
5 months:
thrombus

2) Age 8 years
6 months:
Recanalized vessels

3) Age 14 years 6
months

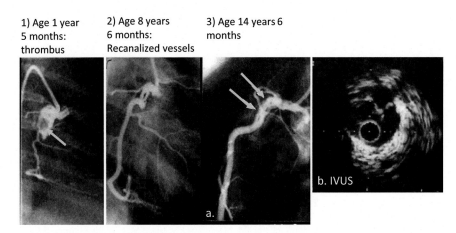

Fig. 3 Membranous tubes in aneurysm. Onset of KD (age 1 year 3 months). CAG at age 1 year 5 months revealed a thrombus in the aneurysm. CAG at age 8 years 8 months detected recanalized vessels. Intravascular ultrasound (IVUS) was performed at age 14 years 6 months, and thin membranous tubes were observed as walls of recanalized vessels. These tubes fluttered in the blood flow

used for Spiral BB have a "partial volume effect" [8], which tends to overestimate the larger solid mass of a thrombus (Fig. 2).

Limitations of MRCA

The number of localized stenoses tends to be overestimated on SSFP. We therefore recommended simultaneous use of black-blood methods [2] and magnetic resonance myocardial imaging in patients with severe stenosis [1].

The quality of MRCA images depends on radiologist skill, and such skill is acquired only with considerable experience. The cost/performance ratio for MRCA assessment of children is poor because examination using all protocols requires more than 1 h and sleeping children must be observed by a doctor during the examination. Only a few hospitals have the resources to provide MRCA for children.

Conclusion

Noninvasive MRCA is a useful method for CAL detection and follow-up, especially for children with severe CAL, which require intensive monitoring. Thrombi in aneurysms are very changeable. MRCA is thus the best method for frequent observation.

References

1. Stuber M, Botnar RM, Danias PG, Sodickson DK, Kissinger KV, Van Cauteren M, et al. Double-oblique free-breathing high resolution three-dimensional coronary magnetic resonance angiography. J Am Coll Cardiol. 1999;34(2):524–31. http://dx.doi.org/10.1016/S0735-1097(99)00223-5 PMID:10440168.
2. Suzuki A, Takemura A, Inaba R, Sonobe T, Tsuchiya K, Korenaga T. Magnetic resonance coronary angiography to evaluate coronary arterial lesions in patients with Kawasaki disease. Cardiol Young. 2006;16(6):563–71. http://dx.doi.org/10.1017/S1047951106001168 PMID:17116270.
3. Takemura A, Suzuki A, Inaba R, Sonobe T, Tsuchiya K, Omuro M, et al. Utility of coronary MR angiography in children with Kawasaki disease. AJR Am J Roentgenol. 2007;188(6):W534–9. http://dx.doi.org/10.2214/AJR.05.1414 PMID:17515343.
4. Ahn CB, Kim JH, Cho ZH. High-speed spiral-scan echo planar NMR imaging-I. IEEE Trans Med Imaging. 1986;5(1):2–7. http://dx.doi.org/10.1109/TMI.1986.4307732 PMID:18243976.
5. Sakurai K, Miura T, Sagisaka T, Hattori M, Matsukawa N, Mase M, et al. Evaluation of luminal and vessel wall abnormalities in subacute and other stages of intracranial vertebrobasilar artery dissections using the volume isotropic turbo-spin-echo acquisition (VISTA) sequence: a preliminary study. J Neuroradiol. 2013;40(1):19–28. http://dx.doi.org/10.1016/j.neurad.2012.02.005 PMID:22633047.
6. Suzuki A. Standardization of the findings of coronary arterial lesions on echocardiography. Pediatric MOOK. 1986;1:160–70.
7. Suzuki A, Kamiya T, Ono Y, Kinoshita Y, Kawamura S, Kimura K. Clinical significance of morphologic classification of coronary arterial segmental stenosis due to Kawasaki disease. Am J Cardiol. 1993;71(13):1169–73. http://dx.doi.org/10.1016/0002-9149(93)90641-O PMID:8480642.
8. González Ballester MA, Zisserman AP, Brady M. Estimation of the partial volume effect in MRI. Med Image Anal. 2002;6(4):389–405. http://dx.doi.org/10.1016/S1361-8415(02)00061-0 PMID:12494949.

CT Coronary and Myocardial Images in Patients with Coronary Artery Lesions

Hiroshi Kamiyama

Abstract Coronary computed tomographic angiography (CCTA) is a next-generation modality that can be used instead of coronary catheterization. It can be useful in evaluating coronary artery lesions after Kawasaki disease (KD) if physicians are mindful of its three drawbacks, namely, the use of beta-blockade, use of contrast medium, and exposure to radioactivity. CCTA has potential advantages in comparison with MR coronary angiography, including better spatial resolution, shorter imaging time, easier operation, and better visualization of collateral circulation characteristic to KD. Myocardial perfusion imaging (MPI) using technetium-labeled agents is practical in assessing coronary perfusion in patients with myocardial ischemia or infarction after KD. Both rest and stress imaging are essential for evaluating myocardial ischemia or infarction by means of a 1-day protocol, but a 2-day protocol should be used when evaluating infants with pharmacologic stress. A comprehensive plan is required, including control of body movement, ensuring a sufficient interval (and a high-fat meal) between administration of agents and acquisition, the use of the Monzen position during acquisition, and ensuring the patient consumes soda water immediately before acquisition. The Japanese Society of Nuclear Medicine proposes using pediatric-appropriate doses of nuclear agents. Combined evaluation with CCTA and MPI is the new standard for managing patients with coronary artery lesions after KD.

Keywords Coronary • Computed tomography • Myocardial perfusion • Nuclear medicine • Radioactive exposure

H. Kamiyama (✉)
Division of Medical Education Planning and Development, Nihon University School of Medicine, 173-8610, 30-1 Oyaguchi Kamicho, Itabashi-ku, Tokyo, Japan

Department of Pediatrics and Child Health, Nihon University School of Medicine, 173-8610, 30-1 Oyaguchi Kamicho, Itabashi-ku, Tokyo, Japan
e-mail: kanamaru.hiroshi@nihon-u.ac.jp

© Springer Japan 2017 285
B.T. Saji et al. (eds.), *Kawasaki Disease*, DOI 10.1007/978-4-431-56039-5_32

Beyond Cardiac Catheterization

Coronary computed tomographic angiography (CCTA) has surpassed selective coronary angiography by cardiac catheterization. Multislice spiral CT was first used, in 2003, to evaluate coronary artery lesions after Kawasaki disease (KD) in adolescents [1]. One report noted that multislice spiral CT had a sensitivity of 100 % in detecting coronary artery aneurysms after KD, as determined by cardiac catheterization [2]. Furthermore, CCTA is less invasive than cardiac catheterization, as advanced CCTA uses satisfactorily low doses of radioactivity. Combined evaluation with CCTA and myocardial perfusion imaging (MPI) promises high diagnostic ability in patients with severe coronary artery lesions after KD.

Coronary Computed Tomographic Angiography

Overview

CCTA is useful for patients with coronary artery lesions after KD and for those with congenital coronary artery abnormalities and congenital heart disease, among other conditions. Recent high-end CT, such as area detector CT, can visualize coronary arteries in patients unable to hold their breath, such as those younger than 5 years. CCTA is indicated for any patient likely to benefit from the procedure.

Indications for CCTA

The Japanese guidelines for diagnosis and management of cardiovascular sequelae in KD [3] specify that coronary artery imaging should be performed for patients with coronary aneurysm in the second year or later after onset or stenosis. CCTA is controversial for patients with regression of coronary artery dilatation after less than 1 year. CCTA can be used to evaluate such patients if the three drawbacks of CCTA are considered, namely, use of beta-blockade, use of contrast medium, and radioactive exposure.

Three Drawbacks of CCTA

The risks and benefits of CT scanning should be evaluated when considering its indications.

Beta-Blockade

Beta-blockade is necessary before CT scanning, to maintain appropriate patient heart rate, which can lower radioactive exposure. However, additional administration of beta-blockade may not be effective in controlling heart rate. For pediatric CCTA, a beta-blocker such as metoprolol should be administered at a dose of 0.6–0.8 mg/kg, without additional use.

Contrast Medium

Iodine concentration and dose of contrast medium should be carefully considered. A low or moderate iodine concentration is sufficient to visualize the coronary artery in CCTA [4], although a high iodine concentration, 350–370 mgI/ml, is usually used for adults [5]. A lower concentration and viscosity of contrast medium at a level of 320 mgI/ml and at a mean dose of 0.8 ml/kg is sufficient to prepare the coronary artery for CCTA in children.

Radioactive Exposure

Radioactive exposure must be carefully considered, in consultation with International Commission on Radiological Protection recommendations. Four factors should be considered in attempting to reduce radioactive dose. (1) Carefully define the target, which could be level of stenosis, aneurysm size, or collateral circulation. The target selected will determine the scanning parameters. (2) Patient age and clinical characteristics should be carefully considered in planning the scan. It might be sufficient for scans of infants to visualize coronary artery lesions favorite sites including each proximal coronary artery. (3) It is important to calculate cumulative radioactive dose, because repeated examinations are needed for patients with coronary artery lesions after KD. (4) We need to carefully consider measures to reduce radioactive exposure.

Advantages of CCTA

Advantages of CCTA as Compared with Magnetic Resonance Coronary Angiography

CCTA is superior to magnetic resonance coronary angiography in (1) spatial resolution—a small slice thickness should be used, to achieve high spatial resolution, (2) imaging time—one volume scan enables short imaging time with a breath-hold of 2–3 s, if area detector CT is used, and (3) ease of operation—specialized technical expertise is not needed for routine CCTA.

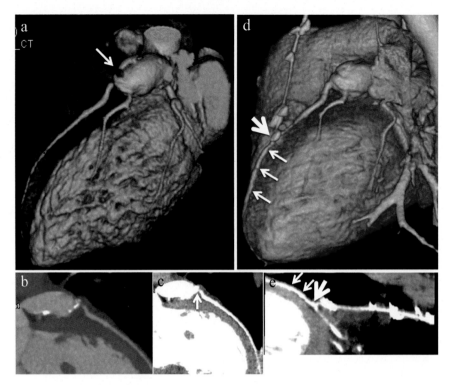

Fig. 1 Giant aneurysm and severe stenotic lesion after KD in a boy aged 6 years. The giant aneurysm (*arrow*) at the proximal left anterior descending coronary artery is visualized in a volume-rendered image (**a**) and is covered with severe calcifications (**b**). A severe stenotic lesion (*arrow*) adjacent to the calcified giant aneurysm is clearly visualized before surgery in a multiplanar reconstructed image (**c**). Bypass graft patency (*large arrow*) with a well developed distal left anterior descending coronary artery (*arrows*) is seen 1 year after surgery (**d**, **e**)

CCTA Advantages in Patients with Coronary Artery Lesions After KD

CCTA can produce excellent images of collateral circulation, a characteristic of KD. High-end CT can eliminate partial volume effects, which sometimes result in false-positive results for culprit lesions with severe concentric calcification, a characteristic of KD. Figures 1 a–e show a series of CCTA images before coronary arterial bypass graft surgery and 1 year after surgery in a 6-year-old boy with a giant aneurysm and severe stenotic lesions after KD.

Cardiac Radionuclide Imaging

Category

Cardiac radionuclide imaging includes myocardial perfusion imaging (MPI), imaging of myocardial fatty acid metabolism using I-123 beta methyl-iodophenyl-pentadecanoic acid (BMIPP), and imaging of cardiac sympathetic nerve function using I-123 metaiodobenzylguanidine (MIBG). Myocardial ischemia or infarction in patients after KD should be evaluated by MPI. Because technetium (Tc)-labeled myocardial perfusion agents (eg, Tc-99m sestamibi and Tc-99m tetrofosmin) have a shorter half-life than thallium-201 chloride, they are very suitable for SPECT imaging and result in far less radioactive exposure, which is particularly important when examining children.

Indications for MPI

MPI is widely used in adult ischemic heart disease and is useful in evaluating coronary perfusion in patients with myocardial ischemia or infarction after KD or due to congenital coronary arterial abnormalities, including anomalous origin of the left coronary artery from the pulmonary artery [6]. The Japanese guidelines for the diagnosis and management of cardiovascular sequelae in KD [3] recommend that MPI should be performed if a patient has trouble with a remaining coronary aneurysm in the second year or later after onset or stenosis. MPI is controversial for patients with regression of coronary arterial dilatation within 1 year. The indications for MPI should be carefully considered for patients with regression.

Planning of Rest and Stress Imaging for MPI

One-Day Protocol

Both rest and stress imaging are essential in the evaluation of ischemia or infarction by MPI. The 1-day protocol is the standard for assessment of patients with coronary artery lesions after KD. In this protocol, Tc-labeled stress imaging is scheduled first, following by rest imaging, in the pediatric population (Fig. 2) [7].

Two-Day Protocol

A 2-day protocol is required for infants who need pharmacologic sedation for imaging, patients with missing data, and patients with possible severe ischemia or

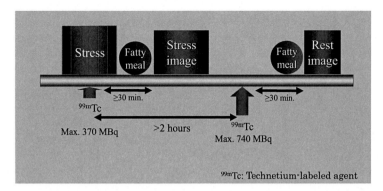

Fig. 2 Schedule for a technetium-labeled stress-first 1-day protocol for myocardial perfusion imaging: institutes will decide whether the first image is a stress or rest image. Exercise or pharmacological stress should be scheduled before the examination, which depends on patient age, physical findings, and background characteristics. The interval between the initial and second administrations of the technetium-labeled agent should be longer than 2 h, and the second dose is 2–3 times the first dose. The time interval should be longer than 30 min between administration of the technetium-labeled agent and image acquisition. A high-fat meal, such as cocoa, cow's milk, or a sandwich with an egg topping, is given to patients during the waiting period between administration of the technetium-labeled agent and image acquisition

infarction. Pharmacologic stress MPI is usually performed for children because it is impossible for infants and children younger than 6 years to undergo exercise stress testing. Rest imaging should be performed first in case of coronary events, followed by stress imaging 2–3 days later.

Outline of Stress Imaging

Exercise Stress Imaging

Exercise is recommended in stress testing for MPI in children and young adults with adequate athletic capability, because exercise stress resembles the conditions of natural stress. A load method including exercise should be performed by ergometer or treadmill, usually until maximum stress is achieved. Maximum stress is determined by evaluating patient heart rate and/or double product and should be continued for at least 1 min after injection of Tc-labeled agents, to obtain optimal stress images.

Pharmacologic Stress Imaging

Adenosine is the only approved agent for pharmacologic stress testing in Japan, although other agents, including dipyridamole [8] and dobutamine [9], have been used. The general protocol recommends adenosine stress to be continued for 6 min at a dose of 140 μg/kg/min [10] or 120 μg/kg/min in Japan. The Tc-labeled agent is administered 3 min after load following 3 min of stress. Bronchial asthma is a possible adverse effect of adenosine, so physicians should auscultate for respiratory sounds. The most common adverse effects—flushing, headache, and asthma attack—usually resolve spontaneously immediately after discontinuation of adenosine administration, because of its short half-life.

Comprehensive Plan for Image Acquisition Using Tc-Labeled Agents

Control of Body Movement

Body movement should be controlled during image acquisition. If excessive body movement is observed, repeat acquisition may be necessary in order to obtain satisfactory images.

Time Interval in Image Acquisition

The time interval between administration of Tc-labeled agents and image acquisition should be longer than 30 min, to promote excretion from the liver and gallbladder.

Monzen Position

The Monzen position [11] resembles the backstroke position, with raised left arm and upper body bent to the right during image acquisition. This position reduces interference from rays scattered by the liver and gallbladder to the posteroinferior wall of the heart, due to descent of the liver.

Soda Water

Soda water should be given to patients immediately before image acquisition, to expand the stomach and reduce interference of rays scattered from the intestine to the posteroinferior wall of the heart.

High-Fat Meal

A high-fat meal should be given to patients during the waiting period between administration of Tc-labeled agents and image acquisition, to promote excretion of

Table 1a Class and baseline activity/minimum activity of radiopharmaceuticals

| | | | Dose | |
| | | | Baseline activity | Minimum activity |
Nuclides	Radiopharmaceuticals	Class	(MBq)	(MBq)
Tc-99 m	MIBI/tetrofosmin (myocardial rest/stress scan 2-day protocol max[a])	B	63.0	80
	MIBI/tetrofosmin (myocardial scan 1-day protocol first[b])	B	28.0	80
	MIBI/tetrofosmin (myocardial scan 1-day protocol second[b])	B	84.0	160

Cited and modified from Koizumi [12]
[a]Dose may be excessive for heavy patients, as compared with conventionally administered dose; therefore, a smaller dose should be considered, as this dose is the maximum
[b]Both rest-first and stress-first protocols are applicable. The second dose is 2–3 times larger than the first dose

Tc-labeled agents and avoid interference of rays scattered from the liver and gallbladder to the posteroinferior wall of the heart.

Appropriate Administration of Nuclear Agents

Appropriate doses of nuclear agents must be considered in pediatric nuclear medicine. In 1988, the Subcommittee for Standardization of Radionuclide Imaging of the Japan Radioisotope Association recommended use of the following formula: Pediatric dose (MBq) = adult dose × (age + 1)/(age + 7). In 2014, the Japanese Society of Nuclear Medicine (JSNM) distributed cards with methods to calculate JSNM pediatric dosage [12]. The method is a modified version of the methods shown on the European Association of Nuclear Medicine (EANM) pediatric dosage card [13–15]. It describes how to calculate pediatric administered dose, as follows: Administered activity (MBq) = baseline activity in Table 1a × weight − dependent multiple in Table 1b. Whenever Tc-labeled agents are used for myocardial scanning, the radiopharmaceutical class should be class B (Tables 1a and 1b). Minimum activity should be maintained, even if the calculated administered activity is lower than the minimum recommended activity. Examples of calculation using Tc-labeled agents are shown as below.

Example 1 Weight 44 kg, Tc-99 m tetrofosmin (myocardial 2-day protocol) $63.0 \times 9.57 = 603 > 592$ (adult administered activity) → 592 MBq should be administered, if the recommended adult administered activity at the institution is 592 MBq.

Example 2 Weight 14 kg, Tc-99 m MIBI (myocardial 1-day protocol first) $28.0 \times 3.57 = 100 > 80$ (minimum activity) → 100 MBq should be administered.

Table 1b Weight-dependent multiples for each class

Body weight	Class		
kg	A	B	C
3	1	1	1
4	1.12	1.14	1.33
6	1.47	1.71	2
8	1.71	2.14	3
10	1.94	2.71	3.67
12	2.18	3.14	4.67
14	2.35	3.57	5.67
16	2.53	4	6.33
18	2.71	4.43	7.33
20	2.88	4.86	8.33
22	3.06	5.29	9.33
24	3.18	5.71	10
26	3.35	6.14	11
28	3.47	6.43	12
30	3.65	6.86	13
32	3.77	7.29	14
34	3.88	7.72	15
36	4	8	16
38	4.18	8.43	17
40	4.29	8.86	18
42	4.41	9.14	19
44	4.53	9.57	20
46	4.65	10	21
48	4.77	10.29	22
50	4.88	10.71	23
52–54	5	11.29	24.67
56–58	5.24	12	26.67
60–62	5.47	12.71	28.67
64–66	5.65	13.43	31
68	5.77	14	32.33

Modified from Koizumi [12]

Example 3 Weight 14 kg, Tc-99 m MIBI (myocardial 1-day protocol second) $84.0 \times 3.57 = 300 > 160$ (minimum activity) $\rightarrow$ 300 MBq should be administered.

Future Directions

Patients with coronary artery lesions after KD should be managed in accordance with current knowledge. It is essential to recover all patients with severe coronary artery lesions who are lost to follow-up. Such patients may return to hospital because of pregnancy, chest pain, or chronic anxiety after surgery. Furthermore, the system and environment for new progress should be re-evaluated. Combined evaluation with CCTA and MPI is likely to be incorporated into the follow-up plan of all institutions, because it yields precise information and is straightforward for physicians.

Acknowledgments The author thanks Drs. Kensuke Karasawa and Mamoru Ayusawa (Department of Pediatrics and Child Health, Nihon University School of Medicine) for their passionate guidance, and all radiologic technicians in the CT and isotope examination rooms at Nihon University Itabashi Hospital for their kind cooperation.

References

1. Sato Y, Kato M, Inoue F, Fukui T, Imazeki T, Mitsui M, et al. Detection of coronary artery aneurysms, stenoses and occlusions by multislice spiral computed tomography in adolescents with kawasaki disease. Circ J. 2003;67(5):427–30. http://dx.doi.org/10.1253/circj.67.427 PMID:12736482.
2. Kanamaru H, Sato Y, Takayama T, Ayusawa M, Karasawa K, Sumitomo N, et al. Assessment of coronary artery abnormalities by multislice spiral computed tomography in adolescents and young adults with Kawasaki disease. Am J Cardiol. 2005;95(4):522–5. http://dx.doi.org/10.1016/j.amjcard.2004.10.011 PMID:15695145.
3. Ogawa S, Ayusawa M, Ishii M, JCS Joint Working Group, et al. Guidelines for diagnosis and management of cardiovascular sequelae in Kawasaki disease (JCS 2013). Circ J. 2014;78 (10):2521–62 http://doi.org/10.1253/circj.CJ-66-0096.
4. Johnson PT, Pannu HK, Fishman EK. IV contrast infusion for coronary artery CT angiography: literature review and results of a nationwide survey. AJR Am J Roentgenol. 2009;192(5): W214–21. http://dx.doi.org/10.2214/AJR.08.1347 PMID:19380526.
5. Miller JM, Dewey M, Vavere AL, Rochitte CE, Niinuma H, Arbab-Zadeh A, et al. Coronary CT angiography using 64 detector rows: methods and design of the multi-centre trial CORE-64. Eur Radiol. 2009;19(4):816–28. http://dx.doi.org/10.1007/s00330-008-1203-7 PMID:18998142.
6. Kanamaru H, Karasawa K, Ichikawa R, Matsumura M, Miyashita M, Taniguchi K, et al. Dual myocardial scintigraphy mismatch in an infant with Bland-White-Garland syndrome. Int J Cardiol. 2009;135(1):e1–3. http://dx.doi.org/10.1016/j.ijcard.2008.03.021 PMID:18597871.
7. Karasawa K, Ayusawa M, Noto N, Sumitomo N, Okada T, Harada K. Optimum protocol of technetium-99 m tetrofosmin myocardial perfusion imaging for the detection of coronary stenosis lesions in Kawasaki disease. J Cardiol. 1997;30(6):331–9. PMID:9436075.
8. Kondo C, Hiroe M, Nakanishi T, Takao A. Detection of coronary artery stenosis in children with Kawasaki disease. Usefulness of pharmacologic stress 201Tl myocardial tomography. Circulation. 1989;80(3):615–24. http://dx.doi.org/10.1161/01.CIR.80.3.615 PMID:2788529.
9. Ogawa S, Fukazawa R, Ohkubo T, Zhang J, Takechi N, Kuramochi Y, et al. Silent myocardial ischemia in Kawasaki disease: evaluation of percutaneous transluminal coronary angioplasty by dobutamine stress testing. Circulation. 1997;96(10):3384–9. http://dx.doi.org/10.1161/01.CIR.96.10.3384 PMID:9396431.
10. Prabhu A, Singh T, Morrow W, Muzik O, Di Carli M. Safety and efficacy of intravenous adenosine for pharmacologic stress testing in children with aortic valve disease or Kawasaki disease. Am J Cardiol. 1999;83(2):284–6, A6. http://dx.doi.org/10.1016/S0002-9149(98)00841-8.
11. Monzen H, Hara M, Hirata M, Nakanishi A, Ogasawara M, Suzuki T, et al. Exploring a technique for reducing the influence of scattered rays from surrounding organs to the heart

during myocardial perfusion scintigraphy with technetium-99m sestamibi and technetium-99m tetrofosmin. Ann Nucl Med. 2006;20(10):705–10. http://dx.doi.org/10.1007/BF02984684 PMID:17385311.

12. Koizumi K, Masaki H, Matsuda H, Uchiyama M, Okuno M, Oguma E, et al. Japanese Society of Nuclear Medicine; Optimization Committee for Pediatric Nuclear Medicine Studies. Japanese consensus guidelines for pediatric nuclear medicine. Part 1: Pediatric radiopharmaceutical administered doses (JSNM pediatric dosage card). Part 2: Technical considerations for pediatric nuclear medicine imaging procedures. Ann Nucl Med. 2014;28(5):498–503. http://dx.doi.org/10.1007/s12149-014-0826-9 PMID:24647992.

13. Piepsz A, Hahn K, Roca I, Ciofetta G, Toth G, Gordon I, et al. Paediatric Task Group European Association Nuclear Medicine. A radiopharmaceuticals schedule for imaging in paediatrics. Eur J Nucl Med. 1990;17(3–4):127–9. http://dx.doi.org/10.1007/BF00811439 PMID:2279492.

14. Jacobs F, Thierens H, Piepsz A, Bacher K, Van de Wiele C, Ham H, et al. European Association of Nuclear Medicine. Optimised tracer-dependent dosage cards to obtain weight-independent effective doses. Eur J Nucl Med Mol Imaging. 2005;32(5):581–8. http://dx.doi.org/10.1007/s00259-004-1708-5 PMID:15619101.

15. Lassmann M, Biassoni L, Monsieurs M, Franzius C, Jacobs F. EANM Dosimetry and Paediatrics Committees. The new EANM paediatric dosage card. Eur J Nucl Med Mol Imaging. 2007;34(5):796–8. http://dx.doi.org/10.1007/s00259-007-0370-0 PMID:17406866.

Long-Term Follow-Up and Education Regarding Daily Life Activities, School Life, and Guidelines After Acute KD

Mamoru Ayusawa

Abstract Almost all patients with Kawasaki disease take aspirin for 2–3 months after disease onset. During and after such treatment, patients without coronary artery lesions (CAL) are not restricted with respect to sports, vaccination, or normal daily life activities. Management of daily life activities of patients with CAL depends on individual risk of cardiac events, as determined by appropriate assessment techniques. If the patient requires anticoagulant and/or antiplatelet treatment, external injuries should be avoided and participation in contact sports restricted. When warfarin is used, the dose needs to be carefully monitored by blood testing, and the patient should be informed about foods that increase vitamin K levels. Angiograms obtained by computed tomography or magnetic resonance are beginning to supplant catheter angiograms in the morphological evaluation of CAL; however, these modalities have advantages and disadvantages. Echocardiography and scintigraphy with pharmacological or exercise stress testing is useful in functional studies. However, an experienced examiner must be available to conduct and evaluate the results of such tests. As patients age, they must be made aware of the possibility of cardiac sequelae and the need for transition to an adult cardiologist.

Keywords Anticoagulation • Antiplatelet • Sports restriction • Transition • Vaccination • School life

Two to 3 Months After Onset

After recovery from acute KD, almost all patients receive 3–5 mg/kg of aspirin as antiplatelet therapy. Platelet count and coagulation activity increase until 2–3 months after onset of acute KD [1]. After discharge from hospital, at around the second week from onset, some patients may complain of mild bruising or epistaxis as their activity level improves. Aspirin may cause allergic eruptions or anorexia with liver dysfunction. In rare cases, infection with influenza or varicella virus may

M. Ayusawa (✉)
Department of Pediatrics and Child Health, Nihon University School of Medicine, 30-1, Oyaguchi Kami-cho, Itabashi-ku, Tokyo 173-8610, Japan
e-mail: ayusawa.mamoru@nihon-u.ac.jp

© Springer Japan 2017
B.T. Saji et al. (eds.), *Kawasaki Disease*, DOI 10.1007/978-4-431-56039-5_33

cause Reye syndrome during this stage; thus, patients and their families are commonly instructed on prevention of these infections. When a patient taking aspirin is infected with influenza or varicella, aspirin is usually discontinued or changed to ticlopidine or dipyridamole.

Vaccination After KD

Inactivated vaccines are not prohibited, even immediately after recovery; however, live attenuated vaccines are not given until at least 6 months from KD onset in most Japanese outpatient clinics. This practice is based on studies by the Japan Ministry of Health of antibody acquisition after measles vaccination [2, 3]. Miura et al. proposed a 9-month interval after KD onset for patients who received additional IVIG due to ineffectiveness of standard therapy with 2 g/kg of IVIG [4]. In the US population, Mason et al. proposed that a longer interval was necessary [5]. Miura et al. is currently conducting a further study for uncertain effect of varicella and mumps vaccine, and the results will be reported.

After 2–3 Months from Onset

Patients without CAL need not restrict daily life activities or exercise during school. Patients who have CAL with a diameter ≤ 5 mm need to continue aspirin or other antiplatelet drugs such as dipyridamole or ticlopidine and to undergo CAL assessment by echocardiography every 1–3 months. It is important for patients to be aware of foods that increase levels of vitamin K, as it inhibits the effect of warfarin. In Japan, fermented soybean (i.e., *natto*) is prohibited for this reason, as are seaweed, broccoli, and spinach.

Patients with CAL ≥ 6 mm need the antithrombotic drug warfarin in addition to antiplatelet drugs. The effect of warfarin needs to be assessed and controlled by evaluating prothrombin time (PT) and its international normalized ratio (PT-INR). The target value for PT-INR in children is 1.8–2.5, although this may be adjusted depending on patient sex, age, and activity. Use of protective headwear is advised if the child is likely to fall. Contact sports are prohibited. Despite the difficulties in dose control and food restriction and the risk of hemorrhagic complications, warfarin clearly increases cardiac event–free survival in patients with giant aneurysm [6]. The feasibility of recently developed "novel oral anticoagulants" for children is currently being investigated.

Evaluation and Management of Patients with CAL

After acute KD, patients with aneurysms >5 mm in diameter, as estimated by echocardiography, must be evaluated with coronary artery angiography by cardiac catheterization. Evaluation of small aneurysms by catheter angiography depends on an individualized safety assessment, particularly in infants. In morphological studies, angiography by computed tomography or magnetic resonance is beginning to supplant catheter angiography; however, these techniques have their respective advantages and disadvantages.

Medical prevention of thrombosis in coronary arteries in patients with CAL depends on whether CAL induce ischemia during exercise. Echocardiography and scintigraphy with pharmacological or exercise stress testing is quite useful for functional study in such cases, but an experienced examiner must be available to conduct and evaluate the results of such tests.

Management of the daily life activities of patients with CAL depends on ischemia severity, including the risk of a cardiac event as determined by appropriate methods. If a patient requires anticoagulant and/or antiplatelet medication, activities that increase the risk of external injury and contact sports must be restricted, and PT-INR should be monitored.

Management of School Life in Japan

In Japan, all students are screened using a questionnaire on heart disease, which includes past history of Kawasaki disease and its complications, and electrocardiography. If a student has CAL and is restricted from certain activities, the referring physician must submit a "Table for Management of School Life", which shows the allowed and prohibited school activities. One table is designed for use for primary school students, and another is used for junior and senior high school students. These tables can be downloaded from the website of Japanese Society of Pediatric Cardiology and Cardiac Surgery.

Preparation for Transition to Adult Cardiologists

After symptoms resolve and patients resume daily life, they and their parents should be educated about the particulars of daily life activities. The long-term effects of KD on vascular health have been discussed extensively in the guidelines of the Japanese Circulation Society [2] and American Heart Association [7]. Patients with CAL have varying risks of arteriosclerosis. A recent study reported that carotid artery stiffness, intima–media thickness, and the endothelial pulsatile index in KD patients with normal coronary arteries or mildly ectatic CAL were normal at an average of 12 years after onset, which provides some reassurance regarding peripheral vascular health [8]. The mechanism by which inflammation from KD vasculitis causes coronary artery sclerosis probably differs from that responsible for aging-related atherosclerosis; however, there are concerns regarding long-term sclerotic change in coronary arteries in persons with a history of KD [9–11]. Although long-term outcomes (>20 years after onset) are still a matter of debate, it is prudent to advise KD patients to be careful of risk factors for metabolic syndrome, including obesity, diabetes mellitus, and smoking.

Loss to follow-up when children become independent of their parents is a serious concern. As most KD patients are not fully aware of their history, detailed instruction on KD and its sequelae is necessary before high school graduation because of the risk of smoking or pregnancy among women, regardless of marriage. Successful transition to an adult cardiologist is one of the most important issues in the management of KD. Patients need to be aware of the possibility of cardiac sequelae and the importance of proper adult care.

References

1. Yamada K, Fukumoto T, Shinkai A, Shirahata A, Meguro T. The platelet functions in acute febrile mucocutaneous lymph node syndrome and a trial of prevention for thrombosis by antiplatelet agent. Nihon Ketsueki Gakkai Zasshi. 1978;41(4):791–802. PMID:716791.
2. Joint Working Group JCS. Guidelines for diagnosis and management of cardiovascular sequelae in Kawasaki disease (JCS 2013). Digest version. Circ J. 2014;78(10):2521–62. http://dx.doi.org/10.1253/circj.CJ-66-0096 PMID:25241888.
3. Sonobe T. Practice of immunization: High-dose gamma-globulin therapy and immunization. Shoni naika. 1994;26:1929–33 (in Japanese).
4. Miura M, Katada Y, Ishihara J. Time interval of measles vaccination in patients with Kawasaki disease treated with additional intravenous immune globulin. Eur J Pediatr. 2004;163(1):25–9. http://dx.doi.org/10.1007/s00431-003-1335-3 PMID:14624356.
5. Mason W, Jordan S, Sakai R, Takahashi M. Lack of effect of gamma-globulin infusion on circulating immune complexes in patients with Kawasaki syndrome. Pediatr Infect Dis J. 1988;7(2):94–9. http://dx.doi.org/10.1097/00006454-198802000-00006 PMID:2449651.
6. Suda K, Kudo Y, Higaki T, Nomura Y, Miura M, Matsumura M, et al. Multicenter and retrospective case study of warfarin and aspirin combination therapy in patients with giant coronary aneurysms caused by Kawasaki disease. Circ J. 2009;73(7):1319–23. http://dx.doi.org/10.1253/circj.CJ-08-0931 PMID:19436123.
7. Newburger JW, Takahashi M, Gerber MA, Gewitz MH, Tani LY, Burns JC, American Academy of Pediatrics, et al. Diagnosis, treatment, and long-term management of Kawasaki disease: a statement for health professionals from the Committee on Rheumatic Fever, Endocarditis and Kawasaki Disease, Council on Cardiovascular Disease in the Young, American Heart Association. Circulation. 2004;110(17):2747–71. http://dx.doi.org/10.1161/01. CIR.0000145143.19711.78 PMID:15505111.
8. Selamet Tierney ES, Gal D, Gauvreau K, Baker AL, Trevey S, O'Neill SR, et al. Vascular health in Kawasaki disease. J Am Coll Cardiol. 2013;62(12):1114–21. http://dx.doi.org/10. 1016/j.jacc.2013.04.090 PMID:23835006.
9. Noto N, Okada T, Yamasuge M, Taniguchi K, Karasawa K, Ayusawa M, et al. Noninvasive assessment of the early progression of atherosclerosis in adolescents with Kawasaki disease

and coronary artery lesions. Pediatrics. 2001;107(5):1095–9. http://dx.doi.org/10.1542/peds. 107.5.1095 PMID:11331692.

10. Cheung YF, Yung TC, Tam SC, Ho MH, Chau AK. Novel and traditional cardiovascular risk factors in children after Kawasaki disease: implications for premature atherosclerosis. J Am Coll Cardiol. 2004;43(1):120–4. http://dx.doi.org/10.1016/j.jacc.2003.08.030 PMID:14715193.

11. Mitani Y, Okuda Y, Shimpo H, Uchida F, Hamanaka K, Aoki K, et al. Impaired endothelial function in epicardial coronary arteries after Kawasaki disease. Circulation. 1997;96 (2):454–61. PMID:9244212.

Assessment of Cardiac Ischemia During Acute and Long-Term Follow-Up and Rheologic Assessment of Coronary Artery Lesions After Kawasaki Disease

Shunichi Ogawa

Abstract Cardiac ischemia is important for the prognosis of Kawasaki disease (KD) in patients with coronary artery lesions. Assessment of cardiac ischemia requires exercise stress testing, which young children may not be able to tolerate. Therefore, pharmacologic stress tests using adenosine, dipyridamole, or dobutamine have primarily been used for young children. Stress myocardial single-photon emission computed tomography is another important method for diagnosing coronary stenotic lesions due to KD. Treadmill and ergometer stress electrocardiography, pharmacologic stress body surface potential mapping, signal-averaged electrocardiography, and echocardiography are also useful for detecting cardiac ischemia. Rheologic indices such as coronary flow reserve (CFR) and myocardial fractional flow reserve (FFRmyo) can also be helpful in detecting cardiac ischemia. Shear stress and CFR significantly decrease in areas with giant aneurysms and in patients with vessels distal to a giant aneurysm. FFRmyo, CFR, and shear stress also decrease in areas distal to a significant stenotic lesion. These findings suggest that vascular endothelial dysfunction, cardiac ischemia, and coronary microcirculation disorder due to decreased perfusion may also be present.

Keywords Cardiac ischemia • Coronary artery lesions • Shear stress • Coronary flow reserve • Myocardial fractional flow reserve

Assessment of Cardiac Ischemia During Short- and Long-Term Follow-Up

Cardiac ischemia is an imbalance between myocardial oxygen supply and demand. Cardiac ischemia seriously affects outcomes of Kawasaki disease (KD) patients with coronary artery lesions (CAL), which include severe stenosis, giant coronary

S. Ogawa, M.D. (✉)
Department of Pediatrics, Nippon Medical School, 1-1-5 Sendagi Bunkyo-ku, Tokyo 113-8603, Japan
e-mail: boston@nms.ac.jp

© Springer Japan 2017
B.T. Saji et al. (eds.), *Kawasaki Disease*, DOI 10.1007/978-4-431-56039-5_34

aneurysm with or without coronary stenosis, and coronary microcirculatory disturbances without coronary stenosis. Exercise stress tests are necessary for the assessment of cardiac ischemia; however, young children may not be able to tolerate such
tests. Thus, pharmacologic stress tests using adenosine, dipyridamole, or
dobutamine have been primarily used to assess young children.

Exercise Electrocardiography

Because electrocardiography (ECG) is not sensitive for detecting cardiac ischemia
in patients with KD at rest, exercise or pharmacologic stress tests should instead be
used. Treadmill and ergometer stress tests can be administered to school-age or
older children, although these tests are less sensitive than myocardial scintigraphy
in detecting ischemic findings. To increase the detection rate, pharmacologic stress
tests are therefore recommended.

Treadmill Stress and Ergometer Stress ECG

A stress treadmill test and ergometer stress test (ST) at an intensity greater than
10 metabolic equivalent units (MET) may detect cardiac ischemia in some patients.
Subendocardial or transmural cardiac ischemia affects ST changes. Subendocardial
ischemia, the most common type, shows horizontal or down-slope ST depression.
In contrast, transmural-type ischemia is rare and presents as ST elevation. On an
ECG, ST depression or elevation greater than 0.1 mV indicates cardiac ischemia.
The location of the ischemic area can be determined by the placement of the surface
ECG, as follows: inferior—leads II · III · aVF; anterior—leads V2–V6; anterior-
septal—leads V1–V3; lateral—leads I · aVL; posterior—leads V1 · V2 with a tall
R wave.

Pharmacologic Stress Body Surface Potential Mapping

The dipyridamole stress test using body surface potential mapping is highly sensitive and specific for the presence of ischemia and is a useful method for diagnosing
cardiac ischemia, including in young children [1]. This method is also useful for
identifying and localizing silent myocardial ischemia in children with KD, especially those who cannot perform tests involving physical exercise [2].

Signal-Averaged ECG

The results of ECGs from patients with coronary dilatation, with and without
stenosis, during acute KD exhibit a larger proportion of high-frequency

components, suggesting the presence of myocardial involvement [3]. The presence of late ventricular potentials, evaluated by criteria adjusted to body surface area, are highly specific for cardiac ischemia and previous myocardial infarction [4]. Use of dobutamine stress test readings containing signal-averaged ventricular late potentials may improve detection of these signals in children who cannot undergo exercise stress tests [5].

Stress Echocardiography

Stress echocardiography, especially dobutamine stress echocardiography, is an established diagnostic method for ischemic heart diseases [6]. It is also a useful noninvasive method to diagnose and follow-up myocardial ischemia due to KD.

Radionuclide Imaging

To minimize radioactive exposure for children, technetium (Tc)-labeled myocardial perfusion agents (eg, Tc-99 m sestamibi and Tc-99 m tetrofosmin) are commonly used [7, 8]. Stress myocardial single-photon emission computed tomography (SPECT) is an important method for diagnosing coronary stenotic lesions due to KD, and pharmacologic-stress SPECT is commonly performed for children who cannot undergo exercise-stress SPECT [9–14]. When myocardial ischemia is detected in patients without coronary stenosis and myocardial perfusion imaging produces a false-positive result, coronary microcirculation disorder is suspected [15]. The availability of 3D automatic quantitative analysis of ECG-gated myocardial perfusion SPECT (quantitative gated SPECT [QGS]) [16] has allowed physicians to detect postischemic myocardial stunning [17] and determine the viability of infarcted myocardium in patients with severe coronary artery lesions due to KD [18, 19].

Pharmacologic Stress Myocardial Perfusion Scintigraphy

In Japan, adenosine has been approved as a nuclear medicine agent, and it is expected that pharmacologic stress myocardial perfusion scintigraphy using adenosine will soon be common. Adenosine should not be administered with dipyridamole, which potentiates the action of adenosine. Adenosine may induce asthma attacks, but its half-life is short, and most adverse reactions resolve after discontinuation of the drug [20].

Cardiac Ischemia Assessed by Rheologic Index

See sections "Hemodynamics in vessels distal to an aneurysm" and "Hemodynamics in the area distal to a stenotic lesion".

Rheologic Assessment of CAL After KD

Methods and Criteria for Assessment of Coronary Hemodynamics

To evaluate the functional severity of CALs associated with KD, it is useful to determine average peak flow velocity (APV), coronary flow reserve (CFR), myocardial fractional flow reserve (FFRmyo), shear stress, and peripheral vascular resistance, among other measures. Common instruments for assessment include a 0.014-inch guidewire equipped with an ultrasonic probe and a high-sensitivity pressure sensor (Doppler wires or pressure wires). In particular, CFR (ie, [stress APV]/[APV at rest], where APV is the value at peak dilatation after infusion of papaverine injection) (Fig. 1) and FFRmyo (ie, [mean pressure at a site distal to the coronary lesion of interest] − {[mean right atrial pressure]/[mean pressure at the

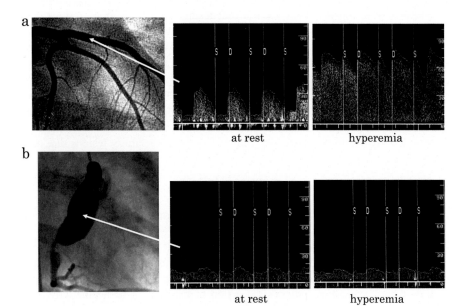

Fig. 1 (**a**) Normal coronary artery. Averaged peak flow velocities (APV) were 20 cm/s at rest and 66 cm/s after hyperemia, and coronary flow reserve (CFR) was 3.3. (**b**) Giant coronary aneurysm. APV at rest and after hyperemia were equal (11 cm/s), and CFR was 1.0

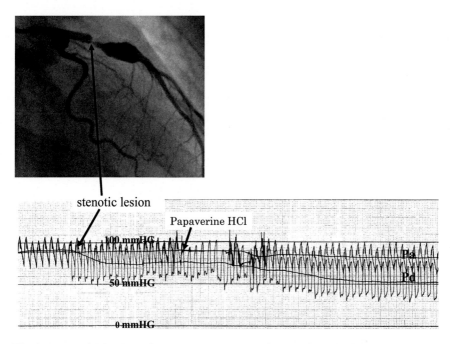

Fig. 2 Myocardial fractional flow reserve (FFRmyo) calculated from simultaneously recorded values of coronary artery ostium pressure (Pa) and intracoronary pressure (Pd) at steady-state maximum hyperemia distal to lesions with greater than 95 % stenosis. Pd and Pa values were 52 mmHg and 80 mmHg, respectively, and FFRmyo was 0.65

coronary ostium]} – [mean right atrial pressure], where these pressures are obtained simultaneously at peak dilatation after infusion of papaverine hydrochloride) are suitable for evaluating presence/absence and severity of myocardial ischemia and presence/absence of peripheral coronary circulatory disorder (Fig. 2). These values are also useful in selecting appropriate treatment strategies (catheter intervention vs. coronary artery bypass grafting [CABG]) and postoperative evaluation.

The reference values in children and adults are 2.0 for CFR and 0.75 for FFRmyo [21–23]. Shear stress induces mechanical stress on vascular endothelial cells and affects hemodynamics through endothelium-derived vasoactive substances. The reference value for shear stress in children [24] (calculated with an approximation formula using APV and lumen diameter) is 40 dyn/cm^2.

The APV determined with the above method represents velocity at the lumen center. Flow velocity near the wall is lower than that at the center; thus, shear stress near the wall is lower than the estimate obtained using this method. Because coronary blood flow correlates fairly well with APV, the ratio of mean coronary blood pressure to APV may be used to calculate total peripheral resistance. The reference values for total peripheral resistance at rest and during vascular dilatation are 4.0 and 2.0, respectively [24].

Measurements obtained with pressure wires are useful in evaluating stenotic lesions, and those obtained with Doppler wires are useful for evaluating dilatation lesions.

Change in Coronary Hemodynamics Associated with CAL

Hemodynamics in Coronary Aneurysms Without Significant Stenosis and in Distal Vessels

Hemodynamics in Aneurysms

A turbulent blood flow pattern, reduced flow velocity, and reduced CFR are present in coronary artery aneurysms, especially giant aneurysms. Reduced CFR indicates cardiac ischemia in the distal area of giant aneurysms. Although there is no decrease in perfusion pressure, a significant decrease in shear stress, which is known to damage vascular endothelial cells, is present. It is assumed that endothelial cells in giant aneurysms are seriously damaged by vasculitis and hemodynamic change. Vascular endothelial dysfunction promotes vasoconstriction and increases susceptibility to thrombogenesis, inflammation, fibrosis, oxidation, and atherosclerosis. In giant aneurysms caused by KD, thrombogenesis is the most important concern, since thrombi readily form in giant aneurysms in which accelerated platelet aggregation, hypercoagulation, and hypofibrinolysis are present. Some aneurysms with an internal diameter greater than 8 mm retain a normal blood flow waveform, APV, and CFR. Because some giant aneurysms have normal hemodynamics, functional assessment of aneurysms is necessary in order to identify risky aneurysms.

Hemodynamics in Vessels Distal to an Aneurysm

Blood flow waveform, APV, CFR, and peripheral vascular resistance in vessels distal to an aneurysm are similar to values in the aneurysm itself. Shear stress is higher in the distal area than in the aneurysms with a significantly large luminal diameter.

In contrast, FFRmyo in the distal area is within the normal range, regardless of the size or shape of the aneurysm, unless significant stenoses are present. Such findings suggest that vascular endothelial dysfunction, myocardial ischemia, and coronary microcirculation disorder due to decreased perfusion may be present in the area distal to a giant coronary aneurysm, even when significant stenosis is not present.

Hemodynamics in the Area Distal to a Stenotic Lesion

In the region distal to a coronary stenosis causing myocardial ischemia, CFR, FFRmyo, shear stress, and peripheral vascular resistance significantly differ from values obtained in a normal segment, and results outside reference ranges are obtained for many of these measurements [24]. The volume of blood perfusing this region is small, which suggests the presence of endothelial dysfunction and myocardial ischemia. Perfusion pressure is also low, but peripheral vascular resistance is rather high, as the effect of decreased blood perfusion volume is larger than that of decreased perfusion pressure in this region.

References

1. Matsuda M, Shimizu T, Oouchi H, Saito S, Kawade M, Arakaki Y, et al. Diagnosis of myocardial ischemia using body surface electrocardiographic mapping with intravenous dipyridamole in children who have a history of Kawasaki disease [in Japanese]. J Jpn Pediatr Soc. 1995;99:1618–27.
2. Takechi N, Seki T, Ohkubo T, Ogawa S. Dobutamine stress surface mapping of myocardial ischemia in Kawasaki disease. Pediatr Int. 2001;43(3):218–25. http://dx.doi.org/10.1046/j. 1442-200x.2001.01384.x PMID:11380912.
3. Takeuchi M, Matsushita A, Tsuda E, Kurotobi S, Kogaki S. Clinical assessment of ventricular late potential in children with Kawasaki disease: frequency analysis and its clinical significance [in Japanese]. Prog Med. 1994;14:1828–32.
4. Ogawa S, Nagai Y, Zhang J, Yuge K, Hino Y, Jimbo O, et al. Evaluation of myocardial ischemia and infarction by signal-averaged electrocardiographic late potentials in children with Kawasaki disease. Am J Cardiol. 1996;78(2):175–81. http://dx.doi.org/10.1016/S0002-9149(96)90392-6 PMID:8712139.
5. Genma Y, Ogawa S, Zhang J, Yamamoto M. Evaluation of myocardial ischemia in Kawasaki disease by dobutamine stress signal-averaged ventricular late potentials. Cardiovasc Res. 1997;36(3):323–9. http://dx.doi.org/10.1016/S0008-6363(97)00196-X PMID:9534852.
6. Noto N, Ayusawa M, Karasawa K, Yamaguchi H, Sumitomo N, Okada T, et al. Dobutamine stress echocardiography for detection of coronary artery stenosis in children with Kawasaki disease. J Am Coll Cardiol. 1996;27(5):1251–6. http://dx.doi.org/10.1016/0735-1097(95) 00570-6 PMID:8609352.
7. Hijazi ZM, Udelson JE, Snapper H, Rhodes J, Marx GR, Schwartz SL, et al. Physiologic significance of chronic coronary aneurysms in patients with Kawasaki disease. J Am Coll Cardiol. 1994;24(7):1633–8. http://dx.doi.org/10.1016/0735-1097(94)90167-8 PMID:7963108.
8. Paridon SM, Galioto FM, Vincent JA, Tomassoni TL, Sullivan NM, Bricker JT. Exercise capacity and incidence of myocardial perfusion defects after Kawasaki disease in children and adolescents. J Am Coll Cardiol. 1995;25(6):1420–4. http://dx.doi.org/10.1016/0735-1097(95) 00003-M PMID:7722143.
9. Miyagawa M, Mochizuki T, Murase K, Tanada S, Ikezoe J, Sekiya M, et al. Prognostic value of dipyridamole-thallium myocardial scintigraphy in patients with Kawasaki disease. Circulation. 1998;98(10):990–6. http://dx.doi.org/10.1161/01.CIR.98.10.990 PMID:9737519.
10. Kondo C, Hiroe M, Nakanishi T, Takao A. Detection of coronary artery stenosis in children with Kawasaki disease. Usefulness of pharmacologic stress 201Tl myocardial tomography. Circulation. 1989;80(3):615–24. http://dx.doi.org/10.1161/01.CIR.80.3.615 PMID:2788529.

11. Ogawa S, Fukazawa R, Ohkubo T, Zhang J, Takechi N, Kuramochi Y, et al. Silent myocardial ischemia in Kawasaki disease: evaluation of percutaneous transluminal coronary angioplasty by dobutamine stress testing. Circulation. 1997;96(10):3384–9. http://dx.doi.org/10.1161/01. CIR.96.10.3384 PMID:9396431.
12. Karasawa K, Ayusawa M, Noto N, Yamaguchi H, Okada T, Harada K. The dobutamine stress T1-201 myocardial single photon emission computed tomography for coronary artery stenosis caused by Kawasaki disease [in Japanese]. Ped Cardiol Card Surg. 1994;9:723–33.
13. Prabhu AS, Singh TP, Morrow WR, Muzik O, Di Carli MF. Safety and efficacy of intravenous adenosine for pharmacologic stress testing in children with aortic valve disease or Kawasaki disease. Am J Cardiol. 1999;83:284–6, A286. http://dx.doi.org/10.1016/S0002-9149(98) 00841-8
14. Kinoshita S, Suzuki S, Shindou A, Watanabe K, Muramatsu T, Ide M, et al. The accuracy and side effects of pharmacologic stress thallium myocardial scintigraphy with adenosine triphosphate disodium (ATP) infusion in the diagnosis of coronary artery disease [in Japanese]. Kaku Igaku. 1994;31(8):935–41. PMID:7933682.
15. Hamaoka K, Kamiya Y, Sakata K, Fukumochi Y, Ohmochi Y. Coronary reserve in children of Kawasaki disease with ischemic findings on exercise ECG and myocardial SPECT but angiographically no stenotic lesion. Evaluation of coronary hemodynamics and myocardial metabolism during atrial pacing [in Japanese]. J Jpn Pediatr Soc. 1991;95:145–51.
16. Germano G, Erel J, Lewin H, Kavanagh PB, Berman DS. Automatic quantitation of regional myocardial wall motion and thickening from gated technetium-99 m sestamibi myocardial perfusion single-photon emission computed tomography. J Am Coll Cardiol. 1997;30 (5):1360–7. http://dx.doi.org/10.1016/S0735-1097(97)00276-3 PMID:9350940.
17. Johnson LL, Verdesca SA, Aude WY, Xavier RC, Nott LT, Campanella MW, et al. Postischemic stunning can affect left ventricular ejection fraction and regional wall motion on post-stress gated sestamibi tomograms. J Am Coll Cardiol. 1997;30(7):1641–8. http://dx.doi.org/10.1016/S0735-1097(97)00388-4 PMID:9385888.
18. Ishikawa Y, Fujiwara M, Ono Y, Tsuda E, Matsubara T, Furukawa S, et al. Exercise- or dipyridamole-loaded QGS is useful to evaluate myocardial ischemia and viability in the patients with a history of Kawasaki disease. Pediatr Int. 2005;47(5):505–11. http://dx.doi. org/10.1111/j.1442-200x.2005.02102.x PMID:16190955.
19. Karasawa K, Miyashita M, Taniguchi K, Kanamaru H, Ayusawa M, Noto N, et al. Detection of myocardial contractile reserve by low-dose dobutamine quantitative gated single-photon emission computed tomography in patients with Kawasaki disease and severe coronary artery lesions. Am J Cardiol. 2003;92(7):865–8. http://dx.doi.org/10.1016/S0002-9149(03)00903-2 PMID:14516896.
20. Yamazaki J, Nishimura T, Nishimura S, Kajiya T, Kodama K, Kato K. The diagnostic value for ischemic heart disease of thallium-201 myocardial scintigraphy by intravenous infusion of SUNY4001 (adenosine) – the report of clinical trial at multi-center: phase III [in Japanese]. Kaku Igaku. 2004;41(2):133–42. PMID:15354726.
21. Ogawa S, Ohkubo T, Fukazawa R, Kamisago M, Kuramochi Y, Uchikoba Y, et al. Estimation of myocardial hemodynamics before and after intervention in children with Kawasaki disease. J Am Coll Cardiol. 2004;43(4):653–61. http://dx.doi.org/10.1016/j.jacc.2003.10.032 PMID:14975478.
22. Donohue TJ, Kern MJ, Aguirre FV, Bach RG, Wolford T, Bell CA, et al. Assessing the hemodynamic significance of coronary artery stenoses: analysis of translesional pressure-flow velocity relations in patients. J Am Coll Cardiol. 1993;22(2):449–58. http://dx.doi.org/10. 1016/0735-1097(93)90049-7 PMID:8335814.
23. Pijls NH, van Son JA, Kirkeeide RL, De Bruyne B, Gould KL. Experimental basis of determining maximum coronary, myocardial, and collateral blood flow by pressure measurements for assessing functional stenosis severity before and after percutaneous transluminal coronary angioplasty. Circulation. 1993;87(4):1354–67. http://dx.doi.org/10.1161/01.CIR.87. 4.1354 PMID:8462157.
24. Ogawa S. Rheologic and hemodynamic characteristics of coronary arteries [in Japanese]. J Jpn Pediatr Soc. 2009;113:1769–78.

Promising Biomarkers in Acute Kawasaki Disease and Acute Coronary Ischemia

Ryuji Fukazawa

Abstract There are no specific biomarkers to confirm a diagnosis of Kawasaki disease (KD) or predict nonresponse to immunoglobulin therapy (IVIG) or development of coronary artery lesions (CAL). Among the many abnormal laboratory findings in acute KD, only some biomarkers are useful for diagnosis, assessment of the risk of IVIG nonresponse, and determining the likelihood of CAL formation. Instead of a single marker, characteristic profiles may be examined. High levels of C-reactive protein (CRP), pentraxin-3, serum amyloid A, urinary beta microglobulin, brain natriuretic protein (BNP), and N-type (NT)-pro BNP and low serum albumin and sodium levels are together suggestive of KD and a high likelihood of IVIG nonresponse and CAL formation. In addition, levels of many inflammatory cytokines are elevated in acute KD. Simultaneous evaluation of multiple cytokines has recently become possible. Some characteristic cytokine expression patterns for auto-inflammatory diseases such as KD, systemic juvenile arteritis, and periodic fever syndrome have been described. An IL-6–dominant cytokine profile pattern is characteristic of KD, and cytokine profiling is promising in KD diagnosis. However, several days are required to obtain the results of these tests, and this is a significant drawback for a potential biomarker. There are, however, reliable biomarkers for detecting myocardial injury. Creatine kinase (CK), CK-MB, myoglobin, heart-type fatty acid–binding protein, myocardial troponin I and T, and myosin light chain are established markers of myocardial injury in adults and can be also be used in the assessment of children. Myocardial infarction without specific symptoms sometimes occurs in children. In such cases, cytokine markers are useful for detecting early myocardial infarction. Although no specific biomarkers are present for KD, some characteristic overall laboratory findings are useful for clinical decision-making and are considered relevant biomarkers. To select appropriate treatment strategies, it is important to assess a patient's condition by incorporating multiple laboratory findings with physical findings.

R. Fukazawa, M.D. (✉)
Department of Pediatrics, Nippon Medical School, 1-1-5 Sendagi, Bunkyo-ku, Tokyo 113-8603, Japan
e-mail: oraora@nms.ac.jp

© Springer Japan 2017
B.T. Saji et al. (eds.), *Kawasaki Disease*, DOI 10.1007/978-4-431-56039-5_35

311

Keywords Biomarker • Immunoglobulin therapy nonresponse • Risk scoring •
Coronary artery lesions • Myocardial infarction

Introduction

Kawasaki disease (KD) is a systemic vasculitis that often affects midsized arteries.
This is important, as severe coronary arteritis can lead to coronary artery lesions
(CALs). Research has focused on minimizing CAL formation and identifying
additional biomarkers that predict immunoglobulin therapy (IVIG) nonresponse,
CAL formation, vasculitis severity, and early atherosclerosis progression. Although
the cause of KD is unknown, and there are no specific biomarkers for KD diagnosis,
some characteristic laboratory findings, including cytokine evaluation, are helpful
for diagnosis. While diagnostic biomarkers are not entirely specific or infallible,
comprehensive evaluation of biomarkers might be a reliable clinical diagnostic
method. This chapter describes biomarkers that are clinically helpful in diagnosing
acute KD and acute coronary ischemia.

Predicting Nonresponse to Immunoglobulin Therapy

IVIG is the most effective standard treatment for acute KD. Unfortunately, 20–30 %
of patients do not respond to IVIG, and CALs are likely to develop among these
patients. Predicting nonresponse to IVIG is very important in designing an effective
individualized KD treatment strategy, but there is no specific biomarker that predicts IVIG nonresponse. Instead, Japanese researchers have established scoring
systems that use laboratory data and clinical findings of KD. The Egami score
[1], Sano score [2], and Kobayashi score [3] all attempt to predict nonresponse to
IVIG by stratifying patients according to the risk of nonresponse (Table 1). Total
scores greater than 2, 1, or 4, respectively, indicate high risk of IVIG nonresponse.
Using these criteria, clinicians select combined therapy with steroid and IVIG for
treatment of high-risk KD, and this regimen has proven effective for preventing
CAL formation [4, 5]. The sensitivity and specificity of these scoring systems are
75–80 %, and these values are reproducible in the Japanese population. In North
America, however, the sensitivity and specificity of the Kobayashi score are 33 %
and 87 %, respectively [6]. Thus, it is unclear whether these scoring systems can be
used in non-Japanese populations. One potential factor, "day of treatment start",
depends on the medical and insurance systems in the country. This variation may
increase the range of error in these point-scoring systems. Clearly, a more accurate
and objective scoring system is necessary in order to standardize prediction of IVIG
nonresponse.

Table 1 Scoring systems used to predict IVIG nonresponse

Kobayashi score (cutoff: ≥5 points; sensitivity 76 %, specificity 80 %)

	Threshold	Points
Na	≤133 mmol/l	2
AST	≥100 IU/l	2
Day of treatment start (or diagnosis)	Day 4 of illness or earlier	2
Neutrophils	≥80 %	2
CRP	≥10 mg/dl	1
Platelet count	≤300,000/μl	1
Age	≤12 months	1

Egami score (cutoff: ≥3 points; sensitivity 76 %, specificity 80 %)

	Threshold	Points
ALT	≥80 IU/l	2
Day of treatment start (or diagnosis)	Day 4 of illness or earlier	1
CRP	≥8 mg/dl	1
Platelet count	≤300,000/μl	1
Age	≤6 months	1

Sano score (cutoff: ≥2 points; sensitivity 77 %, specificity 86 %)

	Threshold	Points
AST	≥200 IU/l	1
Total bilirubin	≥0.9 mg/dl	1
CRP	≥7 mg/dl	1

Kobayashi, Egami, and Sano scores of ≥5, ≥3, and ≥2, respectively, indicate potential IVIG nonresponse

AST aspartate aminotransferase, *CRP* C-reactive protein, *ALT* alanine aminotransferase

Diagnosis and Evaluation of the Severity and Likelihood of CAL Formation in KD

Inflammatory Proteins

CRP

CRP is markedly elevated at KD onset, and levels decrease with clinical improvement. The liver produces CRP, which is largely induced by inflammatory cytokines such as tumor necrosis factor-alpha (TNF-α) and interleukin (IL)-6. CRP level reflects the severity of KD vasculitis, and a high CRP level suggests greater risk of CAL formation.

Pentraxin-3 (PTX3)

Structurally in the same family as CRP and serum amyloid protein, PTX3 is produced locally at the inflammation site by endothelial cells, macrophages, fibroblasts, smooth muscle cells, and dendritic cells and activates leukocytes. PTX3 is a promising biomarker of vascular damage, like that observed in vasculitis [7] and other cardiovascular diseases [8]. Preliminary findings suggest that it is a good biomarker for predicting IVIG nonresponse and CAL formation.

Serum Amyloid A (SAA)

SAA is an acute inflammatory protein produced by endothelium. It catalyzes high-density lipoprotein cholesterol into apolipoprotein A-1. SAA levels are significantly higher in patients with acute and chronic KD [9, 10].

General Laboratory Variables

Total Protein and Albumin

Although total protein levels are almost normal or slightly decreased at KD onset, serum albumin levels decrease because of increased vascular permeability caused by vasculitis. In addition, IL-6 depresses albumin synthesis in liver. A lower serum albumin level reflects severe vasculitis and is regarded as a risk factor in CAL formation.

Serum Transaminase

Increased aspartate aminotransferase (AST) and alanine aminotransferase (ALT) levels are often observed in acute KD. Extremely high levels (>500 IU/L) are rare, and AST and ALT return to normal levels within 2–3 weeks in most patients. High AST is considered a strong risk factor for IVIG nonresponse and is used to predict IVIG nonresponse in the 3 scoring systems described above.

Serum Electrolyte

Serum sodium level decreases in severe KD. A low sodium level is thought to reflect increased vascular permeability due to vasculitis and is regarded as a risk factor for IVIG nonresponse and CAL formation.

Urinary Beta-2 Microglobulin (u-β2MG)

Levels of u-β2MG are thought to reflect serum cytokine level. Interferon gamma (INF-γ) induces HLA class I molecules on endothelial cell surfaces, causing overtranscription of HLA class I L chain or u-β2MG. Overproduction of BMG increases u-β2MG levels. A high u-β2MG level suggests hypercytokinemia and is useful for KD diagnosis.

Brain Natriuretic Peptide (BNP) and N-Terminal proBNP (NT-proBNP)

BNP is a diuretic peptide secreted mainly from cardiac ventricles. Levels of BNP and its N-terminal moiety, NT-proBNP, are thought to reflect ventricular dysfunction. Levels of BNP and NT-proBNP are elevated in acute KD, despite preservation of global left ventricular function. Severe coronary inflammation and increased vascular permeability may contribute to these elevations. Some reports suggest that NT-proBNP is more useful than BNP as a biomarker in the diagnosis of KD and incomplete KD and in identifying potential IVIG nonresponse [11–13].

An important aspect of biomarkers is their sensitivity and specificity for determining the risk of developing a given KD type. Another important feature of successful biomarkers is the speed with which results can be obtained. Physicians select a treatment strategy according to the patient's risk. Treatment for acute KD should not be delayed by the need to wait for examination results; ideally, biomarker examination results should be available within a few hours. Unfortunately, there is no rapid diagnosis kit for some of the above-described markers, such as PTX3 or SAA. However, because PTX3 and SAA are promising markers, development of rapid diagnosis kits for these markers is expected.

Inflammatory Cytokines

Almost all inflammatory cytokines are elevated during acute KD; hence, KD is sometimes called a "cytokine storm" disease. Among cytokines, TNF-α, IL-1, IL-6, IL-8, MCP-1, G-CSF, M-CSF and IP-10 are particularly elevated in acute KD [14–17] and are indicative of vasculitis and CAL formation.

Cytokine storm is a characteristic of many autoinflammatory diseases, including KD, systemic juvenile rheumatoid arthritis (sJRA), and periodic fever syndrome. The symptoms of KD and sJRA are very similar, and differential diagnosis is thus sometimes difficult. Almost all inflammatory cytokines are similarly elevated in KD and sJRA. Currently, more than 30 types of cytokines can be evaluated simultaneously. Because cytokine profiles are characteristic of certain autoinflammatory diseases, they can be very useful in differential diagnoses. According to cytokine profiling, IL-6 elevation is dominant in KD, and IL-18 elevation is dominant in sJRA [18]. Thus, multiple cytokines should be examined in order to accurately diagnose KD.

Currently, the most difficult aspect of evaluating cytokine levels for KD diagnosis is that it takes several days to 1 week to obtain results. Because KD is an acute disease, cytokine profiling is the decisive criterion for treatment. Despite the time

Table 2 Blood biochemical markers of myocardial infarction

Marker	Clinical use	Limitations
CK-MB	Principal biochemical marker; can be used as standard test at almost all institutions	Low myocardial specificity
		Low detection rate within 6 h after onset
Myoglobin	Because of poor myocardial specificity, AMI cannot be diagnosed with myoglobin alone	Poor myocardial specificity
		No use for diagnosis of late MI after AMI onset
H-FABP	Rapid test kits are available and useful in early diagnosis	Highly sensitive for early AMI diagnosis, but specificity relatively low
TnT	High sensitivity and specificity	Sensitivity low within 6 h after onset
	Rapid test kits available; TnT is a principal biochemical marker	Sensitivity for late-onset small reinfarction is low
MLC	Rapid diagnostic tests not available	Sensitivity relatively low
		MLC level may be abnormal in patients with renal failure

CK-MB creatine kinase-MB, *H-FABP* heart-type fatty acid binding protein, *TnT* troponin T, *MLC* myosin light chain

lag, comprehensive evaluation of cytokines is essential in the diagnosis and treatment of patients with an ambiguous presentation suggestive of KD.

Acute Coronary Ischemia

There are no baseline biomarker values for children at risk for severe coronary ischemia or myocardial infarction. Instead, adult values are used. Biochemical biomarkers for diagnosing myocardial injury are myocardial cytoplasm type (creatine kinase [CK], CK-MB, myoglobin, heart-type fatty acid–binding protein [H-FABP]) and myocardial structural protein type (myocardial troponin T and I [TnT and TnI] and myosin light chain [MLC]). In children, myocardial infarction sometimes occurs without specific symptoms. These biomarkers are very helpful in detecting myocardial infarction from the early phase of onset, in the absence of other clinical signs (Table 2).

Markers in Myocardial Cytoplasm

CK and CK-MB

CK and CK-MB levels increase during the 4–6 h after myocardial infarction and normalize within 2–3 days. CK and CK-MB levels strongly correlate with the extent of myocardial necrosis. Furthermore, CK-MB is a useful indicator of myo-cardial reperfusion and reinfarction and is the marker of choice for assessing myocardial damage [19]. Among CK-MB isoforms, increases in CK-MB2 and MB2/MB1 ratio may be detected within 4 h after onset of myocardial infarction. CK-MB levels are also elevated in skeletal muscle diseases, however, and are less specific for the diagnosis of myocardial infarction.

Myoglobin

Myoglobin levels increase during the 1–2 h after onset of myocardial infarction, reach their peak in about 10 h, and normalize within 1–2 days. Myoglobin is useful for early diagnosis of myocardial infarction and is a good indicator of reperfusion. However, it is not specific to the myocardium, as it is present in all skeletal muscle.

H-FABP

H-FABP level increases during the 1–2 h after onset of myocardial damage and is useful in early diagnosis of myocardial infarction, estimation of infarct size, and detection of reperfusion. The cutoff level for diagnosis of myocardial infarction is 6.2 ng/ml [20].

Myocardial Structural Proteins as Markers

TnT and TnI

The biomarkers TnT and TnI are specific to the myocardium, reach peak levels at 12–18 h and 90–120 h, respectively, after onset of myocardial infarction, and may be used as markers of reperfusion. TnT is a highly sensitive and specific marker for detecting onset of myocardial infarction and is useful in the diagnosis and prog-nostic assessment of non-ST elevation myocardial infarction. In a whole-blood rapid assay for TnT, a positive test is defined as a level ≥ 0.10 ng/ml. When a negative result is obtained within 6 h after onset of symptoms, the test should be repeated 8–12 h after onset to ensure absence of myocardial infarction

MLC

Plasma MLC level reflects the process of myofibrillar necrosis. Increased MLC levels are detected in blood at 4–6 h after onset, reach a peak level in 2–5 days, and remain high for 7–14 days. Tests for both MLC1 and MLC2 are available. The cutoff level for acute myocardial infarction is 2.5 ng/ml. Peak MLC1 level reflects infarct size, and a result of ≥ 20 ng/ml is defined as major infarction [21].

The characteristics of the above-mentioned markers indicate that myoglobin and H-FABP are useful in detecting early myocardial infarction, and that CK-MB and TnT are beneficial in diagnosing myocardial infarction ≥ 6 h after onset. The primary markers for acute myocardial infarction are CK-MB and TnT.

References

1. Egami K, Muta H, Ishii M, Suda K, Sugahara Y, Iemura M, et al. Prediction of resistance to intravenous immunoglobulin treatment in patients with Kawasaki disease. J Pediatr. 2006;149 (2):237–40. http://dx.doi.org/10.1016/j.jpeds.2006.03.050 PMID:16887442.
2. Sano T, Kurotobi S, Matsuzaki K, Yamamoto T, Maki I, Miki K, et al. Prediction of non-responsiveness to standard high-dose gamma-globulin therapy in patients with acute Kawasaki disease before starting initial treatment. Eur J Pediatr. 2007;166(2):131–7. http://dx.doi.org/ 10.1007/s00431-006-0223-z PMID:16896641.
3. Kobayashi T, Inoue Y, Takeuchi K, Okada Y, Tamura K, Tomomasa T, et al. Prediction of intravenous immunoglobulin unresponsiveness in patients with Kawasaki disease. Circulation. 2006;113(22):2606–12. http://dx.doi.org/10.1161/CIRCULATIONAHA.105.592865 PMID:16735679.
4. Kobayashi T, Saji T, Otani T, Takeuchi K, Nakamura T, Arakawa H, et al. RAISE study group investigators. Efficacy of immunoglobulin plus prednisolone for prevention of coronary artery abnormalities in severe Kawasaki disease (RAISE study): a randomised, open-label, blinded-endpoints trial. Lancet. 2012;379(9826):1613–20. http://dx.doi.org/10.1016/S0140-6736(11) 61930-2 PMID:22405251.
5. Ogata S, Ogihara Y, Honda T, Kon S, Akiyama K, Ishii M. Corticosteroid pulse combination therapy for refractory Kawasaki disease: a randomized trial. Pediatrics. 2012;129(1):e17–23. http://dx.doi.org/10.1542/peds.2011-0148 PMID:22144699.
6. Sleeper LA, Minich LL, McCrindle BM, Li JS, Mason W, Colan SD, et al., Pediatric Heart Network Investigators. Evaluation of Kawasaki disease risk-scoring systems for intravenous immunoglobulin resistance. J Pediatr. 2011;158(5):831–5.e3. http://dx.doi.org/10.1016/j. jpeds.2010.10.031 PMID:21168857.
7. Monach PA. Biomarkers in vasculitis. Curr Opin Rheumatol. 2014;26(1):24–30. http://dx.doi. org/10.1097/BOR.0000000000000009 PMID:24257367.
8. Bonacina F, Baragetti A, Catapano AL, Norata GD. Long pentraxin 3: experimental and clinical relevance in cardiovascular diseases. Mediat Inflamm. 2013;2013:725102.
9. Cabana VG, Gidding SS, Getz GS, Chapman J, Shulman ST. Serum amyloid A and high density lipoprotein participate in the acute phase response of Kawasaki disease. Pediatr Res. 1997;42(5):651–5. http://dx.doi.org/10.1203/00006450-199711000-00017 PMID:9357939.
10. Mitani Y, Sawada H, Hayakawa H, Aoki K, Ohashi H, Matsumura M, et al. Elevated levels of high-sensitivity C-reactive protein and serum amyloid-A late after Kawasaki disease: association between inflammation and late coronary sequelae in Kawasaki disease. Circulation. 2005;111 (1):38–43. http://dx.doi.org/10.1161/01.CIR.0000151311.38708.29 PMID:15611368.
11. Iwashima S, Ishikawa T. B-type natriuretic peptide and N-terminal pro-BNP in the acute phase of Kawasaki disease. World J Pediatr. 2013;9(3):239–44. http://dx.doi.org/10.1007/s12519-013-0402-8 PMID:23335186.
12. Dahdah N, Siles A, Fournier A, Cousineau J, Delvin E, Saint-Cyr C, et al. Natriuretic peptide as an adjunctive diagnostic test in the acute phase of Kawasaki disease. Pediatr Cardiol. 2009;30(6):810–17. http://dx.doi.org/10.1007/s00246-009-9441-2 PMID:19365652.

13. McNeal-Davidson A, Fournier A, Spigelblatt L, Saint-Cyr C, Mir TS, Nir A, et al. Value of amino-terminal pro B-natriuretic peptide in diagnosing Kawasaki disease. Pediatr Int. 2012;54 (5):627–33. http://dx.doi.org/10.1111/j.1442-200X.2012.03609.x PMID:22414326.

14. Suzuki H, Uemura S, Tone S, Iizuka T, Koike M, Hirayama K, et al. Effects of immunoglobulin and gamma-interferon on the production of tumour necrosis factor-alpha and interleukin-1 beta by peripheral blood monocytes in the acute phase of Kawasaki disease. Eur J Pediatr. 1996;155(4):291–6. http://dx.doi.org/10.1007/BF02002715 PMID:8777922.

15. Furukawa S, Matsubara T, Jujoh K, Yone K, Sugawara T, Sasai K, et al. Peripheral blood monocyte/macrophages and serum tumor necrosis factor in Kawasaki disease. Clin Immunol Immunopathol.   1988;48(2):247–51.   http://dx.doi.org/10.1016/0090-1229(88)90088-8 PMID:3390972.

16. Lin CY, Lin CC, Hwang B, Chiang B. Serial changes of serum interleukin-6, interleukin-8, and tumor necrosis factor alpha among patients with Kawasaki disease. J Pediatr. 1992;121 (6):924–6. http://dx.doi.org/10.1016/S0022-3476(05)80343-9 PMID:1447658.

17. Ko T, Kuo H, Chang J, Chen S, Liu Y, Chen H, et al. CXCL10/IP-10 is a biomarker and mediator for Kawasaki disease. Circ Res. 2015;116:876–83.

18. Shimizu M, Yokoyama T, Yamada K, Kaneda H, Wada H, Wada T, et al. Distinct cytokine profiles of systemic-onset juvenile idiopathic arthritis-associated macrophage activation syndrome with particular emphasis on the role of interleukin-18 in its pathogenesis. Rheumatology (Oxford). 2010;49(9):1645–53. http://dx.doi.org/10.1093/rheumatology/keq133 PMID:20472718.

19. Alpert JS, Thygesen K, Antman E, Bassand JP. Myocardial infarction redefined – a consensus document of The Joint European Society of Cardiology/American College of Cardiology Committee for the redefinition of myocardial infarction. J Am Coll Cardiol. 2000;36 (3):959–69. http://dx.doi.org/10.1016/S0735-1097(00)00804-4 PMID:10987628.

20. Okamoto F, Sohmiya K, Ohkaru Y, Kawamura K, Asayama K, Kimura H, et al. Human heart-type cytoplasmic fatty acid-binding protein (H-FABP) for the diagnosis of acute myocardial infarction. Clinical evaluation of H-FABP in comparison with myoglobin and creatine kinase isoenzyme MB. Clin Chem Lab Med. 2000;38(3):231–8. http://dx.doi.org/10.1515/CCLM. 2000.034 PMID:10905760.

21. Isobe M, Nagai R, Ueda S, Tsuchimochi H, Nakaoka H, Takaku F, et al. Quantitative relationship between left ventricular function and serum cardiac myosin light chain I levels after coronary reperfusion in patients with acute myocardial infarction. Circulation. 1987;76 (6):1251–61. http://dx.doi.org/10.1161/01.CIR.76.6.1251 PMID:3677350.

Coronary Artery Diameter Z Score Calculator

Shigeto Fuse

Abstract The author has developed accurate coronary artery diameter Z score curves and a Z score calculator for children. The figures and tables show Z scores for males and females. Z scores should be used in the assessment and treatment of coronary artery dilatation and aneurysms in Kawasaki disease.

Keywords Coronary artery • Z score • LMS method • Kawasaki disease • Children

Introduction

For more than 30 years, researchers have been attempting to determine normal coronary artery diameter in children and to develop quantitative criteria for assessing dilatation and aneurysm in coronary arteries of Kawasaki disease (KD) patients. However, curves for normal coronary artery diameter in growing children are extremely difficult to produce, both theoretically and technically. Fortunately, progress in statistical techniques has enabled development of precise and clinically useful normal curves and a Z score calculator.

History

Kamiya et al. (1983) were pioneers in developing dilatation criteria on echocardiography for coronary arteries in KD patients. They wrote that:

> although quantitative measurement of dilated lesions is desirable, sufficient data on echocardiographic measurements of normal coronary artery size are not available at this time. For the time being...an increase in coronary internal diameter to more than 1.5 times the adjacent vessel diameter should be considered a dilated lesion. For children under 5 years of age, coronary arteries with a diameter of 3 mm or greater should be regarded as dilated lesion. [1]

S. Fuse (✉)

Department of Pediatrics, NTT Sapporo Medical Center, South 1 West 15, Chuo-ku, Sapporo, Hokkaido 060-0061, Japan

e-mail: shigeto_fuse@east.ntt.co.jp

© Springer Japan 2017

B.T. Saji et al. (eds.), *Kawasaki Disease*, DOI 10.1007/978-4-431-56039-5_36

It was difficult to develop curves for normal coronary artery diameter in growing children. There were problems with the spatial resolution of echo devices, echocardiographic techniques, and the statistical methods used to create curves of normal values.

Arjunan et al. [2] studied the calibers of right and left coronary arteries in 42 normal subjects and 68 KD patients in 6 age groups and noted that coronary artery caliber ranged from 2 mm in infants to 5 mm in teenagers. Oberhoffer et al. [3] found a relation between right coronary artery (RCA) and left coronary artery (LCA) diameters and age, height, and weight in 100 healthy children. Dajani et al. [4] noted that normal coronary artery size was 1–2 mm in newborns and infants and 4.5–5.0 mm in teenagers. Durongpisikul et al. [5] proposed that dilatation be defined as a diameter of at least 3 mm in children younger than 5 years and 4 mm in children aged 5 years or older.

De Zorzi et al. [6] were the first to use Z scores to evaluate coronary artery dilatation. They used linear regression models to analyze the association between coronary artery diameter and body surface area (BSA) in 89 subjects. Kurotobi et al. [7] also used linear regression analysis of the association between coronary artery diameter and BSA in 71 healthy children. Tan et al. [8] used linear regression analysis of age and BSA in 214 males and 176 females. Newburger et al. [9] suggested that coronary artery Z scores be incorporated into recommendations regarding evaluation and treatment of KD and provided Z score curves of 2 and 3 standard deviations (SD) according to BSA. Newburger et al. [10] used a coronary artery Z score of 2.5 or more for the RCA and left anterior descending coronary artery as part of diagnostic inclusion criteria in their clinical study of KD.

McCrindle et al. [11] produced the first exponential regression equations, and the associated SDs of the predicted value were obtained by solving the second linear regression equation based on BSA from 221 healthy children. Olivieri et al. [12] developed an exponential approximation model incorporating BSA in 432 echocardiographically normal subjects. They also developed an equation for Z score calculation. Using the LMS method, Fuse et al. [13] generated smoothing Z score curves with age and BSA [14] that adequately fit skewed distribution data from 544 healthy children. Using the square root model, Dallaire and Dahdah [15] developed equations for Z score calculation with BSA from 1033 echocardiographic studies.

Recent Advances

The author and colleagues designed and conducted a multicenter prospective study to develop highly reliable normal and Z score curves. To reduce error caused by echocardiographic measurement, standard methods of echocardiographic measurement of coronary arteries were established [16] and pediatric cardiologists and sonographers were trained to evaluate coronary artery diameter (CAD). All observers were then subject to quality control of CAD measurement. Sample sizes were calculated to yield groups large enough to create +2SD curves with CAD and BSA. BSA was classified into 15 classes per 0.1 m^2 (range, 0.2–1.6 m^2). Each BSA class required at least 50 samples because the probability frequency over 2SD in the normal distribution is 2.3 %. Minimal sample size was set at 750 (50 × 15 classes), and the target size with a margin was 1500 for both males and females. In total, 2078 males and 1773 females were evaluated. The distribution of biological measurements is usually skewed from a normal distribution. We adopted the LMS method to create Z score curves with CAD and BSA. The LMS method can transform a skewed distribution to a normal distribution and create statistically accurate Z curves. Figure 1 and Tables 36.1 and 36.2 show Z score curves and CAD according to Z score and BSA.

Coronary Artery Diameter Z Score Calculator

Kobayashi et al. created a ready-to-use Microsoft Excel-based Z score calculator to enable straightforward clinical use by physicians (http://raise.umin.jp/zsp/calcula tor/). This calculator can calculate Z scores using a formula by Kobayashi et al. or a new Z score formula. Furthermore, the calculator yields median coronary artery diameter (Z score = 0) and ratio, ie, the measurement value divided by the median.

Meaning of Coronary Artery Diameter Z Scores

A Z score represents the frequency distribution in a population. The frequencies of Z scores >2, >2.5, and >3 are 2.3 %, 0.62 %, and 0.13 %, respectively. The frequency of a Z score greater than 2 or 3 does not mean that these scores are abnormal or unusually large. We should carefully determine the criteria for abnormally large CAD, to obtain consensus. These criteria depend on the purpose of assessment and clinical needs, such as early diagnosis of KD or prognosis prediction for coronary artery aneurysm, ie, determining criteria or guidelines for using Z score to assess dilatation and aneurysm.

In KD, CAD expansion results from pathologic damage to reinforcing structures by coronary arterial pressure. Greater damage to the coronary artery during acute KD results in greater dilatation of CAD. Accurate evaluation of dilatation must reflect the severity of coronary arteritis caused by KD. In the future, CAD Z score might have a role as a marker of coronary arteritis severity.

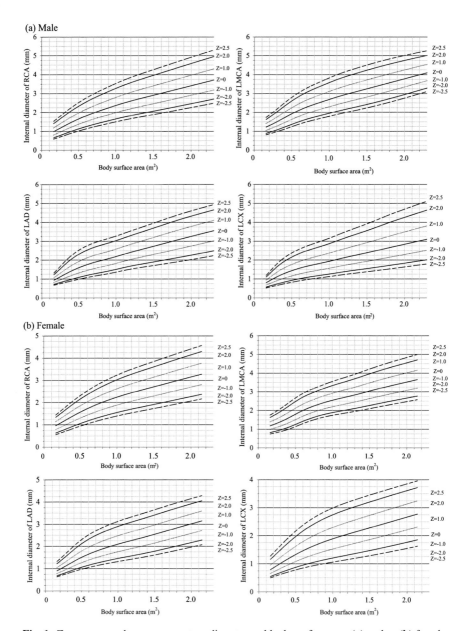

Fig. 1 Z score curves by coronary artery diameter and body surface area (**a**) males, (**b**) females *RCA* proximal right coronary artery, *LMCA* left main coronary artery, *LAD* proximal left anterior descending artery, *LCX* proximal left circumflex artery

Table 36.1 Coronary artery diameter according to Z score and BSA, males

(A) Proximal right coronary artery (mm)

BSA (m²)	Z = −2.5	Z = −2.0	Z = −1.0	Z = 0	Z = 1.0	Z = 2.0	Z = 2.5
0.15	0.59	0.65	0.81	0.98	1.18	1.40	1.52
0.20	0.65	0.73	0.90	1.09	1.31	1.55	1.69
0.25	0.71	0.79	0.96	1.17	1.40	1.67	1.81
0.30	0.77	0.86	1.05	1.27	1.52	1.81	1.96
0.35	0.83	0.93	1.14	1.37	1.64	1.95	2.11
0.40	0.90	1.00	1.22	1.47	1.76	2.08	2.25
0.45	0.96	1.06	1.30	1.56	1.87	2.21	2.39
0.50	1.02	1.13	1.37	1.65	1.97	2.33	2.52
0.55	1.07	1.19	1.45	1.74	2.07	2.44	2.65
0.60	1.13	1.25	1.52	1.82	2.17	2.55	2.76
0.65	1.18	1.30	1.58	1.90	2.26	2.66	2.87
0.70	1.23	1.36	1.65	1.97	2.34	2.75	2.98
0.75	1.28	1.41	1.71	2.04	2.42	2.85	3.08
0.80	1.32	1.46	1.77	2.11	2.50	2.94	3.17
0.85	1.37	1.51	1.82	2.18	2.58	3.02	3.27
0.90	1.41	1.56	1.88	2.24	2.65	3.11	3.36
0.95	1.46	1.61	1.94	2.31	2.72	3.19	3.45
1.00	1.50	1.65	1.99	2.37	2.80	3.27	3.53
1.05	1.54	1.70	2.04	2.43	2.87	3.35	3.62
1.10	1.59	1.75	2.10	2.49	2.94	3.43	3.70
1.15	1.63	1.79	2.15	2.55	3.00	3.51	3.78
1.20	1.67	1.83	2.20	2.61	3.07	3.58	3.85
1.25	1.71	1.87	2.24	2.66	3.13	3.65	3.93
1.30	1.74	1.91	2.29	2.71	3.19	3.71	4.00
1.35	1.78	1.95	2.33	2.76	3.24	3.78	4.07
1.40	1.82	1.99	2.38	2.81	3.30	3.84	4.14
1.45	1.85	2.03	2.42	2.86	3.36	3.91	4.20
1.50	1.89	2.07	2.47	2.91	3.41	3.97	4.27
1.55	1.92	2.11	2.51	2.96	3.47	4.03	4.33
1.60	1.96	2.15	2.55	3.01	3.52	4.09	4.40
1.65	2.00	2.19	2.60	3.06	3.58	4.15	4.46
1.70	2.03	2.22	2.64	3.11	3.63	4.22	4.53
1.75	2.07	2.26	2.69	3.16	3.69	4.28	4.59
1.80	2.11	2.30	2.73	3.21	3.75	4.34	4.66

(B) Left main coronary artery (mm)

BSA (m²)	Z = −2.5	Z = −2.0	Z = −1.0	Z = 0	Z = 1.0	Z = 2.0	Z = 2.5
0.15	0.81	0.89	1.05	1.22	1.41	1.62	1.73
0.20	0.86	0.94	1.11	1.30	1.51	1.73	1.86
0.25	0.91	1.00	1.19	1.39	1.62	1.87	2.01
0.30	0.97	1.07	1.27	1.49	1.74	2.02	2.16
0.35	1.04	1.14	1.36	1.60	1.87	2.17	2.33

(continued)

Table 36.1 (continued)

(B) Left main coronary artery (mm)

BSA (m^2)	Z = −2.5	Z = −2.0	Z = −1.0	Z = 0	Z = 1.0	Z = 2.0	Z = 2.5
0.40	1.10	1.21	1.45	1.71	2.00	2.32	2.49
0.45	1.17	1.29	1.54	1.82	2.12	2.46	2.65
0.50	1.24	1.36	1.63	1.92	2.24	2.60	2.79
0.55	1.31	1.44	1.71	2.02	2.36	2.73	2.93
0.60	1.38	1.51	1.79	2.11	2.46	2.85	3.06
0.65	1.44	1.57	1.87	2.20	2.56	2.96	3.18
0.70	1.50	1.64	1.94	2.28	2.66	3.07	3.29
0.75	1.55	1.69	2.01	2.36	2.74	3.16	3.39
0.80	1.60	1.75	2.07	2.43	2.82	3.25	3.48
0.85	1.65	1.80	2.13	2.49	2.89	3.33	3.57
0.90	1.70	1.85	2.19	2.56	2.97	3.42	3.66
0.95	1.74	1.90	2.24	2.62	3.04	3.50	3.74
1.00	1.79	1.95	2.30	2.69	3.11	3.58	3.83
1.05	1.84	2.00	2.36	2.75	3.18	3.66	3.91
1.10	1.89	2.05	2.41	2.81	3.25	3.73	3.99
1.15	1.93	2.10	2.47	2.87	3.32	3.81	4.07
1.20	1.98	2.15	2.52	2.93	3.38	3.87	4.14
1.25	2.02	2.20	2.57	2.99	3.44	3.94	4.20
1.30	2.07	2.24	2.62	3.04	3.50	4.00	4.27
1.35	2.11	2.29	2.67	3.09	3.56	4.06	4.33
1.40	2.15	2.33	2.72	3.15	3.61	4.12	4.39
1.45	2.20	2.38	2.77	3.20	3.67	4.18	4.45
1.50	2.24	2.43	2.82	3.25	3.72	4.24	4.51
1.55	2.29	2.47	2.87	3.31	3.78	4.29	4.57
1.60	2.34	2.52	2.92	3.36	3.83	4.35	4.62
1.65	2.39	2.57	2.97	3.41	3.89	4.40	4.68
1.70	2.44	2.63	3.03	3.46	3.94	4.46	4.73
1.75	2.49	2.68	3.08	3.52	3.99	4.51	4.78
1.80	2.54	2.73	3.13	3.57	4.05	4.56	4.83

(C) Proximal left anterior descending artery (mm)

BSA (m^2)	Z = −2.5	Z = −2.0	Z = −1.0	Z = 0	Z = 1.0	Z = 2.0	Z = 2.5
0.15	0.67	0.71	0.81	0.93	1.07	1.22	1.31
0.20	0.71	0.76	0.88	1.02	1.18	1.37	1.48
0.25	0.76	0.82	0.96	1.12	1.32	1.55	1.68
0.30	0.80	0.87	1.04	1.23	1.46	1.73	1.88
0.35	0.85	0.93	1.11	1.33	1.59	1.89	2.07
0.40	0.89	0.98	1.18	1.42	1.71	2.04	2.24
0.45	0.94	1.03	1.25	1.51	1.82	2.18	2.39
0.50	0.98	1.08	1.32	1.59	1.92	2.31	2.52
0.55	1.02	1.13	1.38	1.67	2.01	2.41	2.64
0.60	1.07	1.18	1.44	1.74	2.10	2.51	2.74

(continued)

Table 36.1 (continued)

(C) Proximal left anterior descending artery (mm)

BSA (m²)	Z = −2.5	Z = −2.0	Z = −1.0	Z = 0	Z = 1.0	Z = 2.0	Z = 2.5
0.65	1.10	1.22	1.49	1.81	2.17	2.59	2.83
0.70	1.14	1.27	1.54	1.87	2.24	2.67	2.91
0.75	1.18	1.30	1.59	1.92	2.30	2.73	2.97
0.80	1.21	1.34	1.63	1.97	2.36	2.79	3.03
0.85	1.24	1.38	1.68	2.02	2.41	2.85	3.09
0.90	1.28	1.42	1.72	2.07	2.47	2.91	3.15
0.95	1.32	1.46	1.77	2.13	2.52	2.97	3.21
1.00	1.36	1.50	1.82	2.18	2.58	3.03	3.27
1.05	1.40	1.55	1.87	2.24	2.65	3.09	3.34
1.10	1.44	1.59	1.93	2.30	2.71	3.16	3.40
1.15	1.48	1.64	1.98	2.36	2.77	3.23	3.47
1.20	1.52	1.68	2.03	2.42	2.84	3.30	3.54
1.25	1.56	1.72	2.08	2.47	2.90	3.37	3.61
1.30	1.59	1.76	2.12	2.52	2.96	3.43	3.68
1.35	1.62	1.79	2.17	2.58	3.02	3.50	3.75
1.40	1.65	1.83	2.21	2.63	3.08	3.56	3.82
1.45	1.68	1.86	2.26	2.68	3.14	3.63	3.89
1.50	1.71	1.90	2.30	2.73	3.20	3.70	3.96
1.55	1.74	1.93	2.34	2.79	3.26	3.76	4.02
1.60	1.77	1.97	2.39	2.84	3.32	3.83	4.09
1.65	1.80	2.00	2.43	2.89	3.38	3.89	4.16
1.70	1.83	2.04	2.48	2.94	3.44	3.96	4.23
1.75	1.86	2.07	2.52	3.00	3.50	4.02	4.29
1.80	1.89	2.11	2.57	3.05	3.56	4.08	4.36

(D) Proximal left circumflex artery (mm)

BSA (m²)	Z = −2.5	Z = −2.0	Z = −1.0	Z = 0	Z = 1.0	Z = 2.0	Z = 2.5
0.15	0.52	0.57	0.68	0.80	0.94	1.10	1.18
0.20	0.56	0.62	0.75	0.89	1.06	1.25	1.36
0.25	0.61	0.68	0.83	1.00	1.21	1.45	1.58
0.30	0.65	0.73	0.90	1.10	1.34	1.63	1.78
0.35	0.70	0.78	0.97	1.20	1.47	1.78	1.96
0.40	0.74	0.83	1.04	1.28	1.58	1.92	2.11
0.45	0.78	0.88	1.10	1.36	1.67	2.04	2.25
0.50	0.82	0.92	1.15	1.43	1.76	2.15	2.37
0.55	0.86	0.97	1.21	1.50	1.84	2.25	2.47
0.60	0.90	1.01	1.26	1.56	1.91	2.33	2.57
0.65	0.93	1.04	1.30	1.61	1.98	2.41	2.66
0.70	0.96	1.08	1.35	1.66	2.04	2.49	2.74
0.75	0.99	1.11	1.38	1.71	2.10	2.56	2.81
0.80	1.02	1.14	1.42	1.76	2.15	2.62	2.88
0.85	1.04	1.17	1.46	1.80	2.20	2.68	2.95

(continued)

Table 36.1 (continued)

(D) Proximal left circumflex artery (mm)

BSA (m²)	Z = −2.5	Z = −2.0	Z = −1.0	Z = 0	Z = 1.0	Z = 2.0	Z = 2.5
0.90	1.07	1.20	1.49	1.84	2.25	2.74	3.01
0.95	1.10	1.23	1.53	1.88	2.31	2.80	3.08
1.00	1.12	1.26	1.56	1.93	2.36	2.87	3.16
1.05	1.15	1.29	1.60	1.98	2.42	2.94	3.23
1.10	1.18	1.32	1.64	2.02	2.48	3.01	3.31
1.15	1.20	1.35	1.68	2.07	2.54	3.08	3.39
1.20	1.23	1.38	1.72	2.12	2.60	3.16	3.47
1.25	1.26	1.41	1.75	2.17	2.65	3.23	3.55
1.30	1.28	1.44	1.79	2.21	2.71	3.29	3.62
1.35	1.31	1.46	1.82	2.25	2.76	3.36	3.69
1.40	1.33	1.49	1.86	2.30	2.81	3.42	3.77
1.45	1.35	1.52	1.89	2.34	2.87	3.49	3.84
1.50	1.38	1.54	1.93	2.38	2.92	3.56	3.92
1.55	1.40	1.57	1.96	2.43	2.98	3.63	3.99
1.60	1.43	1.60	2.00	2.47	3.04	3.70	4.07
1.65	1.45	1.63	2.03	2.52	3.10	3.77	4.15
1.70	1.48	1.66	2.07	2.57	3.15	3.85	4.24
1.75	1.50	1.69	2.11	2.61	3.21	3.92	4.32
1.80	1.53	1.71	2.15	2.66	3.27	3.99	4.39

Table 36.2 Coronary artery diameter according to Z score and BSA, females

(A) Proximal right coronary artery (mm)

BSA (m²)	Z = −2.5	Z = −2.0	Z = −1.0	Z = 0	Z = 1.0	Z = 2.0	Z = 2.5
0.15	0.57	0.64	0.80	0.98	1.16	1.36	1.47
0.20	0.63	0.71	0.88	1.07	1.27	1.49	1.60
0.25	0.68	0.77	0.96	1.16	1.38	1.61	1.73
0.30	0.74	0.83	1.03	1.25	1.48	1.73	1.86
0.35	0.80	0.90	1.11	1.34	1.59	1.85	1.99
0.40	0.85	0.96	1.18	1.43	1.69	1.97	2.12
0.45	0.91	1.02	1.26	1.52	1.79	2.09	2.24
0.50	0.96	1.08	1.33	1.60	1.89	2.20	2.36
0.55	1.01	1.14	1.40	1.68	1.98	2.30	2.47
0.60	1.06	1.19	1.46	1.76	2.07	2.40	2.58
0.65	1.11	1.25	1.53	1.83	2.16	2.50	2.68
0.70	1.16	1.30	1.59	1.90	2.24	2.59	2.77
0.75	1.21	1.35	1.65	1.97	2.31	2.68	2.87
0.80	1.25	1.39	1.70	2.03	2.38	2.76	2.95
0.85	1.29	1.44	1.75	2.09	2.45	2.84	3.04
0.90	1.33	1.48	1.81	2.15	2.52	2.91	3.11
0.95	1.37	1.52	1.85	2.21	2.58	2.98	3.19
1.00	1.41	1.57	1.90	2.26	2.64	3.05	3.26
1.05	1.44	1.60	1.95	2.31	2.70	3.12	3.33
1.10	1.48	1.64	1.99	2.36	2.76	3.18	3.40
1.15	1.51	1.68	2.03	2.41	2.81	3.24	3.46
1.20	1.55	1.72	2.07	2.46	2.87	3.30	3.52
1.25	1.58	1.75	2.12	2.50	2.92	3.36	3.58
1.30	1.61	1.79	2.16	2.55	2.97	3.41	3.64
1.35	1.65	1.82	2.20	2.60	3.02	3.47	3.70
1.40	1.68	1.86	2.24	2.64	3.07	3.52	3.76
1.45	1.71	1.89	2.27	2.68	3.12	3.58	3.82
1.50	1.74	1.93	2.31	2.73	3.17	3.63	3.87
1.55	1.78	1.96	2.35	2.77	3.22	3.69	3.93
1.60	1.81	2.00	2.39	2.82	3.27	3.74	3.99
1.65	1.84	2.03	2.43	2.86	3.32	3.79	4.04
1.70	1.88	2.07	2.47	2.91	3.36	3.85	4.10
1.75	1.91	2.10	2.51	2.95	3.41	3.90	4.16
1.80	1.94	2.14	2.55	2.99	3.46	3.95	4.21

(B) Left main coronary artery (mm)

BSA (m²)	Z = −2.5	Z = −2.0	Z = −1.0	Z = 0	Z = 1.0	Z = 2.0	Z = 2.5
0.15	0.75	0.83	1.00	1.19	1.41	1.65	1.78
0.20	0.79	0.88	1.06	1.27	1.50	1.75	1.89
0.25	0.84	0.93	1.12	1.34	1.59	1.87	2.02
0.30	0.89	0.98	1.19	1.43	1.69	1.99	2.15
0.35	0.95	1.05	1.27	1.52	1.80	2.12	2.29

(continued)

Table 36.2 (continued)

(B) Left main coronary artery (mm)

BSA (m²)	Z = −2.5	Z = −2.0	Z = −1.0	Z = 0	Z = 1.0	Z = 2.0	Z = 2.5
0.40	1.01	1.12	1.35	1.62	1.92	2.25	2.43
0.45	1.08	1.20	1.45	1.73	2.04	2.39	2.58
0.50	1.16	1.28	1.54	1.83	2.16	2.52	2.71
0.55	1.24	1.36	1.63	1.93	2.27	2.64	2.84
0.60	1.32	1.44	1.72	2.03	2.37	2.74	2.95
0.65	1.39	1.52	1.80	2.11	2.46	2.84	3.04
0.70	1.46	1.59	1.87	2.19	2.54	2.92	3.13
0.75	1.52	1.65	1.94	2.26	2.62	3.00	3.21
0.80	1.58	1.71	2.01	2.33	2.69	3.08	3.29
0.85	1.63	1.77	2.06	2.39	2.76	3.15	3.36
0.90	1.67	1.81	2.12	2.45	2.82	3.22	3.44
0.95	1.71	1.86	2.17	2.51	2.88	3.29	3.51
1.00	1.75	1.90	2.21	2.56	2.94	3.36	3.58
1.05	1.79	1.94	2.26	2.61	3.00	3.42	3.65
1.10	1.82	1.97	2.30	2.66	3.05	3.48	3.71
1.15	1.86	2.01	2.34	2.70	3.10	3.54	3.77
1.20	1.89	2.05	2.38	2.75	3.16	3.60	3.83
1.25	1.93	2.08	2.42	2.80	3.21	3.66	3.90
1.30	1.96	2.12	2.47	2.85	3.27	3.72	3.96
1.35	2.00	2.16	2.51	2.90	3.32	3.79	4.03
1.40	2.03	2.20	2.56	2.95	3.38	3.85	4.10
1.45	2.07	2.24	2.60	3.00	3.44	3.92	4.18
1.50	2.11	2.28	2.65	3.06	3.50	3.99	4.25
1.55	2.15	2.32	2.70	3.11	3.56	4.05	4.32
1.60	2.19	2.36	2.74	3.16	3.62	4.12	4.38
1.65	2.23	2.41	2.79	3.21	3.67	4.18	4.45
1.70	2.26	2.45	2.83	3.26	3.73	4.24	4.51
1.75	2.30	2.48	2.88	3.31	3.78	4.30	4.57
1.80	2.34	2.52	2.92	3.36	3.83	4.35	4.63

(C) Proximal left anterior descending artery (mm)

BSA (m²)	Z = −2.5	Z = −2.0	Z = −1.0	Z = 0	Z = 1.0	Z = 2.0	Z = 2.5
0.15	0.64	0.69	0.80	0.92	1.07	1.25	1.35
0.20	0.70	0.75	0.87	1.01	1.18	1.38	1.49
0.25	0.75	0.81	0.94	1.10	1.29	1.51	1.64
0.30	0.80	0.86	1.01	1.19	1.40	1.65	1.79
0.35	0.85	0.92	1.08	1.28	1.51	1.78	1.93
0.40	0.90	0.97	1.15	1.37	1.61	1.91	2.08
0.45	0.94	1.03	1.22	1.45	1.72	2.03	2.21
0.50	0.99	1.08	1.29	1.53	1.82	2.15	2.34
0.55	1.03	1.13	1.35	1.61	1.91	2.26	2.45
0.60	1.07	1.17	1.41	1.68	1.99	2.35	2.56

(continued)

Table 36.2 (continued)

(C) Proximal left anterior descending artery (mm)							
BSA (m²)	Z = −2.5	Z = −2.0	Z = −1.0	Z = 0	Z = 1.0	Z = 2.0	Z = 2.5
0.65	1.10	1.21	1.46	1.74	2.07	2.44	2.65
0.70	1.14	1.25	1.51	1.80	2.14	2.52	2.73
0.75	1.17	1.29	1.56	1.86	2.21	2.60	2.81
0.80	1.21	1.33	1.60	1.92	2.27	2.67	2.89
0.85	1.24	1.37	1.65	1.97	2.33	2.74	2.96
0.90	1.27	1.40	1.69	2.02	2.39	2.80	3.02
0.95	1.30	1.43	1.73	2.07	2.44	2.86	3.09
1.00	1.33	1.47	1.77	2.11	2.49	2.92	3.14
1.05	1.36	1.50	1.81	2.16	2.54	2.97	3.20
1.10	1.38	1.53	1.85	2.20	2.59	3.02	3.25
1.15	1.41	1.56	1.88	2.24	2.64	3.07	3.30
1.20	1.44	1.59	1.92	2.29	2.69	3.12	3.36
1.25	1.47	1.62	1.96	2.33	2.74	3.17	3.41
1.30	1.50	1.66	2.00	2.37	2.78	3.23	3.46
1.35	1.53	1.69	2.04	2.42	2.83	3.28	3.51
1.40	1.56	1.72	2.08	2.47	2.88	3.33	3.56
1.45	1.59	1.76	2.12	2.51	2.93	3.38	3.62
1.50	1.62	1.80	2.16	2.56	2.98	3.43	3.67
1.55	1.66	1.83	2.21	2.61	3.03	3.49	3.72
1.60	1.69	1.87	2.25	2.66	3.09	3.54	3.77
1.65	1.73	1.91	2.29	2.70	3.14	3.59	3.82
1.70	1.76	1.95	2.34	2.75	3.19	3.64	3.88
1.75	1.80	1.99	2.38	2.80	3.23	3.69	3.93
1.80	1.83	2.03	2.43	2.85	3.28	3.74	3.97
(D) Proximal left circumflex artery (mm)							
BSA (m²)	Z = −2.5	Z = −2.0	Z = −1.0	Z = 0	Z = 1.0	Z = 2.0	Z = 2.5
0.15	0.51	0.56	0.67	0.81	0.98	1.18	1.30
0.20	0.56	0.61	0.74	0.89	1.08	1.31	1.44
0.25	0.60	0.66	0.80	0.97	1.18	1.43	1.58
0.30	0.64	0.71	0.86	1.05	1.28	1.55	1.71
0.35	0.68	0.76	0.93	1.13	1.38	1.67	1.84
0.40	0.72	0.80	0.99	1.21	1.47	1.79	1.97
0.45	0.76	0.85	1.05	1.28	1.56	1.90	2.09
0.50	0.80	0.89	1.10	1.35	1.65	2.01	2.20
0.55	0.83	0.93	1.15	1.42	1.74	2.11	2.31
0.60	0.86	0.97	1.21	1.49	1.82	2.20	2.42
0.65	0.89	1.00	1.25	1.55	1.89	2.29	2.51
0.70	0.92	1.04	1.30	1.61	1.96	2.37	2.60
0.75	0.95	1.07	1.34	1.66	2.03	2.45	2.68
0.80	0.97	1.10	1.39	1.72	2.09	2.52	2.75
0.85	1.00	1.13	1.43	1.77	2.15	2.59	2.83

(continued)

Table 36.2 (continued)

(D) Proximal left circumflex artery (mm)

BSA (m²)	Z = −2.5	Z = −2.0	Z = −1.0	Z = 0	Z = 1.0	Z = 2.0	Z = 2.5
0.90	1.02	1.16	1.47	1.81	2.21	2.65	2.89
0.95	1.05	1.19	1.50	1.86	2.26	2.71	2.95
1.00	1.07	1.21	1.54	1.90	2.31	2.77	3.01
1.05	1.09	1.24	1.57	1.95	2.36	2.82	3.06
1.10	1.11	1.27	1.61	1.99	2.41	2.87	3.11
1.15	1.14	1.29	1.64	2.03	2.45	2.92	3.16
1.20	1.16	1.32	1.68	2.07	2.50	2.96	3.21
1.25	1.18	1.35	1.71	2.11	2.54	3.01	3.26
1.30	1.20	1.37	1.74	2.14	2.58	3.05	3.30
1.35	1.23	1.40	1.77	2.18	2.62	3.09	3.34
1.40	1.25	1.43	1.81	2.22	2.66	3.14	3.38
1.45	1.27	1.46	1.84	2.26	2.71	3.18	3.43
1.50	1.30	1.48	1.88	2.30	2.75	3.22	3.47
1.55	1.32	1.51	1.91	2.34	2.79	3.26	3.51
1.60	1.35	1.54	1.94	2.37	2.83	3.30	3.55
1.65	1.37	1.57	1.98	2.41	2.87	3.34	3.59
1.70	1.40	1.60	2.01	2.45	2.91	3.38	3.63
1.75	1.42	1.63	2.05	2.49	2.95	3.43	3.67
1.80	1.45	1.66	2.08	2.53	2.99	3.47	3.71

References

1. Kamiya T, Kawasaki T, Ookuni M, Katoh H, Baba K, Nakano H. Report of subcommittee on standardization of diagnostic criteria and reporting of coronary artery lesions in Kawasaki disease. Diagnostic criteria of cardiovascular lesions in Kawasaki Disease. Research Committee on Kawasaki Disease (Committee Chairman: T. Kawasaki). Tokyo: Ministry of Health and Welfare; 1983. pp. 1–10. Available from http://www.niph.go.jp/wadai/mhlw/ssh_1983_05. htm and select first report or http://www.niph.go.jp/wadai/mhlw/1983/s5805004.pdf (in Japanese) 1984. pp. 55–66. Available from http://www.niph.go.jp/wadai/mhlw/ssh_1984_06.htm and select 8th report, or http://www.niph.go.jp/wadai/mhlw/1984/s5906011. pdf (in English). Accessed 28 July 2014.
2. Arjunan K, Daniels SR, Meyer RA, Schwartz DC, Barron H, Kaplan S. Coronary artery caliber in normal children and patients with Kawasaki disease but without aneurysms: an echocardiographic and angiographic study. J Am Coll Cardiol. 1986;8(5):1119–24. http://dx.doi.org/10.1016/S0735-1097(86)80390-4. PMID:3760385.
3. Oberhoffer R, Lang D, Feilen K. The diameter of coronary arteries in infants and children without heart disease. Eur J Pediatr. 1989;148(5):389–92. http://dx.doi.org/10.1007/BF00595893. PMID:2920744.
4. Dajani AS, Taubert KA, Gerber MA, Shulman ST, Ferrieri P, Freed M, et al. Diagnosis and therapy of Kawasaki disease in children. Circulation. 1993;87(5):1776–80. http://dx.doi.org/10.1161/01.CIR.87.5.1776. PMID:8491037.
5. Durongpisitkul K, Gururaj VJ, Park JM, Martin CF. The prevention of coronary artery aneurysm in Kawasaki disease: a meta-analysis on the efficacy of aspirin and immunoglobulin treatment. Pediatrics. 1995;96(6):1057–61. PMID:7491221.

6. de Zorzi A, Colan SD, Gauvreau K, Baker AL, Sundel RP, Newburger JW. Coronary artery dimensions may be misclassified as normal in Kawasaki disease. J Pediatr. 1998;133(2):254–8. http://dx.doi.org/10.1016/S0022-3476(98)70229-X. PMID:9709715.

7. Kurotobi S, Nagai T, Kawakami N, Sano T, Sano T. Coronary diameter in normal infants, children and patients with Kawasaki disease. Pediatr Int. 2002;44(1):1–4. http://dx.doi.org/10.1046/j.1442-200X.2002.01508.x. PMID:11982862.

8. Tan TH, Wong KY, Cheng TK, Heng JT. Coronary normograms and the coronary-aorta index: objective determinants of coronary artery dilatation. Pediatr Cardiol. 2003;24(4):328–35. http://dx.doi.org/10.1007/s00246-002-0300-7. PMID:12360388.

9. Newburger JW, Takahashi M, Gerber MA, Gewitz MH, Tani LY, Burns JC, American Academy of Pediatrics, et al. Diagnosis, treatment, and long-term management of Kawasaki disease: a statement for health professionals from the Committee on Rheumatic Fever, Endocarditis and Kawasaki Disease, Council on Cardiovascular Disease in the Young, American Heart Association. Circulation. 2004;110(17):2747–71. http://dx.doi.org/10.1161/01.CIR.0000145143.19711.78. PMID:15505111.

10. Newburger JW, Sleeper LA, McCrindle BW, Minich LL, Gersony W, Vetter VL, et al. Randomized trial of pulsed corticosteroid therapy for primary treatment of Kawasaki disease. N Engl J Med. 2007;356(7):663–75.

11. McCrindle BW, Li JS, Minich LL, Colan SD, Atz AM, Takahashi M, Pediatric Heart Network Investigators, et al. Coronary artery involvement in children with Kawasaki disease: risk factors from analysis of serial normalized measurements. Circulation. 2007;116(2):174–9. http://dx.doi.org/10.1161/CIRCULATIONAHA.107.690875. PMID:17576863.

12. Olivieri L, Arling B, Friberg M, Sable C. Coronary artery Z score regression equations and calculators derived from a large heterogeneous population of children undergoing echocardiography. J Am Soc Echocardiogr. 2009;22(2):159–64. http://dx.doi.org/10.1016/j.echo.2008.11.003. PMID:17576863.

13. Fuse S, Morii M, Ooyanagi R, Kuroiwa Y, Hotsubo T, Mori T. Generation of coronary arterial inner diameter standards by echocardiography using the LMS method in children. J Jpn Pediatr Soc. 2009;113:928–34.

14. Cole TJ, Green PJ. Smoothing reference centile curves: the LMS method and penalized likelihood. Stat Med. 1992;11(10):1305–19. http://dx.doi.org/10.1002/sim.4780111005. PMID:1518992.

15. Dallaire F, Dahdah N. New equations and a critical appraisal of coronary artery Z scores in healthy children. J Am Soc Echocardiogr. 2011;24(1):60–74. http://dx.doi.org/10.1016/j.echo.2010.10.004. PMID:21074965.

16. Fuse S, Kobayashi T, Arakaki Y, Ogawa S, Katoh H, Sakamoto N, et al. Standard method for ultrasound imaging of coronary artery in children. Pediatr Int. 2010;52(6):876–82. http://dx.doi.org/10.1111/j.1442-200X.2010.03252.x. PMID:21166948.

Evidence of Endothelial Damage in Acute KD

Keiichi Hirono and Fukiko Ichida

Abstract Although the cause of Kawasaki disease (KD) is unknown, endothelial dysfunction is a key event in atherogenesis associated with KD. Systemic endothelial dysfunction in KD in reflected by flow-mediated dilation of the brachial artery, particularly in children with coronary artery lesions. Nitric oxide has a key role in maintaining the vascular wall, especially endothelial cells. Nitric oxide synthase (NOS) function is disrupted in patients with KD, and a genetic link exists in the form of NOS gene polymorphisms. Levels of endothelial microparticles, circulating markers of endothelial cell damage, are significantly higher during acute KD and lower during convalescence of KD. Levels of endothelial progenitor cells, which contribute to endothelial repair and neovascularization, are lower in KD patients with coronary artery lesions. These measures of endothelial function yield important evidence regarding vascular biology in KD and may help uncover the mechanisms of and new therapies for KD.

Keywords Endothelial dysfunction • NO • FMD • EMP • EPC

Abbreviations

KD: Kawasaki disease
CAL: coronary artery lesion
FMD: flow-mediated dilation
EMP: Endothelial microparticles
EPC: Endothelial progenitor cell

K. Hirono, M.D., PhD • F. Ichida, M.D., PhD (✉)
Department of Pediatrics, Graduate School of Medicine, University of Toyama, 2630 Sugitani,
Toyama City, Toyama 930-0194, Japan
e-mail: fukiko@med.u-toyama.ac.jp

© Springer Japan 2017   335
B.T. Saji et al. (eds.), *Kawasaki Disease*, DOI 10.1007/978-4-431-56039-5_37

Introduction

Kawasaki disease (KD) is an acute inflammatory syndrome that manifests as systemic vasculitis. Acute inflammation and the subsequent reparative processes may lead to permanent changes in arterial structures and hemodynamics—even during convalescence of KD—including increased carotid arterial intima-media thickness, endothelial dysfunction, and increased arterial stiffness. Repairing damaged endothelial cells is therefore essential in preventing the development and progression of vascular lesions.

The present review summarizes the present understanding of endothelial dysfunction in KD and the strengths, weaknesses, and potential clinical applications of current testing methods.

The Endothelium and Endothelial Injury and Repair

The endothelium is a thin layer of cells that lines the interior surface of blood vessels and lymphatic vessels, forming an interface between circulating blood or lymph in the lumen and the rest of the vessel wall. Although only a simple monolayer, the healthy endothelium is optimally placed and is able to respond to physical and chemical signals by producing a wide range of factors that regulate vascular tone, cellular adhesion, thromboresistance, smooth muscle cell proliferation, and vessel wall inflammation.

Endothelial dysfunction is a systemic pathologic state of the endothelium and can be broadly defined as an imbalance between vasodilating and vasoconstricting substances produced by the endothelium. Normal functions of endothelial cells include mediation of coagulation, platelet adhesion, immune function, and control of volume and content of electrolyte in intravascular and extravascular spaces. A key quantifiable feature of endothelial dysfunction is the inability of arteries and arterioles to dilate fully in response to an appropriate stimulus that triggers release of vasodilators from the endothelium, like nitric oxide (NO). NO helps keep the vascular wall in a quiescent state by inhibiting inflammation, cellular proliferation, and thrombosis. Endothelial dysfunction is commonly associated with decreased NO bioavailability, which is due to impaired NO production by the endothelium and/or increased inactivation of NO by reactive oxygen species (ROS).

Clinical Assessment of Endothelial Function and KD

A noninvasive method to measure endothelial dysfunction is %flow-mediated dilation (FMD) on brachial artery ultrasound imaging. A negative correlation between FMD and baseline artery size is recognized as a fundamental scaling problem, leading to biased estimates of endothelial function. Several previous reports have shown that there is systemic endothelial dysfunction late after KD onset, as reflected in FMD of the brachial artery, particularly in children with CAL [1, 2]. However, other reports found that systemic endothelial dysfunction was not present late after KD and that there was no relationship with coronary artery involvement [1, 3]. These discrepancies may be related to variations in the racial and KD characteristics of patient and normal control subject populations, acute-stage therapeutic regimens, and length of follow-up, or to small sample sizes and problems in ultrasonographic assessment. Additional long-term international studies are needed in order to assess the impact of KD on vascular health. Recently, Huang et al. reported that ongoing chronic vascular inflammation and endothelial dysfunction were present in children with CAL late after KD, as reflected by increased high-sensitivity c-reactive protein (hs-CRP) level and reduced FMD [4].

Interestingly, Kurio et al. studied acetylcholine-induced vasodilatation of the microcirculation, as determined by laser Doppler fluximetry (LDF) [5]. Transient endothelial dysfunction of the microvasculature was documented during acute KD, but microvascular endothelial function was similar to controls after recovery from KD. These findings suggest that endothelial damage in KD is confined to medium-size or larger arteries and does not involve the microcirculation.

Circulating Markers of Endothelial Function and KD

The numerous functions of the endothelium can be better appreciated by studying the levels of molecules of endothelial origin in circulating blood. These include direct products of endothelial cells that change when the endothelium is activated, such as measures of NO biology, inflammatory cytokines, adhesion molecules, and regulators of thrombosis, as well as markers of endothelial function.

NO is synthesized by two NOS isoforms, termed endothelial NOS (eNOS) and inducible NOS (iNOS), and has diverse roles in the physiology and pathophysiology of the cardiovascular system. Yu et al. demonstrated that neutrophils, monocytes, and endothelial cells express iNOS at different stages in acute KD and that iNOS expression in neutrophils was maximal and restricted to the very early stage [6]. They suggested that NO synthesized by iNOS in neutrophils has a role in triggering early endothelial dysfunction in acute KD. The degree of iNOS expression in response to inflammatory stimuli in KD might differ from that in bacterial infection, and this discrepancy may be due to gene polymorphisms in the iNOS promoter, leading to increased iNOS expression. Recently, Yoshimura et al. reported that in acute KD neutrophils generate both NO and ROS [7]. NO production by neutrophils was increased only during early KD and decreased after IVIG treatment, while ROS production increased to the same level as that in febrile controls [7]. These findings suggest that immune system abnormalities in KD might be caused by NO overproduction; however, the role of NO in endothelial damage remains to be elucidated.

Endothelial microparticles (EMPs) are vesicles formed by the cell membrane after endothelial activation. The details of EMP composition can be used to characterize the status of the parent endothelial cell. The characteristics of circulating EMPs during the different stages of KD in children are not well understood. Guiducci et al. reported increased numbers of microparticles in KD patients, mainly from endothelial cells and T cells, after IVIG therapy [8]. Tan et al. found elevated EMP levels in KD patients, a positive correlation with tumor necrosis factor-α, and a negative correlation with albumin, suggesting involvement of EMPs in the development of vasculitis in children with KD [9]. Recently, Ding et al. reported that EMP levels were higher in plasma of patients with acute or subacute KD and were lower during convalescence, suggesting that endothelial damage persists during convalescence of KD [10].

Endothelial progenitor cells (EPCs) in postnatal bone marrow and peripheral blood may contribute to endothelial repair and neovascularization. Nakatani et al. reported that the number of EPCs was elevated during acute KD in patients with CAL, which contradicts very recent findings regarding the convalescent phase [11, 12]. This apparent contradiction suggests that EPC mobilization may be biphasic, ie, that there is an increase during acute KD and a decrease during convalescence. In the early phase, EPCs are increased, reflecting bone marrow response to diffuse, severe endothelial damage. During convalescence, increased consumption of EPCs may decrease circulating EPCs. It is generally believed that a reduction in the number of EPCs is a result of exhaustion of the pool of progenitor cells available in bone marrow [13]. Several recent studies reported that KD patients with CALs, irrespective of persistence of coronary aneurysms, have fewer circulating EPCs and arterial dysfunction during late convalescence. The decrease in circulating EPCs, with subsequent impairment of endothelial cell repair and function, may be at least partially related to arterial dysfunction [12, 14].

Furui et al. investigated the relationship between plasma levels of soluble forms of the selectin family and incidence of CALs in patients with KD [15]. Before intravenous immunoglobulin treatment, plasma levels of E- and P-selectin were significantly higher in patients with CALs than in those without CALs.

Strategies to reverse endothelial function are now being evaluated in patients with KD. Benefits have been seen with a number of pharmacologic interventions, including drugs that lower lipids and blood pressure and with novel therapies based on a new understanding of endothelial biology. Matrix metalloproteinase (MMP)-9 is a member of the MMP family that has elastolytic activity and is involved in cardiac remodeling. A recent study found that MMP-9 was involved in coronary artery aneurysm formation in KD patients [16, 17]. Inoue et al. reported that MMP-9 was inhibited by captopril in KD patients [18]. Hamaoka et al. showed that short-term statin therapy improved chronic vascular inflammation and endothelial dysfunction in these patients [4, 19]. Statins may prove to be a potent therapy for chronic vascular inflammation and endothelial dysfunction with no adverse effects in children with CAL late after KD.

Recent Advances

Assessment of endothelial function shows great promise because it reflects important aspects of vascular biology, is associated with disease burden and outcome, and responds to interventions. Furthermore, as with other biomarkers used in research, clinical usefulness will depend on obtaining more information on the quantitative relationship between measures of endothelial function and outcomes, not merely associations shown in cohorts.

A comprehensive approach that involves measurement of genetic predisposition, risk factors, endothelial function, and structural arterial disease is likely to be the best way to evaluate new treatment strategies, particularly in the early preclinical phase of KD.

References

1. Dhillon R, Clarkson P, Donald AE, Powe AJ, Nash M, Novelli V, et al. Endothelial dysfunction late after Kawasaki disease. Circulation. 1996;94(9):2103–6. http://dx.doi.org/10.1161/01.CIR.94.9.2103. PMID:8901658.
2. Ikemoto Y, Ogino H, Teraguchi M, Kobayashi Y. Evaluation of preclinical atherosclerosis by flow-mediated dilatation of the brachial artery and carotid artery analysis in patients with a history of Kawasaki disease. Pediatr Cardiol. 2005;26(6):782–6. http://dx.doi.org/10.1007/s00246-005-0921-8. PMID:16132279.
3. McCrindle BW, McIntyre S, Kim C, Lin T, Adeli K. Are patients after Kawasaki disease at increased risk for accelerated atherosclerosis? J Pediatr. 2007;151(3):244–8. http://dx.doi.org/10.1016/j.jpeds.2007.03.056. PMID:17719931.
4. Huang SM, Weng KP, Chang JS, Lee WY, Huang SH, Hsieh KS. Effects of statin therapy in children complicated with coronary arterial abnormality late after Kawasaki disease: a pilot study. Circ J. 2008;72(10):1583–7. http://dx.doi.org/10.1253/circj.CJ-08-0121. PMID:18758088.
5. Kurio GH, Zhiroff KA, Jih LJ, Fronek AS, Burns JC. Noninvasive determination of endothelial cell function in the microcirculation in Kawasaki syndrome. Pediatr Cardiol. 2008;29(1):121–5. http://dx.doi.org/10.1007/s00246-007-9077-z. PMID:17891433.
6. Yu X, Hirono KI, Ichida F, Uese K, Rui C, Watanabe S, et al. Enhanced iNOS expression in leukocytes and circulating endothelial cells is associated with the progression of coronary artery lesions in acute Kawasaki disease. Pediatr Res. 2004;55(4):688–94. http://dx.doi.org/10.1203/01.PDR.0000113464.93042.A4. PMID:14764920.
7. Yoshimura K, Tatsumi K, Iharada A, Tsuji S, Tateiwa A, Teraguchi M, et al. Increased nitric oxide production by neutrophils in early stage of Kawasaki disease. Eur J Pediatr. 2009;168(9):1037–41. http://dx.doi.org/10.1007/s00431-008-0872-1. PMID:19020897.
8. Guiducci S, Ricci L, Romano E, Ceccarelli C, Distler JH, Miniati I, et al. Microparticles and Kawasaki disease: a marker of vascular damage? Clin Exp Rheumatol. 2011;29(1 Suppl 64):S121–5. PMID:21385556.
9. Tan Z, Yuan Y, Chen S, Chen Y, Chen TX. Plasma endothelial microparticles, TNF-a and IL-6 in Kawasaki disease. Indian Pediatr. 2013;50(5):501–3. http://dx.doi.org/10.1007/s13312-013-0152-7. PMID:23255681.
10. Ding YY, Ren Y, Feng X, Xu QQ, Sun L, Zhang JM, et al. Correlation between brachial artery flow-mediated dilation and endothelial microparticle levels for identifying endothelial dysfunction in children with Kawasaki disease. Pediatr Res. 2014;75(3):453–8. http://dx.doi.org/10.1038/pr.2013.240. PMID:24336465.

11. Nakatani K, Takeshita S, Tsujimoto H, Kawamura Y, Tokutomi T, Sekine I. Circulating endo-thelial cells in Kawasaki disease. Clin Exp Immunol. 2003;131(3):536–40. http://dx.doi.org/10.1046/j.1365-2249.2003.02091.x. PMID:12605708.
12. Liu XQ, Huang GY, Liang XV, Ma XJ. Endothelial progenitor cells and arterial functions in the late convalescence period of Kawasaki disease. Acta Paediatr. 2009;98(8):1355–9. http://dx.doi.org/10.1111/j.1651-2227.2009.01334.x. PMID:19438842.
13. Heiss C, Keymel S, Niesler U, Ziemann J, Kelm M, Kalka C. Impaired progenitor cell activity in age-related endothelial dysfunction. J Am Coll Cardiol. 2005;45(9):1441–8. http://dx.doi.org/10.1016/j.jacc.2004.12.074. PMID:15862416.
14. Kuroi A, Imanishi T, Suzuki H, Ikejima H, Tsujioka H, Yoshikawa N, et al. Clinical charac-teristics of patients with Kawasaki disease and levels of peripheral endothelial progenitor cells and blood monocyte subpopulations. Circ J. 2010;74(12):2720–5. http://dx.doi.org/10.1253/circj.CJ-10-0317. PMID:20921814.
15. Furui J, Ishii M, Ikeda H, Muta H, Egami K, Sugahara Y, et al. Soluble forms of the selectin family in children with Kawasaki disease: prediction for coronary artery lesions. Acta Paediatr. 2002;91(11):1183–8. http://dx.doi.org/10.1111/j.1651-2227.2002.tb00126.x. PMID:12463316.
16. Takeshita S, Tokutomi T, Kawase H, Nakatani K, Tsujimoto H, Kawamura Y, et al. Elevated serum levels of matrix metalloproteinase-9 (MMP-9) in Kawasaki disease. Clin Exp Immunol. 2001;125(2):340–4. http://dx.doi.org/10.1046/j.1365-2249.2001.01608.x. PMID:11529928.
17. Gavin PJ, Crawford SE, Shulman ST, Garcia FL, Rowley AH. Systemic arterial expression of matrix metalloproteinases 2 and 9 in acute Kawasaki disease. Arterioscler Thromb Vasc Biol. 2003;23(4):576–81. http://dx.doi.org/10.1161/01.ATV.0000065385.47152.FD. PMID:12692003.
18. Inoue N, Takai S, Jin D, Okumura K, Okamura N, Kajiura M, et al. Effect of angiotensin-converting enzyme inhibitor on matrix metalloproteinase-9 activity in patients with Kawasaki disease. Clin Chim Acta. 2010;411(3–4):267–9. http://dx.doi.org/10.1016/j.cca.2009.11.020. PMID:19945447.
19. Hamaoka A, Hamaoka K, Yahata T, Fujii M, Ozawa S, Toiyama K, et al. Effects of HMG-CoA reductase inhibitors on continuous post-inflammatory vascular remodeling late after Kawasaki disease. J Cardiol. 2010;56(2):245–53. http://dx.doi.org/10.1016/j.jjcc.2010.06.006. PMID:20678900.

Oxidative Stress in Kawasaki Disease

Tomoyo Yahata and Kenji Hamaoka

Abstract Because inflammation and oxidative stress are closely related, oxidative stress cannot be ignored when considering pathologic conditions associated with inflammation-based Kawasaki disease (KD). KD pathogenesis is triggered by certain unknown infectious factors that activate one or multiple inflammation pathways via intricately intertwined cytokine cascades. Overproduction of reactive oxygen species from activated inflammation pathways increases oxidative stress in the body and results in an endless vicious cycle between inflammation reactions and reactive oxygen, which presumably underlies the diffuse vasculitis formed during acute KD. Although vascular inflammation and oxidative stress can be rapidly suppressed by treatment during the acute phase, they may persist in various forms for a long time. This has recently been identified as a concern in late KD. Generally, the presence of vascular inflammation and oxidative stress impairs blood vessels, leading to atherosclerosis onset, a widely recognized risk (Li et al., Atherosclerosis 237(1):208–219, 2014). This chapter will focus on determining whether the same is valid for blood vessels in late KD.

Keywords Oxidative stress • Reactive oxygen species • NAD(P)H • Hydroperoxide • Endothelial dysfunction • Arteriosclerosis • Atherosclerosis

What Is Oxidative Stress?

The redox system is one of the body's regulation systems to maintain homeostasis against external stress. Reactive oxygen species (ROS) produced by internal or external factors are normally reduced by the ROS elimination system of the body. However, when the elimination system is overwhelmed by overproduction of ROS, excessive ROS accumulate inside the body or are converted to further reactive ROS, resulting in a state of oxidative stress [1] (Fig. 1).

T. Yahata (✉) • K. Hamaoka
Department of Pediatric Cardiology and Nephrology, Kyoto Prefectural University of Medicine, Graduate School of Medical Science, Kawaramachi-Hirokoji, Kamigyo-ku, Kyoto 602-8566, Japan
e-mail: tomoya@koto.kpu-m.ac.jp

© Springer Japan 2017
B.T. Saji et al. (eds.), *Kawasaki Disease*, DOI 10.1007/978-4-431-56039-5_38

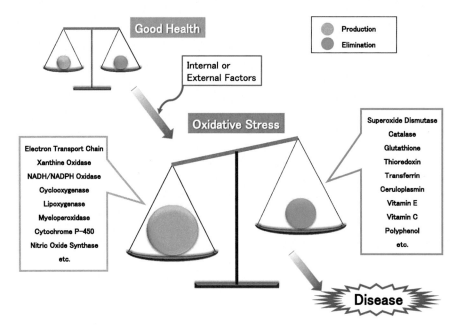

Fig. 1 What is oxidative stress? When the elimination system is overwhelmed by overproduction of ROS, excessive ROS accumulate inside the body or are converted to further reactive ROS, causing oxidative stress

Phagocytes are at the forefront of innate immunity and are part of the biological defense mechanism. NAD(P)H oxidase controls the ROS production system in cells. When inflammation is triggered, NAD(P)H oxidase in neutrophils and macrophages rapidly produces large quantities of ROS as a biological defense mechanism. If the reaction is impaired, the body fails to kill bacteria and other pathogens and thus becomes more susceptible to infection. Therefore, oxidative stress can be regarded as a defensive reaction of the body and is not always harmful. However, excessive ROS can target any organic substances in the body, including lipids, proteins, amino acids, and nucleic acids, causing oxidative damage to these substances. This induces lipid peroxidation, protein denaturation, and oxidative DNA damage. Thus, oxidative stress is a double-edged sword in maintaining homeostasis.

Inflammation and Oxidative Stress

During acute Kawasaki disease (KD), monocyte/macrophage–dominant inflammatory cell infiltration is observed in all layers of arteries, exhibiting an "inflammation" condition [2]. These cells are activated by proinflammatory cytokines (known as priming), resulting in their migration and infiltration. The primed inflammatory cells are irritable and can easily show reactions such as ROS production.

Factors involved in ROS production at the time of inflammation are diverse, including infiltrating neutrophils and macrophages, xanthine oxidase in vascular endothelial cells, arachidonic acid metabolism initiated by the activation of phospholipase A2, and intracellular mitochondria. Among these factors, infiltrating inflammatory cells are believed to be the main source of ROS production, as mentioned above, and large quantities of ROS produced by NAD(P)H oxidase [3] on the cell membrane are also involved in priming neutrophils. Intranuclear NF-κB in inflammatory cells is activated by increased oxidative stress, thus facilitating production of various cytokines and expression of cell adhesion molecules. Moreover, arachidonic acid, which is released from the cell membrane during inflammation, has various functions, from producing ROS during its metabolic pathway to regulating NAD(P)H oxidase activation, and acts as an inflammatory agent. Furthermore, inducible NO synthase (iNOS) is expressed not only in infiltrating and accumulating inflammatory cells but also in vascular smooth muscle cells, leading to production of large amounts of NO. NOs derived from iNOS are unstable radicals, quickly reacting with superoxide under oxidative stress to form ONOO−, which then produces radicals that are even more reactive. These radicals have a strong propensity to impair vascular tissues [4].

Oxidative Stress During Acute KD

Because the main pathologic condition of KD is vascular inflammation, it is possible that oxidative stress is increased during acute KD. Some recent reports support this view [5]. We also simultaneously measured blood reactive oxygen metabolites (ROM), an indicator for the ROS production system, and blood biological antioxidant potential (BAP), an indicator for the ROS elimination system, to assess oxidative stress in patients with the acute KD (Fig. 2) [6].

We examined 19 patients with acute KD, among whom 13 responded well to initial IVIG therapy (2 g/kg, single dose) and 6 were poor responders. All patients were tested for blood ROM and BAP immediately before IVIG therapy, 24 h after completion of IVIG administration, and 2 weeks after the end of IVIG therapy. The poor responders to IVIG subsequently underwent additional IVIG or steroid therapy after initial IVIG therapy to lower fever within 1 week. Among the IVIG responders, blood ROM levels were very high immediately before IVIG therapy but decreased during the initial IVIG treatment. In contrast, blood ROM levels in the nonresponders were very high immediately before IVIG, as in the responders, remained high after initial IVIG therapy, and were significantly lower 2 weeks thereafter. BAP levels in the IVIG responders did not change much before and after IVIG therapy and tended to gradually increase 2 weeks after IVIG therapy. In contrast, BAP did not significantly change during the disease course in

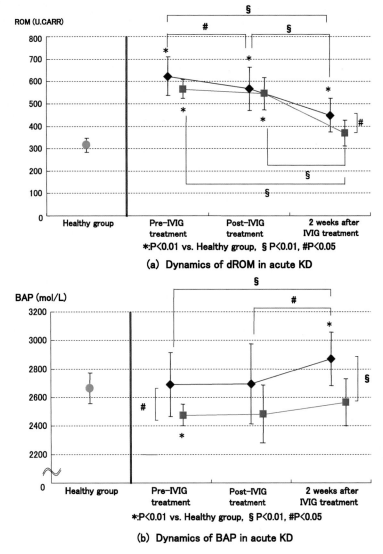

Fig. 2   (a) Dynamics of dROM in acute KD, (b) Dynamics of BAP in acute KD

nonresponders. In addition, BAP immediately before IVIG therapy was significantly lower in nonresponders than in responders ($p < 0.01$).

These findings suggest that ROS production is significantly increased during acute KD and then promptly decreases as inflammation resolves by an IVIG-independent mechanism. Thus, ROM level was useful for assessing therapeutic effects. Because the ROS elimination system changes somewhat later than the production system, the ROS elimination system may use stimulation from increased ROS as a trigger to gradually enhance its function. Nevertheless, our results suggest that the functional capacity of the elimination system determines responsiveness to IVIG therapy and, by extension, the ability to recover from acute-phase damage.

Although there seems to be general agreement that oxidative stress is increased during acute KD, it remains unclear whether oxidative stress is involved in KD pathogenesis. Some researchers argue that it is merely a by-product of vasculitis formation process during the acute phase, and thus antioxidative therapy is not actively considered as a treatment option for acute disease. However, one study found that administration of vitamins E and C was effective for coronary arteritis [7]. In addition, recent studies showed an antioxidant effect for aspirin, which is listed in the acute-phase treatment guideline and is often used accordingly, for its pleiotropic effects [8]. Although some clinicians disagree on the effectiveness of aspirin administration for acute KD, we must remember that aspirin should, at a minimum, be part of the treatment regimen during acute KD, when oxidative stress is clearly increased.

The current acute-phase treatment regimen focuses on anti-inflammation. There is wide agreement on the use of IVIG as the first-line therapy. Recent large-scale studies showed that steroid [9], cyclosporine A [10], and anti-TNFα antibodies [11] are also effective as anti-inflammatory agents for acute KD. Therefore, the strategy for medical treatment of acute KD has been gradually diversifying. Along with this diversification, the incidence of coronary artery lesions, the most worrisome complication during acute KD, is decreasing but not yet zero. Under these circumstances, the presence of increased oxidative stress during the acute phase represents an important foothold for creating new treatment strategies in the future, because controlling oxidative stress, which is closely linked to inflammation, is expected to be very useful in ensuring prompt resolution of inflammation during the acute phase.

Involvement of Oxidative Stress in Vascular Illnesses After the Acute Phase

What happens to blood vessels after the acute phase of KD? Unless a lethal complication such as coronary artery aneurysm rupture or thromboembolism occurs, intense systemic vasculitis subsides as a result of anti-inflammation therapy indicated in the guidelines for acute-phase treatment. Patients with severe inflammation resulting in destruction of vascular structures develop coronary artery lesions (CAL) to varying degrees. Because of the subsequent prolonged repair process of vascular remodeling, fibrosis and other inflammation scars remain. Patients with mild inflammation are not complicated by CAL and seemingly have no scarring. Therefore, patients without CAL are usually deemed cured during the period from a few months to a few years after KD onset and do not undergo further follow-up observation. However, recent controversial studies reported that blood vessel impairment might be present during the late phase, even in patients without CAL [12]. Advanced examination methods can now detect intimal hypertrophy in blood vessels that were judged to be morphologically normal by conventional examination methods. Moreover, many studies have found evidence of blood vessel impairment, such as deterioration of vascular endothelial function and elevated high-sensitivity CRP values. If these reports are accurate, it would be risky to terminate follow-up observation. Evaluation of blood vessels after acute KD, when inflammation subsides, is an important issue because it can greatly affect the prognosis of late-phase KD.

In general, oxidative stress is theoretically and naturally involved in the presence of vascular endothelial function impairment and chronic inflammation. The links among these three factors have been detailed in a number of studies, particularly in Ross's response-to-inflammation hypothesis [13] and Steinberg's oxidation hypothesis [14], and are widely accepted.

Specifically, when vascular endothelial cells are impaired, the production of ROS increases. Subsequently, ROS activate NF-κB, triggering the release of various proinflammatory cytokines. Then, immunocompetent cells activated by cytokines adhere to endothelial cells and migrate subendothelially. Vascular smooth muscle cells and fibroblasts then migrate subendothelially and thrombi adhere, further impairing endothelial cells. This constitutes positive feedback. Previous studies have reported various sources of ROS production in vascular endothelial cells. Mitochondria and xanthine oxidase are reported as sources involved in hypoxia and hypercholesterolemia, respectively. In any case, this vicious cycle is believed to eventually lead to arteriosclerosis.

In response, vascular endothelial cells constitutively express endothelial NO synthase (eNOS) to produce NO, thereby eliminating ROS. NO has other effects, such as vascular dilatation and platelet aggregation suppression effects, and suppresses vascular remodeling and arteriosclerosis. It is worth noting that eNOS requires tetrahydrobiopterin (BH4) as a coenzyme to produce NO, and that when BH4 declines eNOS starts producing O_2- rather than NO, reversing the pathway to produce ROS. The present evidence supports the hypothesis that eNOS is as an ROS production source in certain diseases, such as arteriosclerosis and diabetes [15, 16]. Therefore, treatments to suppress vascular remodeling should consider both increasing eNOS and supplementing BH4.

To discuss arteriosclerosis during late KD, one must first define the term arteriosclerosis. In general contexts, arteriosclerosis simply refers to atherosclerosis, whereas arteriosclerosis during late KD refers to the presence of postinflammatory arteriosclerotic lesions. We need to clearly distinguish the two because they differ histologically [17]. Moreover, a study examined CAL in cases of adolescent KD, using a recently developed examination method called virtual histology intravascular ultrasound, which is capable of detailed pathological examination. The results showed that patients with regressed aneurysms and coronary artery aneurysms mainly had fibrotic lesions, whereas intimal hypertrophy entailed a certain level of calcification. Moreover, more-severe lesions had more uneven components other than fibrotic hypertrophy, along with calcification, similar to

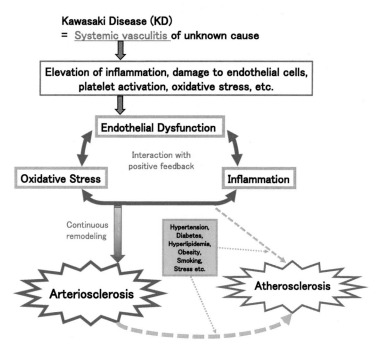

Fig. 3 Hypothetical mechanism of onset and progression of atherosclerosis in KD. Arteriosclerosis during late KD refers to postinflammatory arteriosclerotic lesions. We need to clearly distinguish arteriosclerosis from atherosclerosis because they are histologically different. There are limited data on atherosclerosis in KD, even now

general arteriosclerosis lesions [18]. Vascular calcification during late KD has previously been considered to be all-round calcification in the tunica adventitia and tunica media, unlike calcification observed in arteriosclerosis. However, the new method enabled reporting of atherosclerosis-like calcification lesions. Furthermore, another study reported that atherosclerosis developed in an animal model of KD-like vasculitis after challenge with a hypercholesterolemic diet [19]. This implies that atherosclerosis can develop and progress in young adults when other risk factors for arteriosclerosis, such as hyperlipidemia, are present during late KD. Additional studies will be necessary in order to address the issue, including the involvement of oxidative stress (Fig. 3).

Real Picture of Oxidative Stress During Late KD

To date, very few studies have examined oxidative stress during late KD. Our group measured urine 8-isoprostane, a sensitive marker of oxidative stress, and found that it was markedly increased in patients with a history of KD, regardless of the presence of CAL (Fig. 4). Thus, patients with a history of KD were under oxidative

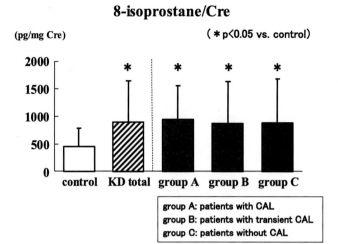

Controls: n=367 (males: n=192; females: n=175), average 15.3 years
KD patients: n=149 (males: n=91; females: n=58), average 15.6 years
group A: n=32, group B: n=21, group C: n=96

Fig. 4 8-isoprostane in chronic KD

stress even during the late phase, indicating the possible involvement of oxidative stress in the onset and development of vascular endothelial cell impairment [12]. Among these patients, those with CAL were treated with fluvastatin. We examined the vascular protective effects of this agent because statins have vascular protective effects mediated by increased eNOS production and activation as well as anti-oxidative effects, including suppression of NAD(P)H oxidase activity. The results showed improvement in %FMD, baPWV, and urine NOx, all of which are markers of vascular functions, as well as in highly sensitive CRP and urine 8-isoprostane. These findings indicate that statins have vascular protective effects and improve vascular endothelial function as well as chronic inflammation (Fig. 5) [20].

Before our report, an article reported that late-phase KD patients with reduced FMD showed FMD improvement after receiving the antioxidant vitamin C [21]. This suggests that oxidative stress is closely involved in the impairment of vascular endothelial cells during late KD and strongly supports the feasibility of improving vascular endothelial function by anti-oxidative therapy.

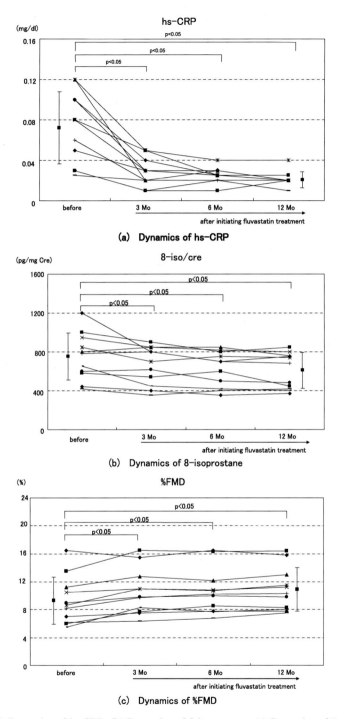

Fig. 5 (**a**) Dynamics of hs-CRP, (**b**) Dynamics of 8-isoprostane, (**c**) Dynamics of %FMD, (**d**) Dynamics of baPWV, (**e**) Dynamics of NOx

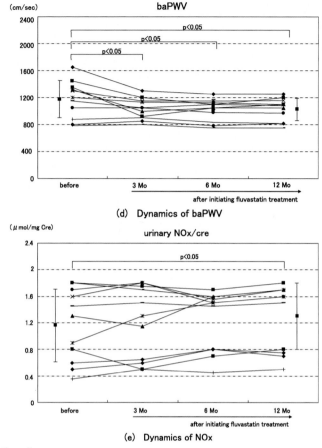

(d) Dynamics of baPWV

(e) Dynamics of NOx

Fig. 5 (continued)

Conclusion

As described above, oxidative stress is very likely involved in the pathology of acute and late KD in many ways and is not just a consequence of the pathologic processes. Therefore, oxidative stress should be regarded as a future therapeutic target for KD. This approach has already been gradually initiated. However, oxidative stress is involved in many signaling pathways, including the defense system against infections, and is not entirely harmful. Therefore, we must reconsider whether ROS should be simply eliminated to prevent blood vessel impairment. Oxidative therapies, in which oxidative stress is given to activate antioxidative functions, are frequently administered in Germany and the United States. This illustrates that oxidative stress is difficult to manage because it is both harmful and beneficial. At what times, how, and to what extent should oxidative stress be suppressed? The continued development of anti-oxidative therapies will likely yield answers to these questions.

References

1. Sies H. What is oxidative stress? In: Kency Jr JF, editor. Oxidative stress and vascular disease. Boston: Kluwer Academic Publishers; 2000. p. 1–8. 10.1007/978-1-4615-4649-8_1.

2. Takahashi K, Oharaseki T, Naoe S, Wakayama M, Yokouchi Y. Neutrophilic involvement in the damage to coronary arteries in acute stage of Kawasaki disease. Pediatr Int. 2005;47 (3):305–10. http://dx.doi.org/10.1111/j.1442-200x.2005.02049.x. PMID:15910456.

3. Griendling KK, Sorescu D, Ushio-Fukai M. NAD(P)H oxidase: role in cardiovascular biology and disease. Circ Res. 2000;86(5):494–501. http://dx.doi.org/. 10.1161/01.RES.86.5.494. PMID:10720409.

4. Kumar U, Chen J, Sapoznikhov V, Canteros G, White BH, Sidhu A. Overexpression of inducible nitric oxide synthase in the kidney of the spontaneously hypertensive rat. Clin Exp Hypertens. 2005;27(1):17–31. http://dx.doi.org/10.1081/CEH-200044249. PMID:15773227.

5. Takatsuki S, Ito Y, Takeuchi D, Hoshida H, Nakayama T, Matsuura H, Saji T. IVIG reduced vascular oxidative stress in patients with Kawasaki disease. Circ J. 2009;73(7):1315–8. http://doi.org/10.1253/circj.CJ-07-0635. PMID:19436119.

6. Yahata T, Suzuki C, Hamaoka A, Fujii M, Hamaoka K. Dynamics of reactive oxygen metabolites and biological antioxidant potential in the acute stage of Kawasaki disease. Circ J. 2011;75(10):2453–9. http://dx.doi.org/10.1253/circj.CJ-10-0605. PMID:21785226.

7. Shen CT, Wang NK. Antioxidants may mitigate the deterioration of coronary arteritis in patients with Kawasaki disease unresponsive to high-dose intravenous gamma-globulin. Pediatr Cardiol. 2001;22(5):419–22. http://dx.doi.org/10.1007/s002460010268. PMID:11526424.

8. Steer KA, Wallace TM, Bolton CH, Hartog M. Aspirin protects low density lipoprotein from oxidative modification. Heart. 1997;77(4):333–7. http://dx.doi.org/10.1136/hrt.77.4. 333. PMID:9155612.

9. Kobayashi T, Saji T, Otani T, Takeuchi K, Nakamura T, Arakawa H, RAISE study group investigators, et al. Efficacy of immunoglobulin plus prednisolone for prevention of coronary artery abnormalities in severe Kawasaki disease (RAISE study): a randomised, open-label, blinded-endpoints trial. Lancet. 2012;379(9826):1613–20. http://dx.doi.org/10.1016/S0140-6736(11)61930-2. PMID:22405251.

10. Suzuki H, Terai M, Hamada H, Honda T, Suenaga T, Takeuchi T, et al. Cyclosporin A treatment for Kawasaki disease refractory to initial and additional intravenous immunoglobulin. Pediatr Infect Dis J. 2011;30(10):871–6. http://dx.doi.org/10.1097/INF.0b013e318220c3cf. PMID:21587094.

11. Tremoulet AH, Jain S, Jaggi P, Jimenez-Fernandez S, Pancheri JM, Sun X, et al. Infliximab for intensification of primary therapy for Kawasaki disease: a phase 3 randomised, double-blind, placebo-controlled trial. Lancet. 2014;383(9930):1731–8. http://dx.doi.org/10.1016/S0140-6736(13)62298-9. PMID:24572997.

12. Niboshi A, Hamaoka K, Sakata K, Yamaguchi N. Endothelial dysfunction in adult patients with a history of Kawasaki disease. Eur J Pediatr. 2008;167(2):189–96. http://dx.doi.org/10. 1007/s00431-007-0452-9. PMID:17345094.

13. Ross R. The pathogenesis of atherosclerosis: a perspective for the 1990s. Nature. 1993;362 (6423):801–9. http://dx.doi.org/10.1038/362801a0. PMID:8479518.

14. Steinberg D, Parthasarathy S, Carew TE, Khoo JC, Witztum JL. Beyond cholesterol. Modifications of low-density lipoprotein that increase its atherogenicity. N Engl J Med. 1989;320 (14):915–24. PMID:2648148.

15. Kawashima S, Yokoyama M. Dysfunction of endothelial nitric oxide synthase and atherosclerosis. Arterioscler Thromb Vasc Biol. 2004;24(6):998–1005. http://dx.doi.org/10.1161/01. ATV.0000125114.88079.96. PMID:15001455.

16. Guzik TJ, Mussa S, Gastaldi D, Sadowski J, Ratnatunga C, Pillai R, et al. Mechanisms of increased vascular superoxide production in human diabetes mellitus: role of NAD(P)H oxidase and endothelial nitric oxide synthase. Circulation. 2002;105(14):1656–62. http://dx. doi.org/10.1161/01.CIR.0000012748.58444.08. PMID:11940543.

17. Takahashi K, Oharaseki T, Naoe S. Pathological study of postcoronary arteritis in adolescents and young adults: with reference to the relationship between sequelae of Kawasaki disease and atherosclerosis. Pediatr Cardiol. 2001;22(2):138–42. http://dx.doi.org/10.1007/s002460010180. PMID:11178671.

18. Mitani Y, Ohashi H, Sawada H, Ikeyama Y, Hayakawa H, Takabayashi S, et al. In vivo plaque composition and morphology in coronary artery lesions in adolescents and young adults long after Kawasaki disease: a virtual histology-intravascular ultrasound study. Circulation. 2009;119(21):2829–36. http://dx.doi.org/10.1161/CIRCULATIONAHA.108.818609. PMID:19451352.

19. Liu Y, Onouchi Z, Sakata K, Ikuta K. An experimental study on the role of smooth muscle cells in the pathogenesis of atherosclerosis of the coronary arteritis. J Jpn Pediatr Soc. 1996;100:1453–8.

20. Hamaoka-Okamoto A, Suzuki C, Yahata T, Ikeda K, Nagi-Miura N, Ohno N, et al. The involvement of the vasa vasorum in the development of vasculitis in animal model of Kawasaki disease. Pediatr Rheumatol Online J. 2014;12(1):12. http://dx.doi.org/10.1186/1546-0096-12-12. PMID:24678599.

21. Deng YB, Xiang HJ, Chang Q, Li CL. Evaluation by high-resolution ultrasonography of endothelial function in brachial artery after Kawasaki disease and the effects of intravenous administration of vitamin C. Circ J. 2002;66(10):908–12. http://dx.doi.org/10.1253/circj.66. 908. PMID:12381083.

Part V
Catheter Intervention and Surgery

Antiplatelet and Anticoagulant Therapies for Kawasaki Disease: Theory and Practice

Masato Takahashi

Abstract Antiplatelet and anticoagulant therapies are important elements in the medical management of Kawasaki disease (KD). Both the enzymatic coagulation cascade and platelets are activated on a systemic scale. Experimental evidence from *in vitro* models suggests that disturbed blood flow induces a coagulation cascade resulting in thrombin production. This line of evidence is relevant for KD patients with large coronary aneurysms. This chapter discusses antiplatelet and anticoagulant drugs and examines evidence related to their use. Regarding thrombolytic therapy, the evidence suggests that intravenous therapy is equal to or better than an intracoronary approach in achieving desired therapeutic goals. Unresolved issues for improving the quality of antithrombotic therapies will require multicenter clinical research programs.

Keywords Antiplatelet drugs • Anticoagulants • Aspirin • Aspirin resistance • Clopidogrel • Abciximab • Warfarin • Unfractionated heparin (UFH) • Low-molecular-weight heparin (LMWH) • tPA

Introduction

Because of the rarity of thromboembolism in children, we owe most of our knowledge to the extensive experience in adults. The concept of arterial thrombosis suggests coronary artery plaque rupture, which induces platelet adhesion. We conceptualize deep vein thrombosis in an immobile postoperative adult who develops venous thrombosis and pulmonary embolism. Kawasaki disease (KD) is a very different scenario that challenges us to think more critically, build our own hypothesis, and draw on innovative research ideas and results, with the hope of finding optimal, individualized therapies. This chapter describes salient points of KD pathophysiology and offers evidence-based recommendations for antiplatelet, anticoagulant, and thrombolytic therapies.

M. Takahashi (✉)
Heart Center, Seattle Children's Hospital, 4800 Sand Point Way NE, Seattle, WA 98105, USA
e-mail: masato.takahashi@seattlechildrens.org

© Springer Japan 2017   355
B.T. Saji et al. (eds.), *Kawasaki Disease*, DOI 10.1007/978-4-431-56039-5_39

Historical Review

During the time since Kawasaki's original description, KD has become a world-wide health problem, and a series of changes have occurred in its treatment. Kawasaki felt that the new disease combined features of infection and collagen disease. His first 50 cases were treated with antibiotics and/or corticosteroids. None of these 50 patients died, and the disease was thus characterized as a self-limited process with benign outcomes. However, shortly after publication of his report, a number of patients with identical signs and symptoms died suddenly during convalescence. Postmortem examinations of these patients showed thrombotic occlusion of coronary arteries. Imaging studies of living patients with KD also showed coronary artery aneurysms. At this point use of aspirin as an antithrombotic gained acceptance. Periodic nationwide surveys of KD showed that, by 1979, KD patients were treated predominantly with aspirin. Around the year 1982, intravenous immunoglobulin (IVIG) gained acceptance from clinicians. A dramatic decline in KD fatality rate, from 2 % to less than 0.5 %, occurred between 1975 and 1980. This coincided with the increased use of aspirin but was well before widespread acceptance of IVIG. The fatality rate has further declined during the IVIG era, to 0.2 % [1]. Earlier IVIG treatment and wider use of warfarin or heparin for large aneurysms probably contributed to improved mortality.

The Procoagulant State in KD

Traditionally, thrombosis is dichotomized into arterial and venous thrombosis, which differ in pathogenesis, risk factors, and treatments [2]. Arterial thrombosis is initiated at the site of vascular damage by activated platelets expressing a large array of membrane receptors that bind to collagen fibers and von Willebrand factor (vWF). Apropos of KD, inflammatory cytokines such as tumor necrosis factor induce endothelium to express adhesion molecules such as intercellular adhesion molecule 1 and P-selectin to capture leukocytes, and platelets initiate thrombosis. As the clot matures, various growth factors come into play to stimulate cellular migration and proliferation, resulting in vascular remodeling.

In contrast, venous thrombosis is mainly driven by enzyme-based cascades of reactions, culminating in the action of tenase (the enzyme that activates factor X). The previous concept of coequal intrinsic and extrinsic pathways has been supplanted by a newer concept. The enzymatic cascade begins with an omnipresent tissue factor, which is activated by vascular injury. This activation is amplified by thrombin and factor XI through positive feedbacks, and may be mitigated by tissue factor inhibitor, antithrombin, and protein C [3]. The fibrinolytic system represented by plasmin may reverse nascent thrombus. Another important factor is blood flow abnormalities, including turbulence and stagnation. Disturbed flow can activate endothelium, which then interacts with monocytes and platelets, thereby promoting the coagulation cascade.

Vasculitis as the Basis for Hypercoagulability

Acute KD is unique in that the hypercoagulable state is created through simultaneous activation of platelets and the enzymatic cascade. The third element of hypercoagulability is decreased fibrinolytic function, which is poorly understood in the context of KD. The intrinsically low levels of plasminogen in young infants may be important. In a prospective evaluation of coagulation status in 31 KD patients, Burns and colleagues found simultaneous increases in factor VIII activity, fibrinogen level, and thrombocytosis. Elevated plasma β-thromboglobulin was noted in KD patients with coronary artery abnormalities, indicating platelet activation [4].

Pathologically, acute KD is characterized by immune-mediated panvasculitis with necrosis of endothelium and reduced synthesis of nitric oxide and prostacyclin (PGI_2), and release of inflammatory markers such as tumor necrosis factor α, interleukin-1, interleukin-6, CD84, and anticardiolipin immune complex, all indicating a procoagulant state. Although clinically acute clinical symptoms subside within 1–2 weeks in most patients, there are signs that the chronic procoagulant state and endothelial dysfunction persist much longer.

Flow Disturbance and Stagnation Stimulate Coagulation

Recently, a series of bioengineering studies used *in vitro* models to evaluate disturbed flow in monolayers of cultured endothelium. These studies allowed measurement of shear stress at multiple points and the assay of biological markers of endothelial dysfunction. Endothelial cells exposed to disturbed flow showed increased intracellular levels of transcription factors (such as nuclear factor-KB) and surface expression of adhesion molecules (such as intercellular adhesion molecule 1 and E-selectin). There was enhanced adhesion of monocytes at a point downstream where laminar flow reemerged [5]. In another study, Fallon and colleagues used models of complex orifice geometry with changing lumen diameters to map blood velocity and shear stress profiles. Blood samples were tested for thrombin–antithrombin complex and platelet factor four levels. They showed that small changes in geometry affected the propensity for blood coagulation by increasing thrombin generation [6]. Using a murine model of blood stagnation by ligating the carotid artery, Kawasaki et al. induced tissue factor expression in luminal leukocytes initiating coagulation cascade, fibrin formation, and neointimal formation [7]. Sengupta et al. used computed tomographic angiograms to create a model of the aneurysmal coronary arteries of KD patients and found marked flow disturbances, namely, wall shear stress values that were an order of magnitude less than those seen in normal arteries. Particle residence times (a measure of stagnation) in some cases spanned five cardiac cycles. Such abnormal rheology, when combined with procoagulant endothelium and activated platelets, would pose substantial short- and long-term risks of thrombosis [8].

Platelet Activation, Adhesion, and Aggregation in KD

Inactive platelets are discoid and about one-third the size of erythrocytes. The membrane is studded with many types of receptors, and the cytoplasm contains storage granules (α-granules and dense granules) that are connected with the open canalicular system. In a typical arterial lumen with a laminar flow profile, larger erythrocytes tend to flow in the center of the lumen, while smaller platelets tend to move near the arterial wall. When platelets are activated, their shapes become irregular. Platelet activation is mainly mediated by thrombin and ADP. The open canalicular system becomes externalized, and granular contents are easily discharged. Cell deformations are caused by increases in intracellular calcium concentration. Platelet activation often follows localized injury of the endothelial layer, such as in atherosclerotic plaque rupture, trauma, or surgical or catheter interventions. In contrast to adult-onset coronary atherosclerosis, platelets are activated on a systemic scale rather than locally during acute Kawasaki disease, although the exact molecular crosstalk leading to such systemic activation has not been elucidated. The hypothesis that platelet activation is widespread in acute KD is supported by several lines of evidence. Burns et al. reported increased β-thromboglobulin, a chemokine released by α granules [4]. Using a particle counting method, Taki and colleagues demonstrated spontaneous platelet aggregation in the blood of KD patients [9]. Using ELISA, Yahata et al. measured platelet-derived microparticles (diameter, 0.02–0.1 μm), a marker of platelet activation. They incorporate phospholipids on their surface and platelet granule components within and possess intrinsic procoagulant activity and the capacity for adhesion with heterogeneous cells. Strikingly, levels of platelet-derived microparticles rebounded in patients for whom aspirin therapy was discontinued 2–3 months after treatment initiation, raising some questions about duration of aspirin treatment [10]. The mechanism of platelet activation was studied using analytical cytology and cytometry with fluorescent staining. KD patients had markers indicating a high level of platelet aggregation, including heterotopic (platelet-leukocyte-erythrocyte) aggregation (Fig. 1), degranulation, externalization of phosphatidylserine, and decreased intracellular p-selectin [11]. Another study showed that epinephrine-induced platelet aggregation rates remained accelerated long after acute KD [12]. Activated platelets undergo adhesion to injured vascular tissues, through the actions of primary agonists: vWF and collagen. vWF is a particularly important platelet ligand in arteries exposed to high shear rates. In contrast, only under low shear-rate conditions in the vein, and possibly within the lumen of a giant coronary aneurysm, can fibrinogen and fibrin bind platelets. Aggregation of platelets is primarily caused by thromboxane A2 and ADP. Activation of integrin receptor G

Platelets features

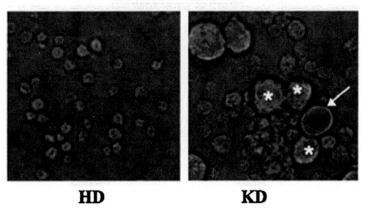

HD   **KD**

Fig. 1 Two representative light photomicrographs showing plates obtained from peripheral blood samples of a healthy donor (HD – *left* panel) and a KD patient (*right* panel) (To note: clusters of platelets with leukocytes (*asterisks*) and red blood cells (*arrow*) in a KD patient (*right* panel) Courtesy of Elsevier Inc, from Straface E, et al Biochem Biophys Research Communication 392: p. 428)

IIb/IIIa allows stronger binding of platelets to vWF, thus stabilizing anchoring of the thrombus. The G IIb/IIIa receptor also has a central role in platelet aggregation, by signaling crosslinking of vWF and fibrinogen molecules to form a stronger union of platelets.

Antiplatelet Drugs

Aspirin

We rely heavily on aspirin both for its anti-inflammatory effect during acute KD and for its antiplatelet effect. However, there is limited understanding of its optimal dose and duration and the prevalence and severity of aspirin resistance.

Pharmacodynamics Aspirin irreversibly blocks cyclooxygenase (COX)-1, resulting in inhibition of thromboxane A2 (TXA2) release from platelets and prostaglandin (PG) I_2 release from endothelial cells. The antiplatelet effect of aspirin lasts for the lifetime of the affected platelet (10–12 days). There is some evidence that the antiplatelet effect of aspirin is caused not only by its inhibition of TXA2 and that platelets under the influence of aspirin could still be activated under conditions of high shear stress, due to activation by thrombin, but that much higher doses of aspirin may suppress such platelet reactivity [13].

Platelets in Neonates As compared with adult controls, platelets of neonates are hyporeactive to agonists such as thrombin, ADP, and thromboxane A_2 [14]

Pharmacokinetics Once ingested, aspirin is easily converted to salicylic acid. Most salicylic acid is metabolized in the liver. The rest is eliminated by the kidneys, with an elimination half-life of about 2.0–4.5 h. Renal excretion of salicylic acid is facilitated by alkalinized urine pH.

Current Uses in KD Use of aspirin for KD varies by country. In Japan it is generally agreed that the antiplatelet effect of aspirin, as opposed to its anti-inflammatory effect, is the main benefit. Thus, in Japan the usual dose is 30–50 mg/kg per day for the duration of active KD. In patients who develop persistent coronary artery abnormalities, the same dose is continued. However, in the United States and Canada most practitioners believe in the value of a high anti-inflammatory dose (80–100 mg/kg per day divided into four equal doses every 6 h, until defervescence). The dose is then reduced to an antiplatelet dose of 3–5 mg/kg per day. This dose is continued for 6–8 weeks, until clinical symptoms and signs resolve and a sense of well-being has returned. In some cases, termination of aspirin is guided by the decline in acute reactants (mainly C-reactive protein). If the patient has persistent coronary artery dilatation or aneurysm, low-dose aspirin is continued much longer. The duration of aspirin therapy is a subject of controversy.

Aspirin Resistance A number of studies have investigated aspirin resistance in adults. Most enrolled a relatively small number of patients (range, 39–325). The prevalence of aspirin resistance ranged from 8 to 56 %. Prevalence tended to be higher if platelet function was assessed by the Platelet Function Analyzer-100 (PFA-100) as compared with light transmission aggregometry (35.8 ± 15.1 % vs. 15.9 ± 10.6 %, respectively). Patients receiving higher aspirin doses are less likely to develop resistance than those on low doses. Even so, among patients on 1500 mg/day, 8 % developed resistance. Some patients who were aspirin-sensitive at the beginning of follow-up later became resistant [15]. Few studies have investigated aspirin resistance in children. In an unpublished study of 30 children with KD, the PFA-100 showed aspirin resistance in 9 of 28 (32 %), and thromboelastography (TEG) showed resistance in 8 of 30 (26 %). However, there was poor concordance in the results of the two tests (personal communication).

Drug–Drug Interaction According to a warning by the US Food and Drug Administration, the antiplatelet effect of aspirin may be negated by ibuprofen (a nonselective COX inhibitor) taken 8 h or less before the aspirin dose. In addition, patients were advised against taking ibuprofen within 30 min of taking aspirin.

Adverse Effects The major adverse effects of aspirin are gastrointestinal irritation (nausea, vomiting, indigestion) and bleeding tendency. Reye syndrome is now uncommon and appears more likely with large anti-inflammatory doses than with antiplatelet doses.

Recommendations

For the purpose of offering recommendations, the author will refer only to antiplatelet aspirin therapy and not to anti-inflammatory therapy. The current antiplatelet regimen for KD patients, whether 30 mg/kg per day in Japan or 3–5 mg/kg per day in the United States, is empirical rather than evidence-based. However, it seems safe and effective in all but a few patients, who might have increased thrombotic risks due to the presence of unequivocal coronary artery lesions.

1. In KD patients with normal coronary arteries or mild ectasia in the proximal RCA, LMCA, or proximal LAD (Z-score <2.5), it is reasonable to continue the antiplatelet aspirin regimen for that country. (Class IIa, B)
2. Antiplatelet aspirin therapy should be continued for at least 8 weeks or until transient coronary dilatation has regressed to normal dimensions. (Class IIa, B)
3. In patients with unequivocal coronary artery lesions and greater than minimal risk of thrombosis, aspirin may be initiated at a conventional dosage. Within 6 months of starting the therapy the patient should undergo a platelet function study including but not limited to PFA-100. If the results show suboptimal flow-mediated platelet aggregation against a collagen/epinephrine agonist, a coagulation specialist should be consulted regarding aspirin dose adjustment or addition of another antiplatelet drug and future follow-up. (Class IIa, C)

Thienopyridine ADP Receptor Blockers (Ticlopidine and Clopidogrel)

Pharmacodynamics Ticlopidine and clopidogrel selectively inhibit platelet aggregation by irreversibly blocking ADP-receptor $P2Y_{12}$ on platelets. Clopidogrel has not been evaluated in a rigorous randomized clinical trial but has been investigated in the PICOLO study and a dosage-escalation study (for pharmacokinetics and pharmacodynamics) using ADP-induced light-transmission aggregometry concurrently with adult control samples. The authors concluded that a dose of 0.2 mg/kg per day on average would produce 30–50 % platelet aggregation (which occurred in adults receiving 75 mg/day), but the drug effect was highly variable, possibly because of the high variability of CYP3A4 enzyme among individuals, especially in young infants [16].

Pharmacokinetics Ticlopidine is the shorter acting of the two and must be administered twice daily; clopidogrel can be administered once daily at the dose suggested above.

Current Uses in KD Despite the dosing challenges caused by the fact that clopidogrel is dispensed only as a 75-mg tablet, its use in tertiary care pediatric hospitals in the US has increased 15-fold during the 10-year period between 2000 and 2009, from 6 to 89.5 per 100,000 admissions according to an analysis of the Pediatric Health Information Database by Gentilomo et al. However, most of these patients had congenital heart disease, and about 10 % had KD [17]. Because of the absence of data suggesting otherwise, the recommended starting dose for children is 0.2 mg/kg per day.

Adverse Effects To date, all public reports of adverse effects involve adult patients. Bleeding is the most frequently reported adverse effect. According to data collected by Gentilomo et al. bleeding occurred in 14.6 % of total clopidogrel admissions. Bleeding events were most frequently associated with procedures (35 %), followed by gastrointestinal (21 %), intracranial (16 %), and mucocutaneous (14 %) complications [15]. Ticlopidine has been associated with aplastic anemia and neutropenia. Both agents have been associated with thrombotic thrombocytopenic purpura, which is a rare but serious, potentially life-threatening, complication [18].

Recommendations

1. Ticlopidine may be considered as an antiplatelet drug for KD, and patients should be monitored for possible drug toxicity. (Class IIb, B)
2. Clopidogrel can be selected as an alternative or supplementary antiplatelet drug for moderately high-risk KD patients, after the patient and family are informed of its limited dosing flexibility, individual variability in dose effect, and the possibility of thrombotic thrombocytopenic purpura. The patient should be monitored for bleeding, thrombocytopenia, hemolytic anemia, and decreased renal function. (Class IIa, B)

Dipyridamole

Pharmacodynamics Dipyridamole is a phosphodiesterase inhibitor and thus increases the level of adenyl cyclase. However, its antiplatelet effect is weak and short-lived. Dipyridamole has a more profound vasodilatory effect, especially in coronary arteries, and is frequently used as a pharmacological stress agent in myocardial perfusion imaging.

Current Uses in KD Dipyridamole was used in place of or in combination with aspirin before the availability of thienopyridines. Currently, it is not considered a first- or second-line antiplatelet drug.

Adverse Effects Dizziness, headache, chest pain (angina pectoris), nausea.

Recommendations

1. The antiplatelet effect of dipyridamole is relatively weak and its safety profile is unfavorable for young children. Therefore, it is not recommended as an antiplatelet drug for children. (Class III, C)

Abciximab (Glycoprotein IIb/IIIa Inhibitor)

Pharmacodynamics Abciximab is the first commercially produced human–murine chimeric monoclonal antibody. Its Fab segments bind to glycoprotein IIb/IIIa receptors on human platelets, which are considered the final common pathway for platelet aggregation. It inhibits platelet aggregation by preventing binding of fibrinogen and vWF to platelets. It has other inhibitory effects on receptors on smooth muscle cells and macrophages. The product was marketed primarily as an adjunct to coronary angioplasty in patients who are at high risk of sudden closure of revascularized coronary arteries.

Current Uses in KD Abciximab was initially used in KD patients with large coronary artery aneurysms with thrombosis. Williams et al. later reported that a reduction in aneurysm size was more likely among patients with acute KD who received abciximab in addition to IVIG and aspirin (13 of 19 patients) than among those who received standard treatment only (7 of 19 patients) during a follow-up period of 4–6 months.

Adverse Effects Bleeding is the foremost concern. Abciximab should not be given to patients with bleeding tendency or those still under the effects of other anti-coagulant(s).

Recommendations

1. This drug may be considered in patients who are at high risk of coronary thrombosis. (Class IIa, B)
2. Its efficacy in promoting coronary artery aneurysm regression needs to be verified.

Anticoagulant Drugs

Warfarin

Pharmacodynamics Warfarin, the most widely used vitamin K antagonist (VKA), inhibits synthesis of vitamin K–dependent coagulation factors II, VII, IX, and X, as well as anticoagulant factors C and S. Some of these factors are naturally reduced in newborns to levels that are frequently achieved in adults receiving therapeutic amounts of warfarin with a target international normalized ratio (INR) of 2–3.

Dietary and Drug Interactions The effect of warfarin is blunted by foods such as dark-green vegetables (eg, broccoli and spinach), soy products, and infant formulas rich in vitamin K and by interactions with diet and other drugs. Warfarin consists of two optically active isomers. The S-enantiomer is five times as active as the

R-enantiomer. Many food and drug interactions with warfarin have been reported, although relatively few are based on scientifically verified mechanisms. Some but not all drug interactions involve stereo-selective clearance. There are many reports of drug interactions citing COX-2–selective nonsteroidal anti-inflammatory drugs, antibiotics (particularly the macrolides azithromycin, erythromycin, and clarithromycin), azoles (fluconazole and miconazole), amoxicillin, and quinolones (ciprofloxacin and levofloxacin). For more detailed information, readers are advised to consult the review by Holbrook et al., which analyzed data from 184 reports [19] Among the reports reviewed, 70 % described potentiation of warfarin, 15 % inhibition, and 15 % no effect. Of interest are the "no effect" drugs, including clopidogrel, losartan, and vitamin E.

Pharmacokinetics and Dose Monitoring Onset of action occurs in 24 h, whether the drug is given orally or intravenously. The effect peaks in 4 h if given orally, faster when given intravenously. Drug half-life is 20–60 h. The anticoagulant effect is monitored by prothrombin time converted to INR, using the formula:

$$\text{INR} = \left[\frac{\text{PT measured}}{\text{PT control}} \right]^{\text{ISI}}$$

ISI = international sensitivity index, an estimate of the sensitivity of thromboplastin; the higher the ISI, the less sensitive the agent

Dose Adjustment A practical guide to warfarin dosing in children was published by Andrew et al. [20]. An initial dose of 0.2 mg/kg was followed by subsequent dose adjustments, according to a nomogram using INR values. Children vary greatly in the dosage required to maintain a therapeutic INR range. The largest cohort study (319 patients), by Streif et al., found that to maintain a target INR of 2–3, infants required 0.33 mg/kg warfarin, and teenagers required 0.09 mg/kg.

Home INR Monitoring Recently, home monitoring of INR by finger stick blood sampling has become available. Among adults, those who utilized home INR monitoring as compared with high-quality laboratory testing had moderately higher costs but better quality of life. The incidences of bleeding and thrombotic complications were not higher than those of patients who received laboratory INR measurements. No data are available on home monitoring for pediatric patients.

Adverse Effects Bleeding is the main complication. The incidence of bleeding is estimated to be 0.5 per patient-year. Among young active children, the INR value is not necessarily related to bleeding risk.

Vitamin K may be given to patients with a high INR and no significant bleeding. In patients with clinically significant bleeding, immediate reversal using fresh-frozen plasma or other procoagulant factors may be required, at the discretion of a hematologist. In pregnant women, warfarin has a teratogenic effect on about 5 % of fetuses. The risk is highest during the first trimester. One should test for pregnancy before starting warfarin in women of childbearing age. If a patient who is already on warfarin becomes pregnant, the drug should be discontinued and an alternate drug should be started. When appropriate, a physician familiar with management of anticoagulation during pregnancy should be consulted.

Current Uses in KD Although aspirin treatment appears to protect KD patients from coronary thrombosis, those with giant coronary artery aneurysms are particularly vulnerable to coronary thrombosis because of their severe endothelial dysfunction combined with an abnormal flow profile in diseased coronary arteries. In the present author's two decades of experience, those patients with giant coronary artery aneurysms who received warfarin (target INR 2.0–2.5) in combination with aspirin had more stable long-term outcomes, with fewer cardiovascular events such as acute myocardial infarction and occlusive coronary artery thrombosis, as compared with those who received aspirin only. It should be remembered, however, that despite the best efforts of providers to ensure compliance of the family and patient, giant aneurysms will develop stenoses, thromboses, and calcifications and may require revascularizing procedures during the patient's lifetime (Fig. 2). Suda and colleagues, in Japan, reported their experience with 83 patients who were treated with warfarin (target INR, 1.5 to >2.5) and aspirin [21].

The median follow-up period was 6.0 years. Survival without cardiac events was 92.5 % at 1 year and 91 % at 10 years. Eight patients developed myocardial infarction, two died, and three required emergency intracoronary thrombolytic therapy. Levy et al., in Toronto, followed 39 patients with giant aneurysm (2.2 % of their total KD patients), from 1990 to 2000 [22]. The patients were allocated to two groups: one group received warfarin and an antiplatelet drug and the other received an antiplatelet drug only. Of the tests done in the warfarin group, 52 % were within the target INR range of 2.0–3.0. Three patients developed acute nonfatal myocardial infarction within the first year after onset, all of whom had received warfarin. The authors were cautious about the value of warfarin given in combination with an antiplatelet drug. The pathophysiology of giant coronary aneurysms combines markedly activated platelets, dysfunctional endothelium, and severely disturbed rheology, which results in an acutely procoagulant state. In this setting, combining antiplatelet therapy with a therapy to mitigate thrombin production makes a great deal of sense. Unfortunately, the present supporting data are retrospective and not from a randomized clinical trial.

Recommendations

1. In KD patients with giant coronary aneurysm or rapidly enlarging aneurysm, it is reasonable to start combined warfarin and antiplatelet therapy. (Class IIa B)
2. Healthcare centers that administer warfarin to patients must have a proper laboratory for checking prothrombin/INR with approved quality control and staff who can educate families about possible complications, dose changes, diet modifications, and dose adjustments for concomitant medications and management of unforeseen bleeding. (Class I B)

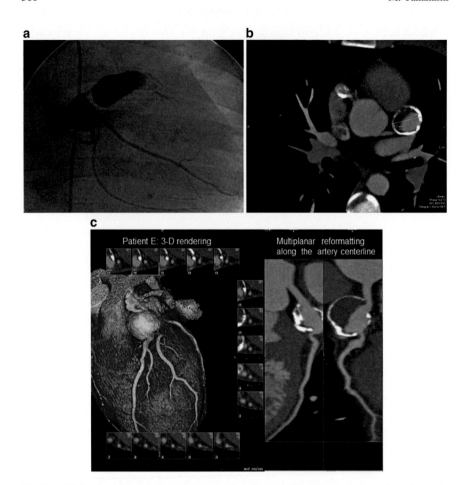

Fig. 2 (a) Selective left coronary arteriogram at age 2 years. The patient was treated continuously with warfarin and aspirin since diagnosis of giant aneurysm. Note the smooth contour of the aneurysm in the left anterior descending artery and the absence of a filling defect. (b) CT angiogram of the left coronary artery at age 22 years showing a heavily calcified secular aneurysm with a nonocclusive thrombus occupying about 40 % of the lumen. (c) CT angiogram of the left coronary artery at age 24 years, including 3D reconstruction (*left panel*) and multiplanar reformatting to demonstrate patency of the LAD channel (Note that the amount of thrombus has increased since the previous angiogram. This patient was highly compliant with his medications and his INR had remained within the target range >90 % of the time for 24 years)

Unfractionated Heparin

Unfractionated heparin (UFH) is widely used as a first-line anticoagulant because of its immediate onset of action in acutely ill patients with venous access. A 1996 meta-analysis showed that a heparin/aspirin combination was superior to aspirin alone in reducing the risk of ischemic events in adults with unstable angina [23].

Pharmacodynamics Heparin inhibits thrombin and factor Xa by binding to anti-thrombin through a high-affinity pentasaccharide. Because of its longer molecular chain, UFH can bind thrombin more tightly than the shorter low-molecular-weight heparin (LMWH).

Pharmacokinetics UFH has several unfavorable properties, including a short half-life (2–4 h), unpredictable pharmacokinetics, and a narrow therapeutic range.

Current Uses in KD UFH is often begun in an inpatient setting as a short-term lead-in to long-term oral anticoagulation with warfarin. It can effectively prevent or even reverse thrombosis while warfarin is being up-titrated, using the INR as a guide. A dose of 75–100 units/kg brings 90 % of children to a therapeutic activated partial thromboplastin time (aPTT) value (1.5–2 times the control value). The maintenance dose is age-dependent. Infants ≥ 2 months on average require 28 U/kg/h, while children >1 year require 20 U/kg/h [24].

Adverse Effects In the event of an excessively high aPTT value or bleeding, heparin may have to be reversed with protamine. The protamine dose depends on the last heparin dose and the interval since the previous heparin dose. In general, 1 mg protamine/100 U heparin is given if it has been <30 min. The dose is scaled down inversely with greater passage of time [24].

Heparin-induced thrombocytopenia (HIT) occurs in about 3 % of adults treated with unfractionated heparin, which is frequently associated with venous or arterial thrombosis. This phenomenon is attributed to platelet activation by heparin-dependent IgG antibodies. HIT incidence in children is less well documented. One study reported an incidence after cardiopulmonary bypass of 0.33 % (95 % confidence interval, <0.01–2.04).

Recommendations

1. To achieve maximum safety and efficacy, UFH should be given intravenously under supervision, with close clinical and laboratory monitoring and a well-defined aPTT target. (Class I, A)

LMWH

Because of the above-mentioned disadvantages of UFH, LMWH was developed using chemical and enzymatic depolymerization of UFH. LMWH is an oligosaccharide containing about 18 residues. There are several types of LMWH, but enoxaparin is the most widely used type in the United States.

Pharmacokinetics LMWH has a plasma half-life two to four times that of UFH and therefore has more predictable therapeutic effects and requires intermittent rather than continuous administration and less frequent factor Xa monitoring. In general, the peak anti-FXa level is 2–6 h after subcutaneous injection.

Pharmacodynamics As is the case with UFH, LMWH inhibits thrombin and factor Xa by binding to antithrombin. It has less interaction with endothelial cells and platelets. A randomized comparison trial showed that the risk of HIT was much lower for LMWH than for UFH [25].

Current Uses in KD Manlhiot et al. compared the anticoagulant effects of LMWH and warfarin in 38 KD patients with coronary artery aneurysms. In an early phase of the study, patients were stratified by age: older patients received warfarin and younger patients were given LMWH. Later in the study, all participants were started on LMWH and then warfarin 12–18 months later. The investigators noted that patients on LMWH more rapidly achieved the predefined optimal anticoagulation level (factor Xa level of 0.5–1.0 U/mL) and more predictably remained in range with fewer dose changes, as compared with the warfarin group [26]. Infants younger than 3 months or with a body weight <5 kg tend to have a higher requirement per kilogram. The recommended initial treatment dose is 1.5 mg/kg for infants weighing <2.5 kg and 1.0 mg/kg for infants and children weighing >2.5 kg. The prophylactic dose is 50 % of the treatment dose [24].

Adverse Effects HIT among patients who received LMWH is about one tenth that of UFH-treated patients. Estimated incidence is <0.5 %.

Recommendations

1. It is reasonable to use LMWH in lieu of oral VKA in combination with an antiplatelet agent in patients at high risk of coronary thrombosis for whom anticoagulation is difficult to manage due to age or location of residence (Class IIa, B)

Thrombolytic Therapy

Historical Background Kato et al. investigated intracoronary urokinase in 15 children with thrombotic occlusion of coronary arteries due to KD [27]. They achieved either partial or complete recanalization but noted recurrent thrombosis in four of 15 patients but no recurrent myocardial infarction or death in up to 8 years of follow-up.

Pharmacodynamics Thrombolytic agents mediate conversion of endogenous plasminogen into plasmin. Plasminogen level in KD is reduced to about 50 % of the adult level. Some workers add extrinsic plasminogen, abciximab, or fresh-frozen plasma to thrombolytic agent to boost its effect. Regarding the selection of agents, tissue-type plasmin activator (tPA) has become the agent of choice, and is preferred over streptokinase and urokinase in pediatric patients because of a US Food and Drug Administration warning and the fact that in vitro comparisons of the three agents showed improved clot lysis by tPA. However, there are no comparative studies of the clinical efficacy and safety of the three agents. The frequently quoted general thrombolytic regimen of tPA is 0.5 mg/kg/h for 6 h concurrent with heparin infusion at 10 U/kg/h. In most cases, a minimum of partial thrombus clearing is attained in 20–65 % of patients [24].

Current Uses in KD Because of the rarity of acute coronary thrombosis, studies of thrombolysis have been case series with small numbers of KD cases, with one notable exception. Harada et al. reported the results of a national Japanese survey of thrombolytic therapy encompassing 23 patients in 14 centers. In a comparison of intracoronary (ICT) and intravenous (IVCT) administration routes, ICT was effective for relatively small clots ($\leq$10 mm), while IVCT was effective even for giant thrombi (>10 mm). An increasing number of adults with a definite or probable history of KD unexpectedly develop ischemic symptoms. The youngest KD patient to undergo thrombolysis in this series was 27 days of age [28].

Adverse Effects Bleeding is the most serious complication and appears to be dose-related. Thus, it is prudent to start with relatively low doses. Irritation of the local site of infusion is another concern.

Recommendations

1. Intravenous thrombolytic therapy is indicated when there is clear evidence of thrombus within a major coronary artery. (Class I, B)

Future Directions in Antiplatelet and Anticoagulant Therapies for KD

Initiative Toward Evidence-Based Uses of Antiplatelet Agents

Currently, aspirin dosage varies by country and practitioner, as does duration of therapy. Some evidence shows that platelet activation persists for 1 year or longer after acute onset. The frequency of aspirin resistance, the best method for detecting it, its dose-relatedness, and its natural progression are unclear. These issues demand evidence-based solutions. ADP-receptor antagonists, especially clopidogrel, singly or in combination with aspirin, are promising but need stronger evidential support. Commercially available pediatric clopidogrel formulations are needed. International multicenter randomized clinical trials are required in order to settle these issues.

Randomized Clinical Trials of New Oral Direct Anticoagulants

Although warfarin remains the primary oral anticoagulant, it has several important drawbacks. Newer, direct thrombin or FXa inhibitors are now becoming accepted by adult cardiologists for deep vein thrombosis and non–valve-related atrial fibrillation. Clinical research on the efficacy and safety of this class of drugs in children is at a nascent stage. A meta-analysis comparing these agents with VKA in adults showed noninferiority to warfarin in efficacy and slight superiority in safety (i.e, decreased bleeding risk) [29]. It is generally believed that optimal control of INR and avoidance of bleeding complications are more difficult in infants and children than in adults. It is hoped that pediatric application of these newer agents will soon be explored in a multicenter RCT comparing them with warfarin or LWMH.

References

 1. Yanagawa H, Nakamura Y, Yashiro M, Kawasaki T, editors. Epidemiology of Kawasaki disease – a 30-year achievement. Shindan to Chiryo Company Tokyo; 2002 [in Japanese]
 2. Martinelli I, Bucciarelli P, Mannucci PM. Thrombotic risk factors: basic pathophysiology. Crit Care Med. 2010;38(2 Suppl):S3–9. http://dx.doi.org/10.1097/CCM.0b013e3181c9cbd9. PMID:20083911.
 3. Lijnen HR, Panekoek H, Vermylen J. Thrombosis and thrombolytic therapy. In: Chien KR, editor. Molecular basis of cardiovascular disease. 2nd ed. Philadelphia: WB Saunders; 2004. p. 519–38.
 4. Burns JC, Glode MP, Clarke SH, Wiggins Jr J, Hathaway WE. Coagulopathy and platelet activation in Kawasaki syndrome: identification of patients at high risk for development of coronary artery aneurysms. J Pediatr. 1984;105(2):206–11. http://dx.doi.org/10.1016/S0022-3476(84)80114-6. PMID:6235335.
 5. Chiu JJ, Chien S. Effects of disturbed flow on vascular endothelium: pathophysiological basis and clinical perspectives. Physiol Rev. 2011;91(1):327–87. http://dx.doi.org/10.1152/physrev.00047.2009. PMID:21248169.
 6. Fallon AM, Dasi LP, Marzec UM, Hanson SR, Yoganathan AP. Procoagulant properties of flow fields in stenotic and expansive orifices. Ann Biomed Eng. 2008;36(1):1–13. http://dx.doi.org/10.1007/s10439-007-9398-3. PMID:17985244.
 7. Kawasaki T, Dewerchin M, Lijnen HR, Vreys I, Vermylen J, Hoylaerts MF. Mouse carotid artery ligation induces platelet-leukocyte-dependent luminal fibrin, required for neointima development. Circ Res. 2001;88(2):159–66. http://dx.doi.org/10.1161/01.RES.88.2.159. PMID:11157667.
 8. Sengupta D, Kahn AM, Burns JC, Sankaran S, Shadden SC, Marsden AL. Image-based modeling of hemodynamics in coronary artery aneurysms caused by Kawasaki disease. Biomech Model Mechanobiol. 2012;11(6):915–32. http://dx.doi.org/10.1007/s10237-011-0361-8. PMID:22120599.
 9. Taki M, Kobayashi M, Ohi C, Shimizu H, Goto K, Aso K, et al. Spontaneous platelet aggregation in Kawasaki disease using the particle counting method. Pediatr Int. 2003;45(6):649–52. http://dx.doi.org/10.1111/j.1442-200X.2003.01810.x. PMID:14651534.
10. Yahata T, Suzuki C, Yoshioka A, Hamaoka A, Ikeda K. Platelet activation dynamics evaluated using platelet-derived microparticles in Kawasaki disease. Circ J. 2014;78(1):188–93. http://dx.doi.org/10.1253/circj.CJ-12-1037. PMID:24152721.

11. Straface E, Gambardella L, Metere A, Marchesi A, Palumbo G, Cortis E, et al. Oxidative stress and defective platelet apoptosis in naïve patients with Kawasaki disease [BBRC]. Biochem Biophys Res Commun. 2010;392(3):426–30. http://dx.doi.org/10.1016/j.bbrc.2010.01.040. PMID:20079717.

12. Shirahata A, Nakamura T, Asakura A. Studies on blood coagulation and antithrombotic therapy in Kawasaki disease. Acta Paediatr Jpn. 1983;25(2):180–91. http://dx.doi.org/10.1111/j.1442-200X.1983.tb01685.x.

13. Ratnatunga CP, Edmondson SF, Rees GM, Kovacs IB. High-dose aspirin inhibits shear-induced platelet reaction involving thrombin generation. Circulation. 1992;85(3):1077–82. http://dx.doi.org/10.1161/01.CIR.85.3.1077. PMID:1537105.

14. Rajasekhar D, Kestin AS, Bednarek FJ, Ellis PA, Barnard MR, Michelson AD. Neonatal platelets are less reactive than adult platelets to physiological agonists in whole blood. Thromb Haemost. 1994;72(6):957–63. PMID:7740470.

15. Macchi L, Sorel N, Christiaens L. Aspirin resistance: definitions, mechanisms, prevalence, and clinical significance. Curr Pharm Des. 2006;12(2):251–8. http://dx.doi.org/10.2174/138161206775193064. PMID:16454741.

16. Li JS, Yow E, Berezny KY, Bokesch PM, Takahashi M, Graham Jr TP, PICOLO Investigators, et al. Dosing of clopidogrel for platelet inhibition in infants and young children: primary results of the Platelet Inhibition in Children On cLOpidogrel (PICOLO) trial. Circulation. 2008;117 (4):553–9. http://dx.doi.org/10.1161/CIRCULATIONAHA.107.715821. PMID:18195173.

17. Gentilomo C, Huang YS, Raffini L. Significant increase in clopidogrel use across U.S. children's hospitals. Pediatr Cardiol. 2011;32(2):167–75. http://dx.doi.org/10.1007/s00246-010-9836-0. PMID:21132568.

18. Zakarija A, Kwaan HC, Moake JL, Bandarenko N, Pandey DK, McKoy JM, et al. Ticlopidine- and clopidogrel-associated thrombotic thrombocytopenic purpura (TTP): review of clinical, laboratory, epidemiological, and pharmacovigilance findings (1989–2008) [NIH Public Access]. Kidney Int Suppl. 2009;112(112):S20–4. http://dx.doi.org/10.1038/ki.2008.613. PMID:19180126.

19. Holbrook AM, Pereira JA, Labiris R, McDonald H, Douketis JD, Crowther M, et al. Systematic overview of warfarin and its drug and food interactions. Arch Intern Med. 2005;165(10):1095–106. http://dx.doi.org/10.1001/archinte.165.10.1095. PMID:15911722.

20. Andrew M, Marzinotto V, Brooker LA, Adams M, Ginsberg J, Freedom R, et al. Oral anticoagulation therapy in pediatric patients: a prospective study. Thromb Haemost. 1994;71(3):265–9. PMID:8029786.

21. Suda K, Kudo Y, Higaki T, Nomura Y, Miura M, Matsumura M, et al. Multicenter and retrospective case study of warfarin and aspirin combination therapy in patients with giant coronary aneurysms caused by Kawasaki disease. Circ J. 2009;73(7):1319–23. http://dx.doi.org/10.1253/circj.CJ-08-0931. PMID:19436123.

22. Levy DM, Silverman ED, Massicotte MP, McCrindle BW, Yeung RSM. Longterm outcomes in patients with giant aneurysms secondary to Kawasaki disease. J Rheumatol. 2005;32: 928–34.22.

23. Oler A, Whooley MA, Oler J, Grady D. Adding heparin to aspirin reduces the incidence of myocardial infarction and death in patients with unstable angina. A meta-analysis. JAMA. 1996;276(10):811–5. http://dx.doi.org/10.1001/jama.1996.03540100055028. PMID:8769591.

24. Monagle P, Chan A, Massicotte P, Chalmers E, Michelson AD. Antithrombotic therapy in children: the seventh ACCP Conference on Anthithrombotic and Thrombolytic Therapy. Chest. 2004;126(3 Suppl):645S–87. http://dx.doi.org/10.1378/chest.126.3_suppl.645S. PMID:15383489.

25. Warkentin TE, Levine MN, Hirsh J, Horsewood P, Roberts RS, Gent M, et al. Heparin-induced thrombocytopenia in patients treated with low-molecular-weight heparin or unfractionated heparin. N Engl J Med. 1995;332(20):1330–5. http://dx.doi.org/10.1056/NEJM199505183322003. PMID:7715641.

26. Manlhiot C, Brandão LR, Somji Z, Chesney AL, MacDonald C, Gurofsky RC, et al. Long-term anticoagulation in Kawasaki disease: initial use of low molecular weight heparin is a viable option for patients with severe coronary artery abnormalities. Pediatr Cardiol. 2010; 31(6):834–42. http://dx.doi.org/10.1007/s00246-010-9715-8. PMID:20431996.

27. Kato H, Inoue O, Ichinose E, Akagi T, Sato N. Intracoronary urokinase in Kawasaki disease: treatment and prevention of myocardial infarction. Acta Paediatr Jpn. 1991;33(1):27–35. http://dx.doi.org/10.1111/j.1442-200X.1991.tb01516.x. PMID:1853711.

28. Harada M, Akimoto K, Ogawa S, Kato H, Nakamura Y, Hamaoka K, et al. National Japanese survey of thrombolytic therapy selection for coronary aneurysm: intracoronary thrombolysis or intravenous coronary thrombolysis in patients with Kawasaki disease. Pediatr Int. 2013; 55(6):690–5. http://dx.doi.org/10.1111/ped.12187. PMID:23919576.

29. Gómez-Outes A, Terleira-Fernandez AI, Lucumberri R, Suárez-Gea ML, Vargas-Cashtrillôn E. Direct oral anticoagulants in the treatment of acute venous thromboembolism: a systematic review and meta-analysis. Thromb Res. 2014;134(4):774–82. http://dx.doi.org/10.1016/j.thromres.2014.06.020. PMID:25037495.

Guideline for Catheter Intervention in Coronary Artery Lesion in Kawasaki Disease

Masahiro Ishii, Takafumi Ueno, Teiji Akagi, Kiyoshi Baba,
Kensuke Harada, Kenji Hamaoka, Hitoshi Kato, Etsuko Tsuda,
Shigeru Uemura, Tsutomu Saji, Shunichi Ogawa, Shigeyuki Echigo,
Tetsu Yamaguchi, and Hirohisa Kato

The guidelines in this chapter are reprinted with permission from *Pediatrics International*, John
Wiley & Sons, Inc., 2001.

M. Ishii, M.D., FACC (✉)
Department of Pediatrics and The Cardiovascular Research Institute, Kurume University
School of Medicine, 67 Asahi-machi, Kurume 830, Japan

Department of Pediatrics, Kitasato University School of Medicine, Sagamihara, Kanagawa
228-0855, Japan
e-mail: ishiim@med.kitasato-u.ac.jp

T. Ueno, M.D.
The Third Department of Medicine, Kurume University School of Medicine, Kurume, Japan

T. Akagi • H. Kato, M.D., FACC
Department of Pediatrics and The Cardiovascular Research Institute, Kurume University
School of Medicine, 67 Asahi-machi, Kurume 830, Japan

K. Baba, M.D. • K. Harada, M.D.
Division of Pediatrics, Kurashiki Central Hospital, Okayama, Japan

Department of Pediatrics, Nihon University School of Medicine, Tokyo, Japan

K. Hamaoka, M.D.
Department of Pediatrics, Kyoto Prefectural University of Medicine, Kyoto, Japan

H. Kato, M.D.
Department of Pediatrics, The University of Tokyo School of Medicine, Tokyo, Japan

E. Tsuda, M.D. • S. Echigo, M.D.
Department of Pediatrics, National Cardiovascular Center, Suita, Osaka, Japan

S. Uemura, M.D.
Department of Pediatrics, Wakayama Medical University, Wakayama, Japan

T. Saji, M.D.
Department of Pediatrics, Toho University School of Medicine, Tokyo, Japan

S. Ogawa, M.D.
Department of Pediatrics, Nippon Medical School, Tokyo, Japan

T. Yamaguchi, M.D., FACC
Third Department of Internal Medicine, Toho University School of Medicine, Tokyo, Japan

Research Group of Ministry of Health, Labour and Welfare "Study of treatment and long-term management in Kawasaki disease".

Chairman
Hirohisa Kato, MD, FACC
 Department of Pediatrics, Kurume University School of Medicine

Group Members
Kiyoshi Baba, MD
 Division of Pediatrics, Kurashiki Central Hospital
Kensuke Harada, MD
 Department of Pediatrics, Nihon University School of Medicine
Kenji Hamaoka, MD
 Department of Pediatrics, Kyoto Prefectural University of Medicine
Hitoshi Kato, MD
 Department of Pediatrics, The University of Tokyo School of Medicine
Etsuko Tsuda, MD
 Department of Pediatrics, National Cardiovascular Center
Shigeru Uemura, MD
 Department of Pediatrics, Wakayama Medical University
Tsutomu Saji, MD
 Department of Pediatrics, Toho University School of Medicine

Collaborators
Teiji Akagi, MD
 Department of Pediatrics, Kurume University School of Medicine
Masahiro Ishii, MD
 The Cardiovascular Research Institute Kurume University
Shunichi Ogawa, MD
 Department of Pediatrics, Nippon Medical School
Shigeyuki Echigo, MD
 Department of Pediatrics, National Cardiovascular Center

External Evaluation Committee
Tetsu Yamaguchi, MD, FACC
 Third Department of Internal Medicine, Toho University School of Medicine
Takafumi Ueno, MD
 The Third Department of Medicine, Kurume University School of Medicine

Contents

III. Catheter intervention for patients with Kawasaki disease

  1) Indication of catheter intervention
  2) Types of procedures, and their indication and care

    (1) Percutaneous transluminal coronary revascularization (PTCR)
    (2) Percutaneous transluminal coronary balloon angioplasty
    (3) Stent implantation
    (4) Rotational ablation (Rotablator)
    (5) Intravascular ultrasound imaging

  3) Institute and backup system

IV. The management after procedure and evaluation, and follow-up
 V. Prospects, especially relation to bypass surgery
VI. References

I. Background

Catheter intervention in coronary artery lesions is generally performed in adult patients with ischemic heart diseases and has provided satisfactory therapeutic results. The coronary artery stenotic lesions in Kawasaki disease commonly involves severe calcification. These findings are different from adult coronary artery lesions mainly consisting of atherosclerosis. Therefore, indication of catheter intervention for adult patients can not be directly employed in Kawasaki disease patients and, in some cases, could be risky. There are serious issues how to prevent the ischemic heart diseases or how to treat myocardial infarction due to Kawasaki disease, but there is insufficiently established therapeutic procedures including thrombolysis, catheter intervention, and bypass surgery. In particular, catheter intervention in Kawasaki disease has not been introduced long, and long-term prognosis is mostly unclear. This guideline is an update summary of the group members' opinions on how to effectively and appropriately perform catheter intervention in coronary artery lesion in Kawasaki disease on the basis of the information regarding evaluation of the diagnosis and the therapy reported in Japan and overseas. Therefore, therapeutic strategy is not conventionally decided according to only this guideline but should be arranged by sufficient consideration about appropriate therapies in each patient. It is thought that this guideline should be revised following future progression.

II. Natural history of coronary artery lesion in Kawasaki disease

The long-term consequences and the natural history of the cardiovascular sequelae in Kawasaki disease remain uncertain. In the previous report by Kato et al., the natural history of coronary artery lesions was examined in a follow-up study conducted during 10 to 21 years (mean: 13.6 years) in 594 patients with Kawasaki disease. In all the patients, coronary artery lesions were evaluated by coronary angiography just after the acute stage, within 3 months from the onset of Kawasaki disease. One hundred and forty-six patients (24.6%) of the 594 patients were diagnosed as having coronary aneurysms. The second angiogram was performed in 1 to 2 years later in all 146 patients who previously had coronary aneurysm, which demonstrated that 72 (49.3%) of these 146 had regression in the coronary aneurysm. A third angiogram was performed for 62 patients, a fourth for 29, and a fifth for 17. By 10 to 21 years after the onset of the illness, stenosis in the coronary aneurysm had developed in 28 patients (4.7%). Myocardial infarction occurred in 11 patients(1.9%), 5 of whom died. In the 26 patients with giant coronary aneurysms, stenotic lesion developed in 12, and no regression occurred. Systemic artery aneurysms developed in 13 patients (2.2%), and valvular heart disease appeared in 7 (1.2%). Ninety percent of cases with coronary aneurysm regression were observed within 2 years after the onset. The ratio of cases observed stenotic lesions within 2 years after the onset was 50 %, thereafter gradually increased, and in the longest case, stenotic lesions was observed after 17 years after the onset. In pathological findings, stenotic lesions are mainly composed of afferent intima hyperplasia within 2 years after the onset. Lesions of calcification are observed from approximately 5 years after the onset and are noticeable at 10 years after the onset.

III. Catheter intervention for patients with Kawasaki disease

1) Indication of catheter intervention

a. Consideration of indication in patient's conditions

1. Patients presenting ischemic symptoms.
2. Patients presenting no ischemic symptom but having ischemic findings detected by several stress tests, i.e. dipyridamole stress myocardial scintigraphy, and dobutamine stress echocardiography.
3. Patients having no ischemic finding detected by any stress tests but 75% or more of stenotic lesions in the left anterior descending coronary artery possibly causing a sudden death by its obstruction. In these cases, selection of catheter

intervention can be considered. It is decided in each patient which is selected surgical therapy, catheter intervention, or observation of the course.
4. Patients having severe left ventricular dysfunction. In these cases, catheter intervention should not be selected, but bypass surgery would be applied.

b. Consideration of indication in lesion sites

1. Severe stenotic lesions (75% or more)
2. Localized lesions: Contraindication for cases with multiple vessel lesions.
3. No ostial lesion.
4. No long segmental lesion.

2) Types of procedures, and their indications and precautions

(1) Percutaneous transluminal coronary revascularization (PTCR)

Acute myocardial infarction is most frequently occured within 2 years of the onset of Kawasaki disease and is mainly caused by fresh thrombus. The PTCR and intravenous thrombolysis in this time are thought to be significant in prevention and therapy of myocardial infarction. In particular, frequent and careful observation with echocardiography is required in such a case as giant coronary aneurysms having high risk of thrombus formation. In PTCR, 10,000 U/kg of urokinase or 25,000 U/kg of tissue plasminogen activator (t-PA, tisokinase; Hapase Kowa ®) is administered. Injection of these thrombolytic agents direct into coronary artery and intravenous thrombolysis occasionally causes cerebral hemorrhage. Repeated doses of the thrombolytic agents should be carefully performed in pediatric patients having predisposing factors for hemorrhage. After PTCR, 500 U/kg/day of heparin is intravenously infused for 12 hours, thereafter, a small oral dose of aspirin or warfarin is administered in order to prevent thrombus formation. Because t-PA is allowed to be intravenously injected, we recommend that hospital where cardiac catheterization can not be performed, to intravenously treatment with 250,000 U/kg of t-PA in acute myocardial infarction in pediatric patients with Kawasaki disease, thereafter to immediately transport to the hospital where cardiac catheterization can be performe. However, it is required to take sufficient measures against cerebral hemorrhage and arrhythmia possibly caused by the systemic administration. Most of myocardial infarction occured within 2 years of the onset of Kawasaki disease is caused by obstruction with fresh thrombus in coronary aneurysms. PTCR or intravenous thrombolysis in acute myocardial infarction is effective only within 6 hours of the onset. PTCR or intravenous thrombolysis may be indicated for fresh thrombus in giant coronary aneurysms detected by serial echocardiography. A success rate for recanalization using thrombolytic agents would be low in such a case of asymptomatic myocardial infarction as chronic obstruction with thrombus.

(2) Percutaneous transluminal coronary balloon angioplasty (PTCA)

Pathological changes in Kawasaki disease are mainly the afferent intima hyperplasia in early stage. The lesions of calcification are observed from approximately 5 years of the onset. PTCA is useful only stenotic lesion with mild calcification or without calcification within 6 years of the onset. Appearance of new coronary aneurysms, however, is observed by the follow-up angiography at higher rate (16.6%) after PTCA in the patients with Kawasaki disease than adult patients with atherosclerosis. The appearance of the new aneurysms is considered to be depended upon high pressure of balloon (≥ 10 atm). Balloon pressure is recommended to be less than 8–10 atm in PTCA. For a case, in which more balloon pressure (≥ 10 atm) is needed, rotational ablation or bypass surgery is advisable as an alternative procedure. Additionally, when PTCA is defensively performed in young children, short balloon length should be selected.

(3) Stent implantation

Stent implantation is useful for old children (≥ 13 years) in whom calcification is mild and stent can be implanted in coronary artery. The stent implantation is also effective in patients, in whom blood flow is unbalanced by giant aneurysms, because blood vessel diameter can be extended as large as the stent diameter compared to other procedures. The incidence of new aneurysms is lower in the stent implantation than PTCA only, even if high-balloon pressure was applied. Balloon pressure, however, is recommended to be 14 atm or less. Because higher pressure than 14 atm may cause severe calcification, rotational ablation is alternatively indicated for a case in which the higher pressure is needed. The stent implantation is ineffective on a case having severe calcification ($\geq 75\%$ of total circumference). Heparin is infused at 800 to 1,000 U/hr. Activated clotting time is maintained at 200 seconds or more. Thrombolytic therapy with aspirin and ticlopidine is carried out for 2 months from a day of post procedure. Attention should be paid for the occurrence of granulocytopenia during ticlopidine treatment.

(4) Rotational ablation (Rotablator)

Rotablator consists of an abrasive tiny diamond coated burr, remove the lesion with rotation at 200,000 rpm, and allows the lumen dilated. Rotational ablation is also effective on a case having severe calcification. Requiring 6F guiding catheter even minimum, the rotablation is difficult to be performed in small children. Enlargement is possible by 2.5 mm. Combination of the rotational ablation and stent implantation allows the coronary aeterial diameter to further enlarge. As the stent implantation, heparin is infused at 800 to 1,000 U/hr. Activated clotting time is maintained at 200 seconds or more. Aspirin should be administered for 2 months from a day of post-procedure.

(5) Intravascular ultrasound imaging

Histopathological findings of stenotic lesions in Kawasaki disease change with the number of years after the onset. In particular, in a long-term case (≥ 6 years), calcification is observed. It is important that the severity and the extent of calcification are exactly assessed before catheter intervention, and suitable therapeutic procedures are selected. Intravascular ultrasound imaging allows of detailed structural observation of a coronary artery wall. In particular, the extent of calcification can be precisely evaluated. The intravascular ultrasound imaging is desirable to perform after consideration of body size of patients and coronary angiographic finding.

3) Institute and backup system

Catheter intervention for coronary artery lesion in Kawasaki disease is allowed by assistance of cardiac surgeons as well as cooperation of adult cardiologists experienced in catheter intervention and pediatric cardiologists skilled in natural history and pathology of cardiac consequence in Kawasaki disease. The treatment, therefore, is desirable to be carried out in such an institute as a general cardiovascular center where there are adult cardiologist skilled in the catheter intervention, pediatric cardiologist, and cardiac surgeon experienced in coronary bypass surgery.

IV. The management of post-procedure and evaluation, and follow-up

As follow-up, selective coronary angiography is performed in 4 to 6 months after all catheter intervention. Restenosis is defined as developing 50% or more of stenosis assessed by quantitative coronary angiography. The rate of restenosis in follow-up period in Kawasaki disease is unclear at that time, however, is thought to be lower than that in adults on the basis of updated information. Thereafter, the follow-up was continued by non-invasive method, i.e. chest x ray, electrocardiogram, echocardiography, myocardial scintigraphy.

V. Prospects: especially relation to bypass surgery

A decrease in mortality associated with acute myocardial infarction is expected following progression of catheter intervention in coronary artery lesion after Kawasaki disease. However, long-term follow-up study of the procedure is required, because it is quite new. Bypass surgery is indicated in small pediatric patients, in whom catheter intervention is impossible, cases with multiple vessel lesions, cases with severe valvular disease, and cases with severe left ventricular dysfunction. However, occurrence of bypass occlusion and string phenomena by competition of blood flow are known in cases comparatively maintaining native flow despite of severe stenosis. For these cases, catheter intervention is indicated. In current status, many institute have little experience of catheter intervention in coronary artery lesion in Kawasaki disease. Additionally, the treatment is allowed by assistance of cardiac surgeons as well as cooperation of pediatric cardiologists skilled in natural history and pathology of cardiac consequence in Kawasaki disease and adult cardiologists experienced in catheter intervention. Therefore, it is essential for performance of catheter intervention and bypass surgery to scrupulously discuss about validity and indication in each pediatric patient on a joint conference of pediatric cardiologists, adult cardiologist specialized in the catheterization, and cardiac surgeons. Furthermore, in future, combination of catheter intervention with either bypass surgery being minimam invasive or without cardiopulmonary bypass provides a low invasive treatment and probably improves "quality of life" in patients with Kawasaki disease.

※ This guideline is summary of the group members' current opinions on how to effectively and appropriately perform catheter interventional treatment in coronary artery lesion in Kawasaki disease on the basis of the information regarding evaluation of the diagnosis and the therapy reported in Japan and overseas. It also includes a tentative standard such a dosage of drugs. Consequently, the therapeutic strategy is not conventionally decided according to only this guideline but should be done by sufficient consideration of appropriate treatment in each patient referring to this guideline.

References (suggested reading)

I. The natural history and pathology of cardiac consequence in Kawasaki disease

1. Kato H, Ichinose E, Yoshioka F, Takechi T, Matsunaga S, Suzuki K, Rikitake N. Fate of coronary aneurysms in Kawasaki disease: serial coronary angioplasty and long-term follow-up study. Am J Cardiol 1981;49:1758–1766.
2. Kato H, Ichinose E, Kawasaki T. Myocardial infarction in Kawasaki disease: Clinical analyses in 195 cases. J Pediatr 1986;108:923–927.
3. Fujiwara H, Hamashima Y. Pathology of the heart in Kawasaki disease. Pediatrics 1978;61:17–27.
4. Tanaka N, Naoe S, Masuda H, Ueno T. Pathological study of sequelae of Kawasaki disease (MCLS). With special reference to the heart and coronary arterial lesions. Acta Pathol Jpn 1986;36:1513–1527.
5. Suzuki A, Kamiya T, Arakaki Y, Kinoshita Y, Kimura K. Fate of coronary arterial aneurysms in Kawasaki disease. Am J Cardiol 1994;74:822–824
6. Suzuki A, Yamaguchi M, Kimura K, Sugiyama H, Arakaki Y, Kamiya T, miyatake K. Functional behavior and morphology of the coronary artery

wall in patients with Kawasaki disease assessed by intravascular ultrasound. J Am Coll Cardiol 1996;27:291–296.

7. Naoe S, Takahashi K, Masuda H, Tanaka N. Kawasaki disease. With particular emphasis on arterial lesions. Acta Pathol Jpn 1991;41:785–797.

8. Kato H, Sugimura T, Akagi T, Sato N, Hashino K, Hashino Y, Maeno Y, Kazue T, Eto G, Yamakawa R. Long-term consequences of Kawasaki disease: a 10 - to 21 year follow-up study of 594 patients. Circulation 1996;94:1379–1385.

9. Yamakawa R, Ishii M, Sugimura T, Akagi T, Eto G, Iemura M, Tsutsumi T, Kato H: Coronary endothelirum dysfunction after Kawasaki disease: Evaluation by intracoronary injection of acetylcholine. J Am Coll Caridol, 1998;31:1074–1080

10. Iemura M, Ishii M, Sugimura T, Akagi T, Kato H. Long-term consequences of regressed coronary aneurysms after Kawasaki Disease: vascular wall morphology and function. Heart 2000;83:307–311.

II. Catheter intervention for Kawasaki disease

11. Kato H, Inoue O, Ichinose E, Akagi T, Sato N. Intracoronary urokinase in Kawasaki disease: treatment and prevention of myocardial infraction. Acta Paediatr Jpn 1991;33:27–35.

12. Ino T, Nishimoto K, Akimoto K, Park I, Shimazaki S, Yabuta K, Yamaguchi H. Percutaneous transluminal coronary angioplasty for Kawasaki disease: a case report and literature. Pediatr Cardiol 1991;12:33–35.

13. Satler LF, Leon MB, Kent KM, Pichard AD, Martin GR. Angioplasty in a child with Kawasaki disease. Am Heart J 1992;124:216–219.

14. Nishimura H, Sawada T, Azuma A, Kohno Y, Katsume H, Nakagawa M, Sakata K, Hamaoka K, Onouchi Z. Percutaneous transluminal coronary angioplasty in a patient with Kawasaki disease: a case report of an unsuccessful angioplasty. J Heart J 1992;33:869–873.

15. Kawata T, Hasegawa J, Yoshida Y, Yoshikawa Y, Kawachi K, Kitamura S. Percutaneous transluminal coronary angioplasty of the left internal thoracic artery graft: a case report in a child. Cathet Cardiovasc Diagn 1994;32:340–342.

16. Tsubata S, Ichida F, Hamamichi Y, Miyazaki A, Hashimoto T, Okada T. Successthrombolytic thrapy using tissue-type plasminogen activator in Kawasaki disease. Pediatr Cardiol 1995;16:186–189.

17. Ino T, Akimoto K, Ohkubo M, Nishimoto K, Yabuta K, Takaya J, Yamaguchi H. Application of percutaneous transluminal coronary angioplasty to coronary arterial stenosis in Kawasaki disease. Circulation 1996;93:1709–1715.

18. Oda H, Miida T, Ochiai Y, Toeda T, Higuma N, Ito E. Successful stent implantation in acute myocardial infarction and successful directional coronary atherectomy of a stenotic lesion involving an aneurysm in a woman with Kawasaki disease of adult onset. J Interven Cardiol 1997;10:375–380.

19. Hijazi ZM, Smith JJ, Fulton DR. Stent implantation for coronary artery stenosis after Kawasaki disease. J Invasive Cardiology 1997;9:534–536.

20. Sugimura T, Yokoi H, Sato N, Akagi T, Kimura T, Iemura M, nobuyoshi M, Kato H. Interventional treatment for children with severe coronary artery stenosis with calcification after long-term Kawasaki disease. Circulation 1997;96:3928–3933.

21. Ogawa S, Fukazawa R, Ohkubo T, Zhang J, Takechi N, Kuramochi Y, Hino Y, Jimbo O, Katsube Y, Kamisago M, Genma Y, Yamamoto M. Silent myocardial ischemia in Kawasaki disease: evaluation of percutaneous transluminal coronary angioplasty by dobutamine stress testing. Circulation 1997;96:3384–3389.

22. Kato H, Ishii M, Akagi T, Eto G, Iemura M, Tsutsumi T, Ueno T. Interventional catheterization in Kawasaki disease. J Interven Cardiol 1998;11:355–361.

23. Moore JW, Buchbinder M. Successful coronary stenting in a 4-year-old child. Cathet. Cardiovasc. Diagn 1998;44:202–205.

24. Min JH, Huh J, Kim YW, Kim HS, Noh CI, Choi JY, Yun YS, Lee MM. Percutaneous transluminal coronary angioplasty in child with Kawasaki disease. J Korean Med Sci 1998;13:693–695.

25. Hijazi ZM. Coronary arterial stenosis after Kawasaki disease: role of catheter intervention. Catheter Cardiovasc Interv 1999;46:337.

26. Ueno T, Kai H, Ikeda H, Hashino T, Imaizumi T. Coronary stent deployment in a young adult with Kawasaki disease and recurrent myocardial infarction. Clin Cardiol 1999;22:147–149.

27. Hashmi A, Lazzam C, McCrindle BW, Benson LN. Stenting of coronary artery stenosis in Kawasaki disease. Cathet. Cardiovasc. Intervent 1999;46:333–336

28. Akagi T, Ogawa S, Ino T, Iwasa M, Echigo S, Kishida K, Baba K, Matsushima M, Hamaoka K, Tomita H, Ishii M, Kato H. Catheter interventional treatment in Kawasaki disease: a report from the japanese pediatric interventional cardiology investigation group. J Pediatr 2000;137:181–18

Long-Term Clinical Follow-Up After Rotational Atherectomy for Coronary Arterial Stenosis in Kawasaki Disease

Hiroyoshi Yokoi

Abstract During acute KD, the coronary artery lesions most frequently observed in pediatric Kawasaki disease (KD) patients are giant arterial aneurysms. Severely stenotic calcified lesions appear near the aneurysms when patients reach school age. Traditional balloon catheter treatment of stenotic lesions is hampered by the presence of calcification, which makes balloon expansion difficult. In addition, long-term patency is a problem for bypass surgery. Hence, standard treatment has been medical therapy with restrictions on physical activity. Rotablation has made it possible to safely perform catheterization of lesions in pediatric KD patients for which balloon catheter treatment is not indicated. The effects are maintained over the long term and provide benefits as the child grows and develops.

Keywords Kawasaki disease • Coronary artery disease • PCI • Rotablator • Coronary aneurysm

Clinical Outcomes for Rotablation for Kawasaki Disease Coronary Artery Lesions

We used rotablation to treat 33 lesions from 26 patients between May 1993 and December 2002.

Patients, Lesions, and Information on the Procedures

Patient age ranged from 8 to 28 years, and the average age was young, 15 years. Kawasaki disease (KD) was generally diagnosed between age 0 and 8 years, and average age at diagnosis was 2 years. Males represented 77 % of patients; 31 % of patients had multivessel disease, 8 % had a previous myocardial infarction (MI),

H. Yokoi (✉)
Cardiovascular Center, Fukuoka Sanno Hospital, 3-6-45 Momochihama, Sawara-ku, Fukuoka 814-0001, Japan
e-mail: hiroyokoi@circus.ocn.ne.jp

© Springer Japan 2017   383
B.T. Saji et al. (eds.), *Kawasaki Disease*, DOI 10.1007/978-4-431-56039-5_41

and all patients were either asymptomatic or had only mild stable-effort angina. Lesion morphology was highly complex: 100 % had calcified lesions, 85 % had coronary aneurysms, 22 % had ostial lesions, and 100 % had lesions that were not balloon-expandable. The target vessel was the LAD in 58 %, RCA in 36 %, and LCX in 6 %. Average lesion length was 4.7 mm (vessel diameter, 3.82 mm). In other words, there were many focal lesions in large-diameter vessels and very few diffuse lesions, which made these patients suitable for rotablation. The average minimum vessel diameter was 1.26 mm, and average stenosis was 66 %. The number of burrs used per lesion was 1.5, and the final burr-to-artery ratio was 0.61. Because these patients had large-diameter vessels, the burrs used were larger than those used for adult patients. The final average burr size was 2.23 mm, and the largest burr size, 2.5 mm, was used for 37 % of the lesions. All patients underwent additional post-rotablation balloon dilatation, which was performed at a relatively low average of 9.5 ATM, although some patients required dilatation at high pressure, 20 ATM. Stents were implanted in only 9 % of patients, for whom coronary artery dissection led to decreased blood flow.

Acute Outcomes

The lesion dilatation technical success rate and clinical success rate were both 100 %. The procedures were conducted quite safely, and there were no primary complications, including death, emergency bypass, Q-wave MI, or acute coronary occlusion. The incidence rate of post-dilatation balloon rupture was 8 %, and complete expansion by balloon was possible in only 35 % of cases. Minimum vessel diameter increased from a pre-procedural 1.26 mm to a post-procedural 2.57 mm, and restenosis decreased from 66 to 33 %. There were no cases of coronary perforation, no-reflow, or spasm, which are complications particular to rotablation. There was one case in which the burr became trapped in the lesion but was subsequently removed. The diamond particles on the Rotablator are only attached to the front end of the burr, so if the burr passes the lesion without sufficient cutting, it sometimes get trapped in heavily calcified stenotic areas. To avoid this, it is important to cut in several steps, starting with a small burr, and to avoid using excessive pressure when advancing the burr. In contrast to treatment of atherosclerotic lesions in adults, we found that rotablation could be performed quite safely for these young patients, most likely because KD coronary artery lesions were focal, vessel diameters were large, and tortuous lesions were uncommon. We also found that, because high-pressure balloon post-dilatation could lead to balloon rupture, it is advisable to avoid excessively high pressures and to increase burr size as necessary. In children younger than 10 years, 6-Fr is the largest sheath that can be used, so only burrs smaller than 2 mm may be used. In some cases we waited 5 years for a child to grow enough to permit use of a 10-Fr sheath and 2.5-mm burr, for re-treatment.

Late Restenosis

Follow-up angiography was performed for 33 lesions (100 %) 3–6 months post-procedure. Minimum vessel diameter was 1.25 mm pre-procedure, 2.57 mm post-procedure, and 2.32 mm in the late phase. Late restenosis ($\geq$50 %) was noted in 9 (27 %) lesions. Restenosis occurred in 17 % of cases for which the final burr size was 2.5 mm and 33 % of cases for which the burr was less than 2.5 mm. Although the difference was not statistically significant, there was less restenosis among patients for whom the largest possible size burr was used and the greatest diameter gained.

Late lumen loss was 0.25 mm, clearly lower than that for adult elective percutaneous coronary intervention (PCI), for which average late lumen loss is 0.90–1.00 mm. Restenosis is determined by initial diameter gain and late lumen loss, the latter of which is caused by neointimal hyperplasia triggered by inflammation resulting from vessel injury. Drug-eluting stents, which are coated with a drug meant to inhibit this, have dramatically reduced post-PCI restenosis and are used in clinical settings. It may be that in KD coronary lesions, because young coronary arteries are pathologically subject to severe inflammation, both the normal media and intima structures are destroyed, and the neointimal hyperplasia caused by smooth muscle cell proliferation and migration that is seen in adult atherosclerotic lesions does not occur so easily. The late lumen loss ratio, calculated by dividing late lumen loss by initial lumen gain, is 0.4 for balloon angioplasty, 0.6 for stenting, and 0.7 for rotablation when performed on adult atherosclerotic lesions. In contrast, the ratio for Rotablator-treated KD coronary artery lesions is 0.2, almost as low as the 0.1 ratio for drug-eluting stenting in adults. Therefore, in contrast to adult patients, restenosis prevention in KD artery lesions depends greatly on initial gain; thus, it is necessary to use as large a burr as possible. Vessel diameters of 3.8 mm and comparatively large lesions are common, so even using the largest burr size of 2.5 mm, the burr-to-artery ratio is 0.6, which suggests little risk of perforation.

Catheterization was repeated in 8 (24 %) patients with restenotic lesions. Of these, 44 % underwent repeat rotablation, 22 % received stents, 33 % were treated with balloon dilatation, and 11 % were treated conservatively. No patient who underwent repeat rotablation had received treatment using the largest (2.5 mm) burr during their initial rotablation. There was no repeat restenosis after the second rotablation.

New Coronary Aneurysms in the Late Period

In follow-up angiography performed 3–6 months post-procedure on all 33 lesions (100 %), four (12 %) patients had new coronary aneurysms at the treatment site; 60 % of these occurred in lesions with sufficient post-procedural stenosis (<25 %). This proportion was significantly higher than that for lesions with post-procedural stenosis of 25 % or greater (4 %). While there were no new coronary artery aneurysms found in lesions where intravascular ultrasound revealed circumferential calcification, aneurysms did develop in lesions in which high-pressure balloon dilatation caused cracks in post-procedural circumferential calcification. Because young coronary arteries are subject to pathologically severe inflammation in KD, the normal media and intima structures are destroyed, so it is likely that dilatation force from the vessel lumen reaches the adventitia, which may trigger coronary aneurysm formation.

While we recommend using the largest possible burr, to prevent restenosis, we believe that post-dilatation should be performed at a comparatively low pressure, aiming at 30–50 % post-procedural stenosis and refraining from excessively high-pressure dilatation. Furthermore, the development of new aneurysms is a phenomenon particular to KD patients [1]. Stent use may result in late-stage stent malapposition, so stenting should be undertaken only when absolutely necessary, and limited to bail-out situations.

Long-Term Prognosis for Patients Undergoing PCI on KD Coronary Artery Lesions

We investigated long-term outcomes (follow-up period: 13 years) for initial elective PCI in 39 KD pediatric patients (44 lesions). The mean age at time of treatment was 16 years. In 37 stenotic lesions (90 %) with marked calcification near the coronary aneurysm, we performed rotablation and POBA (balloon dilatation); bare metal stents were placed in 4 lesions (10 %). The rate of reintervention for restenosis was 35 % during a period of 5 years, and most of these procedures were performed within 1 year of the initial intervention. No reinterventions were performed during years 5 through 15. These patients continued periodic follow-up during their school years and were maintained on aspirin and warfarin (in cases of residual aneurysm); almost none required repeat (non-medical) treatment for the initially treated area during adulthood. Additionally, no aneurysm progression or rupture was seen, and, as reported by Suda et al. [2], outcomes were good for giant aneurysms as well. Only two patients (5.6 %) had cardiac-vessel events in adulthood, after the 10-year mark. The first patient, who underwent stent placement at age 27 years, did not undergo regular check-ups thereafter and developed recurrent chest pain at age 38 years. A new lesion was found in a location different from that of the previously treated lesion and the patient underwent stent placement. The second patient did not undergo regular check-ups after rotablation and POBA treatment, at age 14 years, and experienced cardiopulmonary arrest during exercise, at age 25 years. The patient was rushed to the hospital, where targeted temperature management and coronary bypass saved his life. This patient also presented with a new lesion in a location different from that of the previously treated lesion.

The above findings suggest that while restenosis can occur within 1 year of PCI treatment in school-aged patients, re-treatment prognosis is good, aneurysms do not progress even as the patient enters adulthood, and lesions remain stable. However, these findings do indicate that continued antiplatelet therapy and anticoagulant therapy (in patients with aneurysms) are necessary, that new lesions appear earlier than in non-KD patients of similar age, and that medical therapy is required for more stringent atherosclerosis prevention. For these reasons it seems that ongoing medical observation, even into adulthood, is necessary. In their 30-year follow-up of 60 pediatric KD patients with a history of MI, Tsuda et al. [3] found that many patients with low cardiac function had died from life-threatening ventricular arrhythmias, which led the authors to stress the importance of rigorous control.

Summary

Catheter-based treatment of KD coronary artery lesions can be performed safely with a Rotablator, and the effects are maintained over the long-term. Furthermore, the effects were not limited to treatment of focal coronary lesions but extend over time as KD patients mature. As long as a guidewire can cross the lesion, KD coronary artery lesions should be treated with less invasive catheter treatment rather than by surgery.

References

1. Akagi T. Interventions in Kawasaki disease. Pediatr Cardiol. 2005;26(2):206–12. http://dx.doi.org/10.1007/s00246-004-0964-2. PMID:15868317.
2. Suda K, Iemura M, Nishiono H, Teramachi Y, Koteda Y, Kishimoto S, et al. Long-term prognosis of patients with Kawasaki disease complicated by giant coronary aneurysms: a single-institution experience. Circulation. 2011;123(17):1836–42. http://dx.doi.org/10.1161/CIRCULATIONAHA.110.978213. PMID:21502578.
3. Tsuda E, Hirata T, Matsuo O, Abe T, Sugiyama H, Yamada O. The 30-year outcome for patients after myocardial infarction due to coronary artery lesions caused by Kawasaki disease. Pediatr Cardiol. 2011;32(2):176–82. http://dx.doi.org/10.1007/s00246-010-9838-y. PMID:21120463.

Long-Term Outcomes of Pediatric Coronary Artery Bypass Grafting and Down-Sizing Operation for Giant Coronary Aneurysms

Yuji Maruyama and Masami Ochi

Abstract There are several concerns regarding surgical revascularization for Kawasaki coronary disease, including the choice of conduit, optimal timing, and indications for coronary artery bypass grafting (CABG). The internal thoracic artery is the best conduit for pediatric CABG because of its favorable growth potential and long-term patency. Use of a saphenous vein graft should be avoided unless the internal thoracic artery is unavailable. Indications for CABG for Kawasaki coronary disease have not yet been established. In principle, coronary aneurysms should be observed continuously for 1–2 years under restrictive anticoagulation therapy, because coronary aneurysms regress in 50 % of patients within 1–2 years. Presence of severe ischemia with giant coronary aneurysms involving obstructive lesions of the left main trunk or left anterior descending artery (LAD) is an unequivocal indication for CABG. In addition, a giant aneurysm with recurrent thrombosis under restrictive anticoagulation therapy or with severely delayed flow without significant localized stenosis may be an indication for CABG. However, determining surgical indications is difficult, especially for younger children, because of technical challenges. To prevent fatal complications, CABG might be indicated at a young age for patients with severe ischemia, because a history of myocardial infarction and impaired cardiac function affect prognosis. Down-sizing operation for giant aneurysms of non-LAD lesions without significant stenosis and severe calcification may be a good choice to improve coronary circulation and allow discontinuation of warfarin, if indications for this procedure can be established.

Keywords Coronary artery bypass grafting • Down-sizing operation • Internal thoracic artery • Giant coronary aneurysm

Y. Maruyama (✉) • M. Ochi
Department of Cardiovascular Surgery, Nippon Medical School, 1-1-5 Sendagi, Bunkyo-ku, Tokyo 113-0022, Japan
e-mail: maruyamayuji@nms.ac.jp

© Springer Japan 2017
B.T. Saji et al. (eds.), *Kawasaki Disease*, DOI 10.1007/978-4-431-56039-5_42

Long-Term Outcomes of Pediatric CABG

Introduction

The long-term outcomes for coronary artery bypass grafting (CABG) for patients with Kawasaki disease (KD) remain uncertain. Issues involved in improving long-term outcomes for pediatric CABG include conduit choice and the optimal timing and correct indications for CABG. These issues will be discussed in the next section.

The characteristics of pediatric CABG need to be considered for patients with Kawasaki coronary disease. KD coronary artery lesions are quite different from those seen in adult atherosclerotic disease. First, patients with atherosclerotic coronary disease occasionally have multivessel and/or diffuse stenotic lesions and require multivessel revascularization, whereas patients with Kawasaki coronary disease usually have coronary aneurysms and subsequent obstructive changes in only the proximal portion of the left anterior descending artery (LAD) or right coronary artery (RCA) and require 1- or 2-vessel revascularization. Second, the mean age of patients with atherosclerotic disease undergoing CABG is 60–70 years, whereas that of patients undergoing pediatric CABG is around 10 years. Hence, patients undergoing pediatric CABG have a longer life expectancy, and quality-of-life considerations are more important than for adult patients. Third, off-pump technique is not applicable in pediatric CABG because young patients do not have the usual risk factors for cardiopulmonary bypass, such as diabetes or failure of other organs, including cerebrovascular disease, peripheral vascular disease, or chronic kidney disease. Reliable conduits with expected long-term patency thus need to be anastomosed accurately under on-pump arrest conditions in pediatric CABG.

Choice of Conduit

Kitamura et al. reported the first pediatric CABG using the saphenous vein graft (SVG), in 1976, [1] and the internal thoracic artery (ITA), in 1985 [2]. Their results showed a significantly higher actuarial patency rate for the ITA than for the SVG, and this difference was even greater in young children [3–7]. They reported that the actuarial patency of SVG for patients aged ≤10 years was extremely poor, 25 % at 3 years postoperatively, and most patients with patent SVG had various degrees of degenerative change [3]. Moreover, late cardiac death was strongly related to absence of an ITA graft [4, 5]. They therefore recommended avoiding the use of SVG unless the ITA is unavailable [3–6].

The ITA appears to be the best conduit for pediatric CABG because of its growth potential, excellent long-term patency [8], and biological characteristics [9]. A Japanese national survey of multiple centers found that ITA patency for patients aged ≤ 12 years was less favorable than for those >12 years, and this difference appeared to be mainly due to technical difficulties encountered in younger children [7]. Moreover, late death was strongly related to younger age at the time of surgery, and the absence of ITA grafts, in a previous multicenter study [4]. However, Kitamura et al. later showed that ITA patency did not depend on patient age at surgery [3]. We believe that left internal thoracic artery (LITA)-to-LAD grafting is the gold standard even in children >1 year of age or >10 kg in body weight.

Use of the right internal thoracic artery (RITA) is recommended as a second arterial conduit. Kitamura et al. first reported bilateral ITA use for pediatric CABG in 1990 [10] and concluded that it should be used whenever indicated [3, 4, 10]. The superiority of bilateral ITA over single ITA was confirmed in adult patients over a 10-year period after CABG [11]. KD patients may benefit much more than adult patients from bilateral ITA grafting because of their longer life expectancy. However, the usefulness of RITA is less than ideal because of the short length of the ITA graft available from the flat, short chest of young children. Moreover, the RITA is often not long enough to reach the LAD, left circumflex artery (LCx), or distal RCA, even in adult patients. A Y-composite graft using bilateral ITA grafts is useful for multivessel CABG in adult patients [12]. However, mild stenosis of the native coronary artery is a significant predictor of competitive flow and graft occlusion for Y-composite grafts [13]. In KD patients, evaluating the degree of localized stenosis around giant aneurysms may be difficult because of severe flow turbulence [14]. A complicated graft design, such as the Y-composite graft, should therefore be avoided in pediatric CABG for Kawasaki coronary disease.

The right gastroepiploic artery (GEA) was first used for pediatric CABG in 1990 [15] and has also been used recently by others, with favorable early results [3]. However, the long-term patency of GEA in young children has not been assessed in a large series. Routine use of the GEA may not be practical for young children because its size depends on the patient. In addition, the risk of flow competition is greater for the GEA than for the ITA because the GEA is the fourth branch of the abdominal aorta. The GEA can thus only be used in large, older children. The radial artery (RA) has been used only in redo cases [3], and long-term patency of the RA has not been assessed in pediatric CABG.

CABG Timing and Indications

The indications for CABG in Kawasaki coronary disease were described in the "Guidelines for diagnosis and management of cardiovascular sequelae in Kawasaki disease (JCS 2008) [16]" (Table 1), which is based on a guideline published two decades ago [17]. CABG is considered when there are (1) severe occlusive lesions in the left main trunk (LMT), (2) severe occlusive lesions in multiple vessels, (3) severe occlusive lesions in the proximal portion of the LAD, or (4) jeopardized collaterals. In addition, indications for younger children are described [16]. Whether CABG is indicated should be considered carefully in younger children, and the

Table 1 Indications of coronary artery bypass grafting for Kawasaki coronary disease [16]

Coronary artery bypass grafting (CABG) is indicated for patients with angiographically evident severe occlusive lesions of the coronary arteries and viability of myocardium in the affected area. Viability should be evaluated comprehensively, based on the presence/absence of angina and findings of ECG, thallium myocardial scintigraphy, two-dimensional echocardiography (regional wall movement), and other techniques
The following findings of coronary angiography are most important. When one of the following findings is present, consider surgical treatment
1. Severe occlusive lesions in the left main trunk
2. Severe occlusive lesions in multiple vessels
3. Severe occlusive lesions in the proximal portion of the left anterior descending artery
4. Jeopardized collaterals
In addition, the following conditions should also be considered in determining treatment strategy
1. When the event is considered a second or third infarction due to the presence of chronic infarct lesions, surgery may be indicated. For example, surgery may be considered to treat lesions limited to the right coronary artery
2. Lesions associated with recanalization of the occluded coronary artery or formation of collateral vessels should be evaluated especially carefully. Surgery may be considered for patients with findings of severe myocardial ischemia
3. Whether CABG is indicated should be considered carefully in younger children based on long-term patency of grafts. In general, young children controllable with medical therapy are followed carefully with periodic coronary angiography to allow them to grow, while patients with severe findings have undergone surgery at 1–2 years of age. It is recommended that pedicle internal mammary artery grafts can be used in such cases as well

decision should be based on long-term graft patency. In general, young children controllable with medical therapy are followed carefully with periodic coronary angiography (CAG) to allow growth, while those with severe disease undergo surgery at age 1–2 years.

In addition to the above guideline, CABG indications in Kawasaki coronary disease are also described in the American Heart Association (AHA) scientific statement [18]. Indications for coronary bypass procedures in children have yet to be established in clinical trials, but such surgery should be considered when reversible ischemia is present on stress-imaging test results, the myocardium to be perfused through the graft is still viable, and no appreciable lesions are present in the artery distal to the planned graft site (evidence level C). However, these indications are ambiguous and impractical in clinical situations.

The surgical indications for Kawasaki coronary disease in our center are listed in Table 2. In principle, coronary aneurysms should be carefully observed for 1–2 years under restrictive anticoagulation therapy, because coronary aneurysms regress in 50 % of patients within 1–2 years [17, 19]. The presence of a giant aneurysm ($\geq$8 mm in diameter) is a risk factor for thrombotic occlusion and progression of obstructive lesions [17, 20], and aneurysms $\geq$5 mm in diameter may become stenotic [21]. Giant aneurysms involving the LMT or both the LAD and RCA can cause fatal complications, whereas single-vessel obstruction of the RCA is often accompanied by marked development of collateral vessels without symptoms [22–24]. Single-vessel obstruction of the RCA is therefore not a basic surgical indication [23]. The presence of severe ischemia in giant coronary aneurysms involving obstructive lesions of the LMT or LAD is an unequivocal indicator for CABG at our center. Kitamura et al. limited their surgical indications to angiographically significant obstructive lesions (usually stenosis >75 %, and preferably >90 %), with ischemia [3, 5, 14]. In addition, giant aneurysms with recurrent thrombosis under restrictive anticoagulation therapy, or giant aneurysms with severely delayed flow without significant localized stenosis, are not indications for CABG, because they experienced early occlusion of the ITA graft due to competitive flow [14]. However, we consider that these conditions are indications for CABG when ischemia is obvious, because these conditions increase the risk of myocardial infarction. Use of a Doppler wire or pressure wire to measure average peak flow velocity (APV), coronary flow reserve (CFR), and myocardial functional flow reserve (FFRmyo) is useful in determining the functional severity of coronary artery stenosis and myocardial ischemia [25]. Nevertheless, surgical indications for giant aneurysm without significant stenosis should be considered carefully, because evaluating the degree of localized stenosis around giant aneurysms is difficult, owing to severe flow turbulence.

Early detection and treatment of myocardial ischemia is essential to prevent myocardial infarction and fatal complications. However, determining surgical indications for younger children is particularly difficult because of the technical difficulties involved. About one-third of KD patients who develop myocardial infarction have no obvious symptoms, probably because infants and younger children do not complain of chest pain [22]. Comprehensive evaluation of CABG candidates should comprise clinical signs and symptoms and findings from CAG, exercise electrocardiography (ECG), echocardiography, stress myocardial scintigraphy, left ventriculography (LVG), and other modalities [16]. In particular, pharmacological stress tests are useful for young children, who may not be able to tolerate exercise stress tests for evaluation of myocardial ischemia [26]. Surgical treatment is strongly recommended for children with a history of myocardial infarction and impaired left ventricular ejection fraction (LVEF), because about 60 % of survivors of first myocardial infarction have some degree of cardiac dysfunction [22], and impaired LVEF adversely affects prognosis [7]. In addition, patients who underwent surgical intervention soon after KD onset had fewer episodes of preoperative myocardial infarction and a lower incidence of postoperative cardiac events than did those who underwent surgical intervention later [27]. A recent report showed that CABG can be performed safely even in young children, in contrast to previous indications [3]. Application of plain old balloon angioplasty (POBA) for anastomotic stenosis of ITA grafts has improved graft patency in young children [28]. CABG may thus be indicated for severe ischemia in patients aged 1–2 years [16]. ITA grafts have also been used for congenital cardiac surgery in infants and young children [29, 30]. We believe that LITA-to-LAD grafting is the gold standard, even in children >1 year in age or >10 kg in body weight.

Table 2 Surgical indications for Kawasaki coronary disease at our center

1. Deliberate observation for 1–2 years, under restrictive anticoagulation therapy
2. Surgical indications: positive ischemia with giant aneurysms involving the left main trunk or left anterior descending artery
2.1 Stenotic or occluded coronary artery
2.1 Giant aneurysm with recurrent thrombosis under restrictive anticoagulation therapy
2.3 Giant aneurysm with severely delayed flow

CABG at Our Center

Patients and Methods

Forty-one children and adolescents underwent CABG for Kawasaki coronary disease between 1991 and 2014 at Nippon Medical School Hospital in Japan, on the basis of our surgical indications. Mean age at surgery was 12.7 ± 8.9 years (range, 1–37 years); 32 (78 %) were male and nine (22 %) were female. There were 26 patients (63 %) aged ≤ 12 years and seven patients (17 %) aged ≥ 20 years. Mean age at KD onset was 3.5 ± 2.8 years (range, 4 months to 12 years; no data for 3 patients). Twelve patients (29 %) had a history of myocardial infarction and a preoperative LVEF of $<35 \%$ was noted in one patient (2 %). Four patients (10 %) had a history of percutaneous coronary intervention (PCI), including percutaneous transluminal coronary rotational ablation (PTCRA) in two patients (5 %). One patient with a history of PTCRA was eventually referred to our hospital after she had undergone PCI four times at another hospital. Two patients (5 %) had severe mitral regurgitation. The preoperative characteristics of the patients are summarized in Table 3.

Surgical indications at our center are listed in Table 2 and discussed in the previous section. Severe ischemia in a giant coronary aneurysm involving obstructive lesions of the LMT or LAD is an unequivocal indication for CABG. In addition, when obvious ischemia is detected, a giant aneurysm with recurrent thrombosis or severely delayed flow, without significant obstructive lesions, is an indication for CABG. Giant aneurysms were identified in 40 patients (98 %) by CAG. In the remaining patient without obvious coronary aneurysm, an occlusive lesion was found at the LMT. The aneurysms were located at the LMT in 17 patients (41 %), the LAD in 40 (98 %), the LCx in 16 (39 %), and the RCA in 38 patients (93 %) (Fig. 1). Most patients for whom CABG was indicated had aneurysms in both the LAD and RCA. Obstructive lesions developed at the inflow or outflow sites of coronary aneurysms in 31 patients (76 %) and at the LMT in three (7 %), LAD in 29 (71 %), LCx in six (15 %), and RCA in 21 patients (51 %). CABG was indicated for the remaining 10 patients (24 %) without obstructive lesions, because of giant aneurysms of the LMT or LAD with recurrent thrombosis or severely delayed flow. In all patients, we detected clinical signs of myocardial ischemia or positive signs of ischemia on ECG, echocardiography, or myocardial scintigraphy during exercise or pharmacological interventions.

Table 3 Preoperative characteristics of patients

	Value
Males	32 (78 %)
Age at surgery, y (range)	12.7 ± 8.9 (1–37)
Age ≤12 years	26 (63 %)
Age ≥20 years	7 (17 %)
Age at KD onset, y	3.5 ± 2.8
Prior myocardial infarction	12 (29 %)
Low LVEF	1 (2 %)
Previous PCI	4 (10 %)
Severe MR	2 (5 %)

KD Kawasaki disease, *LVEF* left ventricular ejection fraction, *PCI* percutaneous coronary intervention, *MR* mitral regurgitation

Fig. 1 Distribution of coronary aneurysms in 41 patients undergoing CABG. Aneurysms were located at the LMT in 17 patients (41 %), LAD in 40 (98 %), LCx in 16 (39 %), and RCA in 38 patients (93 %)

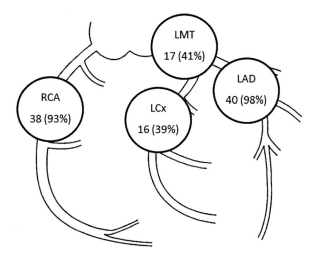

Operative Procedure

All patients underwent initial CABG. Thirty-nine (95 %) underwent conventional CABG under cardiopulmonary bypass and cardioplegic arrest. Among the remaining two patients, one (age 29 years) underwent on-pump beating CABG and the other (age 37 years) underwent off-pump CABG. Two patients (5 %) underwent concomitant mitral valve repair for coexisting severe mitral regurgitation. Nine patients (22 %) underwent concomitant down-sizing operation for giant aneurysms of non-LAD lesions.

The 41 patients received a mean of 1.6 ± 0.7 grafts: one graft for 20 patients (49 %), two grafts for 17 (41 %), and three grafts for four patients (10 %). Most patients (90 %) underwent revascularization of only one or two vessels. Forty patients (98 %) underwent ITA-to-LAD grafting (LITA in 37; RITA in 3) exclusively. The remaining patient, who had a history of successful PTCRA for the LAD, underwent two-vessel revascularization for the LCx and RCA, using the RITA and

Table 4 Details of surgical procedures for CABG

Type of CABG	
Conventional CABG	39 (95 %)
On-pump beating CABG	1 (2 %)
Off-pump CABG	1 (2 %)
Concomitant procedure	
Mitral valve repair	2 (5 %)
Down-sizing operation	9 (22 %)
No. of distal anastomoses	1.6 ± 0.7
Single/double/triple	20 (49 %)/17 (41 %)/4 (10 %)
Conduits used	
LITA/RITA/GEA	40 (98 %)/14 (34 %)/3 (7 %)
ITA to LAD grafting	40 (98 %)
Sequential grafting	9 (22 %)
Y-composite graft	2 (5 %)
Target coronary arteries	
LAD/Dx/LCx/RCA	40/11/7/8

CABG coronary artery bypass grafting, *LITA* left internal thoracic artery, *RITA* right internal thoracic artery, *GEA* right gastroepiploic artery, *ITA* internal thoracic artery, *LAD* left anterior descending artery, *Dx* diagonal branch, *LCx* left circumflex artery, *RCA* right coronary artery

GEA to preserve the LITA for a forthcoming obstructive lesion of the LAD. All operations were completed using only arterial grafts, comprising the LITA in 40 patients (98 %), RITA in 14 (34 %), and GEA in three (7 %); no SVG was used. A total of 66 distal anastomoses were placed, for the LAD in 40, the diagonal branch (Dx) in 11, the LCx in seven, and the RCA in eight. Revascularization for the RCA was not completed in some patients in whom obstructive lesions in the RCA accompanied marked development of collateral vessels without ischemia. Sequential grafting, such as LITA-Dx-LAD, was performed in nine patients (22 %). A Y-composite graft was used in two patients (5 %). However, we avoided complicated graft designs, such as the Y-composite graft, since we have encountered graft occlusion due to a string phenomenon of the LITA graft in a Y-composite graft using bilateral ITA grafts. Details of the surgical procedure for CABG are summarized in Table 4.

Results

There were no operative or hospital deaths, and no late deaths occurred during follow-up (mean duration, 10.9 ± 6.3 years). The cardiac event-free rate at 23 years after first-time CABG was 91.1 % (Fig. 2). Cardiac events occurred three times, in three patients. Two patients underwent redo CABG; the GEA as a free graft was anastomosed to the LAD at 1 year after primary surgery in one patient, because of occlusion of the LITA graft (used as a Y-composite graft) anastomosed to the LAD.

Fig. 2 Cardiac event–free rate in the 41 patients. The cardiac event-free rate at 23 years postoperatively was 91.1 %. Cardiac events occurred in three patients, including redo CABG in two patients (for graft occlusion in one patient and for a new obstructive lesion in one patient) and ICD implantation for VT in one patient

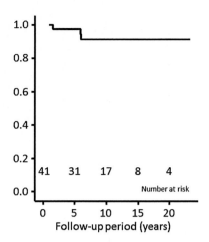

The GEA as an in-situ graft was anastomosed to the RCA at 5 years after primary surgery in another patient, because of a new obstructive lesion. One patient received an implantable cardioverter-defibrillator (ICD) for ventricular tachycardia (VT) at 7 years after primary surgery. No patient suffered myocardial infarction postoperatively. All patients were symptom-free with no obvious restrictions in daily life.

Graft patency was evaluated postoperatively in all patients (by CAG in 40 patients; by multidetector-row computed tomography (MDCT) in one patient aged 37 years). Most patients underwent CAG postoperatively within 6 months after the primary operation, and about half underwent sequential CAG to evaluate mid- and long-term graft patency. The early graft patency rate was 98 % (65/66 anastomoses). The LITA graft (used as a Y-composite graft with the RITA) anastomosed to the LAD was occluded and required redo CABG at 1 year after primary operation, as described previously. No PCI was needed postoperatively.

Case Presentations

Case 1 (Fig. 3)

A 1-year-old boy with a giant aneurysm of the LMT to the proximal LAD (with severely delayed flow) underwent CABG (LITA-LAD). The patency of the LITA graft was confirmed by CAG at 1 month postoperatively, and growth of the LITA graft was confirmed by CAG at 1 year postoperatively, suggesting that the ITA represented a "live conduit".

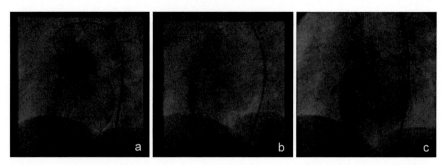

Fig. 3 A 1-year-old boy underwent CABG (LITA-LAD) for a giant aneurysm of the LMT to proximal LAD, with severely delayed flow. (**a**) Preoperative CAG shows a giant aneurysm of the LMT to proximal LAD, with severely delayed flow. (**b**) Patency of the LITA graft is confirmed on CAG at 1 month postoperatively. (**c**) Growth of the LITA graft is confirmed on CAG at 1 year postoperatively

Case 2 (Fig. 4)

A 27-year-old man with giant aneurysms of the proximal LAD (with total occlusion) and proximal RCA (with segmental stenosis) and severe mitral regurgitation underwent CABG (LITA-Dx-LAD and RITA-RCA) and mitral valve annuloplasty. Patency of the LITA and RITA grafts and absence of mitral regurgitation were confirmed by CAG and LVG at 1 month postoperatively.

Down-Sizing Operation for Giant Coronary Aneurysms

Introduction

Giant aneurysms often develop at the proximal portion of the LAD and RCA [19, 22]. LITA-to-LAD grafting is the gold standard, whereas surgical revascularization for giant aneurysms of non-LAD lesions is controversial, particularly for young children, because of the lack of reliable grafts. Giant aneurysms impair coronary circulation with reduced APV, CFR and shear stress and a turbulent flow pattern [31–33]. This can induce thrombus formation inside aneurysms, which may predispose the patient to acute thrombosis, leading to myocardial ischemia and infarction.

Combination therapy using warfarin and aspirin reduces the risk of myocardial infarction in KD patients with giant aneurysms [34, 35], but several arguments against anticoagulation treatment have been raised, especially for young children. First, anticoagulation therapy in an infant obviously increases the risk of hemorrhagic complications, although a multicenter study revealed that hemorrhagic complications associated with combination therapy for KD patients were acceptably low, at 1.7 % per patient-year [34]. Second, the optimal duration of warfarin treatment has not been determined. Lifelong anticoagulation treatment is

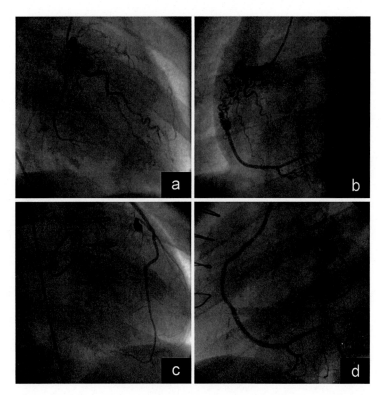

Fig. 4 A 27-year-old man with giant aneurysms of the proximal LAD (with total occlusion) and proximal RCA (with segmental stenosis) and severe mitral regurgitation underwent CABG (LITA-Dx-LAD and RITA-RCA) and mitral valve annuloplasty. (**a** and **b**) Preoperative CAG shows giant aneurysms of the proximal LAD (with total occlusion) and proximal RCA (with segmental stenosis). (**c** and **d**) Postoperative CAG shows patency of the LITA and RITA grafts

recommended as long as giant aneurysms are present, unless regression of aneurysms is detected [34]. In addition, thrombus formation was observed in most giant aneurysms despite adequate anticoagulation [31].

The extent of flow disturbances associated with coronary artery aneurysms correlates with aneurysm size [31–33]. On the basis of this rheological finding, we have adopted a down-sizing operation for giant aneurysms of non-LAD lesions without stenosis and severe calcification, concomitant with CABG, to improve coronary circulation and allow discontinuation of warfarin.

Surgical Procedure of Down-Sizing Operation

The procedure in the down-sizing operation for a giant aneurysm of the proximal RCA is shown in Fig. 5. After cardioplegic arrest, the giant aneurysm is exposed along its entire length, using an ultrasound scalpel, and incised longitudinally. Care is taken not to injure the right ventricular branches, to avoid perioperative right ventricular dysfunction. Fresh and old thrombi located on the posterior side of the distal aneurysm are carefully removed with a No. 15 knife and forceps. Interrupted mattress monofilament sutures are placed on the bottom of the aneurysm to make a "new" posterior wall for the RCA. The anterior wall of the "new" RCA is tailored with interrupted mattress monofilament sutures. A soft tube 5 mm in diameter is inserted into the internal lumen to maintain the appropriate size. Finally, the roof of

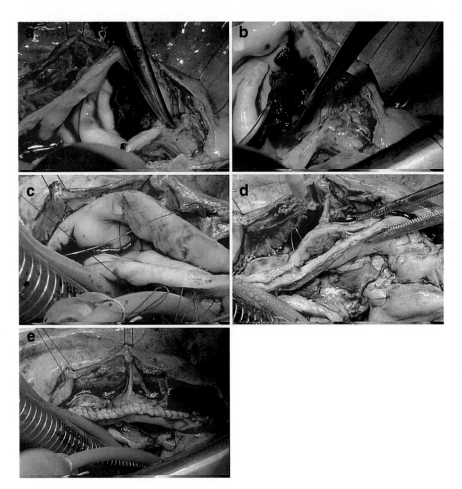

Fig. 5 Surgical procedure in a down-sizing operation for giant aneurysm of the proximal RCA. (**a**) The giant aneurysm is exposed along its entire length and incised longitudinally to maintain an adequate distance to the ostium of the right ventricular branch. (**b**) Fresh and old thrombi located on the posterior side of the distal aneurysm are carefully removed using a No. 15 knife and forceps. (**c**) Interrupted mattress monofilament sutures are placed at the bottom of the aneurysm to form a new posterior wall for the RCA. (**d**) The anterior wall of the new RCA is tailored with interrupted mattress monofilament sutures, to reconstruct an internal lumen of appropriate size. (**e**) The roof of the RCA is closed by continuous monofilament sutures, to ensure hemostasis

the RCA is closed using continuous monofilament over-and-over sutures, to ensure hemostasis. Care should be taken to avoid stenosis around the transition between the aneurysm and "intact" RCA. To ensure an appropriate internal diameter around the transitional area, a small pericardial patch may be preferable.

Down-Sizing Operation at Our Center

Nine patients underwent down-sizing operation for giant aneurysms of non-LAD lesions concomitant with conventional CABG. Mean age at surgery was 7.1 ± 3.7 years (range, 1–11 years). There were seven males (78 %) and two females (22 %). Mean age at KD onset was 4.4 ± 2.9 years (range, 1–9 years). Mean interval from KD onset to surgery was 3.2 ± 3.6 years (range, 4 months to 10 years). Giant aneurysms were located at the RCA in eight patients (proximal RCA in 7; distal RCA in 1) and at the proximal LCx in one patient. This procedure was applied mainly to sausage-like giant aneurysms in the proximal RCA. Surgical indications for a down-sizing operation were giant aneurysms without significant stenosis and severely calcified lesions. The degree of calcification was evaluated preoperatively by CAG and CT, and indication for down-sizing operation was decided based on operative findings (finger palpation). In addition, measurement of APV, CFR, and flow pattern by Doppler flow wire is essential to evaluate the functional severity of myocardial ischemia (as described in [25]). These parameters (APV ≥ 15 cm/s, CFR ≥ 2.0, and pulsatile flow pattern) were also measured postoperatively as an indicator of coronary circulation improvement and to evaluate the possibility of warfarin discontinuation.

The size of giant aneurysms was adequately reduced in five patients, who were able to discontinue warfarin due to improved parameters. Two patients continued warfarin because they could not complete the down-sizing operation sufficiently due to severe calcification. The intervals from KD onset to surgery in these two patients were 8 years and 10 years. Occlusion occurred in two patients. One patient underwent a down-sizing operation within 5 months after onset of KD. Occlusion was confirmed by CAG at 1 month postoperatively, without cardiac events. In the other patient, preoperative CFR was extremely low, indicating a disturbance of microcirculation. Patency of the RCA, with reduced size, was confirmed on CAG at 1 month postoperatively, but occlusion and collateral vessels were identified on CAG at 6 months postoperatively, without cardiac events. On the basis of these findings, we believe that conditions such as acute phase or existence of micro-circulatory disturbance may be contraindications for a down-sizing operation. The down-sizing operation for giant aneurysms of non-LAD lesions may be a good choice to improve coronary circulation and allow warfarin discontinuation, if suitable indications for this procedure can be established. Long-term patency of coronary arteries after a down-sizing operation should be assessed in the future study.

Case Presentation

Case 3 (Fig. 6)

An 11-year-old boy with giant aneurysms of the proximal LAD (with severely delayed flow) and the proximal RCA (without significant stenosis) underwent CABG (LITA-LAD) and down-sizing operation of the RCA. Postoperative CAG at 1 month postoperatively showed patency of the LITA graft and adequate

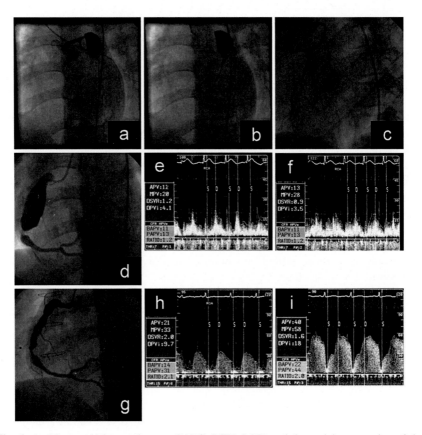

Fig. 6 An 11-year-old boy underwent CABG (LITA-LAD) and down-sizing operation of the RCA for treatment of giant aneurysms of the proximal LAD (with severely delayed flow) and proximal RCA (without significant stenosis). (**a** and **b**) Preoperative CAG shows a giant aneurysm of the proximal LAD, with severely delayed flow (**a**: early phase; **b**: delayed phase). (**c**) Patency of the LITA graft is confirmed on CAG at 1 month postoperatively. Preoperative CAG shows giant aneurysm of the proximal RCA, without significant stenosis. (**e** and **f**) Coronary blood flow velocity is measured by Doppler flow wire. APV is 11 cm/s, CFR is 1.2, and the flow pattern is turbulent (**e**: at rest; **f**: after papaverine hydrochloride infusion). (**g**) Postoperative CAG at 1 month postoperatively shows that the size of the giant aneurysm of the RCA has been adequately reduced. (**h** and **i**) After down-sizing operation, APV is 21 cm/s, CFR is 2.0, and the flow pattern is pulsatile (**h**: at rest; **i**: after papaverine hydrochloride infusion)

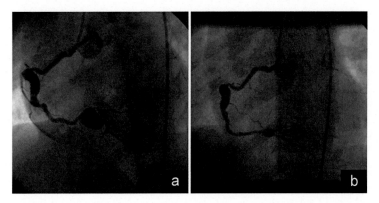

Fig. 7 A 4-year-old boy with giant aneurysms of the proximal LAD (with severely delayed flow) and distal RCA (without significant stenosis) underwent CABG (LITA-LAD) and down-sizing operation of the giant aneurysm of the distal RCA. (**a**). Preoperative CAG shows a giant aneurysm of the distal RCA, without significant stenosis. (**b**). Postoperative CAG at 1 month postoperatively shows that the size of the giant aneurysm of the distal RCA has been adequately reduced

reduction in the size of the giant aneurysm of the RCA. Coronary blood flow velocity was measured by Doppler flow wire. Preoperatively, APV was 11 cm/s, CFR was 1.2, and the flow pattern was turbulent. After down-sizing operation, APV was 21 cm/s, CFR was 2.0, and the flow pattern was pulsatile. The patient was able to discontinue warfarin, due to these improved measurements. RCA patency was confirmed by CAG at 4 years postoperatively.

Case 4 (Fig. 7)

A 4-year-old boy with giant aneurysms of the proximal LAD (with severely delayed flow) and distal RCA (without significant stenosis) underwent CABG (LITA-LAD) and down-sizing operation of the distal RCA. Postoperative CAG at 1 month postoperatively showed patency of the LITA graft and adequate reduction of the size of the giant aneurysm of the distal RCA. He was able to discontinue warfarin. RCA patency was confirmed by CAG at 1 year postoperatively.

References

1. Kitamura S, Kawashima Y, Fujita T, Mori T, Oyama C. Aortocoronary bypass grafting in a child with coronary artery obstruction due to mucocutaneous lymphnode syndrome: report of a case. Circulation. 1976;53(6):1035–40. http://dx.doi.org/10.1161/01.CIR.53.6. 1035. PMID:1083781.

2. Kitamura S, Kawachi K, Oyama C, Miyagi Y, Morita R, Koh Y, et al. Severe Kawasaki heart disease treated with an internal mammary artery graft in pediatric patients. A first successful report. J Thorac Cardiovasc Surg. 1985;89(6):860–6. PMID:3873581.

3. Kitamura S, Tsuda E, Kobayashi J, Nakajima H, Yoshikawa Y, Yagihara T, et al. Twenty-five-year outcome of pediatric coronary artery bypass surgery for Kawasaki disease. Circulation. 2009;120(1):60–8. http://dx.doi.org/10.1161/CIRCULATIONAHA.108.840603, PMID:19546384.

4. Kitamura S, Kameda Y, Seki T, Kawachi K, Endo M, Takeuchi Y, et al. Long-term outcome of myocardial revascularization in patients with Kawasaki coronary artery disease. A multicenter cooperative study. J Thorac Cardiovasc Surg. 1994;107(3):663–73. PMID:8127095.

5. Kitamura S. The role of coronary bypass operation on children with Kawasaki disease. Coron Artery Dis. 2002;13(8):437–47. http://dx.doi.org/10.1097/00019501-200212000-00009. PMID:12544719.

6. Yoshikawa Y, Yagihara T, Kameda Y, Taniguchi S, Tsuda E, Kawahira Y, et al. Result of surgical treatments in patients with coronary-arterial obstructive disease after Kawasaki disease. Eur J Cardiothorac Surg. 2000;17(5):515–9. http://dx.doi.org/10.1016/S1010-7940(00)00355-9. PMID:10814912.

7. Tsuda E, Kitamura S, Cooperative Study Group of Japan. National survey of coronary artery bypass grafting for coronary stenosis caused by Kawasaki disease in Japan. Circulation. 2004; 110(11 Suppl 1):II61–6. PMID:15364840.

8. Kitamura S, Seki T, Kawachi K, Morita R, Kawata T, Mizuguchi K, et al. Excellent patency and growth potential of internal mammary artery grafts in pediatric coronary artery bypass surgery. New evidence for a "live" conduit. Circulation. 1988;78(3 Pt 2):I129–39. PMID:3261649.

9. He GW. Arterial grafts for coronary artery bypass grafting: biological characteristics, functional classification, and clinical choice. Ann Thorac Surg. 1999;67:277–84.

10. Kitamura S, Kawachi K, Seki T, Morita R, Nishii T, Mizuguchi K, et al. Bilateral internal mammary artery grafts for coronary artery bypass operations in children. J Thorac Cardiovasc Surg. 1990;99(4):708–15. PMID:2319795.

11. Lytle BW, Blackstone EH, Loop FD, Houghtaling PL, Arnold JH, Akhrass R, et al. Two internal thoracic artery grafts are better than one. J Thorac Cardiovasc Surg. 1999;117(5): 855–72. http://dx.doi.org/10.1016/S0022-5223(99)70365-X. PMID:10220677.

12. Ochi M, Hatori N, Bessho R, Fujii M, Saji Y, Tanaka S, et al. Adequacy of flow capacity of bilateral internal thoracic artery T graft. Ann Thorac Surg. 2001;72(6):2008–11. http://dx.doi.org/10.1016/S0003-4975(01)03201-5. PMID:11789785.

13. Nakajima H, Kobayashi J, Toda K, Fujita T, Shimahara Y, Kasahara Y, et al. A 10-year angiographic follow-up of competitive flow in sequential and composite arterial grafts. Eur J Cardiothorac Surg. 2011;40(2):399–404. PMID:21236696.

14. Tsuda E, Fujita H, Yagihara T, Yamada O, Echigo S, Kitamura S. Competition between native flow and graft flow after coronary artery bypass grafting. Impact on indications for coronary artery bypass grafting for localized stenosis with giant aneurysms due to Kawasaki disease. Pediatr Cardiol. 2008;29(2):266–70. http://dx.doi.org/10.1007/s00246-007-9114-y. PMID:17917764.

15. Takeuchi Y, Gomi A, Okamura Y, Mori H, Nagashima M. Coronary revascularization in a child with Kawasaki disease: use of right gastroepiploic artery. Ann Thorac Surg. 1990;50 (2):294–6. http://dx.doi.org/10.1016/0003-4975(90)90754-T. PMID:2383118.

16. JCS Joint Working Group. Guidelines for diagnosis and management of cardiovascular sequelae in Kawasaki disease (JCS 2008)—digest version. Circ J. 2010;74(9):1989–2020. http://dx.doi.org/10.1253/circj.CJ-10-74-0903. PMID:20724794.

17. Subcommittee of Cardiovascular Sequelae SoST, Kawasaki Disease Research Committee. Guidelines for treatment and management of cardiovascular sequelae in Kawasaki disease. Heart Vessels 1987;3(1):50–4. http://dx.doi.org/10.1007/BF02073648. PMID:3624163

18. Newburger JW, Takahashi M, Gerber MA, Gewitz MH, Tani LY, Burns JC et al.; Committee on Rheumatic Fever, Endocarditis and Kawasaki Disease; Council on Cardiovascular Disease

in the Young; American Heart Association; American Academy of Pediatrics. Diagnosis, treatment, and long-term management of Kawasaki disease: a statement for health professionals from the Committee on Rheumatic fever, Endocarditis and Kawasaki disease, council on cardiovascular disease in the young, American Heart Association. Circulation 2004; 110(17):2747–71. http://dx.doi.org/10.1161/01.CIR.0000145143.19711.78. PMID:15505111

19. Kato H, Sugimura T, Akagi T, Sato N, Hashino K, Maeno Y, et al. Long-term consequences of Kawasaki disease. A 10- to 21-year follow-up study of 594 patients. Circulation. 1996;94 (6):1379–85. http://dx.doi.org/10.1161/01.CIR.94.6.1379. PMID:8822996.

20. Nakano H, Ueda K, Saito A, Nojima K. Repeated quantitative angiograms in coronary arterial aneurysm in Kawasaki disease. Am J Cardiol. 1985;56(13):846–51. http://dx.doi.org/10.1016/ 0002-9149(85)90767-2. PMID:4061324.

21. Suzuki A, Kamiya T, Arakaki Y, Kinoshita Y, Kimura K. Fate of coronary arterial aneurysms in Kawasaki disease. Am J Cardiol. 1994;74(8):822–4. http://dx.doi.org/10.1016/0002-9149 (94)90446-4. PMID:7942561.

22. Kato H, Ichinose E, Kawasaki T. Myocardial infarction in Kawasaki disease: clinical analyses in 195 cases. J Pediatr. 1986;108(6):923–7. http://dx.doi.org/10.1016/S0022-3476(86)80928- 3. PMID:3712157.

23. Suzuki A, Kamiya T, Ono Y, Takahashi N, Naito Y, Kou Y. Indication of aortocoronary by-pass for coronary arterial obstruction due to Kawasaki disease. Heart Vessels. 1985;1 (2):94–100. http://dx.doi.org/10.1007/BF02066356. PMID:3879490.

24. Suzuki A, Kamiya T, Ono Y, Kinoshita Y, Kawamura S, Kimura K. Clinical significance of morphologic classification of coronary arterial segmental stenosis due to Kawasaki disease. Am J Cardiol. 1993;71(13):1169–73. http://dx.doi.org/10.1016/0002-9149(93)90641-O. PMID:8480642.

25. Ogawa S, Ohkubo T, Fukazawa R, Kamisago M, Kuramochi Y, Uchikoba Y, et al. Estimation of myocardial hemodynamics before and after intervention in children with Kawasaki disease. J Am Coll Cardiol. 2004;43(4):653–61. http://dx.doi.org/10.1016/j.jacc.2003.10.032. PMID:14975478.

26. Ogawa S, Fukazawa R, Ohkubo T, Zhang J, Takechi N, Kuramochi Y, et al. Silent myocardial ischemia in Kawasaki disease: evaluation of percutaneous transluminal coronary angioplasty by dobutamine stress testing. Circulation. 1997;96(10):3384–9. http://dx.doi.org/10.1161/01. CIR.96.10.3384. PMID:9396431.

27. Yamauchi H, Ochi M, Fujii M, Hinokiyama K, Ohmori H, Sasaki T, et al. Optimal time of surgical treatment for Kawasaki coronary artery disease. J Nippon Med Sch. 2004;71(4): 279–86. http://dx.doi.org/10.1272/jnms.71.279. PMID:15329488.

28. Tsuda E, Kitamura S, Kimura K, Kobayashi J, Miyazaki S, Echigo S, et al. Long-term patency of internal thoracic artery grafts for coronary artery stenosis due to Kawasaki disease: comparison of early with recent results in small children. Am Heart J. 2007;153(6): 995–1000. http://dx.doi.org/10.1016/j.ahj.2007.03.034. PMID:17540201.

29. Mavroudis C, Backer CL, Muster AJ, Pahl E, Sanders JH, Zales VR, et al. Expanding indications for pediatric coronary artery bypass. J Thorac Cardiovasc Surg. 1996;111(1): 181–9. http://dx.doi.org/10.1016/S0022-5223(96)70415-4. PMID:8551764.

30. Fortune RL, Baron PJ, Fitzgerald JW. Atresia of the left main coronary artery: repair with left internal mammary artery bypass. J Thorac Cardiovasc Surg. 1987;94(1):150–1. PMID:3496498.

31. Ohkubo T, Fukazawa R, Ikegami E, Ogawa S. Reduced shear stress and disturbed flow may lead to coronary aneurysm and thrombus formations. Pediatr Int. 2007;49(1):1–7. http://dx.doi. org/10.1111/j.1442-200X.2007.02312.x. PMID:17250496.

32. Kuramochi Y, Ohkubo T, Takechi N, Fukumi D, Uchikoba Y, Ogawa S. Hemodynamic factors of thrombus formation in coronary aneurysms associated with Kawasaki disease. Pediatr Int. 2000;42(5):470–5. http://dx.doi.org/10.1046/j.1442-200x.2000.01270.x. PMID:11059533.

33. Hamaoka K, Onouchi Z. Effects of coronary artery aneurysms on intracoronary flow velocity dynamics in Kawasaki disease. Am J Cardiol. 1996;77(10):873–5. http://dx.doi.org/10.1016/ S0002-9149(97)89186-2. PMID:8623744.
34. Suda K, Kudo Y, Higaki T, Nomura Y, Miura M, Matsumura M, et al. Multicenter and retrospective case study of warfarin and aspirin combination therapy in patients with giant coronary aneurysms caused by Kawasaki disease. Circ J. 2009;73(7):1319–23. http://dx.doi. org/10.1253/circj.CJ-08-0931. PMID:19436123.
35. Sugahara Y, Ishii M, Muta H, Iemura M, Matsuishi T, Kato H. Warfarin therapy for giant aneurysm prevents myocardial infarction in Kawasaki disease. Pediatr Cardiol. 2008;29(2): 398–401. http://dx.doi.org/10.1007/s00246-007-9132-9. PMID:18027010.

Long-Term Graft Patency and Surgical Outcomes of Coronary Artery Bypass Surgery in Children with Kawasaki Disease

Soichiro Kitamura

Abstract Pediatric coronary artery bypass surgery gained wide acceptance after the internal thoracic arteries began to be used in bypass operations for post–Kawasaki disease lesions. This technique is now the standard surgical procedure, and safety (even in infants), graft patency, growth potential, graft longevity, and clinical efficacy are well documented. This chapter discusses long-term graft patency and outcomes of pediatric coronary bypass surgery for treatment of coronary lesions caused by Kawasaki disease.

Keywords Aneurysm (coronary) • CABG • Coronary artery disease • Inflammation (systemic) • Pediatric

Introduction

In 1967 Kawasaki [1] reported a previously unrecognized acute febrile illness with muco-cutaneous lesions and lymphadenopathy (MCLS or MLNS), which was later referred to as Kawasaki disease (KD). Death in affected children was soon recognized as being primarily due to formation of inflammatory coronary aneurysms [2]. Rupture of coronary aneurysms in the acute phase, and thrombosis or fibroproliferative narrowing of the coronary artery during convalescence and the late phases of KD, were the main cardiac sequelae and causes of death. Acute myocardial infarction due to KD and the resulting high death rate in children [3] were regarded as a public health crisis in Japan in the 1970s and 1980s; however, there had been no reported attempts at pediatric coronary revascularization surgery, and the prevailing opinion in Japan was that surgery had little to offer for this acute inflammatory condition. This chapter reviews the development of pediatric coronary bypass as the main indication for treatment of coronary lesions caused by KD.

S. Kitamura, MD (✉)
National Cerebral and Cardiovascular Center, President Emeritus, 5-7-1 Fujishirodai, Suita, Osaka 565-8565, Japan
e-mail: skitamur@hsp.ncvc.go.jp

© Springer Japan 2017   407
B.T. Saji et al. (eds.), *Kawasaki Disease*, DOI 10.1007/978-4-431-56039-5_43

Historical Overview

In 1986, Kato et al. [3] published the first evidence that significant coronary artery lesions persisted in children after convalescence of KD. In such children, mortality from acute myocardial infarction approached 65 % after the second or third myocardial infarction. In a study published in the late 1970s, coronary artery imaging depended on aortic root injection of contrast, which provided limited detail. Selective coronary arteriography (sCAG) was not performed in children because of the lack of compelling indications and because of concerns about possible higher complication rates for small children. However, sCAG was considered essential in identifying potential targets for surgical treatment in children.

We started sCAG in small children by using a 4 F or 5 F handmade catheter shaped like a Judkins coronary catheter. Size and curvature were adjusted by superimposing catheters on lateral chest radiographs of the child [4]. Although a variety of coronary lesions were identified among individuals with KD, obstructive lesions most commonly involved the entry or exit portions of coronary aneurysms, which were usually located on the proximal coronary arteries, ie, the left main trunk, particularly in the left coronary system. In contrast, right coronary artery lesions tended to involve more distal areas before and sometimes beyond the bifurcation. These findings contradicted the initial belief that surgical indications would be quite rare in KD. Surgical coronary revascularization and coronary artery bypass grafting (CABG) [5, 6] were soon accepted as having roles in KD management and were included in the treatment guidelines for KD in Japan.

In Japan in the late 1970s and early 1980s, saphenous vein grafts (SVGs) were used exclusively as bypass grafts for adult atherosclerotic coronary artery disease, and SVGs were initially used in bypass surgery for children with KD. Because most KD patients are children, expected graft patency must be long and SVGs soon proved unsatisfactory [7]. Moreover, it was not clear how grafts would respond to somatic growth in children. We decided to use a pedicled internal thoracic artery (ITA), as it is rarely involved in KD arteritis and is expected to grow when used in growing children. We reported the first successful use of ITA grafts in children, in 1985 [8]. In addition, we demonstrated the safety of bilateral ITA use, without visible compromise of thorax growth [9]. Since then, we have promoted ITA grafts as the best option in pediatric CABG.

Operation

The ITA of small children is a short, thin-walled artery with a diameter of 1 mm or less, reflecting the child's small thorax. All pediatric CABG operations were performed under cardiopulmonary bypass and aortic cross-clamping with cardioplegic myocardial protection. The procedure requires meticulous and precise coronary dissection and anastomosis under high-magnification surgical glasses or microscope [10] with 8–0 to 10–0 small needles and sutures. Use of a surgical microscope is uncommon for adult CABG but can be useful in pediatric CABG. Vida et al. [11] recently successfully utilized a microscope for an infant case.

Growth Response of Grafts in Children

We developed a method for evaluating the length and diameter of grafts used in children. As reported previously [12], graft length was measured utilizing the 3-dimensional Pythagorean rule applied to bilateral angiograms. These measurements showed that in children the ITA graft could grow in accordance with somatic growth. In contrast, the SVG, although autologous in origin, had poor long-axis growth potential in proportion to body size in children [13]. For this reason coronary artery distortion due to tenting or traction was observed during the late postoperative period, which obstructed or restricted flow in the coronary artery distal to the anastomotic site, even though the SVG was patent [14].

Disadvantages of the ITA Graft

Flow competition can cause a string phenomenon in ITA grafts. This is well-documented and occurs because of insufficient blood flow through the graft when the recipient coronary artery blood flow is unrestricted [15]. The ITA string phenomenon is clinically benign, with no resulting symptoms, and can be identified only by angiography, computed tomography, and/or Doppler echocardiography. This phenomenon has also been observed in adult CABG for atherosclerotic disease and is the major non-technical cause of ITA graft obstruction (thrombosis). However, in pediatric CABG the incidence of ITA graft recanalization classified as occluded or nonfunctioning after the ITA string phenomenon was 20–25 %[16], higher than in adult CABG cases. This phenomenon is endothelium-dependent, and when flow competition between the graft and recipient coronary artery diminishes due to progression of coronary artery obstructive lesions, the ITA regains its flow and function as a graft unless the lumen is completely thrombosed.

Measurement of fractional flow ratio (FFR) with a pressure guidewire may help avoid the ITA string phenomenon due to flow competition. Ogawa et al. [17] reported that abnormal preoperative FFR normalized after successful CABG in KD patients. The usefulness of FFR in preventing the graft string phenomenon in pediatric coronary artery disease with multiple aneurysms needs further prospective evaluation, preferably in a multicenter trial. Anastomotic ITA stenosis due to technical reasons can be managed easily by simple balloon dilatation, with essentially no recurrence of stenosis [18]. Stenting is unnecessary in this setting and should be avoided in children.

Long-Term Graft Patency and Morphology in Growing Children

When SVG and ITA long-term graft patency in pediatric CABG were compared, patency was far better for ITA than for SVG for both the LAD and non-LAD coronary arteries [16, 19]. Recent studies of the patency of ITA grafts for KD found no significant difference between the LAD and non-LAD target coronary arteries or between younger (<10 years) and older children (≥10 years). ITA grafts patent at 1 year after surgery remain so for up to 25 years, [16] and I believe they will remain patent for the entire life of patients. The ITA string sign followed by occlusion can occur within 1 year after surgery [15, 16]. The SVG may close early, within 1 year, probably due to thrombosis, but can also close late after surgery, due to intimal fibroproliferation that eventually results in premature SVG atherosclerosis [14, 16].

The late postoperative angiographic morphology of SVG and ITA grafts substantially differs (Fig. 1). The wall configuration of the ITA graft is smooth, with no luminal stenosis or dilatation, and well matched in size with the recipient coronary artery area 20 years after surgery [16]. In addition, graft length increased in proportion to patient body growth [12, 18]. In contrast, the SVG was usually dilated with local narrowing and was sometimes aneurysmal, with prominent irregularity of wall contours [14, 16]. Patients aged 20–29 years already exhibited fibroproliferative thickening and atherosclerotic changes of the SVG [14, 16]. The SVG could also be a cause of acute myocardial infarction in the late postoperative period, probably due to embolism formation caused by wall thrombus detachment or thrombosis at the site of intimal thickening. Because of the poor growth potential of SVGs, they can cause traction on the recipient coronary artery, distorting the anastomosis and resulting in poor run-off to the distal artery [13, 14].

With enlarged ITA grafts, either unilateral or bilateral, in association with a patent SVG, five fully grown patients who had had total occlusion of both the left and right coronary ostia are alive and well at present (Fig. 1). In summary, the 25-year patency rate was 87 % for the ITA graft and 42 % for the SVG. When used in children younger than 10 years, ITA graft patency was 86 %, essentially the same as that for the whole age group, as compared with 25 % for the SVG (P < 0.001) [16] (Figs. 2 and 3). Data from the 30-year postoperative follow-up indicate that the pedicled ITA is the conduit of choice for pediatric CABG, as it ensures persistent graft patency, growth potential, and possible metabolic benefits for many decades.

Survival of KD Children Treated by Pediatric CABG

Pediatric coronary bypass surgery using arterial grafts is a safe procedure for children with severe coronary involvement due to KD. Surgical mortality with more than 100 such children has been 0 %, and late mortality during the subsequent

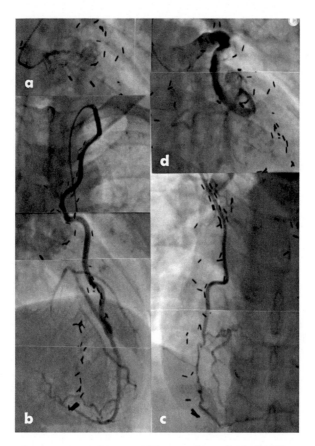

Fig. 1 Postoperative coronary angiograms at 24 years after pediatric CABG surgery for KD. A boy underwent triple bypass grafting at age 12 years for coronary lesions caused by KD. The bilateral coronary ostia and very proximal main trunks were totally obstructed (**a**). Twenty-four years after surgery he developed an acute myocardial infarct due to SVG-LCX artery thrombosis (**d**). Fortunately, bilateral ITAs (LITA-LAD, RITA-RCA) were well patent (**b** and **c**), and the patient survived without complications. Thrombolysis of the SVG was successfully carried out. The configuration and wall characteristics of the ITA (**b** and **c**) and SVG (**d**) are substantially different 24 years after surgery. The presence of old SVG can be a cause of acute myocardial infarction. (**a**): total obstruction of the *left* main trunk, (**b**): left internal thoracic artery (LITA)—left anterior descending artery (LAD), (**c**): right internal thoracic artery (RITA)—right coronary artery (RCA), (**d**): saphenous vein graft (SVG)—left circumflex artery (LCX)

25 years was 5 % (95 % confidence interval [CI], 2–12 %) [16]. Successful surgery may also improve cardiac function [20]. Approximately one-third of surgical subjects had a history of myocardial infarction [16]. Although a strict comparison is impossible, surgery for severe coronary involvement due to KD is likely to improve patient survival. The 30-year survival of KD children with previous myocardial infarction was limited, as low as 49 % (95 % CI, 27–71 %) [21, 22], as compared with 95 % (95 % CI, 88–98 %) survival at 25–30 years with surgical coronary

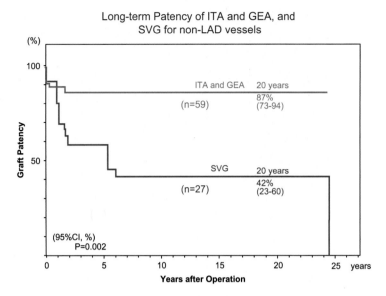

Fig. 2 Long-term patency of ITA, GEA, and SVG for non-LAD vessels. The ITA was exclusively used for the LAD, and use of SVG was infrequent. The ITA remained continuously patent after 1 year, and there was no difference in ITA patency between any target vessels, including the LAD and non-LAD target vessels: 87 % (95 % CI, 78–93 %) vs 87 % (95 % CI, 73–94 %). In contrast, SVG patency progressively declined over 20 years. The difference in patency between these two graft types was significant (p = 0.002). *GEA* gastroepiploic artery; see legend for Fig. 1 for other abbreviations (Copyright permission obtained from the American Heart Association for reference 16)

revascularization [16]. Late death after CABG for KD children was rare, but usually resulted from sudden death of children with both reduced LV function and a history of ventricular tachycardia [16, 21]. Therefore, it may be important to consider early management strategies such as early reintervention for graft failure and electro-physiologic studies with early ablation therapy or ICD implantation for ventricular tachycardia.

Event Incidence After Pediatric Bypass Surgery for KD

Cardiac events were precipitated by (1) ITA graft stenosis at the anastomosis, (2) graft obstruction of any cause, including the string phenomenon of ITA grafts, (3) fibroproliferative intimal thickening and atherosclerosis of the SVG, (4) late thrombosis of the remaining coronary aneurysms, (5) postinflammatory progression of coronary artery fibro-obstructive disease, (6) left ventricular dysfunction, and (7) episodes of ventricular tachyarrhythmias. The incidences of these cardiac events rose as the postoperative period increased, and the total cardiac event–free rates at 5, 10, 20, and 25 postoperative years were 87 %, 81 %, 70 %, and 62 % (95 % CI,

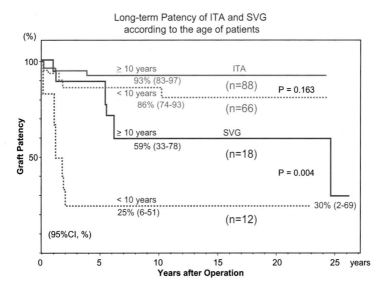

Fig. 3 Difference in graft patency according to patient age (≥10 or <10 years) at surgery. Long-term patency for the ITA did not significantly differ (p = 0.163) between patients aged ≥10 years (93 %) and <10 years (86 %); however, SVG patency was significantly lower (p = 0.004) for patients aged <10 years (25 %) than for those aged ≥10 years (58 %) (Copyright permission obtained from the American Heart Association for reference 16)

48–74 %), respectively [16]. Tsuda et al. [22] reported that the 30-year overall cardiac event–free rate was 36 % (95 % CI, 28–45 %; n = 245) in patients with giant aneurysms and 62 % (95 % CI, 48–74 %; n = 114) in those who underwent bypass surgery [16]. Although cardiac event–free rates are not strictly comparable, surgical patients, who almost always had a history of multiple giant aneurysms, did have fewer cardiac events during the next 25–30 years.

Although cardiac events were not uncommon at 25 years, events resulting in death were rare in surgical patients who received early and adequate interventions, either by reoperation or percutaneous coronary intervention (PCI) [16]. Furthermore most patients had reached adulthood when the second intervention was required. Reoperation utilizing either the radial artery, gastroepiploic artery, or both, and PCI using coronary stents is safer and more effective in adults than in children.

Analysis of long-term follow-up data emphasized the need for prolonged close medical supervision of postoperative KD patients with SVGs or persisting patent coronary aneurysms [23, 24]. In contrast, among children with well-functioning grafts, 84 % could participate in athletic programs at school and 16 % participated in sport clubs [16], although preoperatively all these patients had been strictly excluded from school athletic programs because of the fear of sudden collapse or death on the playground. Upon reaching adulthood, many postsurgical patients were successfully employed, and female patients had successful childbirths. The evidence strongly suggests that pediatric coronary bypass surgery with ITA grafts is an effective, long-lasting treatment that improves quality of life for children with coronary lesions due to KD.

PCI for Coronary Obstructive Lesions Due to KD

PCI technology has significantly developed along with that of CABG and has been effective for KD coronary lesions [25]. Rotablation and/or stenting are more often required for hard fibroproliferative intima and sometimes calcific lesions in KD than for atherosclerotic lesions. However, these approaches, particularly stenting, are not suitable for growing children. Muta et al. reported [26] that PCI for KD was less efficacious than CABG because of the increased need for repeat procedures after PCI, particularly when used for children younger than 12 years. Coronary revascularization surgery utilizing ITA should be the gold standard for pediatric patients with KD.

Current Status of Pediatric Coronary Bypass Surgery in the World

Reports of pediatric CABG for KD have been increasing significantly in the United States, Europe, and Asian countries other than Japan [27–31]. Over the last 15 years the author has often been consulted regarding surgical indications for pediatric patients with complications of KD by pediatric cardiologists and surgeons in many regions and countries, including the United States, Canada, South America, Europe, New Zealand, Australia, Turkey, Malaysia, India, China, Taiwan, Korea, and Singapore. Patients often had severe coronary lesions, and many required surgery; however, the exact number of such patients worldwide is unknown.

Mavroudis et al. [28] reported the largest series in the United States and expanded the indications for pediatric CABG to congenital coronary anomalies of infants, with excellent results. Recently, Viola et al. [29] applied CABG with ITA grafts to a variety of pediatric coronary lesions, with no operative deaths. In addition, at present there is essentially no age limitation for this surgery, and pediatric CABG with ITA grafts is now being successfully carried out in infants [11, 30].

The development of pediatric CABG utilizing pedicled ITAs for KD coronary lesions and the excellent late surgical results have contributed to standardization of surgical coronary revascularization procedures for children, and the procedure is now frequently regarded as the treatment of choice for many disease conditions in children. Sir Magdi Yocoub [32] stated that the work has developed "from a mystery to a paradigm" for KD coronary lesions. Vida et al. [11] recently commented that coronary artery bypass graft operations should be regarded as a fundamental part of the training of contemporary congenital heart surgeons. Pediatric CABG utilizing the ITA, either single or bilateral, can be applied safely not only to KD patients but even to infants with a variety of pediatric coronary lesions. Its favorable long-term outcomes with respect to graft patency, growth potential, and long-term clinical, physiological, and perhaps even metabolic measures, [33] is now well documented.

References

1. Kawasaki T, Kosaki F, Okawa S, Shigematsu I, Yanagawa H. A new infantile acute febrile mucocutaneous lymph node syndrome (MLNS) prevailing in Japan. Pediatrics. 1974;54(3): 271–6. PMID:4153258.
2. Fujiwara H, Hamashima Y. Pathology of the heart in Kawasaki disease. Pediatrics. 1978;61 (1): 100–7. PMID:263836.
3. Kato H, Ichinose E, Kawasaki T. Myocardial infarction in Kawasaki disease: clinical analyses in 195 cases. J Pediatr. 1986;108(6):923–7. http://dx.doi.org/10.1016/S0022-3476(86)80928-3. PMID:3712157.
4. Kitamura S, Kawachi K, Shimazaki Y, Fujino M, Yokota K, Ogawa M. [Selective coronary arteriography in pediatric patients] (author's translation). Kokyu To Junkan. 1980;28(9): 1037–40. PMID:7209153.
5. Kitamura S, Kawachi K, Harima R, Sakakibara T, Hirose H, Kawashima Y. Surgery for coronary heart disease due to mucocutaneous lymph node syndrome (Kawasaki disease). Report of 6 patients. Am J Cardiol. 1983;51(3):444–8. http://dx.doi.org/10.1016/S0002-9149 (83)80077-0. PMID:6600576.
6. Kitamura S. Surgical management for cardiovascular lesions in Kawasaki disease. Cardiol Young. 1991;1(03):240–53. http://dx.doi.org/10.1017/S1047951100000445.
7. Kitamura S, Kawashima Y, Fujita T, Mori T, Oyama C. Aortocoronary bypass grafting in a child with coronary artery obstruction due to mucocutaneous lymphnode syndrome: report of a case. Circulation. 1976;53(6):1035–40. http://dx.doi.org/10.1161/01.CIR.53.6.1035. PMID:1083781.
8. Kitamura S, Kawachi K, Oyama C, Miyagi Y, Morita R, Koh Y, et al. Severe Kawasaki heart disease treated with an internal mammary artery graft in pediatric patients. A first successful report. J Thorac Cardiovasc Surg. 1985;89(6):860–6. PMID:3873581.
9. Kitamura S, Kawachi K, Seki T, Morita R, Nishii T, Mizuguchi K, et al. Bilateral internal mammary artery grafts for coronary artery bypass operations in children. J Thorac Cardiovasc Surg. 1990;99(4):708–15. PMID:2319795.
10. Kitamura S, Taniguchi S, Kawata T, Mizuguchi K, Nishioka H, Kameda Y. Coronary artery revascularization. Ann Vasc Dis (Myakkan-Gaku) (English Abstract) 1998;38:85–90.
11. Vida VL, Torregrossa G, De Franceschi M, Padalino MA, Belli E, Berggren H, et al. European Congenital Heart Surgeons Association (ECHSA). Pediatric coronary artery revascularization: a European multicenter study. Ann Thorac Surg. 2013;96(3):898–903. http://dx.doi.org/10. 1016/j.athoracsur.2013.05.006. PMID:23891408.
12. Kitamura S, Seki T, Kawachi K, Morita R, Kawata T, Mizuguchi K et al. Excellent patency and growth potential of internal mammary artery grafts in pediatric coronary artery bypass surgery. New evidence for a "live" conduit. Circulation 1988 78(3 Pt 2 Supp I):I129–I139. PMID:3261649.
13. Kameda Y, Kitamura S, Taniguchi S, Kawata T, Mizuguchi K, Nishioka H, et al. Differences in adaptation to growth of children between internal thoracic artery and saphenous vein coronary bypass grafts. J Cardiovasc Surg (Torino). 2001;42(1):9–16. PMID:11292899.

14. Wakisaka Y, Tsuda E, Yamada O, Yagihara T, Kitamura S. Long-term results of saphenous vein graft for coronary stenosis caused by Kawasaki disease. Circ J. 2009;73(1):73–7. http://dx.doi.org/10.1253/circj.CJ-08-0225. PMID:19047778.

15. Tsuda E, Fujita H, Yagihara T, Yamada O, Echigo S, Kitamura S. Competition between native flow and graft flow after coronary artery bypass grafting. Impact on indications for coronary artery bypass grafting for localized stenosis with giant aneurysms due to Kawasaki disease. Pediatr Cardiol. 2008;29(2):266–70. http://dx.doi.org/10.1007/s00246-007-9114-y. PMID:17917764.

16. Kitamura S, Tsuda E, Kobayashi J, Nakajima H, Yoshikawa Y, Yagihara T, et al. Twenty-five-year outcome of pediatric coronary artery bypass surgery for Kawasaki disease. Circulation. 2009; 120(1):60–8. http://dx.doi.org/10.1161/CIRCULATIONAHA.108.840603. PMID:19546384.

17. Ogawa S, Ohkubo T, Fukazawa R, Kamisago M, Kuramochi Y, Uchikoba Y, et al. Estimation of myocardial hemodynamics before and after intervention in children with Kawasaki disease. J Am Coll Cardiol. 2004;43(4):653–61. http://dx.doi.org/10.1016/j.jacc.2003.10.032. PMID:14975478.

18. Kitamura S. The role of coronary bypass operation on children with Kawasaki disease. Coron Artery Dis. 2002;13(8):437–47. http://dx.doi.org/10.1097/00019501-200212000-00009. PMID:12544719.

19. Tsuda E, Kitamura S, Kimura K, Kobayashi J, Miyazaki S, Echigo S, et al. Long-term patency of internal thoracic artery grafts for coronary artery stenosis due to Kawasaki disease: comparison of early with recent results in small children. Am Heart J. 2007;153(6): 995–1000. http://dx.doi.org/10.1016/j.ahj.2007.03.034. PMID:17540201.

20. Kawachi K, Kitamura S, Seki T, Morita R, Kawata T, Hasegawa J, et al. Hemodynamics and coronary blood flow during exercise after coronary artery bypass grafting with internal mammary arteries in children with Kawasaki disease. Circulation. 1991;84(2):618–24. http://dx.doi.org/10.1161/01.CIR.84.2.618. PMID:1860205.

21. Tsuda E, Hirata T, Matsuo O, Abe T, Sugiyama H, Yamada O. The 30-year outcome for patients after myocardial infarction due to coronary artery lesions caused by Kawasaki disease. Pediatr Cardiol. 2011;32(2):176–82. http://dx.doi.org/10.1007/s00246-010-9838-y. PMID:21120463.

22. Tsuda E, Hamaoka K, Suzuki H, Sakazaki H, Murakami Y, Nakagawa M, et al. A survey of the 3-decade outcome for patients with giant aneurysms caused by Kawasaki disease. Am Heart J. 2014;167(2):249–58. http://dx.doi.org/10.1016/j.ahj.2013.10.025. PMID:24439987.

23. McCrindle BW. Kawasaki disease: a childhood disease with important consequences into adulthood [Editorial]. Circulation. 2009;120(1):6–8. http://dx.doi.org/10.1161/CIRCULATIONAHA.109.874800. PMID:19546382.

24. Gersony WM. The adult after Kawasaki disease the risks for late coronary events. J Am Coll Cardiol. 2009;54(21):1921–3. http://dx.doi.org/10.1016/j.jacc.2009.06.057. PMID:19909871.

25. Ishii M, Ueno T, Ikeda H, Iemura M, Sugimura T, Furui J, et al. Sequential follow-up results of catheter intervention for coronary artery lesions after Kawasaki disease: quantitative coronary artery angiography and intravascular ultrasound imaging study. Circulation. 2002; 105(25):3004–10. http://dx.doi.org/10.1161/01.CIR.0000019733.56553.D8. PMID:12081995.

26. Muta H, Ishii M. Percutaneous coronary intervention versus coronary artery bypass grafting for stenotic lesions after Kawasaki disease. J Pediatr. 2010;157(1):120–6. http://dx.doi.org/10.1016/j.jpeds.2010.01.032. PMID:20304414.

27. Newburger JW, Fulton DR. Coronary revascularization in patients with Kawasaki disease. J Pediatr. 2010;157(1):8–10. http://dx.doi.org/10.1016/j.jpeds.2010.04.008. PMID:20472246.

28. Mavroudis C, Backer CL, Duffy CE, Pahl E, Wax DF. Pediatric coronary artery bypass for Kawasaki congenital, post arterial switch, and iatrogenic lesions. Ann Thorac Surg. 1999; 68(2):506–12. http://dx.doi.org/10.1016/S0003-4975(99)00588-3. PMID:10475420.

29. Viola N, Alghamdi AA, Al-Radi OO, Coles JG, Van Arsdell GS, Caldarone CA. Midterm outcomes of myocardial revascularization in children. J Thorac Cardiovasc Surg. 2010;139(2): 333–8. http://dx.doi.org/10.1016/j.jtcvs.2009.09.005. PMID:20005530.

30. Legendre A, Chantepie A, Belli E, Vouhé PR, Neville P, Dulac Y, et al. Outcome of coronary artery bypass grafting performed in young children. J Thorac Cardiovasc Surg. 2010;139(2): 349–53. http://dx.doi.org/10.1016/j.jtcvs.2009.07.061. PMID:19775706.
31. Coskun KO, Coskun ST, El Arousy M, Aminparsa M, Hornik L, Blanz U, et al. Pediatric patients with Kawasaki disease and a case report of Kitamura operation. ASAIO J. 2006;52(6): e43–7. http://dx.doi.org/10.1097/01.mat.0000249023.21962.ce. PMID:17117047.
32. Yacoub M. Kawasaki disease—from a mystery to a paradigm. Coron Artery Dis. 2002;13(8): 421–2. http://dx.doi.org/10.1097/00019501-200212000-00006.
33. Kitamura S. Physiological and metabolic effects of grafts in coronary artery bypass surgery. Circ J. 2011;75(4):766–72. http://dx.doi.org/10.1253/circj.CJ-10-1302. PMID:21415547.

Part VI
Follow-Up Concerns

Functional and Structural Alterations of Coronary Arteries Late After Kawasaki Disease and the Risk of Acute Coronary Syndrome in Adults

Yoshihide Mitani

Abstract It has been 48 years since Kawasaki first reported Kawasaki disease (KD), in 1967. Among the 270,000 patients with a history of KD as of 2010, more than 110,000 have reached adulthood. Recent reports indicate that an increasing number of adults with a history of KD are developing acute coronary syndrome. Thus, the risk and management of acute coronary syndrome are important concerns. This chapter describes vessel wall function and morphology of coronary arteries long after KD and the characteristics of acute coronary syndrome in adults with a history of KD.

Keywords Kawasaki disease • Acute coronary syndrome • Transition • Endothelial dysfunction

Introduction

It has been 48 years since Kawasaki first reported Kawasaki disease (KD), in 1967. Among the 270,000 persons with a history of KD as of 2010, more than 110,000 have reached adulthood [1]. Recent reports indicate that an increasing number of adults with a history of KD are developing acute coronary syndrome (ACS). Thus, the risk and management of ACS are emerging concerns. Moreover, even after introduction of intravenous immunoglobulin therapy for acute KD, the annual incidence of severe sequelae, i.e., giant coronary aneurysm, has not greatly decreased [2]. Therefore, post-KD coronary sequelae during adulthood are an important issue. This chapter describes vessel wall function and morphology of coronary arteries long after KD and the characteristics of ACS in adults with a history of KD.

Y. Mitani (✉)
Neonatal Intensive Care Unit and Pediatric Cardiology, Mie University Hospital, Mie University Graduate School of Medicine, 2-174 Edobashi, Tsu, Mie 514-8507, Japan
e-mail: ymitani@clin.medic.mie-u.ac.jp

© Springer Japan 2017
B.T. Saji et al. (eds.), *Kawasaki Disease*, DOI 10.1007/978-4-431-56039-5_44

Table 1 Literature review of Kawasaki disease (KD) cases associated with acute coronary syndrome (ACS) during adulthood (33 cases) [3]

Males:females	25:8		
Age at ACS	29 y (median), 23-32 y (interquartile range)		
KD diagnosis during acute illness			
	15 cases		
Coronary artery lesions	3-vessel disease		8
	2-vessel disease		8
	1-vessel disease		14
	No lesions		1
Characteristics of culprit lesions			
	Vessels		
		RCA	14
		LAD	10
		LCX	5
	Thrombus		24
	Significant stenosis		16
	Persistent aneurysm		23
	Regressed aneurysm		7
	(including insignificant stenosis)		2

ACS acute coronary syndrome, *RCA* right coronary artery, *LAD* left anterior descending artery, *LCX* left circumflex artery

Reports of ACS in Adults with a History of Confirmed or Presumed KD

A literature search was performed to identify abstracts from scientific meetings in which adults (age ≥ 20 years) received a diagnosis consistent with ACS after a history of confirmed or unconfirmed KD [3]. Among the 33 adults (25 men, 8 women; median age, 29 years; range, 20–65 years; interquartile range, 23–32 years) identified, 15 received a diagnosis of KD during acute illness and 18 were suspected of having KD on the basis of coronary findings at the time of ACS, as determined by coronary angiography, CT scanning, or autopsy. Eight patients had three-vessel disease, another eight had two-vessel diseases, and 14 had one-vessel disease at the time of ACS. Culprit lesions were located in right coronary arteries ($n = 14$), left anterior descending coronary arteries ($n = 10$), and left circumflex coronary arteries ($n = 5$). Culprit lesions were associated with thrombosis ($n = 24$), severe stenosis ($n = 16$), persistent aneurysm ($n = 23$), and regressed aneurysm ($n = 7$; insignificant stenosis in 2) (Table 1).

These preliminary results suggest that some KD patients are at risk for thrombus-associated ACS in adulthood, which is associated with coronary aneurysms of varying size, various degrees of localized stenosis, and even regressed aneurysms. However, the findings are limited by the fact that most patients were suspected of having a history of KD on the basis of coronary imaging findings, not a KD diagnosis during acute illness.

Vascular Endothelial Function, Chronic Inflammation, and Oxidative Stress in KD

Provocative coronary angiography, peripheral vessel ultrasound study, and positron emission tomography (PET) have confirmed endothelial dysfunction in coronary and peripheral arteries long after KD. Endothelial dysfunction, as indicated by impaired flow-mediated dilatation of vessels, was reported in brachial arteries long after KD in patients with and without coronary sequelae [4]. Coronary endothelial dysfunction, as indicated by acetylcholine-induced vasoconstriction in the presence of preserved nitroglycerin-induced vasodilation, was reported in normal and diseased vessels long after KD in patients with coronary sequelae in any segment [5, 6]. Coronary endothelial dysfunction, as confirmed by provocative PET, was reported long after KD in patients with and without coronary sequelae [7]. Taken together, these reports indicate that endothelial function is impaired in coronary or brachial arteries long after severe KD in patients with coronary sequelae in any segment [8]. Endothelial dysfunction was confirmed in adult KD cases [9]. However, in patients without any coronary artery involvement after KD, it is unclear whether endothelial function is impaired in coronary or brachial arteries. Endothelial function was preserved in coronary [5] and peripheral vessels [6] of such patients [8].

The mechanisms involved in endothelial dysfunction are unknown. However, the process may be mediated by oxidant stress, as endothelial dysfunction was improved in KD patients after pretreatment with the antioxidant vitamin C [10]. In addition, increased levels of high-sensitivity C-reactive protein and urinary 8-isoprostane were found in patients with persistent aneurysms long after KD, which suggests the involvement of chronic low-grade inflammation in endothelial dysfunction [11, 12].

Intravascular Ultrasound Findings in Patients Long After KD

Coronary artery lesions, including persistent and regressed aneurysms and localized stenoses, long after KD are associated with intimal thickening and subluminal calcification in the lesions [13–17]. This is typically observed in localized stenoses. Intimal thickening is seen in regressed coronary aneurysms ≥ 4 mm in diameter during KD convalescence [16]. Subluminal calcification develops in lesions 6 years or later after acute illness [17]. intravascular ultrasound–derived intimal thickening is observed rarely in normal coronary segments from disease onset [13–17]. Intimal lesions in severe coronary artery lesions, including localized stenoses, long after KD are associated with severe calcification and intravascular ultrasound–derived heterogeneous components [15].

Coronary Sequelae in Adults Long After KD and the Risk of ACS

Coronary sequelae long after KD are pathologically distinct from atherosclerosis in the general adult population [18–20]. However, as such coronary sequelae in KD are associated with intimal thickening in pathological and ultrasound studies [12–20], it is unclear whether such coronary lesions are a substrate for development of premature atherosclerosis in adulthood. Because pathological data from adult KD patients are limited [18–20], it is not known whether any atherogenic components are prone to superimposition on established intimal thickening related to the sequelae of KD vasculitis later, in adulthood. Furthermore, even if atherogenic components are superimposed on KD-related intimal lesions, it must be determined whether such atherogenic components on KD vascular sequelae are related to clinical manifestation such as ACS during adulthood. In light of functional and morphological alterations in coronary artery lesions long after KD, present evidence indicates that lifestyle modification to avoid conventional coronary risk factors is recommended for at-risk patients.

References

1. Nakamura Y, Yashiro M. Fatal Kawasaki disease from epidemiology [in Japanese]. Cardiology. 2011;69(4):412–20.
2. Jichi Medical University. Kawasaki Disease Homepage. http://www.jichi.ac.jp/dph/kawasaki. html. Accessed July 2015.
3. Mitani Y. Kawasaki disease and acute coronary syndrome [in Japanese]. Cardiology. 2011;69 (4):366–70.
4. Dhillon R, Clarkson P, Donald AE, Powe AJ, Nash M, Novelli V, et al. Endothelial dysfunction late after Kawasaki disease. Circulation. 1996;94(9):2103–6. http://dx.doi.org/10.1161/ 01.CIR.94.9.2103. PMID:8901658.
5. Yamakawa R, Ishii M, Sugimura T, Akagi T, Eto G, Iemura M, et al. Coronary endothelial dysfunction after Kawasaki disease: evaluation by intracoronary injection of acetylcholine. J Am Coll Cardiol. 1998;31(5):1074–80. http://dx.doi.org/10.1016/S0735-1097(98)00033-3. PMID:9562009.
6. Mitani Y, Okuda Y, Shimpo H, Uchida F, Hamanaka K, Aoki K, et al. Impaired endothelial function in epicardial coronary arteries after Kawasaki disease. Circulation. 1997;96 (2):454–61. PMID:9244212.
7. Furuyama H, Odagawa Y, Katoh C, Iwado Y, Yoshinaga K, Ito Y, et al. Assessment of coronary function in children with a history of Kawasaki disease using (15)O-water positron

emission tomography. Circulation. 2002;105(24):2878–84. http://dx.doi.org/10.1161/01.CIR. 0000018652.59840.57. PMID:12070117.

8. Dietz SM, Tacke CE, Hutten BA, Kuijpers TW. Peripheral endothelial (Dys)function, arterial stiffness and carotid intima-media thickness in patients after Kawasaki disease: a systematic review and meta-analyses. PLoS One. 2015;10(7):e0130913. http://dx.doi.org/10.1371/journal.pone.0130913. eCollection 2015.

9. Niboshi A, Hamaoka K, Sakata K, Yamaguchi N. Endothelial dysfunction in adult patients with a history of Kawasaki disease. Eur J Pediatr. 2008;167(2):189–96. http://dx.doi.org/10.1007/s00431-007-0452-9. PMID:17345094.

10. Deng YB, Xiang HJ, Chang Q, Li CL. Evaluation by high-resolution ultrasonography of endothelial function in brachial artery after Kawasaki disease and the effects of intravenous administration of vitamin C. Circ J. 2002;66(10):908–12. http://dx.doi.org/10.1253/circj.66.908. PMID:12381083.

11. Hamaoka A, Hamaoka K, Yahata T, Fujii M, Ozawa S, Toiyama K, et al. Effects of HMG-CoA reductase inhibitors on continuous post-inflammatory vascular remodeling late after Kawasaki disease. J Cardiol. 2010;56(2):245–53. http://dx.doi.org/10.1016/j.jjcc.2010.06.006. PMID:20678900.

12. Mitani Y, Sawada H, Hayakawa H, Aoki K, Ohashi H, Matsumura M, et al. Elevated levels of high-sensitivity C-reactive protein and serum amyloid-A late after Kawasaki disease: association between inflammation and late coronary sequelae in Kawasaki disease. Circulation. 2005;111 (1):38–43. http://dx.doi.org/10.1161/01.CIR.0000151311.38708.29. PMID:15611368.

13. Sugimura T, Kato H, Inoue O, Fukuda T, Sato N, Ishii M, et al. Intravascular ultrasound of coronary arteries in children. Assessment of the wall morphology and the lumen after Kawasaki disease. Circulation. 1994;89(1):258–65. http://dx.doi.org/10.1161/01.CIR.89.1.258. PMID:8281655.

14. Sugimura T, Yokoi H, Sato N, Akagi T, Kimura T, Iemura M, et al. Interventional treatment for children with severe coronary artery stenosis with calcification after long-term Kawasaki disease. Circulation. 1997;96(11):3928–33. http://dx.doi.org/10.1161/01.CIR.96.11.3928. PMID:9403617.

15. Mitani Y, Ohashi H, Sawada H, Ikeyama Y, Hayakawa H, Takabayashi S, et al. In vivo plaque composition and morphology in coronary artery lesions in adolescents and young adults long after Kawasaki disease: a virtual histology-intravascular ultrasound study. Circulation. 2009;119 (21):2829–36. http://dx.doi.org/10.1161/CIRCULATIONAHA.108.818609. PMID:19451352.

16. Tsuda E, Kamiya T, Kimura K, Ono Y, Echigo S. Coronary artery dilatation exceeding 4.0 mm during acute Kawasaki disease predicts a high probability of subsequent late intima-medial thickening. Pediatr Cardiol. 2002;23(1):9–14. http://dx.doi.org/10.1007/s00246-001-0004-4. PMID:11922521.

17. Ino T, Akimoto K, Ohkubo M, Nishimoto K, Yabuta K, Takaya J, et al. Application of percutaneous transluminal coronary angioplasty to coronary arterial stenosis in Kawasaki disease. Circulation. 1996;93(9):1709–15. http://dx.doi.org/10.1161/01.CIR.93.9.1709. PMID:8653877.

18. Burns JC, Shike H, Gordon JB, Malhotra A, Schoenwetter M, Kawasaki T. Sequelae of Kawasaki disease in adolescents and young adults [Review]. J Am Coll Cardiol. 1996;28 (1):253–7. http://dx.doi.org/10.1016/0735-1097(96)00099-X. PMID:8752822.

19. Takahashi K, Oharaseki T, Naoe S. Pathological study of postcoronary arteritis in adolescents and young adults: with reference to the relationship between sequelae of Kawasaki disease and atherosclerosis. Pediatr Cardiol. 2001;22(2):138–42. http://dx.doi.org/10.1007/s002460010180. PMID:11178671.

20. Orenstein JM, Shulman ST, Fox LM, Baker SC, Takahashi M, Bhatti TR, et al. Three linked vasculopathic processes characterize Kawasaki disease: a light and transmission electron microscopic study. PLoS One. 2012;7(6):e38998. http://dx.doi.org/10.1371/journal.pone.0038998. PMID:22723916.

Psychosocial Effects of Kawasaki Disease and Transition to Adult Care

Annette L. Baker

Abstract Psychosocial outcomes for patients after Kawasaki Disease (KD) have been positive for most patients. However, a common theme after KD is feelings of anxiety and uncertainty regarding long-term outcome, particularly for parents of children with CAA. As we strive to provide optimal medical treatment, healthcare providers need to be aware of the impact of illness and the potential psychosocial outcomes after KD. Patients with coronary sequelae of KD also begin a lifelong interaction with the medical system. The importance of a well-planned transition from pediatric to adult-based care is an integral component in providing care for these patients. Over recent decades, improved longevity for many patients with chronic conditions has highlighted the need for formal programs designed to transition patients from pediatric healthcare systems to adult-based care. Transition programs should involve collaboration between adult cardiologists and pediatric KD specialists. Careful planning and communication is essential, so that patients transition without gaps in medical care.

Keywords Kawasaki disease • Transition to adult care • Psychosocial issues

Psychosocial Issues

Introduction

Historically, studies of Kawasaki disease (KD) have focused primarily on etiology, diagnosis, treatment, and outcomes of patients. Much less has been written about the psychosocial effects of KD on patients and their families. As with many other illnesses, the personal toll that KD has on children and families can be significant. While data support a positive outcome for most patients after KD, a common theme in studies of psychosocial/quality of life in KD is the prevalence of parental anxiety levels and persisting concerns about their child's health. Parental anxiety is not

A.L. Baker, RN, BSN, MSN, CPNP (✉)
Kawasaki Team, Cardiovascular Program, Boston Children's Hospital, 300 Longwood Avenue, Boston, MA 02115, USA
e-mail: annette.baker@cardio.chboston.org

© Springer Japan 2017
B.T. Saji et al. (eds.), *Kawasaki Disease*, DOI 10.1007/978-4-431-56039-5_45

limited to the acute phase of the illness but may continue for years after illness onset [1–3]. This heightened concern is understandably most significant in patients with coronary artery damage, due to future uncertainties [2].

Impact of KD on Families

The initial impact of KD is likely to be similar for all families during the acute illness, with stresses that are inherent to having a child with an illness that can have long-term health sequelae. The family's daily routine is disrupted in order to attend to the sick child. Most patients with KD require repeated visits to healthcare professionals and, ultimately, unanticipated hospitalization(s). Children with KD are typically irritable for a variable period of time, and their recovery is a protracted process, taking place gradually over 1–2 months. An acute illness in the family requires adjustment of schedules, work hours, and childcare for both the ill child and other household members. Studies of factors that impact reactions to illness are not specific to a particular illness but rather are influenced by several factors, including illness severity, parental and patient anxiety levels, and the developmental age of the child, as well as basic coping styles, family functioning, and personal resiliency [4, 5]. Parental anxiety in the initial phase of illness is related both to the child's current condition and uncertainty regarding the potential long-term effects.

Coronary abnormalities, if they occur, evolve during the initial 4–6 weeks of illness, making this a particularly stressful time period. In addition, the diagnosis of KD can be challenging in the absence of a specific diagnostic test. The child may have had multiple visits and lab tests before receiving a final diagnosis, and this may prompt frustration with the medical system [2]. Parents of children who ultimately developed coronary artery aneurysms (CAA) describe a feeling of helplessness, in conjunction with anger and regret, in situations where the diagnosis and subsequent treatment of KD were delayed. Often, these families blame themselves for not being more persistent at the time of diagnosis and wonder whether the outcome might have been different had their child been diagnosed and treated earlier [2].

Current Understanding of Psychosocial Issues

Fortunately, most children who are treated for KD do not develop coronary aneurysms and return to their previously normal baseline state of health, without long-term sequelae. Studies of psychosocial health show that, for most patients, KD does not affect long-term health-related quality of life [3, 6]. Several studies have shown that KD does not have an adverse effect on cognition or academic performance [7, 8]. Patients with KD who did not develop CAA were similar to the general population in measures of general psychosocial and physical health

[3, 6]. Evidence regarding the effects of KD on behavior is inconsistent: some studies report behavioral concerns [8–10], while others found no behavioral problems in children with a history of KD [7, 10].

To date, there has not been an increase in early heart disease in the group of patients without coronary aneurysms. These children are not on long-term medications and should have no activity restrictions. However, many centers worldwide routinely recommend intermittent follow-up for all KD patients, regardless of coronary sequelae. When the clinician recommends routine cardiology follow-up, despite a positive prognosis, it can create feelings of doubt or confusion for patients and families as to long-term issues. Because these patients are only seen infrequently, it is important to update them as to the rationale for follow-up, if indicated, and to make families aware of changes in follow-up protocols and implications for the patient, as they occur. It is important that families know that KD is a relatively new illness and that information continues to evolve.

In contrast to patients who recover from KD without sequelae, a small but significant number of children develop CAA from KD. These patients and their families now have to adjust to living with a chronic, acquired heart condition. The transition from a healthy child to a child with coronary aneurysms is challenging on many levels. The addition of daily medications, as well as repeated medical visits and testing, to the routine of a previously healthy child can have a significant impact on their life. For patients on anticoagulant and/or antiplatelet agents, certain activities, such as contact sports, may have to be avoided, thereby potentially changing family dynamics and affecting the child's social and psychosocial health. This can particularly impact families if other children are involved in activities in which the affected child can no longer participate. Parents of children with aneurysms describe concerns about the uncertainty of long-term outcomes and the fear of future cardiac events. These concerns are valid and should not be minimized or ignored. In a recent qualitative study in Canada, parents of children with aneurysms described the challenge of trying to find a balance between concerns for the future while attempting to maintain a "normal life" for their child.

Psychosocial Issues: Recommendations for Clinicians

Physicians and nurses play an instrumental role in the education, assessment, and support of families during all phases of KD. Providing accurate and current information is particularly important. This is especially true in the current era of the internet, in which information is vast and can be overwhelming and sometimes misleading. Open and honest communication helps to decrease anxiety and increases trust in the healthcare system.

On a practical basis, it is important to make sure that families have the education and knowledge to respond to medical situations if they arise. Patients and families of children with aneurysms should be educated as to the signs, symptoms, and response to coronary ischemia. Education should be ongoing, beginning during the initial illness and reinforced at each clinic visit. Cardiopulmonary resuscitation should be taught to parents of children with coronary abnormalities. In addition, some patients and families may benefit from additional professional psychological support focused on coping with acute and chronic illness.

Transition to Adult Care

Historical Overview

KD was described more than four decades ago in Japan, with cases in the United States reported shortly thereafter. As it has been over 45 years since the first case, there are now a significant number of adult patients with a history of KD. The advent of early intravenous immunoglobulin (IVIG) treatment, in the late 1980s, has led to a decrease in the cardiac morbidity associated with KD [11, 12]. Although the incidence of CAA has decreased since the use of IVIG, KD continues to be the leading cause of acquired heart disease in the developed world [13]. To assure consistent and knowledgeable lifelong care, adolescent and adult patients with cardiac sequelae require a well-planned transition program. In addition to providing optimal clinical care, transition of patients to formalized adult programs with expertise in KD should facilitate the ability to track these patients over their lifespan, with the goal of improving care for future generations.

Over the last few decades, the improved longevity of many patients with chronic conditions has highlighted the need for formal programs that specifically aim at transitioning patients from pediatric-based healthcare systems to adult-based care. An example of this is the increasing number of patients with congenital heart disease who now survive into adulthood. This population has benefited from advances in treatment, and new specialties have evolved in order to provide a continuum of care to these patients throughout their lifespan. Many pediatric centers have paired up with adult centers to provide care to these patients. Training programs have been developed specifically for clinicians caring for adults with congenital heart disease. Guidelines in place in the United States and several other countries recommend optimal transition practices for children with congenital heart disease [14].

To date, however, there are no specific guidelines or recommendations for designing an optimal adult-based program for the care of adult patients with KD. Therefore, current practices vary greatly across centers. Although the basic principles of transition apply to all adolescents and young adults with chronic healthcare needs, patients with KD present some unique challenges. In contrast to those affected by congenital heart disease, survival into adulthood has not been the main issue in KD, as mortality rates are less than 1 %. In addition, although overall morbidity from CAA has decreased since the start of routine use of IVIG, in the

1980s [11, 12], there are still a significant number of young people living with coronary aneurysms, the most common long-term sequela of KD.

Patients who have CAA from KD are a medically intense group. In particular, patients with large or giant aneurysms require daily medications, such as anticoagulants, antiplatelet agents, beta-blockers, or other medications, which may affect overall daily quality of life. These patients require close medical surveillance and management as well as possible interventions (surgical or catheter-based) throughout their lifespan.

During the time period when most adolescents are dealing with the excitement and demands of developing independence, adolescents with chronic health conditions must face additional demands as they begin to assume responsibility for their own, often complex, healthcare needs. Patients, families, and clinicians are all important participants in the transition plan and process [15]. The age of transition to adult clinicians varies greatly between countries and institutions. Some countries, such as Canada, mandate transfer at age 18; others leave the decision to the patient and/or clinician. Barriers to transition are multifaceted and may include both patient factors (attachment to providers, presence of comorbidities, insurance issues) and provider factors (attachment to patients and families) [16–18]. It is common during these transition years for patients to be at risk for interruptions of healthcare (loss to follow-up) [18, 19]. Patients who have lapsed in their medical care may present to healthcare systems again only after symptoms occur. This highlights the importance of developing and discussing transition options before the planned age of transfer.

Existing transition programs in pediatric cardiology have focused on training clinicians to provide healthcare to adults with congenital heart disease across the life spectrum. In contrast, adult cardiologists are generally well versed in atherosclerotic coronary artery disease but may not be familiar with the vascular sequelae of KD, which differs from atherosclerotic heart disease in its characteristics and natural history [20].

Further complicating the issue of follow-up in patients after acute KD is that one cannot consolidate recommendations for all KD patients under one heading, as follow-up depends on the extent of cardiac involvement. Fortunately, most KD patients have no obvious coronary artery sequelae, and these patients have had an excellent prognosis, without evidence of chronic health issues to date [21, 22].

Transition to Adult Care: Current Practices

As healthcare providers began to recognize the symptoms of KD, in the 1970s and 1980s, KD was diagnosed with increasing frequency. These initial patients are now in their early to middle adult years, and therefore the creation of thoughtful transition programs needs to be a true priority in the decades ahead.

For patients without cardiac sequelae, long-term cardiac follow-up is not mandated, although preventive cardiology evaluation is recommended [13].

Nevertheless, many clinicians believe that, to inform the next generation, it is important to have continued organized follow-up of the natural history of these patients. National registries can be instrumental in collecting the relevant follow-up data.

In contrast to patients with normal coronary arteries, patients with CAA require life-long cardiac follow-up and repeated testing. However, even within the group of patients with coronary artery dilation/aneurysm formation, there is substantial variation in the extent of damage. Every case is unique, and some patients are more significantly affected than others.

Even during childhood, many institutions partner with adult cardiologists for their expertise in coronary testing and interventions. As KD patients reach adulthood, it will be important to formalize these relationships and have programs in place so that patients with CAA or other cardiac sequelae can be transitioned to adult cardiology teams that have knowledge of the unique issues related to KD.

Principles of Transition

To make the transition from pediatric to adult care as easy as possible, it is essential to involve the patient and family in the decision. Education and discussion is a dynamic process and can be performed by a physician, nurse practitioner, or physician's assistant with knowledge of KD. Most importantly, issues related to transition should begin to be addressed many years before the actual change in care.

Because most patients are young when they develop KD, much of the initial education related to the illness is appropriately directed to parents. However, as children age, it is important to include them in the discussion and educate them about KD and their specific medical situation. Speaking to the child/adolescent alone for some of the visit helps patients get used to interacting with the healthcare system [15]. Visual aids may be helpful in describing coronary sequelae. When it is developmentally appropriate, teaching and discussion should also include an explanation of any medications the patients take on a regular basis. In addition, as adolescents begin to spend more time outside of their home with friends and extracurricular activities, it is important to discuss and reinforce potential signs and symptoms that may require immediate medical attention.

Patient education and transfer of some of the responsibilities of care can take place well before an actual transition. Assessment of whether adolescents know the names of their medications and rationale for their use should be part of the visit. As they get older, teenagers can be taught to call the provider and the pharmacy to request medication refills. They can also begin to make their own routine appointments. There are several transition tools that have been designed to determine whether an individual seems ready to transition to an adult provider [23].

Lastly, it is important to consider that several transitions may be occurring simultaneously, adding to the inherent stresses of adolescence and young adulthood. In particular, patients requiring anticoagulants may be followed by several clinicians: a pediatrician, a pediatric cardiology practice, and, sometimes, an anticoagulation team, with whom they may have the most frequent contact. Therefore, some young adults with giant aneurysms may need to make multiple transitions: from home to college or work; from a pediatrician to an adult primary care clinician; from a pediatric cardiologist to an adult cardiologist; and from a pediatric anticoagulation team to an adult-based team. In such cases, a staged transition may be preferable so that the individual and family are comfortable with one provider before moving all at once. Discussing and coordinating the transition plan with the patient's primary pediatrician may be helpful, as they have a long-term history with the family and may see the patient on a more frequent basis [24].

Dealing with Grown-Up Issues in KD and CAA

Preventive Cardiology

Patients with KD with CAA are considered a high-risk coronary group, and routine assessment of adult risk factors for coronary artery disease should begin early in life, with updates at all evaluations. Monitoring of coronary risk factors should be performed at each visit, including screening for hypertension, a review of family history, assessment of individual risk factors (body mass index, exercise level), and documentation of a recent lipid profile. A heart-healthy diet is recommended for all these patients, and those with dyslipidemia or obesity should be referred to a registered dietician. Smoking is discouraged in any patient, but especially so in patients with CAA. Most patients do not have significant exercise restrictions and can participate in some form of aerobic exercise. It is important to encourage regular exercise in all patients, within the restrictions of their particular coronary disease/risk level [13]. The threshold for pharmacologic therapy for hyperlipidemia and hypertension is lower for patients with known coronary artery disease. In addition, many practices routinely use statins in these patients for their anti-inflammatory effects, regardless of lipid status.

Risk Behaviors

Common adolescent behaviors, including smoking and use of alcohol, should be discussed, so that patients are aware of possible interactions (eg, with warfarin). The use of some street drugs, such as cocaine, can have serious adverse consequences for patients with heart conditions.

Pregnancy

Counseling regarding birth control and pregnancy in patients with CAA should begin in adolescence. Any restrictions or recommendations for contraception should be discussed early. Close connections should be developed with high-risk obstetric teams, so that patients can be monitored closely during pregnancy. Some medications used for coronary artery disease, such as warfarin, may be teratogenic, and substitutions may be necessary during pregnancy. It is ideal to recommend referral to a high-risk obstetric service before a planned pregnancy, so that the patient has adequate information and prenatal planning before pregnancy. In general, during pregnancy and delivery, care of patients with CAA is managed jointly between a cardiology team and a high-risk obstetric team. Present evidence indicates no increased risk of pregnancy in patients with a history KD but no CAA.

Transition to Adult Care: Summary and Recommendations (Tables 1 and 2)

In summary, substantial numbers of patients who have had KD are now entering or are well into their adult years. For those without CAA, the outlook is bright, without a documented increase in the incidence of early heart disease to date. In the United States, routine surveillance of these patients is left to the individual provider, with a main focus of optimizing cardiovascular health.

Table 1 Summary of recommendations for transition to adult care in patients with KD and CAA

1. Each program should have a formalized plan in place for transition of patients with CAA after KD in their institution
2. Ideally, transition should be made to an adult provider with expertise in CAA in KD, in collaboration with the pediatric KD team
3. The patient's developmental level and ability to assume independent care should determine the timing of transition
4. All stakeholders (patient, parents, and clinicians) should be involved in the decision regarding when to transition care to an adult-based provider/healthcare system
5. Individual cardiac sequelae should be reviewed with the patient in a developmentally appropriate manner, starting at a young age
6. Decreasing additional coronary artery risk factors should be part of routine follow-up care and education, namely, a heart-healthy diet, exercise, lipid screening, and family history
7. The patient's history, previous test results, and transition plan should be communicated verbally and in writing with the new primary care provider as well as with the adult cardiac team and any other involved clinicians (eg, anticoagulation team)
8. Introduce age-appropriate health information related to contraception and pregnancy beginning early in adolescence in patients with CAA, with referral to a high-risk obstetric team, if indicated

Adapted from Best Practices in Managing Transition (guidelines) [14]

Table 2 Patient education topics related to KD

Cardiac sequelae
Spend time reviewing specific coronary artery/cardiac status for each patient
Discuss signs and symptoms of myocardial ischemia and how to respond
Discuss options for ongoing diagnostic testing: include rationale for each
Echocardiogram/EKG
Stress testing
CTA/MRI/Catheterization
Medication
Review all medications; include rationale, dose, and side effects
Encourage responsible self-administration, compliance techniques (such as setting phone alarms)
Assess readiness for transition with parent and patient
Ability for self-care/medication
Understanding of importance of regular follow-up
Knowledge of illness
Healthcare insurance issues
Decreasing Additional Cardiac Risk Factors
Heart-healthy diet
Maintaining optimal body mass index
Regular aerobic fitness, with discussion of limitations and rationale, if necessary
Avoidance of smoking
Regular monitoring of BP, risk for diabetes, lipid profile
Contraception and pregnancy planning
Contraception options/risks
Discussion of pregnancy in the setting of CAA
Use of medications
Referral to high-risk obstetric team, if indicated

Adapted from Best Practices in Managing Transition (guidelines) [14]

As patients with known CAA become adults, collaboration with adult cardiologists or adult/pediatric cardiology teams needs to be established, and transition programs should be developed to continue care into the adult years. Transition to a selected practice(s) that has an interest in and familiarity with the natural history of CAA in KD will help ensure optimal care and inform treatment options.

The basic principles of transition are similar for chronic health conditions that are diagnosed in childhood and include the gradual and repeated preparation of the patient and family before the actual transition to an adult provider/program. Assessment, planning, discussion, and education should begin well before a scheduled transition to an adult-based healthcare provider and system. Most importantly, detailed verbal and written communication between the pediatric and adult provider is necessary, to provide continuity of care. To decrease the chance of a lapse in medical care, an appointment with the new adult provider can be facilitated at the last pediatric visit. Programs with dedicated staff are helpful in assuring that patients are not lost to follow up during this important period.

References

1. Ishikawa S, Inaba Y, Okuyama K, Asakura T, Kim YS, Sasa S. A study of psycho-social effects of chronic MCLS upon mothers. Prog Clin Biol Res. 1987;250:531–3. PMID:3423064.
2. Chahal N, Clarizia NA, McCrindle BW, Boydell KM, Obadia M, Manlhiot C, et al. Parental anxiety associated with Kawasaki disease in previously healthy children. J Pediatr Health Care. 2010;24(4):250–7. http://dx.doi.org/10.1016/j.pedhc.2009.07.002. PMID:20620851.
3. Baker AL, Gauvreau K, Newburger JW, Sundel RP, Fulton DR, Jenkins KJ. Physical and psychosocial health in children who have had Kawasaki disease. Pediatrics. 2003;111 (3):579–83. http://dx.doi.org/10.1542/peds.111.3.579. PMID:12612239.
4. Knapp PK, Harris ES. Consultation-liaison in child psychiatry: a review of the past 10 years. Part II: Research on treatment approaches and outcomes. J Am Acad Child Adolesc Psychiatry. 1998;37(2):139–46. http://dx.doi.org/10.1097/00004583-199802000-00005. PMID:9473909.
5. Baker AL, Baptista Neto L, Newburger JW, DeMaso DR. Psychosocial concerns in children with Kawasaki disease. Prog Pediatr Cardiol. 2004;19(2):189–94. http://dx.doi.org/10.1016/j.ppedcard.2004.08.013.
6. Muta H, Ishii M, Iemura M, Matsuishi T. Health-related quality of life in adolescents and young adults with a history of Kawasaki disease. J Pediatr. 2010;156(3):439–43. http://dx.doi.org/10.1016/j.jpeds.2009.09.041. PMID:19969307.
7. Nishad P, Singh S, Sidhu M, Malhi P. Cognitive and behaviour assessment following Kawasaki disease—a study from North India. Rheumatol Int. 2010;30(6):851–4. http://dx.doi.org/10.1007/s00296-009-1078-1. PMID:19649637.
8. King WJ, Schlieper A, Birdi N, Cappelli M, Korneluk Y, Rowe PC. The effect of Kawasaki disease on cognition and behavior. Arch Pediatr Adolesc Med. 2000;154(5):463–8. http://dx.doi.org/10.1001/archpedi.154.5.463. PMID:10807296.
9. Carlton-Conway D, Ahluwalia R, Henry L, Michie C, Wood L, Tulloh R. Behaviour sequelae following acute Kawasaki disease. BMC Pediatr. 2005;5(1):14. http://dx.doi.org/10.1186/1471-2431-5-14. PMID:15916701.
10. Tacke CE, Haverman L, Berk BM, van Rossum MA, Kuipers IM, Grootenhuis MA, et al. Quality of life and behavioral functioning in Dutch children with a history of Kawasaki disease. J Pediatr. 2012;161(2):314–9.e1. http://dx.doi.org/10.1016/j.jpeds.2012.01.071. PMID:22421262.
11. Newburger JW, Takahashi M, Burns JC, Beiser AS, Chung KJ, Duffy CE, et al. The treatment of Kawasaki syndrome with intravenous gamma globulin. N Engl J Med. 1986;315(6):341–7. http://dx.doi.org/10.1056/NEJM198608073150601. PMID:2426590.
12. Newburger JW, Takahashi M, Beiser AS, Burns JC, Bastian J, Chung KJ, et al. A single intravenous infusion of gamma globulin as compared with four infusions in the treatment of acute Kawasaki syndrome. N Engl J Med. 1991;324(23):1633–9. http://dx.doi.org/10.1056/NEJM199106063242305. PMID:1709446.
13. Newburger JW, Takahashi M, Gerber MA, Gewitz MH, Tani LY, Burns JC, et al., Committee on Rheumatic Fever, Endocarditis, and Kawasaki Disease, Council on Cardiovascular Disease in the Young, American Heart Association. Diagnosis, treatment, and long-term management of Kawasaki disease: a statement for health professionals from the Committee on Rheumatic Fever, Endocarditis, and Kawasaki Disease, Council on Cardiovascular Disease in the Young, American Heart Association. Pediatrics. 2004;114(6):1708–33. http://dx.doi.org/10.1542/peds.2004-2182 PMID:15574639.
14. Sable C, Foster E, Uzark K, Bjornsen K, Canobbio MM, Connolly HM, et al., American Heart Association Congenital Heart Defects Committee of the Council on Cardiovascular Disease in the Young, Council on Cardiovascular Nursing, Council on Clinical Cardiology, and Council on Peripheral Vascular Disease. Best practices in managing transition to adulthood for adolescents with congenital heart disease: the transition process and medical and psychosocial issues: a scientific statement from the American Heart Association. Circulation. 2011;123 (13):1454–85. http://dx.doi.org/10.1161/CIR.0b013e3182107c56 PMID:21357825.

15. Kovacs AH, McCrindle BW. So hard to say goodbye: transition from paediatric to adult cardiology care. Nat Rev Cardiol. 2014;11(1):51–62. http://dx.doi.org/10.1038/nrcardio.2013. 172. PMID:24217158.

16. Fernandes SM, Khairy P, Fishman L, Melvin P, O'Sullivan-Oliveira J, Sawicki GS, et al. Referral patterns and perceived barriers to adult congenital heart disease care: results of a survey of U.S. pediatric cardiologists. J Am Coll Cardiol. 2012;60(23):2411–8. http://dx. doi.org/10.1016/j.jacc.2012.09.015. PMID:23141490.

17. Hilderson D, Saidi AS, Van Deyk K, Verstappen A, Kovacs AH, Fernandes SM, et al. Attitude toward and current practice of transfer and transition of adolescents with congenital heart disease in the United States of America and Europe. Pediatr Cardiol. 2009;30(6):786–93. http://dx.doi.org/10.1007/s00246-009-9442-1. PMID:19365651.

18. Mackie AS, Rempel GR, Rankin KN, Nicholas D, Magill-Evans J. Risk factors for loss to follow-up among children and young adults with congenital heart disease. Cardiol Young. 2012;22(3):307–15. http://dx.doi.org/10.1017/S104795111100148X. PMID:22013913.

19. Gurvitz M, Valente AM, Broberg C, Cook S, Stout K, Kay J, et al., Alliance for Adult Research in Congenital Cardiology (AARCC) and Adult Congenital Heart Association. Prevalence and predictors of gaps in care among adult congenital heart disease patients: HEART-ACHD (The Health, Education, and Access Research Trial). J Am Coll Cardiol. 2013;61(21):2180–4. http://dx.doi.org/10.1016/j.jacc.2013.02.048 PMID:23542112.

20. Gordon JB, Kahn AM, Burns JC. When children with Kawasaki disease grow up: myocardial and vascular complications in adulthood. J Am Coll Cardiol. 2009;54(21):1911–20. http://dx. doi.org/10.1016/j.jacc.2009.04.102. PMID:19909870.

21. McCrindle BW, McIntyre S, Kim C, Lin T, Adeli K. Are patients after Kawasaki disease at increased risk for accelerated atherosclerosis? J Pediatr. 2007;151(3):244–8. http://dx.doi.org/ 10.1016/j.jpeds.2007.03.056. PMID:17719931.

22. Selamet Tierney ES, Gal D, Gauvreau K, Baker AL, Trevey S, O'Neill SR, et al. Vascular health in Kawasaki disease. J Am Coll Cardiol. 2013;62(12):1114–21. http://dx.doi.org/10. 1016/j.jacc.2013.04.090. PMID:23835006.

23. Sawicki GS, Lukens-Bull K, Yin X, Demars N, Huang IC, Livingood W, et al. Measuring the transition readiness of youth with special healthcare needs: validation of the TRAQ—Transition Readiness Assessment Questionnaire. J Pediatr Psychol. 2011;36(2):160–71. http://dx.doi. org/10.1093/jpepsy/jsp128. PMID:20040605.

24. Gurvitz M, Saidi A. Transition in congenital heart disease: it takes a village. Heart. 2014;100 (14):1075–6. http://dx.doi.org/10.1136/heartjnl-2014-306030. PMID:24855319.

Kawasaki Disease: Road Map for the Future

John B. Gordon

Abstract The long-term outcomes of adults who developed KD in childhood have yet to be determined. Those with severe vascular damage will clearly require longitudinal care, and their risk for myocardial ischemia is clear. For those with no vascular changes detected by transthoracic echocardiogram during the acute and subacute phase of their illness, the prognosis is less clear. Longitudinal studies are critical to improving our understanding of the vascular lesions and potential sequelae after KD.

Keywords Adult sequelae • Coronary artery aneurysms • Myocardial infarction

The number of adults with a history of KD in childhood is increasing each year, and these patients are coming to the attention of adult cardiologists, primarily due to acute thrombosis of coronary aneurysms. System dynamic models suggest that by 2030 one in every 1600 adults in the United States will have a history of KD [1]. Longitudinal, randomized trials to guide management of adult patients who had KD in childhood have not yet been performed. Consequently, appropriate management of adults with a history of KD in childhood is uncertain and controversial.

If a diagnosis of KD is missed or delayed, the likelihood of coronary artery injury increases. Coronary aneurysms or moderate coronary dilation may persist or remodel. Left ventricular systolic dysfunction may also normalize on echocardiography during the subacute phase of the illness. Pediatric patients may be discharged from care and lost to follow-up due to the erroneous assumption that remodeled aneurysms pose no future risk. However, after a honeymoon period that may span decades, a subset of these patients may present with acute myocardial infarction (MI) or heart failure in an adult emergency department [2]. The pediatric cardiologist is unaware that the patient had an unexpected adverse outcome, and the adult cardiologist must now manage a complex clinical situation with which most are unfamiliar.

J.B. Gordon, M.D. (✉)
San Diego Cardiac Center, 3131 Berger St, San Diego, CA 92123, USA
e-mail: jgordon552@mac.com

© Springer Japan 2017   439
B.T. Saji et al. (eds.), *Kawasaki Disease*, DOI 10.1007/978-4-431-56039-5_46

KD patients with giant aneurysms (diameter ≥ 8 mm or Z score >10) have a significantly increased risk for ischemic events and require specialized life-long medical management [3, 4]. Giant aneurysms may occlude due to reduced wall sheer stress, leading to thrombosis, or due to luminal myofibroblastic proliferation, leading to critical stenosis [5, 6]. Coronary calcification within the wall and within a layered thrombus is common and may be extremely dense. Most patients with giant aneurysms will develop cardiac complications requiring percutaneous intervention or coronary artery bypass surgery. Suda studied a series of 76 Japanese patients with giant aneurysms; 59 % required percutaneous or surgical intervention during the 25 years of follow-up after KD onset [4].

The severity of non-atherosclerotic coronary disease may be difficult to assess noninvasively in adults with a history of KD in childhood. Coronary calcium volume scoring using low-dose–radiation CT may be a useful tool to distinguish normal patients from those with more severe disease. As part of the San Diego Adult KD Collaborative study, Kahn et al. studied 70 patients with a history of KD (median interval from acute KD to imaging, 14 years) [7]. All patients with a history of normal coronaries, and 11 of 12 patients with coronary dilation, had a calcium score of zero. Ten of 14 patients with aneurysms had mild to severe coronary calcification with calcium scores ranging from zero to >8000 U/mm^3. Of the four patients with aneurysms and negative calcium scores, all were studied less than 10 years after KD onset, whereas those with aneurysms and positive scores were studied at least 10 years after their initial illness. These data support the use of coronary calcium scores as a sensitive screening test to detect patients with severe coronary damage, if performed at least 10 years after KD.

Management of pregnancy in women with coronary artery aneurysms after KD in childhood requires multidisciplinary teamwork. The combined Japanese literature describes the outcomes of 52 women, all but two of whom had aneurysms [8]. Five (9.6 %) had complications but no MI. MI has been reported in pregnant patients with unrecognized aneurysms secondary to KD. Conversely, in the United States, outcomes were excellent for ten patients with 21 pregnancies managed by both a maternal-fetal specialist and cardiologist [9]. No consistent approach to management has been established in prospective trials, but the existing data support multidisciplinary care.

All patients with giant coronary aneurysms should be treated with low-dose aspirin and systemic anticoagulation with warfarin or enoxaparin. Future studies are needed in order to establish the potential role of novel oral anticoagulants (apixaban, dabigatran, or rivaroxaban) that have the advantages of ease of management (no monitoring) and safety (reduced bleeding), as compared to warfarin. Statin therapy for KD has not been established in clinical trials but may be beneficial due to the anti-inflammatory properties of this class of drugs [10].

The interventional cardiologist must consider the likely possibility of a large thrombus burden when considering stenting in the setting of acute myocardial infarction. Intravascular ultrasound to determine vessel diameter and appropriate stent size is mandatory, [11] as stent sizing based on visual assessment may lead to placement of grossly undersized stents. Another potential pitfall is attempted percutaneous transluminal angioplasty in densely calcified arteries that may not be dilatable with balloons unless pretreated with rotational atherectomy [12]. The role of covered stents is not established, but such stents have been successful in selected cases [13].

There is clear evidence that patients with or without remodeling of aneurysms are at increased risk of coronary events in adulthood. A recent study of 50 patients with acute coronary syndrome [14] noted the following clinical features: male predominance (90 %), variable age at the time of the event (age range, 18–69 years; median, 28 years); thrombotic occlusion in 80 %, giant aneurysms in 80 %, and "resolved" aneurysms in 6 % [14].

Currently, there are no evidence-based guidelines for the management of patients with moderate or regressed aneurysms. Unfortunately, it is wishful thinking to assume that "normalization" of the coronary artery lumen by echo indicates a benign clinical course. Autopsy studies of regressed coronary aneurysms show abnormal vessel architecture with marked myointimal proliferation distinct from atherosclerosis [6]. Endomyocardial biopsy studies have demonstrated that all patients have some degree of myocarditis during the acute phase of KD [15, 16]. Because of the documented occurrence of acute thrombotic events, it is reasonable to treat these patients with low-dose aspirin and perform periodic stress echocardiograms to exclude coronary ischemia and assess left ventricular function. Nuclear medicine perfusion testing is an option but has the limitation of high radiation exposure, particularly if the studies are repeated. Magnetic resonance angiography is useful in specialized centers with high-resolution devices. Statin therapy may be considered for its anti-inflammatory benefits, certainly if low-density lipoprotein cholesterol is high.

Mid-term follow-up data indicate that KD patients with no evidence of coronary or myocardial injury at the time of the acute illness appear to have an excellent prognosis, no different from the general population. At this time, no specific therapy or regular evaluation appears to be necessary. However, definitive recommendations must await longitudinal studies that follow large populations of KD patients into the fourth and fifth decades of life.

When the first series of 50 KD patients was described by Kawasaki in 1967, the syndrome was thought to be a benign, self-limited febrile illness with no sequelae. This may still be true for most patients with no evidence of coronary artery injury at the time of the acute illness. Delayed or missed diagnosis remains an important impediment to prompt treatment with intravenous immunoglobulin. Preventable coronary injury, which may be very severe, is the unfortunate result. Timely diagnosis and treatment remain major challenges for practicing physicians. The challenge for the current generation of biomedical researchers is to determine the etiology of KD and develop a rapid diagnostic test, so that coronary injury can be prevented or reduced.

References

1. Huang SK, Lin MT, Chen HC, Huang SC, Wu MH. Epidemiology of Kawasaki disease: prevalence from national database and future trends projection by system dynamics modeling. J Pediatr. 2013;163:126–131 e121. http://dx.doi.org/10.1016/j.jpeds.2012.12.011
2. Daniels LB, Tjajadi MS, Walford HH, Jimenez-Fernandez S, Trofimenko V, Fick Jr DB, et al. Prevalence of Kawasaki disease in young adults with suspected myocardial ischemia. Circulation. 2012;125(20):2447–53. http://dx.doi.org/10.1161/CIRCULATIONAHA.111. 082107. PMID:22595319.
3. Tsuda E, Hamaoka K, Suzuki H, Sakazaki H, Murakami Y, Nakagawa M, et al. A survey of the 3-decade outcome for patients with giant aneurysms caused by Kawasaki disease. Am Heart J. 2014;167(2):249–58. http://dx.doi.org/10.1016/j.ahj.2013.10.025. PMID:24439987.
4. Suda K, Iemura M, Nishiono H, Teramachi Y, Koteda Y, Kishimoto S, et al. Long-term prognosis of patients with Kawasaki disease complicated by giant coronary aneurysms: a single-institution experience. Circulation. 2011;123(17):1836–42. http://dx.doi.org/10.1161/ CIRCULATIONAHA.110.978213. PMID:21502578.
5. Sengupta D, Kahn AM, Kung E, Esmaily Moghadam M, Shirinsky O, Lyskina GA, et al. Thrombotic risk stratification using computational modeling in patients with coronary artery aneurysms following Kawasaki disease. Biomech Model Mechanobiol. 2014;13 (6):1261–76. http://dx.doi.org/10.1007/s10237-014-0570-z. PMID:24722951.
6. Orenstein JM, Shulman ST, Fox LM, Baker SC, Takahashi M, Bhatti TR, et al. Three linked vasculopathic processes characterize Kawasaki disease: a light and transmission electron microscopic study. PLoS One. 2012;7(6):e38998. http://dx.doi.org/10.1371/journal.pone. 0038998. PMID:22723916.
7. Kahn AM, Budoff MJ, Daniels LB, Jimenez-Fernandez S, Cox AS, Gordon JB, et al. Calcium scoring in patients with a history of Kawasaki disease. JACC Cardiovasc Imaging. 2012;5 (3):264–72. http://dx.doi.org/10.1016/j.jcmg.2011.12.010. PMID:22421171.
8. Tsuda E, Kawamata K, Neki R, Echigo S, Chiba Y. Nationwide survey of pregnancy and delivery in patients with coronary arterial lesions caused by Kawasaki disease in Japan. Cardiol Young. 2006;16(2):173–8. http://dx.doi.org/10.1017/S1047951106000126. PMID:16553980.
9. Gordon CT, Jimenez-Fernandez S, Daniels LB, Kahn AM, Tarsa M, Matsubara T, et al. Pregnancy in women with a history of Kawasaki disease: management and outcomes. BJOG. 2014;121(11):1431–8. http://dx.doi.org/10.1111/1471-0528.12685. PMID:24597833.
10. Blankier S, McCrindle BW, Ito S, Yeung RS. The role of atorvastatin in regulating the immune response leading to vascular damage in a model of Kawasaki disease. Clin Exp Immunol. 2011;164(2):193–201. http://dx.doi.org/10.1111/j.1365-2249.2011.04331.x. PMID:21361911.
11. Suzuki A, Yamagishi M, Kimura K, Sugiyama H, Arakaki Y, Kamiya T, et al. Functional behavior and morphology of the coronary artery wall in patients with Kawasaki disease assessed by intravascular ultrasound. J Am Coll Cardiol. 1996;27(2):291–6. http://dx.doi. org/10.1016/0735-1097(95)00447-5. PMID:8557896.
12. Tsuda E, Miyazaki S, Yamada O, Takamuro M, Takekawa T, Echigo S. Percutaneous transluminal coronary rotational atherectomy for localized stenosis caused by Kawasaki disease. Pediatr Cardiol. 2006;27(4):447–53. http://dx.doi.org/10.1007/s00246-006-1276-5. PMID:16830078.
13. Waki K, Arakaki Y, Mitsudo K. Long-term outcome of transcatheter polytetrafluoroethylene-covered stent implantation in a giant coronary aneurysm of a child with Kawasaki disease. Catheter Cardiovasc Interv. 2013;81(4):713–6. http://dx.doi.org/10.1002/ccd.24486. PMID:22605684.
14. Tsuda E, Abe T, Tamaki W. Acute coronary syndrome in adult patients with coronary artery lesions caused by Kawasaki disease: review of case reports. Cardiol Young. 2011;21(1):74–82.

http://dx.doi.org/10.1017/S1047951110001502. PMID:21070690.

15. Yonesaka S, Nakada T, Sunagawa Y, Tomimoto K, Naka S, Takahashi T, et al. Endomyocardial biopsy in children with Kawasaki disease. Acta Paediatr Jpn. 1989;31 (6):706–11. http://dx.doi.org/10.1111/j.1442-200X.1989.tb01384.x. PMID:2516398.

16. Yutani C, Okano K, Kamiya T, Oguchi K, Kozuka T, Ota M, et al. Histopathological study on right endomyocardial biopsy of Kawasaki disease. Br Heart J. 1980;43(5):589–92. http://dx. doi.org/10.1136/hrt.43.5.589. PMID:6445739.

Appendix: Guidelines for diagnosis and management of cardiovascular sequelae in Kawasaki disease (JCS 2013)

Guidelines for Diagnosis and Treatment of Cardiovascular Diseases (2012 Joint Working Groups Report)[1]

[Digest Version]

Guidelines for diagnosis and management of cardiovascular sequelae in Kawasaki disease (JCS 2013)

This English language document is a revised digest version of Guidelines for diagnosis and management of cardiovascular sequelae in Kawasaki disease reported at the Japanese Circulation Society Joint Working Groups performed in 2012. (Website: http://www.j-circ.or.jp/guideline/pdf/JCS2013_ogawas_d.pdf)

Joint Working Groups: the Japanese Circulation Society, The Japanese Society of Kawasaki Disease, The Japanese Association for Thoracic Surgery, The Japan Pediatric Society, The Japanese Society of Pediatric Cardiology and Cardiac Surgery, The Japanese College of Cardiology

Chair:
Shunichi Ogawa, Department of Pediatrics, Nippon Medical School

Members:
Mamoru Ayusawa, Department of Pediatrics, Nihon University School of Medicine
Masahiro Ishii, Department of Pediatrics, Kitasato University

---

[1] Article Note: The guidelines in this appendix are reprinted with permission from *Circulation Journal*, the Japanese Circulation Society, 2014.

Hirotarou Ogino, Department of Pediatrics, Kansai Medical University

Tsutomu Saji, Department of Pediatrics, Toho University Omori Medical Center

Kazuhiko Nishigaki, Second Department of Internal Medicine, Gifu University

Kenji Hamaoka, Department of Pediatric Cardiology and Nephrology, Graduate School of Medical Science, Kyoto Prefectural University of Medicine

Ryuji Fukazawa, Department of Pediatrics, Nippon Medical School

Collaborators:
Masami Ochi, Department of Cardiovascular Surgery, Nippon Medical School, Graduate School of Medicine

Hiroshi Kamiyama, Department of Pediatrics, Nihon University School of Medicine

Kei Takahashi, Department of Pathology, Toho University School of Medicine, Ohashi Hospital

Etsuko Tsuda, Departments of Pediatric Cardiology, National Cerebral and Cardiovascular Center

Hiroyoshi Yokoi, Department of Cardiology, Kokura Memorial Hospital

Independent Assessment Committee:
Takashi Akasaka, Department of Cardiovascular Medicine, Wakayama Medical University

Soichiro Kitamura, Sakai City Hospital

Tomoyoshi Sonobe, Department of Pediatrics, Japanese Red Cross Medical Center

Toshio Nakanishi, Department of Pediatric Cardiology, Tokyo Women's Medical University

Yoshikazu Nakamura, Department of Public Health, Jichi Medical University
(The affiliations of the members are as of August 2013)

TABLE OF CONTENTS

2. Physiological Examinations
3. Diagnostic Imaging
4. Cardiac Catheterization
5. Summary of Examinations and Diagnosis

IV. Treatment of Cardiovascular Sequelae

1. Pharmacotherapy
2. Non-Pharmacotherapy
3. Summary of Treatment Options

V. Management and Follow-up during Childhood

1. Guidance on Activities of Daily Life and Exercise
2. Follow-up Evaluation
3. Problems in Shifting from Childhood to Adulthood

VI. Problems during Adulthood

1. Progression of Arteriosclerosis: Pathological Features
2. Progression of Arteriosclerosis: Clinical Features

VII. Management of Adults with a History of Kawasaki Disease

1. Diagnosis
2. Treatment
3. Guidance on Lifestyle and Exercise
4. Pregnancy, Labor and Childbirth
5. Healthcare System for Adult Patients

VIII. Summary
References
Appendix
(All Rights Reserved)

Introduction of the Revised Guidelines

Forty-five years have passed since 1967[1], when the first case series of Kawasaki disease was reported. Currently, more than half of the patients diagnosed with Kawasaki disease are 20 years of age or older. As this timeline suggests, it is expected that more than 10,000 patients with cardiovascular sequelae in Kawasaki disease have reached adulthood. However, since Kawasaki disease develops most frequently by around 1 year of age, many internists are still not familiar with it (See **Table 3**). Recent issues on Kawasaki disease include the high percentage of patients who stop visiting their clinic in early adolescence or later, and the occurrence of acute coronary syndrome in adults with a history of Kawasaki disease in whom coronary artery lesions were considered regressed after the acute phase of the disease. We also have to address the problem of susceptibility to atherosclerosis in patients with a history of vasculitis due to Kawasaki disease.

Because the pathophysiology of cardiovascular sequelae in Kawasaki disease changes over time during childhood, adolescence and adulthood, guidance on the diagnosis, treatment and management of cardiovascular sequelae in different ages was required, the Japanese Circulation Society Joint Working Groups published the Guidelines for Diagnosis and Management of Cardiovascular Sequelae in Kawasaki Disease in 2003[2], and the first revision of the guidelines in 2008[3]. The present second revision reflects updates over recent years.

The outline of the present revision is essentially similar to the previous versions. However, the present revision includes detailed descriptions of the pathophysiology of cardiovascular sequelae to provide important information for the diagnosis and treatment of sequelae, and describes genetic background of coronary sequelae and coronary hemodynamics. The chapters on the management and education of children with Kawasaki disease were revised and further segmented to provide more practical information suitable in the clinical setting. Because the susceptibility to atherosclerosis in adults with a history of the disease is expected to become a more important problem in the future, new findings on the pathological and clinical points of view that have been obtained by now are added in this revision.

The Joint Working Groups discussed how to classify coronary aneurysms during the acute phase. Although giant aneurysms were defined as aneurysms with an internal diameter of >8 mm in children under five years of age, and those with the internal diameter of a segment measuring >4 times that of an adjacent segment in children over five years of age, giant aneurysms in children under five years of age are defined as those with the internal diameter of ≥8mm in a currently ongoing national epidemiological survey, recent academic presentations and literature about Kawasaki disease. We thus partly modified the classification of giant aneurysms to fit the clinical practice (See **Table 4**).

Although the present guidelines are based in principle on available evidence, the diagnosis and treatment of cardiovascular sequelae in Kawasaki disease are often based on case reports. Emphasis was therefore placed on case reports in the present guidelines as well. **Table 1** lists the criteria for levels of recommendations on the procedure and treatment of cardiovascular sequelae in Kawasaki disease. We hope this revision will help physicians provide better treatment for their patients.

Table 2 lists abbreviations used in the present guidelines.

Table 1 Levels of Recommendations

Class I	Conditions for which there is evidence for and/or general agreement that the procedure or treatment is useful and effective.
Class II	Conditions for which there is conflicting evidence and/or a divergence of opinion regarding the usefulness/efficacy of a procedure or treatment.
Class III	Conditions for which there is evidence and/or general agreement that the procedure or treatment is not useful/effective and may in some cases be harmful.

Table 2 Abbreviations

3D	three-dimensional	LVEF	left ventricular ejection fraction
ACC	American College of Cardiology	MCLS	infantile acute febrile mucocutaneous lymph node syndrome
ACCP	American College of Chest Physicians	MCP-1	monocyte chemoattractant protein-1
ACE	angiotensin converting enzyme	MDCT	multi-detector row computed tomography
AHA	American Heart Association	MLC	myosin light chain
ALT	alanine aminotransferase	MRA	magnetic resonance angiography
AMI	acute myocardial infarction	MRCA	magnetic resonance coronary angiography
APTT	activated partial thrombo-plastin time	MRI	magnetic resonance imaging
APV	average peak flow velocity	NO	nitric oxide
ARB	angiotensin II receptor blocker	NSAIDs	nonsteroidal antiinflammatory drugs
AST	aspartate aminotransferase	nST	non-stress test
ATP	adenosine triphosphate	OD	once daily
BID	two times a day	PCI	percutaneous coronary intervention
BNP	brain natriuretic peptide	PGI_2	prostacyclin
CABG	coronary artery bypass grafting	POBA	plain old balloon angioplasty
CAG	coronary angiography	pro-UK	pro-urokinase
CASP3	caspase 3	PTCRA	percutaneous transluminal coronary rotational atherectomy
CFR	coronary flow reserve	PVC	premature ventricular contraction
CK	creatine kinase	QGS	quantitative gated SPECT
CK-MB	creatine kinase-myocardial band	QOL	quality of life
CRP	C reactive protein	sc	subcutaneous
ECG	electrocardiography	SCAI	Society for Cardiovascular Angiography and Interventions
EF	ejection fraction	SNP	single nucleotide polymorphism
FFRmyo	myocardial fractional flow reserve	SPECT	single photon emission computed tomography
FMD	flow-mediated dilatation	SSFP	steady-state free precession
% FS	% fractional shortening	TC	total cholesterol
HDL-C	high density lipoprotein cholesterol	Tc	technetium
H-FABP	heart-type fatty acid-binding protein	TG	triglyceride
ICAM-1	intercellular adhesion molecule 1	TID	three times a day
ICT	intracoronary thrombolysis	TnI	troponin I
IgG	immunoglobulin G	TnT	troponin T
I map	isopotential map	t-PA	tissue plasminogen activator

(continued)

Table 2 (continued)

INR	international normalized ratio	TTP	thrombotic thrombocytopenic purpura
ISDN	isosorbide dinitrate	UK	urokinase
ITPKC	inositol 1,4,5-triphosphate 3-kinase C		
iv	intravenous		
IVIG	intravenous immunoglobulin		
IVUS	intravascular ultrasound		
LDL-C	low density lipoprotein cholesterol		
LP	late potential		

I. Epidemiology of Kawasaki Disease, Current Acute-Phase Treatment, and Pathophysiology of Acute-Phase Disease

1. Current Epidemiology

1.1 Number of Patients and Diagnosis (Figure 1)

According to the 21st nationwide survey of Kawasaki disease (2009~2010), the number of patients newly diagnosed with Kawasaki disease was 10,975 (6,249 males and 4,726 females) in 2009, and 12,755 (7,266 males and 5,489 females) in 2010, yielding a total of 23,730 patients, consisting of 13,515 male and 10,215 female patients[4]. The sex ratio (male/female) of patients was 1.32, and that of prevalence was 1.26, suggesting Kawasaki disease is more common among males. The mean prevalence during the 2-year survey period was 222.9 patients/100,000 children 0~4 years of age (247.6 in males and 196.9 in females). The total number of patients with Kawasaki disease reported in the past 20 surveys is 272,749 (157,865 males and 114,884 females).

Figure 1 shows changes over time in the number of patients newly diagnosed with Kawasaki disease each year[4]. In addition nationwide increases occurred in 1979, 1982 and 1986, the number of patients have tended to increase annually. There is a seasonable pattern in the number of new cases. In the recent two years the number of new cases was low in fall (September and October) while high in spring and summer. Patients under three years of age accounted for 66.8%. The incidence rate by age shows a monomodal distribution and is highest in boys 6~8 months of age and girls 9~11 months of age. Kawasaki disease was especially prevalent in Kanagawa, Nagano and Wakayama Prefectures, and there have been sporadic increases in cases in specific areas.

Patients with a family history of Kawasaki disease accounted for 1.6% of all patients. Among the reported cases, 163 patients (0.7% of the reported cases; 0.6% in males and 0.8% in females) had a parent who has suffered from Kawasaki disease

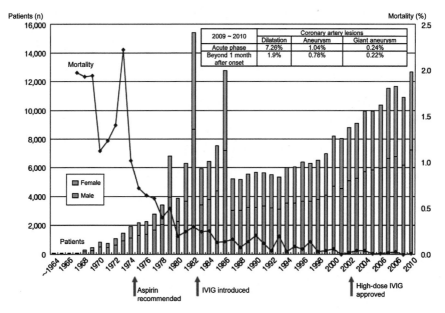

Figure 1 Changes over time in the number of patients with Kawasaki disease and mortality. In the 21st nationwide survey, 1 patient (female) died in 2 years, with a mortality of 0.004%. IVIG, intravenous immunoglobulins. Adapted from Nakamura Y, et al. *J Epidemiol* 2012; 22: 216–221[4)], with modification.

(74 fathers and 69 mothers had the disease). Recurrent cases accounted for 3.6% (3.9% in males and 3.1% in females). In the latest 2 years, one patient died (mortality: 0.004%). The patient had typical Kawasaki disease that occurred at 3 months of age, and died within 2 months after the onset due to cerebral infarction.

Table 3 summarizes guidance for the diagnosis of Kawasaki disease[5)].

1.2 Cardiovascular Complications (Figure 2)

Among the patients assessed in the 21st nationwide survey, 9.3% (11.0% in males and 7.1% in females) experienced acute-phase cardiovascular complications, and 3.0% (3.6% in males and 2.1% in females) experienced cardiovascular sequelae. Acute-phase complications included coronary dilatation in 7.26%, valvular lesions in 1.19%, aneurysms in 1.04%, giant aneurysms in 0.24%, coronary stenosis in 0.03%, and myocardial infarction in 0.01%, which were less prevalent as compared with the previous survey[4)].

Cardiovascular sequelae included coronary dilatation in 1.90%, aneurysms in 0.78%, valvular lesions in 0.29%, giant aneurysms in 0.22%, coronary stenosis in 0.03%, and myocardial infarction in 0.02%. The incidence rate of giant aneurysms was about three-fold higher in males than in females[4)].

Table 3 Diagnostic Guidelines of Kawasaki Disease (MCLS: Infantile Acute Febrile Mucocutaneous Lymph Node Syndrome)

This is a disease of unknown etiology affecting most frequently infants and young children under 5 years of age. The symptoms can be classified into two categories, principal symptoms and other significant symptoms or findings	
A.	Principal symptoms
1.	Fever persisting for 5 days or more (inclusive of those cases in whom the fever has subsided before the 5th day in response to therapy)
2.	Bilateral conjunctival congestion
3.	Changes of lips and oral cavity: Redding of lips, strawberry tongue, diffuse injection of oral and pharyngeal mucosa
4.	Polymorphous exanthema
5.	Changes of peripheral extremities:
	(Acute phase): Redding of palms and soles, indurative edema
	(Convalescent phase): Membranous desquamation from fingertips
6.	Acute nonpurulent cervical lymphadenopathy
At least five items of 1~6 should be satisfied for diagnosis of Kawasaki disease.	
However, patients with four items of the principal symptoms can be diagnosed as Kawasaki disease when coronary aneurysm or dilatation is recognized by two-dimensional (2D) echocardiography or coronary angiography.	
B.	Other significant symptoms or findings
The following symptoms and findings should be considered in the clinical evaluation of suspected patients.	
1.	Cardiovascular: Auscultation (heart murmur, gallop rhythm, distant heart sounds), ECG changes (prolonged PR/QT intervals, abnormal Q wave, low-voltage QRS complexes, ST-T changes, arrhythmias), chest X-ray findings (cardiomegaly), 2D echo findings (pericardial effusion, coronary aneurysms), aneurysm of peripheral arteries other than coronary (e.g., axillary), angina pectoris or myocardial infarction
2.	Gastrointestinal (GI) tract: Diarrhea, vomiting, abdominal pain, hydrops of gallbladder, paralytic ileus, mild jaundice, slight increase of serum transaminase
3.	Blood: Leukocytosis with shift to the left, thrombocytosis, increased erythrocyte sedimentation rate (ESR), positive C reactive protein (CRP), hypoalbuminemia, increased α2-globulin, slight decrease in erythrocyte and hemoglobin levels
4.	Urine: Proteinuria, increase of leukocytes in urine sediment
5.	Skin: Redness and crust at the site of BCG inoculation, small pustules, transverse furrows of the finger nails
6.	Respiratory: Cough, rhinorrhea, abnormal shadow on chest X-ray
7.	Joint: Pain, swelling
8.	Neurological: Cerebrospinal fluid (CSF) pleocytosis, convulsion, unconsciousness, facial palsy, paralysis of the extremities
Remarks	
1.	For item 5 under principal symptoms, the convalescent phase is considered important.
2.	Nonpurulent cervical lymphadenopathy is less frequently encountered (approximately 65%) than other principal symptoms during the acute phase.
3.	Male: Female ratio: 1.3~1.5:1, patients under 5 years of age: 80~85%, mortality: 0.1%
4.	Recurrence rate: 2~3%, proportion of siblings cases: 1~2%
5.	Approximately 10% of the total cases do not fulfill five of the six principal symptoms, in which other diseases can be excluded and Kawasaki disease is suspected. In some of these patients coronary aneurysm or dilatation have been confirmed.

Adapted from Kawasaki Disease Study Group of the Ministry of Health, Labour and Welfare. Guidelines for the Diagnosis of Kawasaki Disease (MCLS, infantile acute febrile mucocutaneous lymph node syndrome), fifth revision. *J Jpn Pediatr Soc* 2002; 106: 836–837[5].

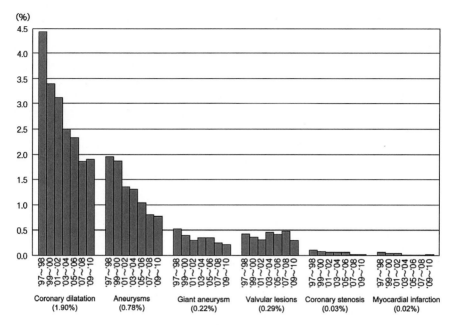

Figure 2 Change over time in the incidence of coronary sequelae in Kawasaki disease. Source: Nakamura Y, et al. *J Epidemiol* 2012; 22: 216–221[4].

Day 4 after onset was the most frequent day of the first visit, and 24.4% of the patients first visited the clinic for Kawasaki disease on day 4 after onset, and 65.9% of the patients visited the clinic by day 4 after onset.

1.3 Treatment[4]

The first administration of intravenous immunoglobulin (IVIG) was given most frequently on day 5 after onset on which 37.4% of the patients received the treatment. Among patients under 2 years of age, 72.8% of them started IVIG therapy by day 5 after onset.

Patients receiving IVIG accounted for 89.5% of the patients assessed in the 21st nationwide survey, and 16.6% of the patients did not respond to the treatment. The daily dose of IVIG was 1,900~2,099mg/kg in 84.5% of the patients receiving the drug, and 900~1,099mg/kg in 13.7%. The duration of treatment was one day in 92.0%, and two days in 7.9%. Additional doses of IVIG were given to 19.1% of the patients. Male patients were dominant in this patient group. Among patients receiving IVIG therapy during the acute phase, 6.5%, 0.9% and 0.8% of the patients received steroids, infliximab and immunosuppressants such as cyclosporine, respectively.

Among patients not responding to IVIG therapy, 29.0%, 4.3%, and 3.7% of them were treated with steroids, infliximab and immunosuppressants, respectively. Plasmapheresis was conducted in 2.2% of the patients.

1.4 Non-Cardiovascular Complications[4)]

Non-cardiovascular complications observed in patients assessed in the 21st nation-wide survey were bronchitis/pneumonia in 2.58%, severe myocarditis in 0.16%, encephalitis/encephalopathy in 0.09%, tachyarrhythmia in 0.07%, and macroscopic hematuria in 0.04%. The incidence rates of encephalitis/encephalopathy, severe myocarditis, vomiting, and diarrhea were higher in female patients than in male patients.

1.5 International Comparison

The prevalence of Kawasaki disease differs substantially among countries. Japan is the highest prevalence of Kawasaki disease in Asia and Oceania. The prevalence of Kawasaki disease in East Asian countries is higher than any other countries, and the number of cases tends to increase in China, Hong Kong, Taiwan and Korea. The prevalences in Korea, Hong Kong, and Taiwan is half, third, and third of that in Japan, respectively. The prevalence in China ranges substantially from 1/100 to 1/7 of that in Japan.

2. Genetic Background of Kawasaki Disease

Although Kawasaki disease is not a genetic disease, the possibility of a genetic predisposition toward it has been suggested by the findings that (1) the incidence of Kawasaki disease in Japan is 10~20-fold that in Western countries, (2) the incidence of Kawasaki disease among siblings of patients is about 10-fold that in the general population, and (3) the incidence in offspring of parents with a history of Kawasaki disease is about twice that in the general population. Although almost all genetic investigation on Kawasaki disease that were available during the preparation of the previous revision were case-control studies that investigated specific genes suspected to be involved in Kawasaki disease, six reports of genome-wide association studies to discover genetic polymorphisms without such hypotheses have been published thereafter[6–11)].

These studies have indicated that the susceptibility to Kawasaki disease may be associated with N-acetylated-α-linked acidic dipeptidase-like 2 (*NAALADL2*)[6)]; zinc finger homeobox 3 (*ZFHX3*)[6)]; pellino homolog 1 (*PELI1*)[7)]; coatomer protein complex beta-2 subunit (*COPB2*)[8)]; endoplasmic reticulum aminopeptidase 1 (*ERAP1*)[8)]; immunoglobulin heavy chain variable region (*IGVH*); Fc fragment of immunoglobulin G (IgG), low affinity IIa, receptor (*FCGR2A*)[9, 11)]; inositol 1,4,5-triphosphate 3-kinase C (*ITPKC*)[9)]; family with sequence similarity 167 member A (*FAM167A*)[10, 11)]; B lymphoid kinase (*BLK*)[10, 11)]; *CD40*[10, 11)]; and human leukocyte antigen (*HLA*)[11)]. Genome-wide linkage disequilibrium analyses have identified *ITPKC* [12], caspase 3 (*CASP3*)[13], ATP (adenosine triphosphate)-binding cassette, sub-family C, member 4 (*ABCC4*)[14], which were then found in case–control studies that these genetic variations are significantly more common in patients with Kawasaki disease than in healthy individuals.

3. Severity Classification

Kawasaki disease is considered severe when coronary artery lesions develop in association with the disease (**Table 4**). As treatment options for Kawasaki disease

Table 4 Severity Classification of Cardiovascular Lesions due to Kawasaki Disease

a. Classification of coronary aneurysms during the acute phase	
- Small aneurysms (ANs) or dilatation (Dil): localized dilatation with ≤4mm internal diameter	
In children ≥5years of age, the internal diameter of a segment measures <1.5 times that of an adjacent segment	
- Medium aneurysms (ANm): aneurysms with an internal diameter from >4mm to <8mm	
In children ≥5years of age, the internal diameter of a segment measures 1.5~4 times that of an adjacent segment	
- Giant aneurysms (ANl): aneurysms with an internal diameter of ≥8mm	
In children ≥5years of age, the internal diameter of a segment measures >4 times that of an adjacent segment	
b. Severity classification	
The severity of Kawasaki disease is classified into the following 5 grades on the basis of findings of echocardiography and selective coronary angiography or other methods:	
I.	No coronary dilatation: patients with no coronary dilatation including those in the acute phase
II.	Transient coronary dilatation during the acute phase: patients with slight and transient coronary dilatation which typically subsides within 30 days after onset
III.	Regression: patients who still exhibit coronary aneurysms meeting the criteria for dilatation or more severe change on day 30 after onset, despite complete disappearance of changes in the bilateral coronary artery systems during the first year after onset, and who do not meet the criteria for Group V
IV.	Remaining coronary aneurysm: patients in whom unilateral or bilateral coronary aneurysms are detected by coronary angiography in the second year or later and who do not meet the criteria for Group V
V.	Coronary stenotic lesions: patients with coronary stenotic lesions detectable by coronary angiography
	(a) Patients without ischemic findings: patients without ischemic signs/symptoms detectable by laboratory tests or other examinations
	(b) Patients with ischemic findings: patients with ischemic signs/symptoms detectable by laboratory tests or other examinations
Other clinical symptoms or findings:	
When patients have moderate or severe valvular disease, heart failure, severe arrhythmia, or other cardiac disease, such conditions should be described in addition to the severity of Kawasaki disease.	

have increased, different scoring systems have been proposed to predict prognosis of patients with coronary artery lesions according to the patient's characteristics, blood test results, and clinical course. The scoring system by Asai and Kusakawa[15] were used widely in the 1970s and 1980s when echocardiography was not common to assess whether coronary angiography (CAG) is indicated for or not. The Iwasa score[16] and the Harada score[17] were developed to assess the indication of IVIG.

In the current situation where the benefits of initial therapy with IVIG have been established, patients at the highest risk of coronary artery lesions are those not responding to IVIG therapy. Unresponsiveness to IVIG therapy is a surrogate endpoint for the development of coronary artery lesions, and represents the severity of Kawasaki disease. In 2006, scoring systems to predict unresponsiveness to IVIG therapy were published[18–20]. These scoring systems are able to predict unresponsiveness to IVIG therapy at a sensitivity of around 80%, and also predict occurrence of coronary artery lesions at a similar sensitivity. The reproducibility of these scoring systems has been demonstrated in Japan[21, 22], while in North America, the sensitivity of these systems is as low as 30~40%[23]. **Table 5** lists commonly used scoring systems[18–20].

Table 5 Scoring Systems to Predict Unresponsiveness to IVIG therapy

Kobayashi score[18] (≥5 points; sensitivity 76%, specificity 80%)	Threshold	Point
Na	≤133mmol/L	2
AST	≥100IU/L	2
Day of starting treatment (or diagnosis)	Day 4 after onset or earlier	2
Neutrophils	≥80%	2
CRP	≥10mg/dL	1
Platelets	≤300,000/μL	1
Age (months)	≤12months	1
Egami score[19] (≥3 points; sensitivity 76%, specificity 80%)	Threshold	Point
ALT	≥80 IU/L	2
Day of starting treatment (or diagnosis)	Day 4 after onset or earlier	1
CRP	≥8 mg/dL	1
Platelets	≤300,000/μL	1
Age (months)	≤6 months	1
Sano score[20] (≥2 points; sensitivity 77%, specificity 86%)	Threshold	Point
AST	≥200 IU/L	1
Total bilirubin	≥0.9 mg/dL	1
CRP	≥7 mg/dL	1

ALT, alanine aminotransferase; AST, aspartate aminotransferase; CRP, C reactive protein; IVIG, intravenous immunoglobulin; Na, sodium.

4. Diagnosis and Treatment of Incomplete Kawasaki Disease

A diagnosis of Kawasaki disease is made according to "Diagnostic Guidelines of Kawasaki Disease (MCLS: Infantile Acute Febrile Mucocutaneous Lymph Node Syndrome)[5]" (**Table 3**) that describes the following six major findings.

1. Fever persisting for 5 days or more (inclusive of those cases in whom the fever has subsided before the 5th day in response to therapy)
2. Bilateral conjunctival congestion
3. Changes of lips and oral cavity: Reddening of lips, strawberry tongue, diffuse injection of oral and pharyngeal mucosa
4. Polymorphous exanthema
5. Changes of peripheral extremities:
   Acute phase: Reddening of palms and soles, indurative edema
   Convalescent phase: Membranous desquamation from fingertips
6. Acute nonpurulent cervical lymphadenopathy

Patients with at least five of the above six major findings are diagnosed as typical Kawasaki disease (described as "level A certainty" in the questionnaires for the nationwide survey[4]). A diagnosis of atypical Kawasaki disease ("level B certainty") is made for patients with four of the six major findings in whom two-dimensional echocardiography or cardioangiography during illness revealed coronary aneurysms or dilatation and other diseases have been excluded. A diagnosis of incomplete Kawasaki disease is made for other patients such as those who meet four of the six findings but do not have coronary aneurysms and those who have three of the six findings and have coronary aneurysms after other diagnoses are excluded.

In the 21st nationwide survey where 23,730 patients were registered during the 2-year survey period, patients with typical, atypical, and incomplete Kawasaki disease accounted for 78.7% (79.0% in males and 78.4% in females), 2.6% (2.7% and 2.5%), and 18.6% (18.3% and 19.0%), respectively[4]. The percentage of incomplete Kawasaki disease has increased over time. Incomplete Kawasaki disease is more prevalent in young children <2years of age, and older children ≥6years of age. Patients with incomplete Kawasaki disease met four, three, two and one of the six major findings in 65.6%, 26.6%, 6.1%, 0.7%, respectively, and the number of criteria met was unknown in 0.9% of them.

A diagnosis of incomplete Kawasaki disease should not be based only on the number of findings observed, and physicians should interpret the clinical picture of individual patients. Redness of the BCG inoculation site in infants and multilocular cervical lymphadenopathy in older children are relatively specific to Kawasaki disease. Physicians should also examine laboratory results for findings typical for Kawasaki disease. Specifically, Kawasaki disease is often associated with increased direct bilirubin, increased hepatic enzyme levels, neutrophilia with left shift, thrombopenia, increased C reactive protein (CRP) and increased brain natriuretic peptide (BNP). Physicians should also observe patients for cardiac complications other than coronary artery lesions, such as cardiac dysfunction, pericardial effusion, and atrioventricular valve regurgitation.

Coronary artery lesions are prevalent in patients with incomplete Kawasaki disease[24–26]. A recent meta-analysis has reported that the risk of occurrence of coronary artery lesions is higher in patients with incomplete Kawasaki disease than in those with typical disease (Odds ratio: 1.45; 95% confidence interval: 1.16~1.81) [27]. Physicians should consider high-dose IVIG therapy for patients with at least four major findings as those for patients with typical Kawasaki disease. Similar treatment equivalent to those for typical cases are also recommended for patients who show only three major findings or less.

II. Genetic Background and Pathology of Cardiovascular Sequelae and Coronary Hemodynamics

1. Genetic Background of Cardiovascular Sequelae

Following the publication of the previous guidelines, genome-wide genetic analysis such as genome-wide SNP (single nucleotide polymorphism) analysis and linkage disequilibrium analysis have been conducted after the release of the previous revision of the guidelines, and genes associated with the susceptibility of Kawasaki disease and coronary artery lesions have been reported[11, 12, 28, 29]. Case-control studies conducted by different study groups have confirmed that *ITPKC* and *CASP3* genes are associated with coronary artery lesions due to Kawasaki disease[11, 13, 30]. *ITPKC* and *CASP3* are among the genes specified in genome-wide gene analyses to be related to the susceptibility of Kawasaki disease. However, as many of these genes have no association with the development of coronary artery lesions due to Kawasaki disease, it is suspected that different genes are playing different roles in the development of Kawasaki disease and the development of coronary artery lesions. Detailed genome-wide SNP analysis should be conducted in a sufficiently large number of patients with coronary artery lesions to clarify these issues.

2. Pathology of Cardiovascular Sequelae

2.1 Coronary Artery Lesions

Kawasaki disease is a systemic vasculitis that often affects coronary arteries. Cardiovascular sequelae is becoming less prevalent due to the advancement in treatment, but it is estimated that in Japan more than 10,000 adults with a history of Kawasaki disease are living with cardiovascular sequelae.

2.1.1 Natural Course of Acute-Phase Coronary Arteritis

Coronary arteritis due to Kawasaki disease develops on day 6~8 after onset when inflammatory cells infiltrate in the intima and adventitia of arteries. This leads to inflammation of all layers of arteries (e.g., panarteritis) around day 10 after onset, and which rapidly progresses to diffuse inflammation affecting the entire circumference of the artery. The cells lining arteries are severely attacked by monocytes, macrophages, neutrophils and other inflammatory cells, and arterial dilatation occurs on around day 12 after onset[31, 32]. Significant infiltration of inflammatory cells continues by around day 25 after onset, and inflammation subsides by around day 40 after onset.

2.1.2 Coronary Sequelae

a. Reduction and Regression of Coronary Aneurysms

Coronary aneurysms remaining ≥30days after the onset of Kawasaki disease typically decrease in size during the convalescent phase or later. "Regression" of coronary aneurysms, i.e., disappearance of abnormal findings on CAG, often occurs within 1~2 years after onset and typically occurs in the case of small or medium aneurysms[33]. Histopathologically, the regression of coronary aneurysms due to Kawasaki disease is an apparent normalization of lumen diameter through circumferential intimal hyperplasia with the migration and proliferation of smooth muscle cells[34]. It has been reported that patients may develop coronary stenosis at the site of regressed coronary aneurysms, a decrease in diastolic function[35], or abnormal vascular endothelial function[36–38] after a long period of time. Patients should thus be followed up even after regression of coronary aneurysms.

b. Arteries with Remaining Aneurysms

Medium or giant aneurysms that remained during the remote phase typically show the following two different pathological features.

The first type is patent aneurysms without regression. The wall of aneurysms consists of hyalinized fibrous tissues with diffuse calcification. At the inlet and outlet of the aneurysm, intimal hyperplasia and/or luminal narrowing due to organized thrombus are noted[39, 40]. There have been reported cases of acute coronary syndrome due to thrombotic occlusion of an aneurysm[41].

The second type is aneurysms with luminal thrombotic occlusion and partial recanalization. The recanalized lumen is surrounded by a thick layer of smooth muscle cells, and the cross-sectional view of the aneurysm shows a lotus-root appearance. Recanalized lumens may become stenotic due to the proliferation of cellular fibrous tissues, and active remodeling is present at the site of aneurysms even during the remote phase[39, 42].

c. Coronary Arteries without Aneurysm Formation

Autopsy of patients with a history of Kawasaki disease who died from causes other than the disease has revealed diverse findings in arteries including clear scars of healed arteritis[43] and no scars[44]. There is no medical consensus about long-term prognosis of coronary artery lesions due to Kawasaki disease. Investigation should be continued to accumulate clinical data.

2.2 Myocardial Disorders

Symptoms of myocarditis often develop during the acute phase of Kawasaki disease, but disappear spontaneously. In a histopathological evaluation of patients who died during the acute phase of Kawasaki disease, all patients showed inflammatory cell infiltration in the myocardium. Characteristic findings included (1) a main finding is infiltration of inflammatory cells into the cardiac interstitium, and myocyte injury is rare; (2) neutrophils are predominant cells at the early phase, but monocytes and macrophages become predominant over time; (3) inflammatory cell infiltration is observed in all regions of the heart during the acute phase, and filtration is gradually localized in the basal area; and (4) inflammatory cells infiltration into the conducting system is also common[45]. Some researchers have reported that interstitial fibrosis as a sequelae of myocarditis persists during the remote phase[46], while others have pointed out that myocardial lesions in this patient population often represent myocardial fibrosis due to previous ischemia in the area perfused by the coronary artery where the aneurysm is present and reported no changes due to myocarditis[47].

2.3 Non-Coronary Arterial Disorders

Kawasaki disease is a systemic vasculitis syndrome that causes vasculitis in a variety of blood vessels including large arteries and small muscular arteries[48-50]. Inflammation occurs in blood vessels located outside the solid organs almost spontaneously[51].

3. Coronary Hemodynamics in Patients with Coronary Sequelae

3.1. Methods and Criteria for Assessment of Coronary Hemodynamics

It is useful to determine average peak flow velocity (APV), coronary flow reserve (CFR), myocardial fractional flow reserve (FFRmyo), shear stress, and peripheral vascular resistance, among other measures, using a 0.014-inch guide wire equipped with an ultrasonic probe and a high-sensitivity pressure sensor (Doppler wires or pressure wires) in order to evaluate the functional severity of coronary artery lesions due to Kawasaki disease. Especially, CFR (CFR=[stress APV]/ [APV at rest], where APV is the value at peak dilatation after infusion of papaverine hydrochloride injection) and FFRmyo (FFRmyo=[Mean pressure at a site distal to the coronary lesion of interest]−{[mean right atrial pressure] / [mean pressure at the coronary ostium]}−[mean right atrial pressure], where these pressures are obtained simultaneously at peak dilatation after infusion of papaverine hydrochloride injection) are suitable for the evaluation of the presence/absence and severity of myocardial ischemia and presence/absence of peripheral coronary circulatory disorder. These values are also useful in selecting appropriate treatment strategies (catheter intervention vs. coronary artery bypass grafting [CABG]) and postoperative evaluation.

The reference values in children are 2.0 for CFR and 0.75 for FFRmyo[52], and identical to those in adults[53–56]. Shear stress induces a mechanical stress on vascular endothelial cells, and affects hemodynamics through endothelium-derived vasoactive substances. The reference value of shear stress in children[57] that is calculated with an approximation formula using APV and lumen diameter is 40dyn/cm^2.

The APV determined with the above method represents the velocity at the center of the lumen, and the flow velocity near the wall is lower than that at the center. Therefore the shear stress near the wall is lower than the APV. As coronary blood flow fairly correlates with APV, a ratio of the mean coronary blood pressure to APV may be used to calculate total peripheral resistance. The reference values of total peripheral resistance at rest and during vascular dilatation are 4.0 and 2.0, respectively[57].

Measurements obtained with pressure wires are useful in the evaluation of stenotic lesions, and those with Doppler wires in the evaluation of dilatation lesions.

3.2 Change in Coronary Hemodynamics Associated with Coronary Artery Lesions

3.2.1 Hemodynamics in Coronary Aneurysms without Significant Stenosis and in the Distal Vessels

a. Hemodynamics in Aneurysms

Turbulent blood flow is present in coronary artery aneurysms, especially giant aneurysms. Although there is no decrease in perfusion pressure, a significant decrease in shear stress, which is known to damage vascular endothelial cells, is noted. It is considered that endothelial cells in giant aneurysms are seriously damaged by vasculitis and hemodynamic change. Vascular endothelial dysfunction promotes vasoconstriction, and increases susceptibility to thrombogenesis, inflammation, fibrosis, oxidation, and atherosclerosis. In giant aneurysms due to Kawasaki disease, thrombogenesis is the biggest problem, because thrombi may be formed readily in giant aneurysms where accelerated platelet aggregation, hypercoagulation and hypofibrinolysis are present. However, some aneurysms with an internal diameter of >8mm have normal blood flow waveform, APV and CFR. Because giant aneurysms with normal hemodynamics may be present, functional assessment of aneurysms should be made to identify aneurysms at risk.

b. Hemodynamics in Vessels Distal to an Aneurysm

Blood flow waveform, APV, CFR and peripheral vascular resistance in vessels distal to an aneurysm are similar to those in the aneurysm. Shear stress is higher in the distal area than in the aneurysms with a significantly large luminal diameter.

On the other hand, FFRmyo in the distal area is within the normal range regardless of the size and shape of aneurysm, unless significant stenoses are present. These findings suggests that vascular endothelial dysfunction, myocardial ischemia and coronary microcirculation disorder due to decreased perfusion may be present in the area distal to a giant coronary aneurysm even when significant stenosis is not present.

3.2.2 Hemodynamics in the Area Distal to a Stenotic Lesion

In the region distal to a coronary stenosis causing myocardial ischemia, CFR, FFRmyo, shear stress, and peripheral vascular resistance are significantly different from those in the control segment, and results outside the reference range are obtained in many of these items[57]. The volume of blood perfusing in this region is small, which suggests the presence of endothelial dysfunction and myocardial ischemia. Perfusion pressure is also low, but peripheral vascular resistance is rather high as the effect of decreased blood perfusion volume is larger than that of decreased perfusion pressure in this region.

III. Examinations and Diagnosis of Cardiovascular Sequelae

1. Blood Test, Biomarkers and Arteriosclerosis

1.1 Blood Test

1.1.1 Myocardial Ischemia, Myocardial Infarction (Table **6**)

a. Markers of Myocardial Cytoplasm

i. CK, CK-MB

Creatine kinase (CK) and CK-myocardial band (MB) levels increase in 4~6 hours after the onset of myocardial infarction and decrease to normal levels in 2~3 days.

Table 6 Blood Biochemical Markers of Acute Myocardial Infarction (AMI)

Marker	Strengths	Weaknesses	Clinical use
CK-MB	- Rapid and accurate test	- Low myocardial specificity (specificity for AMI is low in patients with musculoskeletal disorder)	- CK-MB is one of the principle biochemical markers, and can be used as a standard test in almost all institutions
	- Reinfarction can be detected promptly	- Low detection rate within 6 hours after onset	
Myoglobin	- Detectable 1~2 hours immediately after onset	- Poor myocardial specificity	- Due to poor myocardial specificity, AMI cannot be diagnosed with myoglobin alone
	- Highly sensitive	- Because the level returns to normal in 1~2 days after onset, it cannot be detected in patients who present late after AMI	
	- Reperfusion can be detected		
H-FABP	- Detectable 1~2 hours immediately after onset	- Rapid test kits are available. It is highly sensitive during the early diagnosis, but its specificity is relatively low	- Rapid test kits are available throughout Japan and useful in early diagnosis
	- Infarct size can be estimated		
	- Reperfusion can be detected		
TnT	- Highly sensitive and highly specific	- Sensitivity is low within 6 hours after onset (Retest 8~12 hours after onset)	- Rapid test kits are available throughout Japan, and TnT is a principle biochemical marker
	- Diagnosis is possible 8~12 hours after onset	- Sensitivity to late-onset small reinfarction is low	
	- Diagnosis is possible when testing is performed in the first 2 weeks after onset		
	- Prompt diagnosis is possible with rapid test kits		
	- Reperfusion can be detected		
MLC	- Detectable 4~6 hours after onset	- Sensitivity is relatively low	- Rapid diagnostic tests are not available
	- Diagnosis is possible when testing in the first 2 weeks after onset	- MLC is excreted renally and may be abnormal in patients with renal failure	

CK-MB, creatine kinase-myocardial band; H-FABP, heart-type fatty acid-binding protein; MLC, myosin light chain; TnT, troponin T.

The CK and CK-MB levels correlate well with the volume of myocardial necrosis. CK-MB is also a useful indicator of myocardial reperfusion and reinfarction[58]. Increases in CK-MB2 and MB2/MB1 ratio may be detected within 4 hours after the onset of myocardial infarction[59].

ii. Myoglobin

Myoglobin levels increase in 1~2 hours after the onset of myocardial infarction, reach their peak in about 10 hours, and decrease to a normal level in 1~2 days. Myoglobin is useful in early diagnosis of myocardial infarction, and is also a good indicator of reperfusion[58]. However, it is not specific to myocardium.

iii. Heart-Type Fatty Acid-Binding Protein

Heart-type fatty acid-binding protein (H-FABP) increases in 1~2 hours after the onset of myocardial injury, and is useful in early diagnosis of myocardial infarction, estimating infarct size, and detecting reperfusion[58]. The cut-off level for the diagnosis of myocardial infarction is 6.2ng/mL[60].

b. Markers of Myocardial Structural Proteins

i. Myocardial Troponin T and I

Myocardial troponin T and I (TnT and TnI) are specific to myocardium, and reach peak levels at 12~18 hours and 90~120 hours after the onset of myocardial infarction. These may be used as markers of reperfusion. TnT is highly sensitive and specific in detecting the onset of myocardial infarction, and is useful in the diagnosis and prognosis assessment of non-ST elevation myocardial infarction [58, 61]. In whole-blood rapid assay for TnT, a positive test is defined as ≥ 0.10ng/mL [62]. When a negative result is obtained within 6 hours after the onset of symptoms, the test should be repeated 8~12 hours after onset.

ii. Myosin Light Chain

The plasma myosin light chain (MLC) level reflects the process of myofibrillar necrosis. MLC is detected in blood in 4~6 hours after the onset of myocardial infarction, reaches a peak level in 2~5 days, and maintains high levels for 7~14 days. MLC1 and MLC2 tests are available, but only the MLC1 test is covered with the national health insurance in Japan. The cut-off level for acute myocardial infarction (AMI) is 2.5ng/mL. The peak MLC1 level reflects infarct size, and a result of ≥ 20ng/mL is defined as major infarction[63].

    The above-described features of individual markers indicate that myoglobin and H-FABP are useful in detecting early-phase myocardial infarction, and CK-MB and TnT are beneficial in diagnosing myocardial infarction ≥ 6 hours after onset. Primary markers for AMI are CK-MB and TnT (**Table 6**).

c. Inflammatory Proteins

i. High-Sensitive CRP

High-sensitive CRP is used as an indicator of the presence of coronary arteriosclerotic lesions[64], and it has been reported that elevation of high-sensitive CRP is observed in some patients with late-onset coronary sequelae in Kawasaki disease such as coronary artery lesions and myocardial injury[65, 66]. Elevation of high-sensitive CRP has been reported among patients without coronary sequelae after an average of 8 years after the onset of Kawasaki disease, suggesting that low-grade inflammation continues after healing of Kawasaki disease[67].

ii. Serum Amyloid A Protein

It has been reported that serum amyloid A protein increases during the acute phase of Kawasaki disease. It has been reported that the serum amyloid A protein level remains high even during the remote phase, which suggests the presence of continued inflammation[65].

1.1.2 Arteriosclerosis

A diagnosis of arteriosclerosis should be made after the presence of dyslipidemia and insulin resistance is confirmed. It has been reported that coronary arteriosclerosis as part of metabolic syndrome may develop even during childhood[68]. Researchers are now investigating whether a history of Kawasaki disease and/or coronary artery lesions is a risk factor for the development of arteriosclerosis in children.

a. Dyslipidemia (Table 7)[69]

i. Total Cholesterol

In adults, a total cholesterol (TC) level of <200mg/dL is normal, 200~219mg/dL is borderline, and ≥220mg/dL is abnormal[70].

Table 7 Criteria for Diagnosis of Dyslipidemia during Childhood (Based on Fasting Blood Samples)

Total cholesterol	Normal: <190mg/dL
	Borderline: 190~219mg/dL
	Abnormal: ≥220mg/dL
LDL cholesterol	Normal: <110mg/dL
	Borderline: 110~139mg/dL
	Abnormal: ≥140mg/dL
HDL cholesterol	Cut-off value: 40mg/dL
Triglycerides	Cut-off value: 140mg/dL

HDL, high density lipoprotein; LDL, low density lipoprotein.
Source: Okada T, et al. *Pediatr Int* 2002; 44: 596–601[69].

ii. Serum Low Density Lipoprotein Cholesterol

In adults a serum low density lipoprotein cholesterol (LDL-C) level of <120mg/dL is normal, 120~139mg/dL is borderline, and ≥140mg/dL is abnormal[70].

iii. Serum High Density Lipoprotein Cholesterol

High density lipoprotein cholesterol (HDL-C) prevents arteriosclerosis, and low serum HDL-C levels represent a high risk of arteriosclerosis. In adults, a serum HDL-C level of ≥40mg/dL is normal, and <40mg/dL is defined as hypo HDL cholesterolemia[71]. Low serum HDL-C levels associated with Kawasaki disease are observed not only during the acute phase, but also among patients with coronary artery lesions in the remote phase[72].

iv. Serum Triglycerides

It is known that hypertriglyceridemia promotes the progression of arteriosclerosis. In adults, a serum triglyceride (TG) level of ≥150mg/dL is defined as hypertriglyceridemia[70].

b. Homocysteine

Hyperhomocysteinemia is an independent risk factor for arteriosclerotic disorders such as cerebral infarction and myocardial infarction[73]. The reference value of plasma homocysteine level is 8.2~16.9μmol/L in men and 6.4~12.2μmol/L in women. Plasma homocysteine levels in women increase after menopause[74].

c. Criteria for Diagnosis of Metabolic Syndrome in Children

Table 8 shows the criteria for diagnosis of metabolic syndrome in children in Japan[75].

d. Children in the Remote Phase of Kawasaki Disease

It has been reported that TC and apolipoprotein B levels are higher in individuals who had Kawasaki disease 7~20 years ago than the control group. Children in the remote phase of Kawasaki disease should be observed carefully for the progression of arteriosclerosis[71].

e. Adults in the Remote Phase of Kawasaki Disease

Table 9 shows the reference values for markers of dyslipidemia in Japanese adults[70]. Adults with a history of Kawasaki disease should be instructed to maintain a healthy lifestyle to keep lipid levels within normal ranges[71].

Table 8 Criteria for Diagnosis of Metabolic Syndrome in Japanese Children 6~15 Years of Age (Final Draft In 2006)

Children meeting (1) and at least 2 of items (2)~(4) should be diagnosed with metabolic syndrome.

(1)	Abdominal girth ≥80cm*
(2)	Serum lipid
	Triglyceride ≥120mg/dL and/or HDL cholesterol <40mg/dL
(3)	Blood pressure
	Systolic pressure ≥125mmHg and/or diastolic pressure ≥70mmHg
(4)	Fasting blood glucose ≥100mg/dL

*: Children with an waist-to-height ratio of ≥0.5 fulfill item (1). In elementary school children (6~12 years of age), those with an abdominal girth of ≥75cm should be considered to fulfill item (1).
HDL, high density lipoprotein.
Adapted from Ohzeki T, et al. A cohort study to establish the concept, pathophysiology, and diagnostic criteria of metabolic syndrome in children and design effective interventions: A final report in 2005–2007. 2008: 89–91[75].

Table 9 Criteria for Management of Hyperlipidemia in Adult Japanese for the Prevention and Treatment of Coronary Artery Disease

Hypercholesterolemia	Total cholesterol	≥220mg/dL
Hyper LDL cholesterolemia	LDL cholesterol	≥140mg/dL
Hypo HDL cholesterolemia	HDL cholesterol	<40mg/dL
Hypertriglyceridemia	Triglyceride	≥150mg/dL

HDL, high density lipoprotein; LDL, low density lipoprotein.
Adapted from Japan Atherosclerosis Society (JAS) Guidelines for Diagnosis and Treatment of Atherosclerotic Cardiovascular Diseases, 2002. 2002: 5–7[70].

2. Physiological Examinations

2.1 Electrocardiography at Rest

According to "Diagnostic Guidelines of Kawasaki Disease (MCLS: Infantile Acute Febrile Mucocutaneous Lymph Node Syndrome)" (See **Table 3**), during the acute phase of Kawasaki disease, the electrocardiography (ECG) may show prolonged PR interval, deep Q waves, prolonged QT interval, low voltage, ST-T changes, arrhythmias, and among other findings suggestive of myocardial injury and abnormal repolarization[5, 76]. ECG should be monitored continuously for these changes[77].

It has been reported that QT interval during the acute phase does not clearly correlate with the development of coronary artery lesions[78]; the suggestion that there are relationships between T waveforms and the presence of myocarditis, coronary arteritis, and left ventricular wall movement[79]; and the suggestion that there is a relationship between QT dispersion and coronary artery lesions[80–82]. Premature ventricular contractions (PVCs) are often observed, and the incidence of

PVCs does not differ between patients with and without coronary artery lesions unless coronary stenosis or occlusion is present[83]. When myocardial infarction occurs in patients with giant aneurysms, ST-T changes and abnormal Q waves that are consistent with the lesion of infarction are observed[84].

2.2 Holter ECG

Holter ECG recording is worthwhile in patients complaining of chest pain, chest discomfort, and/or palpitations. Patients with stenosis or giant aneurysms should undergo Holter ECG recording at least once even though it has been reported that the risk of serious arrhythmia and ischemic changes during remote phase is low among those with normal coronary arteries and those who experienced transient coronary artery lesions during the acute phase[83].

2.3 Stress ECG

2.3.1 Exercise ECG

a. Double or Triple Master's Two-Step Test

Although benefits of exercise ECG have been reported, it cannot detect abnormal findings in patients without severe ischemia.

b. Treadmill Test and Ergometer Stress Test

Treadmill test and ergometer stress test can be administered to school-age or older children, though their sensitivity in detecting ischemic findings is less than that of myocardial scintigraphy. It has therefore been recommended that pharmacological stress be added to increase the rate of detection, or that signal-averaged ECG be used.

Treadmill test and ergometer stress test may detect coronary stenosis in some patients. A decrease in coronary reserve due to coronary microcirculation disorder is suspected in patients who have no detectable coronary stenosis but show ST depression during exercise ECG and those with perfusion defect in myocardial scintigraphy[85].

2.3.2 Pharmacological Stress Test and Body Surface Potential Mapping

It has been reported that dipyridamole stress tests using body surface potential mapping is highly sensitive and specific to the presence of ischemia, and is a useful method in diagnosing myocardial ischemia in patients including young children[86]. Also, dobutamine stress test using body surface potential mapping is superior to treadmill test in terms of the sensitivity and specificity for myocardial ischemia, and is reported useful in children[87, 88]. Although magnetocardiography may detect myocardial ischemia[89], this is available only in a limited number of institutions.

2.3.3 Electrophysiological Tests

Life-threatening ventricular arrhythmias may develop in a small number of patients with a history of Kawasaki disease. Studies of patients with cardiovascular sequelae in Kawasaki disease who underwent electrophysiological evaluation[90] have revealed that the prevalence of abnormal sinus or atrioventricular nodal function is significantly higher in patients with cardiac sequelae than in those without them, although the findings of abnormal nodal function were not consistent with the presence of coronary stenosis/occlusion, and are believed to result from myocarditis or abnormal microcirculation in the conducting system.

2.4 Signal-Averaged ECG

During the acute phase, filtered QRS duration changes by $\geq 10\%$[91]. It has been reported that myocardial depolarization becomes inhomogeneous but this change is reversible[92]. It also has been reported that RMS40 during remote phase is significantly lower in patients with coronary artery lesions than without them, and RMS40 is useful as a predictor of ventricular arrhythmias[93]. Signal-averaged ECG is considered highly sensitive for myocarditis due to Kawasaki disease in any phase[94]. Patients with coronary dilatation with and without stenosis during the acute phase contain a larger proportion of high frequency components, suggesting the presence of myocardial involvement[95]. The presence of late ventricular potentials evaluated by criteria with an adjustment to body surface area is highly specific for ischemia and previous myocardial infarction[96]. Dobutamine stress test may improve the detection of these findings in children who cannot undergo exercise stress test[97].

2.5 Summary of Physiological Examinations

Table 10 summarizes the physiological examinations commonly used for patients with Kawasaki disease and their rates of detection of cardiac complications [81, 84, 87, 96, 97].

Because ECG at rest is not sensitive in detecting ischemic lesions in patients in the remote phase of Kawasaki disease, exercise or pharmacological stress tests should be used. Imaging should also be performed to assess ischemic lesions more accurately. Holter ECG and signal-averaged ECG should be performed to assess for ventricular arrhythmia even in patients without ischemic lesions.

Table 10 Detection of Cardiac Complications by Common Physiological Examinations

Investigators	Examination	Target disease	Criteria	N	Sensitivity	Specificity
Osada M, et al[81]	QT dispersion	Coronary artery lesions	QT ≥60ms	56	100% (6/6)	92%
Nakanishi T, et al[84]	12-lead ECG	Inferior wall infarction	deep Q in II, III, aVF	7	86%	97%
		Anterior wall infarction	deep wide Q in V1~6	8	75%	99%
		Lateral wall infarction	deep Q in I, aVL	7	57%	100%
Ogawa S, et al[96]	Signal-averaged ECG	Myocardial ischemia	LP positive	198	69.2%	93.5%
Genma Y, et al[97]	Dobutamine stress signal-averaged ECG	Myocardial ischemia	LP positive	85	87.5%	94.2%
Takechi N, et al[87]	Dobutamine stress body surface potential mapping	Myocardial ischemia	nST >1	115	94.1%	98.9%
			I map ≤4	115	41.7%	96.9%

ECG, electrocardiography; I map, isopotential map; LP, late potential; nST, non-stress test.

3. Diagnostic Imaging

3.1 Chest X-Ray

3.1.1 X-Ray Finding of Calcified Coronary Aneurysms

Pathological investigation has revealed that calcification of aneurysms occurs on day 40 after onset or later[98], but becomes detectable with a chest X-ray 1~6 years after onset[99]. Observation should be made with frontal and lateral projections.

3.1.2 Cardiac Dysfunction Due to Previous Myocardial Infarction
and Enlarged Heart Shadow Due to Valvular Diseases

An enlarged heart shadow is observed in patients with cardiac dysfunction due to previous myocardial infarction, and in patients with volume overload caused by mitral or aortic insufficiency.

3.2 Echocardiography

3.2.1 Echocardiography at Rest

A technique proposed by Fuse et al. has been used to perform coronary echocardiography and determine the intimal diameter of coronary arteries in children[100]. This technique is useful to follow up coronary dilatation[101, 102] and thrombi in coronary aneurysms[103]. Three-dimensional (3D) echocardiography is useful in visualizing the right coronary artery and the circumflex artery, and in visualizing mural thrombi in coronary aneurysms[104]. Echocardiography is the most useful method for evaluation of deterioration of cardiac function due to myocardial injury and the severity of valvular disease[105]. Detailed reports have been published on evaluation of myocardial injury during the acute phase using tissue Doppler imaging[106].

3.2.2 Stress Echocardiography

Stress echocardiography, especially dobutamine stress echocardiography, has been established as a diagnostic method for ischemic heart diseases[107]. It is also a useful noninvasive method to diagnose and follow up myocardial ischemia due to Kawasaki disease.

3.2.3 Myocardial Contrast Echocardiography

The ability of myocardial contrast echocardiography has increased to the level comparable to that of myocardial scintigraphy due to the development and advancement of intravenous contrast agents and the advancement of echocardiography systems[108].

3.3 Radionuclide Imaging

In order to ensure the lowest possible radioactive exposure to children, technetium (Tc)-labeled myocardial perfusion agents (e.g., Tc-99m sestamibi, and Tc-99m tetrofosmin) are commonly used[109, 110]. Stress myocardial single photon emission computed tomography (SPECT) is an important method of diagnosis for coronary stenotic lesions due to Kawasaki disease, and pharmacological stress SPECT is commonly performed for children who cannot undergo exercise stress SPECT [111–116]. When myocardial ischemia is detected in patients without coronary stenoses and there is a false positive result of myocardial perfusion imaging, the presence of coronary microcirculation disorder is suspected[85]. The availability of 3D automatic quantitative analysis of ECG-gated myocardial perfusion SPECT (quantitative gated SPECT, QGS)[117] has allowed physicians to assess for post-ischemic myocardial stunning[118] and the viability of infarcted myocardium in patients with severe coronary artery lesions due to Kawasaki disease[119, 120].

3.3.1 Tc-Labeled Myocardial Perfusion Scintigraphy

Tc-labeled myocardial perfusion scintigraphy is performed under stress at a dose of 10MBq/kg (maximum 370MBq, 10mCi), and the second dose is administered 2~3 hours after the first administration at 2~3 times the first dose (maximum 740MBq, 20mCi)[121]. To obtain clear images, physicians should (1) exercise special caution in avoiding body movement by children during imaging and repeating the imaging when excessive body movement occurs, (2) continue the maximum stress for at least one minute after administration of perfusion agents under stress, (3) promote elimination of perfusion agents from the liver by eating egg products or cocoa, or obtaining images at least 30 minutes after administration of perfusion agents; (4) have the patient maintain the Monzen position (raising the left arm) throughout the procedure to reduce the influence of scattered rays from the liver to the heart[122]; and (5) give the patient soda immediately before the imaging to expand the stomach and reduce the influence of scattered rays from the intestine.

3.3.2 Pharmacological Stress Myocardial Perfusion Scintigraphy

Figure 3 illustrates the outline of pharmacological stress myocardial perfusion scintigraphy[112, 116, 123]. In Japan, adenosine has been approved as a nuclear medicine agent, and it is expected that pharmacological stress myocardial perfusion scintigraphy using adenosine will be a common imaging method. Adenosine should not be administered with dipyridamole, which potentiates the action of adenosine. Adenosine may induce asthmatic attacks, but the half-life of adenosine is short and most of the adverse reactions disappear after discontinuation of the drug[124].

3.3.3 Appropriate Doses of Nuclear Medicine Agents

The Guidelines for Drug Therapy in Pediatric Patients with Cardiovascular Diseases proposed by the Japanese Circulation Society recommend that the dose of nuclear medicine agents for children should be calculated using a formula of "[adult dose]×(years of age+1)/(years of age+7)"[125, 126], while the Committee on Appropriate Use of Nuclear Medicine in Children of the Japanese Society of Nuclear Medicine recommends to determine appropriate doses of agents on the basis of the "dosage card" proposed by the European Association of Nuclear Medicine[127, 128].

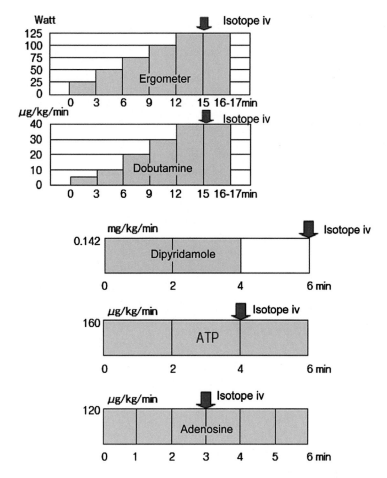

Figure 3 Administration of drugs during myocardial perfusion scintigraphy. ATP, adenosine triphosphate; iv, intravenous.

3.4 Coronary CT and MRCA

3.4.1 Contrast Coronary CT Angiography (MDCT)

Although usefulness of multi-detector row computed tomography (MDCT) in patients with Kawasaki disease has been reported[129], it has drawbacks such as extensive radiation exposure, use of contrast media, and use of β-blockers to control heart rate. However, these drawbacks are being overcome with measures such as decreasing radiation dose to 80kV in infants and young children, and administering contrast media at low or intermediate doses[130].

MDCT has a limitation for visualizing the coronary lumen in segments with calcification, because calcifications cause partial volume effects[131]. It has been reported that the detection rate of stenotic lesions is higher in MDCT than in magnetic resonance coronary angiography (MRCA)[132, 133]. MDCT is superior to MRCA in terms of spatial resolution, image quality, imaging time, and ease of operation. Also, MDCT is useful in visualizing collateral flows that are characteristics to Kawasaki disease.

3.4.2 MRCA

MRCA can be repeatedly performed from the acute phase of Kawasaki disease, because this imaging technique requires neither X-ray exposure nor contrast media, and is useful in screening for mild coronary artery lesions and intimal hyperplasia [134]. Because MRCA can be performed during spontaneous breathing without controlling of the heart rate, infants and young children may undergo it during sleep[135]. There are two imaging techniques of MRCA, the bright blood technique [steady-state free precession (SSFP)] which indicates blood flow as white, and the black blood technique[136, 137], which indicates blood flow as black and occlusions and intimal hyperplasia as gray. MRCA is superior to MDCT as a method to observe thrombi and intimal hyperplasia. Technical expertise is needed to obtain accurate images, and it takes considerable time to create coronary images from data.

3.4.3 Magnetic Resonance Myocardial Imaging

Cine magnetic resonance imaging (MRI) is performed using SSFP without contrast media to acquire images from the left ventricular short axis view, long axis view, and four-chamber view to observe ventricular wall motion, and perfusion MRI is performed after infusion of gadolinium-based contrast media to evaluate the severity of myocardial ischemia by observing the first pass of contrast media in the myocardium during ATP stress and at rest from the left ventricular short axis view[138].

   Delayed-contrast enhanced MRI can visualize the extent and depth of subendocardial infarct lesions by obtaining images 15 minutes after the administration of contrast media with a sequence using T1-weighted gradient echo with myocardial T1 signal suppression. This technique can visualize subendocardial infarct lesions and small infarct lesions in the right ventricle. Because the prevalences of occlusions and recanalization of the right coronary artery are especially high in patients with Kawasaki disease, precise evaluation of the right ventricular myocardium is important[139].

4. Cardiac Catheterization

4.1 CAG

4.1.1 Indications

a. Evaluation of Severity of Coronary Artery Lesions and Patient Follow-Up

Although in the case of adults CAG is indicated for those who exhibit findings of myocardial ischemia, it is recommended for patients with Kawasaki disease that CAG should be performed in those with medium or giant aneurysms during the convalescent phase or later to monitor for the development or progression of localized stenosis, because myocardial ischemia due to Kawasaki disease cannot be fully detected with other types of examinations and myocardial ischemia may manifest as sudden death[140, 141]. The severity classification of cardiovascular lesions due to Kawasaki disease (**Table 4**) is based on the findings of CAG.

b. CAG before and after PCI

CAG is is required before percutaneous coronary intervention (PCI) to determine whether PCI is indicated, during angioplasty to ensure safe and effective intervention, and after angioplasty to evaluate the results of PCI and follow up patients[113, 142, 143].

c. Intracoronary Thrombolysis

Thrombi in coronary aneurysms may sometimes be observed during follow-up of medium to giant aneurysms with echocardiography. In such cases, cardiac catheterization and CAG are performed for intracoronary thrombolysis (ICT).

4.1.2 Coronary Artery Lesions Indicated for CAG

a. Dilatation Lesions

The severity classification of cardiovascular lesions due to Kawasaki disease (**Table 4**), aneurysms with an internal diameter of ≤4mm are defined as small aneurysms, those with from >4mm to <8mm as medium aneurysms, and those with ≥8mm as giant aneurysms. In patients with aneurysms classified as medium or giant, it is desirable to perform CAG during the early part of the convalescent phase for detailed evaluation of the morphology and extent of coronary artery lesions and to specify the methods and duration of follow-up and treatment strategies. Because serious localized stenoses may develop in patients with giant aneurysms in whom examinations have not detected any findings of myocardial ischemia, such patients should undergo CAG every few years[141, 144]. However, as precise evaluation of coronary stenotic lesions is feasible with MRCA and MDCT, it is expected that in the future it will be possible to omit catheterization for the diagnosis of coronary stenotic lesions in some patients[135, 145].

Because the development of stenosis after regression of not only large aneurysms but also smaller ones[146] and the development of arteriosclerotic degeneration[38, 147] have been observed in patients over 10 years after the onset of Kawasaki disease, patients should be followed for a long period of time using coronary imaging techniques such as MRCA and MDCT if follow-up CAG is not feasible.

b. Localized Stenosis

During the remote phase, progressive localized stenosis develop mainly in the inlet and outlet of aneurysms. Multi-directional imaging is required to evaluate stenotic lesions. A significant stenosis is defined as a $\geq 75\%$ stenosis in lumen diameter in the major coronary arteries and a $\geq 50\%$ stenosis in lumen diameter in the left main coronary trunk. Patients with significant stenosis should be followed with angiography[141, 148] or other imaging techniques such as MRCA[135], MDCT[129, 145] at appropriate intervals based on the speed of progression of the stenosis (from 6 months to several years), even when no signs/symptoms of myocardial ischemia are present, and should be considered for aggressive treatment such as CABG[149] and PCI[113] based on the results of the above-described follow-up imaging as well as the results of other studies such as myocardial scintigraphy[150], exercise ECG, and evaluation of CFR.

c. Occlusion

Complete occlusion of a coronary artery is observed in about 16% of patients with coronary artery lesions, and 78% of occlusions are visualized with imaging within 2 years after the onset of Kawasaki disease[141]. It is not uncommon to find coronary occlusive lesions in asymptomatic patients for the first time on routine follow-up imaging. Collateral flows are visualized during angiography in all patients with coronary occlusion. The presence of a well-developed collateral circulation, for which the patient often shows no ischemic findings, is a characteristic feature of occlusive lesions due to Kawasaki disease. Because the extent of collateral flow and growth/development of recanalized vessels differ among individuals and depend on the time after occlusion and cause of occlusion (thrombi vs. intimal hyperplasia), follow-up angiography is required[151].

4.2 Cardiac Function Test

Cardiac function is evaluated by determining ventricular pressure, cardiac output, ventricular volume, ejection fraction (EF), and/or other parameters.

4.3 Intravascular Ultrasound

4.3.1 Morphological Evaluation of Coronary Artery Lesions

Intravascular ultrasound (IVUS) is used to evaluate the severity of intimal hyperplasia, presence/absence of thrombi or calcification, and the severity of luminal narrowing. Severe intimal hyperplasia is observed not only in lesions of localized stenosis but also in aneurysms that have regressed. Intimal narrowing and calcification not detected with angiography may be visualized with IVUS. It has been found that obvious intimal hyperplasia may develop during the remote phase in aneurysms with an internal diameter during the acute phase of >4mm[25]. Evaluation of lesions, and especially quantitative evaluation of calcified lesions with IVUS, is required when the means to be used for PCI are selected[143, 152, 153].

4.3.2 Coronary Arterial Vasodilator Function

It has been reported that the absence of coronary vasodilatation in the coronary artery wall following administration of isosorbide dinitrate (ISDN) or acetylcholine suggests the presence of chronic intimal dysfunction in patients with Kawasaki disease[37, 147, 148]. However, because evaluation of coronary arterial vasodilator function may induce coronary spasm or other adverse reactions, its potential benefits and risks should be carefully weighed before it is performed.

5. Summary of Examinations and Diagnosis (Table 11)

Patients with Class III~V severity of coronary artery lesions should undergo examinations listed in **Table 11** periodically to follow these lesions over time. As the most clinically significant cardiovascular sequelae in Kawasaki disease include coronary stenosis, thrombogenesis in coronary aneurysms, myocardial ischemia, myocardial infarction, vascular endothelial dysfunction, and early progression of arteriosclerosis, and these lesions may develop and progress over time in a considerable number of asymptomatic patients, patients should be followed and evaluated periodically. Recently, MRCA and MDCT have become commonly used as non-invasive methods to delineate coronary artery lesions accurately, and are expected to reduce the mental and physical burden on patients by minimizing the use of invasive catheterization. When these examinations reveal that the lesions have progressed to the point that they require interventions such as PCI and CABG, coronary hemodynamics should also be assessed using stress myocardial perfusion imaging and cardiac catheterization using Doppler flow wire and pressure wire to select appropriate treatment methods.

Table 11 Indications of Imaging Techniques by Severity Classification of Coronary Artery Lesions due to Kawasaki Disease

Blood Test (biomarkers for myocardial ischemia, myocardial infarction, and arteriosclerosis)	
Severity classification IV, V	Class I
Severity classification I, II, III	Class II
None	Class III
Echocardiography at rest, 12-lead ECG	
Severity classification I, II, III, IV, V	Class I
None	Class II
None	Class III
Exercise ECG	
Severity classification III, IV, V	Class I
Severity classification I, II	Class II
None	Class III
Chest X-ray	
Severity classification III, IV, V	Class I
Severity classification I, II	Class II
None	Class III
Holter ECG, signal-averaged ECG	
Severity classification IV, V	Class I
Severity classification I, II, III	Class II
None	Class III
Body surface mapping, pharmacological stress ECG, magnetocardiography	
Severity classification IV, V	Class I
Severity classification I, II, III	Class II
None	Class III
Stress echocardiography, myocardial contrast echocardiography	
Severity classification IV, V	Class I
Severity classification I, II, III	Class II
None	Class III
MRCA, MDCT	
Severity classification IV, V	Class I
Severity classification I, II, III	Class II
None	Class III
Myocardial perfusion imaging, stress myocardial perfusion imaging	
Severity classification IV, V	Class I
Severity classification I, II, III	Class II
None	Class III
Cardiac catheterization	
Severity classification IV, V	Class I
Severity classification III	Class II
Severity classification I, II	Class III

ECG, electrocardiography; MDCT, multi-detector row computed tomography; MRCA, magnetic resonance coronary angiography.

IV. Treatment of Cardiovascular Sequelae

1. Pharmacotherapy

1.1 Treatment Policy

In assessment of cases of death during the remote phase in patients with coronary artery lesions, the major cause of death has been found to be ischemic heart disease due to stenotic lesions resulting from coronary intimal hyperplasia or thrombotic occlusion[40, 154].

In general, treatment of myocardial ischemia is performed to:

- Increase coronary blood flow
- Prevent or relieve coronary spasm
- Prevent the formation of thrombi
- Decrease cardiac work
- Protect myocardium
- Prevent the remodeling of vessel walls

The main purpose of treatment is to decrease the frequency and severity of chest pain attacks, prevent cardiac accidents, and improve the quality of life (QOL) of patients[155]. Drugs used for this purpose include antiplatelet drugs, anticoagulant drugs, calcium channel blockers, nitrates, β-blockers, angiotensin converting enzyme (ACE) inhibitors, angiotensin II receptor blockers (ARBs) and statins (**Table 12**).

Table 12 Guidelines for Long-Term Pharmacotherapy for Patients with Coronary Aneurysms or Dilatation due to Kawasaki Disease

Patients without anginal symptoms
- Patients without demonstrated ischemia: antiplatelet drugs
- Patients with demonstrated ischemia: antiplatelet drugs+calcium channel blockers
Patients with anginal symptoms
In addition to antiplatelet drugs;
- Patients with angina of effort: nitrates and/or calcium channel blockers. If treatment is ineffective, add β blockers.
- Patients with angina at rest or during sleep: calcium channel blockers
- Patients with angina at night: calcium channel blockers+nitrates, or+K-channel openers (nicorandil)
Patients with cardiac dysfunction and those with valvular disease
- Assess the severity of cardiac dysfunction, and use β-blockers, ACE inhibitors, ARBs and/or statins in addition to antianginal drugs.

ACE, angiotensin converting enzyme; ARB, angiotensin II receptor blocker.

1.2 Pharmacotherapy of Vascular Disorders

It has been reported that treatment with the ARB candesartan at a dose of 0.2~0.3mg/kg/day starting within a few days after detecting a coronary aneurysm was effective in preventing stenosis due to intimal hyperproliferation[156]. A recent study has reported that ARBs activate NAD(P)H oxidase, inhibit the expression of monocyte chemoattractant protein-1 (MCP-1) and intercellular adhesion molecule 1 (ICAM-1), and inhibit atherosclerotic changes[157]. It has also been reported that ARBs exert more potent antiatherosclerotic effects when used with statins. These findings suggest that ARBs may also be effective in preventing arteriosclerosis during the remote phase.

1.3 Antiplatelet Drugs and Anticoagulant Drugs

1.3.1 Antiplatelet Drugs (**Table 13**)

Platelet count decreases slightly immediately after the onset of Kawasaki disease (acute phase), and increases during the convalescent phase. Since platelet aggregation activity remains high during the first 3 months after onset and in some cases the first several months to 1 year after onset, it is preferable that patients with Kawasaki disease, including those without coronary sequelae, should be treated with antiplatelet drugs at low doses for about 3 months[158-160].

On the other hand, patients with coronary aneurysm due to Kawasaki disease should receive antiplatelet drugs continuously to prevent ischemic heart disease and prevent the formation or growth of thrombi by platelet activation. This antiplatelet therapy may decrease the incidence of angina and myocardial infarction. Patients who develop AMI should continue treatment with antiplatelet drugs at low doses in combination with anticoagulant drugs from shortly after the onset of infarction until the infarct has healed.

a. Dosage and Administration

It is recommended that children should receive aspirin, a drug inhibiting secondary platelet aggregation, at a low dose (3~5mg/kg/day, once daily). As aspirin inhibits the production of prostacyclin (PGI$_2$), a combination of aspirin with other antiplatelet drugs at low doses may be considered for children. Dipyridamole (2~5mg/kg/day, divided into 3 doses) is expected to potentiate the effect of aspirin, but monotherapy of dipyridamole is not recommended. Ticlopidine is usually administered at a dose of 5~7mg/kg/day, divided into 2 doses, and requires careful observation for major adverse reactions.

Table 13 Antiplatelet Drugs and Anticoagulant Drugs

Drug	Dose	Adverse drug reactions (ADRs) and precautions
Acetylsalicylic acid (Bufferin® or Bayaspirin®)	- 30~50mg/kg/day, divided into 3 doses during the acute phase - 3~5mg/kg/day, once daily after defervescence	- Hepatic dysfunction, gastrointestinal ulcer, Reye syndrome (higher incidence at $\geq$40mg/kg/day), bronchial asthma - Use other drugs during varicella infection and influenza.
Flurbiprofen (Froben®)	- 3~5mg/kg/day, divided into 3 doses	- Hepatic dysfunction, gastrointestinal ulcer - Use when severe hepatic disorder due to aspirin develops.
Dipyridamole (Persantin®, Anginal®)	- 2~5mg/kg/day, divided into 3 doses	- Coronary steal phenomenon, headache, dizziness, thrombocytopenia, hypersensitivity, dyspepsia - May induce angina in patients with severe coronary stenosis.
Ticlopidine (Panaldine®)	- 5~7mg/kg/day, divided into 2 doses	- Thrombotic thrombocytopenic purpura (TTP), leucopenia (granulocytopenia), serious hepatic dysfunction - Blood tests must be performed every other week during the first 2 months of treatment.
Clopidogrel (Plavix®)	- 1mg/kg/day, once daily	- TTP, gastrointestinal symptoms, malaise, myalgia, headache, rash, purpura, pruritus - Bleeding tendency may develop when used with aspirin.
Unfractionated heparin (iv) Low-molecular-weight heparin (sc)	- Loading dose 50 units/kg, maintenance dose 20 units/kg to maintain an APTT of 60~85sec (1.5~2.5 times baseline) - Infants <12months of age Treatment: 3mg/kg/day, divided into 2 doses (every 12 hours) Prevention: 1.5mg/kg/day, as above - Children/adolescents Treatment: 2mg/kg/day, divided into 2 doses (every 12 hours) Prevention: 1mg/kg/day, as above	- Major ADRs: Shock/anaphylactoid reaction, bleeding, thrombocytopenia, thrombocytopenia/thrombosis associated with heparin-induced thrombocytopenia
Warfarin (Warfarin®)	- 0.05~0.12mg/kg/day, once daily (0.05~0.34mg/kg/day in the AHA guidelines)	- Dose should be adjusted to an INR of 2.0~2.5 and a thrombotest value of 10~25%.

(continued)

Table 13 (continued)

Drug	Dose	Adverse drug reactions (ADRs) and precautions
	- 3~7 days required to obtain efficacy	- Sensitivity to this drug, hepatic dysfunction, and bleeding ADRs are possible.
		- The effect of warfarin may be reduced by barbiturates, steroids, rifampicin, bosentan hydrate, and vitamin K-rich foods such as natto, spinach, green vegetables, chlorella, and green juices. The effect of warfarin may be increased by chloral hydrate, NSAIDs, amiodarone, statins, clopidogrel, ticlopidine, antitumor drugs, antibiotics, and antifungal drugs.

The safety and efficacy of the above drugs have not been established in children.
AHA, American Heart Association; APTT, activated partial thromboplastin time; INR, international normalized ratio; iv, intravenous; NSAIDs, nonsteroidal antiinflammatory drugs; sc, subcutaneous.

b. Adverse Drug Reactions

Aspirin may cause adverse drug reactions such as rash, bronchial asthma and hepatic dysfunction. Special care should be taken for bleeding complications. The use of aspirin should be avoided during epidemic of influenza or varicella as aspirin may cause Reye syndrome. Major adverse reactions to ticlopidine include agranulocytosis, serious hepatic dysfunction, and thrombotic thrombocytopenic purpura.

1.3.2 Anticoagulant Drugs (**Table 13**)

Treatment with anticoagulant drugs in patients with Kawasaki disease should be limited for those with medium or giant aneurysms, those with a history of AMI, and those with abrupt dilatation of a coronary artery associated with a thrombus-like echo, among other special cases. Warfarin is often used for these patients. Intravenous heparin should be used in combination with warfarin in emergency cases, and warfarin is used for long-term anticoagulation in patients with chronic conditions. Patients with giant aneurysms should receive a combination of aspirin and warfarin to prevent thrombotic occlusion of aneurysms[162, 163].

a. Dosage and Administration

The maintenance dose of warfarin should be 0.05~0.12mg/kg/day, once daily to achieve an international normalized ratio (INR) of 2.0~2.5, and should be adjusted carefully to prevent bleeding tendency due to excessive warfarin therapy. The recommended dose of unfractionated heparin ranges from 18 units/kg/day for older children to 28 units/kg/day for infants. The activated partial thromboplastin time (APTT) should be maintained at between 60 and 85 seconds.

b. Adverse Drug Reactions and Drug Interactions

As warfarin may cause a severe bleeding tendency, patients should be evaluated carefully for symptoms of bleeding tendency during warfarin therapy. The effects of warfarin are reduced by vitamin K, and are potentiated by aspirin, chloral hydrate, and ticlopidine among other drugs. Vitamin K-rich foods such as natto, green and yellow vegetables, and chlorella reduce the effect of warfarin significantly. Adverse drug reactions to unfractionated heparin include bleeding, hepatic dysfunction, alopecia, and rash.

1.4 Coronary Vasodilators and Antianginal Drugs (Table 14)

1.4.1 Calcium Channel Blockers

In patients with a history of Kawasaki disease, myocardial infarction may occur at rest or during sleep, which suggests the presence of coronary spasm[164, 165]. The addition of amlodipine, a long-acting calcium channel blocker, to the existing regimen may decrease the incidence of cardiovascular events in patients with angina or myocardial ischemia secondary to myocardial infarction. However, amlodipine should not be administered to patients with congestive heart failure and those with atrioventricular block.

1.4.2 β-Blockers

Among patients with Kawasaki disease, β-blockers may be administered to prevent reinfarction or sudden death in those with a history of myocardial infarction and to decrease long-term mortality. However, β-blockers may exacerbate already-existing coronary spasm by blocking β adrenergic receptors to thereby potentiate signaling via α adrenergic receptors.

1.4.3 Nitrates

In a study of the effect of nitrates on coronary arteries in patients with a history of Kawasaki disease who received an intracoronary infusion of ISDN during CAG, the change in diameter after nitrate infusion was significantly lower in arteries with persistent aneurysms and arteries with regressed aneurysms than the control segments, which suggested the presence of endothelial dysfunction. However, the

Table 14 Drugs for the Treatment of Angina, Heart Failure, and Ischemic Attacks

Drug	Dose	Adverse drug reactions and precautions
Drugs for angina		
Nifedipine (Adalat®)	- 0.2~0.5mg/kg/dose, TID (available as 5 and 10mg capsules)	- Hypotension, dizziness, headache
	- Adult dose: 30mg/day, divided into 3 doses	- Care is needed in patients with poor cardiac function.
Slow-release nifedipine (Adalat-CR®, Adalat-L®)	- 0.25~0.5mg/kg/day, OD or BID, maximum dose 3mg/kg/day (Tablets of Adalat-CR® 20mg, L® 10mg, and L® 20mg are available)	Same as above
	- Adult dose: 40mg/kg, OD (Adalat-L® should be divided into 2 doses)	
Amlodipine (Norvasc®)	- 0.1~0.3mg/kg/dose, OD or BID (maximum dose 0.6mg/kg/day)	Same as above
	(Tablets of 2.5mg and 5mg are available)	
	- Adult dose: 5mg/day, OD	
Diltiazem (Herbesser®)	- 1.5~2mg/kg/day, TID (maximum dose 6mg/day) (30mg tablets)	Same as above
	- Adult dose: 90mg/day divided into 3 doses	
Drugs for heart failure		
Metoprolol (Seloken®)	- Start at 0.1~0.2mg/kg/day, divided into 3~4 doses to titrate to 1.0mg/kg/day (40mg tablets)	- Hypotension, cardiac dysfunction, bradycardia, hypoglycemia, bronchial asthma
	- Adult dose: 60~120mg/day, divided into 2~3 doses	
Carvedilol (Artist®)	- Start at 0.08mg/kg/day	Same as above
	- Maintain at 0.46mg/kg/day (average)	
	- Adult dose: 10~20mg/day, OD	
Enalapril (Renivace®)	- 0.08mg/kg/dose, OD (Tablets of 2.5mg and 5mg are available)	- Hypotension, erythema, proteinuria, cough, hyperkalemia, hypersensitivity, edema
	- Adult dose: 5~10mg/day, OD	
Cilazapril (Inhibace®)	- 0.02~0.06mg/kg/day, divided into 1~2 doses (1mg tablets)	Same as above
	- Adult dose: Start at 0.5mg/day, OD and titrate	

(continued)

Table 14 (continued)

Drug	Dose	Adverse drug reactions and precautions
Drugs for angina		
Nitrates		
Isosorbide dinitrate (Nitorol®)	- Sublingual: one-third~one-half tablet/dose (5mg tablets)	- Hypotension, headache, palpitations, dizziness, flushing
	- Oral: 0.5mg/kg/day, divided into 3~4 doses	
	- Adult dose: 1~2 tablets/dose (sublingual)	
	- Frandol tape S® one-eighth~1 sheet	
	- Adult dose: 1 sheet (40mg)/dose	
	- Slow-release tablets (Nitrol-®R, Frandol® tablets) 0.5~1mg/kg/ dose	
	- Adult dose: 2 tablets/day (20mg tablets)	
Nitroglycerin (Nitoropen®)	- One-third~one-half tablet/dose sublingual (0.3mg tablets)	Same as above
	- Adult dose: 1~2 tablets/dose (0.3mg tablets)	

The safety and efficacy of the above drugs have not been established in children. Doses should be determined according to the adult doses.
BID, two times a day; OD, once daily; TID, three times a day.

coronary vasodilative effects of nitrates are not expected to be beneficial in the treatment of acute ischemia due to severe coronary artery lesions. Sublingual or oral spray form of nitrates should be attempted in treating AMI[166, 167].

References

The following guidelines were referred to in the preparation of recommendations for the treatment of patients with cardiovascular sequelae in Kawasaki disease.
  Guidelines proposed by the Japanese Circulation Society:

- Guidelines for diagnostic evaluation of patients with chronic ischemic heart disease (JCS 2010)[168]
- Guidelines for management of anticoagulant and antiplatelet therapy in cardiovascular disease (JCS 2009)[169]
- Guidelines for the primary prevention of ischemic heart disease revised version (JCS 2006)[170]
- Guidelines for management of acute coronary syndrome without persistent ST segment elevation (JCS 2007)[171]
- Guidelines for treatment of chronic heart failure (JCS 2010)[172]

- Guidelines for treatment of acute heart failure (JCS 2011)[173]

Guidelines proposed by the Japanese Society of Pediatric Cardiology and Cardiac Surgery:

- Guidelines for pharmacotherapy of heart failure in children[174]

Guidelines proposed by the American Heart Association (AHA)/American College of Cardiology (ACC):

- Diagnosis, treatment, and long-term management of Kawasaki disease: a statement for health professionals from the Committee on Rheumatic Fever, Endocarditis and Kawasaki Disease, Council on Cardiovascular Disease in the Young, American Heart Association[175]
- AHA/ACC guidelines for secondary prevention for patients with coronary and other atherosclerotic vascular disease: 2006 update: endorsed by the National Heart, Lung, and Blood Institute[176]

1.5 Thrombolytic Therapy and Reperfusion Therapy (Table 15)[126]

1.5.1 Thrombolytic Therapy

Because AMI due to Kawasaki disease is mainly caused by thrombotic occlusion of coronary aneurysms, thrombolytic therapy is of great importance. The sooner thrombolytic therapy is initiated, the better the effect of therapy will be expected. The ACC/AHA/SCAI (Society for Cardiovascular Angiography and Interventions) guidelines recommend that thrombolytic therapy be performed within 12 hours after the onset of AMI[177a].

There are no standard pediatric doses of the drugs used for thrombolytic therapy listed below. Thrombolytic drugs should thus be administered carefully on the basis of the condition of individual patients. It has been reported that the rate of recanalization is 70~80% after intravenous thrombolytic therapy, and may be increased by about 10% when intracoronary administration of thrombolytic drugs (urokinase [UK]) is added to intravenous therapy. Since thrombolytic therapy may be complicated by subcutaneous hemorrhage at the site of catheter insertion, cerebral hemorrhage, and reperfusion arrhythmia, patients should be carefully observed during and following thrombolytic therapy. As tissue plasminogen activators (t-PAs) and pro-urokinase (pro-UK) are proteins and may induce anaphylactic shock, repeated administrations of these drugs should be avoided whenever possible.

Table 15 Thrombolytic Therapy for the Treatment of Thrombotic Occlusion of Coronary Aneurysms due to Kawasaki Disease

Mechanism of action
- Using an enzyme activating the fibrinolytic system to convert plasminogen on the clot into plasmin, which degrades fibrin to dissolve the clot.
Indications
- Dissolution of coronary clots in patients with acute myocardial infarction (within 12 hours after onset).
- Dissolution of clots in coronary aneurysms due to Kawasaki disease.
Drugs (drug classes)
- First-generation thrombolytic drugs: Urokinase (U)
- Second-generation thrombolytic drugs: Alteplase (A), a recombinant tissue plasminogen activator (t-PA)
- Third-generation thrombolytic drugs: Monteplase (M), a modified recombinant t-PA. Indicated only in Japan.
- Drugs indicated for children and adolescents in Japan: None. The safety and efficacy of the above drugs have not been established in this population.
- Use in children: The safety and efficacy of the above drugs in the treatment of acute myocardial infarction in children have not been established.
Method of administration
- Administer intravenously. Consider intracoronary thrombolysis for patients not responding to intravenous thrombolysis.
Doses
Intravenous thrombolysis
- Alteplase: $29.0{\sim}43.5 \times 10^4$ units/kg ($0.5{\sim}0.75$ mg/kg). Administer 10% of the total dose over $1{\sim}2$ minutes intravenously and infuse the remainder over 60 minutes (The recommended dose of alteplase is $0.1{\sim}0.6$ mg/kg/h for 6 hours in ACCP guidelines[177]).
- Monteplase: 2.75×10^4 units/kg. Administer intravenously over $2{\sim}3$ minutes.
- Urokinase: $1.0{\sim}1.6 \times 10^4$ units/kg. Administer intravenously over $30{\sim}60$ minutes.
Intracoronary thrombolysis
- Urokinase: Administer at a dose of 0.4×10^4 units/kg over 10 minutes. Administration may be repeated at most four times.
Precautions for use during pregnancy and effects on fetuses
- Fetal death occurred in animal studies (U, A, M). In rabbit studies, embryos and fetuses died at high doses. It has been suggested these drug may induce premature placental separation through their fibrinolytic activity.
- Major adverse drug reactions: Major bleeding including cerebral hemorrhage, hemorrhagic cerebral infarction, arrhythmias, cardiac rupture, and anaphylactic reactions.
- Thrombolytic drugs are relatively contraindicated for patients with cerebral infarction, transient cerebral ischemia, or other neurological disorders, and those with a history of hypertension.

ACCP, American College of Chest Physicians.
Adapted from Guidelines for Drug Therapy in Pediatric Patients with Cardiovascular Diseases (JCS 2012). Guidelines for Diagnosis and Treatment of Cardiovascular Diseases 2012: 89–301, with modification[126].

a. Intravenous Thrombolysis

i. UK

Infuse at a dose of $1.0 \sim 1.6 \times 10^4$ units/kg (maximum dose 96×10^4 units) over 30~60 minutes.

ii. t-PAs

- Alteplase (Activacin®, Grtpa®): $29.0 \sim 43.5 \times 10^4$ units/kg. Administer 10% of the total dose over 1~2 minutes intravenously and infuse the remainder over 60 minutes.
- Monteplase (Cleactor®): 2.75×10^4 units/kg. Administer intravenously over 2~3 minutes.
- Pamiteplase (Solinase®): 6.5×10^4 units/kg. Administer intravenously over 1 minute.

b. ICT

UK: Administer at a dose of 0.4×10^4 units/kg over 10 minutes. Administration may be repeated at most four times.

1.5.2 Antithrombotic Therapy during PCI

In general, PCI is indicated for patients within ≤12hours after onset. Stenting is the most prevalent PCI technique, and the combination of thrombolysis and stenting is also common. Early treatment with oral antiplatelet drugs (aspirin, clopidogrel [Plavix®], and cilostazol [Pletal®]) or intravenous heparin is promptly begun after PCI to prevent the development of in-stent thrombosis.

1.6 Initial (Medical) Treatment for AMI

1.6.1 General Treatment Policy

The main purpose of treatment of AMI in children is, as in adult patients, to decrease mortality during the acute phase and improve long-term prognosis [178–183]. It has been reported in adults that reperfusion therapy shortly after the onset of AMI decreases mortality. Since AMI in children with a history of Kawasaki disease is caused by thrombotic occlusion of the coronary arteries, it is essential to initiate thrombolytic therapy or PCI as soon as possible to achieve reperfusion, as in the case of AMI in adult patients[184, 185]. During the initial treatment immediately after arrival at the emergency department or admission to hospital, prompt diagnosis and initial treatment should be performed to determine the treatment strategy for AMI and prepare for emergency CAG and reperfusion therapy.

1.6.2 Initial Treatment

a. General Treatment

i. Oxygen Therapy

Oxygen is administered to control myocardial injury.

ii. Establishment of Vascular Access

More than one means of vascular access should be established to ensure prompt treatment of complications possibly associated with AMI.

iii. Pain Control

Morphine hydrochloride (0.1~0.2mg/kg) is the most effective agent, and should be slowly administered intravenously.

iv. Nitrates

Nitroglycerin should be administered intravenously or sublingually.

v. Intravenous Heparin Therapy

Use of heparin therapy prior to reperfusion therapy may increase the rate of recanalization. Heparin should be infused continuously at 10~20 units/kg/hr.

vi. Treatment of Complications

Complications of AMI such as heart failure, cardiogenic shock, and arrhythmia should be treated accordingly.

b. Reperfusion Therapy

Reperfusion therapy is performed to reopen the culprit coronary artery causing thrombotic occlusion shortly after onset in order to avoid the expansion of infarct lesion and maintain cardiac function.

i. Intravenous Thrombolytic Therapy

See Section 1.5.1.a on "Thrombolytic Therapy and Reperfusion Therapy".

c. Anticoagulant Therapy and Antiplatelet Therapy to Prevent Recurrence of AMI

i. Heparin

Heparin should be infused intravenously at a dose of 200~400 units/kg/day, and the dose should be adjusted to maintain an APTT 1.5~2.5 times the baseline value.

ii. Warfarin

Warfarin should be administered at a dose of 0.1mg/kg/day once daily, and the dose should be adjusted to maintain an INR of about 2.0~2.5.

iii. Aspirin

Aspirin should be administered at a dose of 3~5 mg/kg/day once daily (maximum dose of 100mg).

2. Non-Pharmacotherapy

2.1 Catheter-Based Therapy

2.1.1 Indications for Catheter-Based Therapy

The following patients are indicated for catheter-based therapy:

1. Patients with ischemic symptoms caused by coronary stenosis in whom CAG revealed significant stenosis ($\geq$75% luminal diameter).
2. Patients in whom CAG revealed significant stenosis ($\geq$75% luminal diameter), and have no ischemic symptoms during activities of daily living but show ischemic findings during exercise ECG, exercise stress myocardial perfusion scintigraphy, pharmacological stress myocardial perfusion scintigraphy, or other appropriate examinations.
3. Patients with ostial lesions are contraindicated for catheter-based therapy.
4. Catheter-based therapy is contraindicated for patients with multivessel disease and those with significant stenosis ($\geq$75% luminal diameter) or occlusion of the contralateral coronary arteries. However, the latter cases may be treated with catheter-based therapy when bypass surgery is performed for the lesions in the contralateral coronary arteries.

2.1.2 Types of PCI Techniques, Indications, and Precautions

a. PCI

i. Reperfusion Therapy

i-i. ICT

UK should be infused at a dose of 0.4×10^4 units/kg over 10 minutes. Administration may be repeated at most four times.

i-ii. PCI

The guidelines for the management of patients with ST-elevation acute myocardial infarction (JCS 2008) proposed by the Japanese Circulation Society recommend that primary PCI should be considered when it can be performed within 90 minutes (door-to-balloon time) of the first medical contact for patients presenting within 12 hours of symptom onset (**Class I** recommendation)[186]. The guidelines also describe that thrombosuction should be tried first during PCI in order to prevent plaque debris and clots from flowing into peripheral vessels, reduce no-reflow phenomenons, and thereby improve cardiac function after intervention. Stenting is the most prevalent PCI technique. Treatment with oral antiplatelet drugs (aspirin, clopidogrel [Plavix®], and cilostazol [Pletal®]) or intravenous heparin is promptly begun after PCI to prevent the development of in-stent thrombosis.

ii. Plain Old Balloon Angioplasty

In the treatment of coronary artery lesions due to Kawasaki disease, plain old balloon angioplasty (POBA) is effective in the treatment of stenotic lesions that developed ≤ 6 years previously, and becomes less effective as time increases [113, 142, 187–190]. Coronary artery legions due to Kawasaki disease are harder than those observed in adults, a higher balloon pressure is often required, and the risk of development of new aneurysms related to balloon dilatation is higher than in adults. The recommended balloon pressure is ≤ 10 atm.

b. Stenting

Stenting is indicated for older children (≥ 13 years of age) in whom calcification of coronary lesions is relatively mild[152, 153, 191–198]. Stenting can achieve a larger lumen than POBA can. Stenting is also effective in the treatment of coronary arteries in which aneurysms and stenosis are present in succession. The risk of the development of new aneurysms after balloon dilatation is lower in patients receiving balloon dilatation and stenting than those receiving balloon dilatation only, but the balloon pressure should not be higher than 14atm. Lesions that might require a higher balloon pressure require lesion modification using a rotablator. Because surgical treatment of patients with a history of Kawasaki disease is often performed during adolescence, and patients may often receive surgical treatment thereafter, physicians should consider the risk of late-onset thrombosis associated with the discontinuation of antiplatelet therapy. The use of drug-eluting stents should be considered carefully[196].

c. Rotablator (Percutaneous Transluminal Coronary Rotational Atherectomy, PTCRA)

The rotablator uses a rotating metal burr coated with about 2,000 microscopic diamond particles. The burr rotates at high speeds to grind the arteriosclerotic lesion into small fragments, theoretically ≤5µm in diameter, that do not cause peripheral thromboembolism and are degraded in the reticulo-endothelial system. Some physicians do not use balloon dilatation after coronary rotational atherectomy, but many physicians perform balloon dilatation at low pressures after atherectomy.

d. IVUS

In order to ensure successful implementation of PCI, the degree and extent of calcified lesions should be accurately identified to select appropriate procedures. IVUS helps delineate the structure of the coronary artery wall, and determine the percentage of luminal circumference covered with calcification, and the extent of calcified lesions. It is desirable that physicians determine appropriate PCI procedures for children according to the body size, findings of CAG and IVUS[143, 153, 196, 199–201].

2.1.3 Institutions and Backup System Requirements

PCI for patients with coronary artery lesions due to Kawasaki disease is not possible without collaboration between cardiologists with expertise in coronary catheterization and pediatric cardiologists who understand the natural history and pathology of cardiac complications of Kawasaki disease. Support from cardiac surgeons is also essential. It is desirable that PCI for this patient population be performed in cardiovascular centers and other institutions specialized in cardiovascular diseases.

2.1.4 Postoperative Management, Assessment, and Follow-Up

After 4~6 months after PCI, selective CAG should be performed to evaluate the outcome of treatment. A survey has revealed that there is no significant difference between the CAGB and PCI groups in the composite primary endpoint of death or AMI, while the incident of repeated revascularization, a secondary endpoint, is higher in the PCI group[202]. Because surgical treatment for cardiovascular sequelae in Kawasaki disease are typically performed for patients 13~18 years of age, pediatric cardiologists should communicate well with cardiologists to share information and transition the patients to ensure successful long-term management and continued patient education[203].

2.2 Surgical Treatment (Table 16)

Although the prevalence of coronary artery lesions due to Kawasaki disease tends to decrease, there is still a small number of children who have persistent or progressing coronary artery lesions and eventually develop ischemic heart disease during childhood. For such patients who do not respond well to medical treatment, CABG using autologous pedicle internal mammary artery grafts is the most reliable treatment option[204–208]. As the leading causes of death in patients with Kawasaki disease are sudden death and myocardial infarction, the determination of surgical treatment must be made in a timely manner.

2.2.1 Indications for Surgical Treatment of Kawasaki Disease

Table 16 lists the criteria for indications for surgical treatment of cardiovascular sequelae in Kawasaki disease[209]. The nature of coronary artery lesions indicated for surgical treatment in this pediatric population is essentially identical to that in the adult population without Kawasaki disease, and includes (1) severe occlusive lesions in the left main coronary trunk; (2) severe occlusive lesions in multiple vessels (2 or 3 vessels); (3) severe occlusive lesions in the proximal portion of the left anterior descending artery; and (4) jeopardized collaterals. Surgical treatment should be considered as a priority option for patients with a history of myocardial infarction in order to ensure secondary prevention of myocardial infarction. In children, the progression of myocardial ischemia may often occur asymptomatically, and the severity of coronary angiographic findings is often inconsistent with clinical symptoms. Accordingly, candidates for CABG should be comprehensively evaluated on the basis of clinical signs and symptoms as well as findings of CAG, exercise ECG, echocardiography, stress myocardial scintigraphy, left ventriculography, and other techniques to specify the location and viability of ischemic myocardium.

2.2.2 Age at Surgical Treatment

In a survey in Japan, patients undergoing CABG for the treatment of coronary artery lesions due to Kawasaki disease are 11 years of age on average and range between 1 month and 44 years of age at the time of surgery, with children aged 5~12 years predominant[210]. It has been reported that recently CABG can be performed safely even in children younger than those for whom it was previously considered indicated[208, 211, 212]. Surgical treatment during the early phase of the disease is beneficial in avoiding left ventricular hypokinesia, and has a lower incidence of postoperative events than that during later phases of the disease[211].

Table 16 Indications for Surgical Treatment of Kawasaki Disease

Coronary artery bypass grafting (CABG) may be effective in patients who have severe occlusive lesions in main coronary arteries (especially in the central portions of these arteries) or rapidly progressive lesions with evidence of myocardial ischemia. It is preferable to perform CABG using autologous pedicle internal mammary artery grafts regardless of age. Treatment such as mitral valve surgery should be considered when mitral insufficiency not responding to medical treatment is present, although such cases are rare.

CABG

CABG is indicated for patients with angiographically evident severe occlusive lesions of the coronary arteries and viability of myocardium in the affected area. Viability should be evaluated comprehensively, based on the presence/absence of angina and findings of exercise ECG, thallium myocardial scintigraphy, two-dimensional echocardiography, left ventriculography (regional wall movement), and other techniques.

- Findings of coronary angiography:

The following findings are most important. When one of the following findings is present, consider surgical treatment.

1. Severe occlusive lesions in the left main coronary trunk

2. Severe occlusive lesions in multiple vessels (2 or 3 vessels)

3. Severe occlusive lesions in the proximal portion of the left anterior descending artery

4. Jeopardized collaterals

In addition, the following conditions should also be considered in determining treatment strategy.

(1)	When the event is considered a second or third infarction due to the presence of chronic infarct lesions, surgery may be indicated. For example, surgery may be considered to treat lesions limited to the right coronary artery.
(2)	Lesions associated with recanalization of the occluded coronary artery or formation of collateral vessels should be evaluated especially carefully. Surgical treatment may be considered for patients with findings of severe myocardial ischemia.
(3)	Whether CABG is indicated should be considered carefully in younger children based on long-term patency of grafts. In general, young children controllable with medical treatment are followed carefully with periodic coronary angiography to allow them to grow, while patients with severe findings have undergone surgery at 1~2 years of age. It is recommended that pedicle internal mammary artery grafts be used in such cases as well.

- Findings of left ventricular function testing:

It is desirable that patients with favorable left ventricular function be treated with surgery, though patients with regional hypokinesis may also be indicated for surgery. Patients with serious diffuse hypokinesis must be evaluated with particular care and comprehensively based on findings for the coronary arteries and other available data. Heart transplantation may be indicated in rare cases.

Mitral valve surgery

Valvuloplasty and valve replacement may be indicated for patients with severe mitral insufficiency of long duration not responding to medical treatment.

Other surgery

In rare cases, Kawasaki disease has been complicated by cardiac tamponade, left ventricular aneurysm, aneurysms of the peripheral arteries, or occlusive lesion, patients with these conditions may be indicated for surgery.

Adapted from "Study on Kawasaki Disease", the Ministry of Health and Welfare research project on mental and physical disorders. A research report in 1985. 1986: 39–42[209], with modification.

2.2.3 Surgical Techniques

The most desirable surgical technique is CABG using pedicle right or left mammary thoracic artery grafts. It has been reported that the diameter and length of such grafts increase with the somatic growth of children[208, 213]. Large saphenous vein grafts were frequently used in the past, but are no longer used in the present day because of its low long-term patency and the absence of growth after grafting [210, 213, 214]. CABG using right gastroepiploic artery grafts is becoming common [215], but these grafts are not well developed in children, and can be used only in older children with a large body size.

2.2.4 Outcome of Surgery

CABG not only reduces anginal symptoms, but also prevents the occurrence of myocardial infarction and improves prognosis in patients with severe coronary artery legions.

In patients with severe coronary artery lesions due to Kawasaki disease, CABG is also effective in reducing and preventing recurrence of myocardial ischemia and angina. Studies demonstrated the efficacy of CABG, and have revealed that it improved coronary perfusion and left ventricular function during stress testing[216].

a. Graft Patency

The patency of internal thoracic artery grafts, that are the only available grafts for CABG in children, is as high as 87% overall, and 91%, 100%, and 84% when grafted to the left anterior descending artery, the left circumflex artery, and the right coronary artery, respectively, at 20 years after CABG[217].

b. Activities of Daily Life and Problems after Surgery

In a survey of patients with a significant limitation to activities of daily life due to cardiovascular sequelae in Kawasaki disease, 85% of them became able to participate in gym class in school with no limitation, and many patients have a favorable social outcome, including marriage and childbirth[207]. According to a recent report, the 10-, 20- and 25-year survival rates are 98%, 95% and 95%, respectively[217].

2.2.5 Other Surgery

a. Downsizing Operation of Giant Coronary Aneurysms

Blood flow in giant aneurysms is slow and the risk of thrombogenesis is high[218, 219]. Recently, attempts have been made to use the combination of CABG and downsizing operation to treat giant aneurysms to improve flow rate and flow pattern in lesions by decreasing the diameter of the aneurysms, and to prevent the formation of thrombi by increasing shear stress on vessel walls. It has been reported that warfarin therapy could be terminated in some patients treated in this fashion[211, 220].

b. Surgical Treatment of Mitral Valve Insufficiency

Surgical treatment should be considered for patients with severe mitral valve regurgitation due to Kawasaki disease according to the severity of regurgitation, age of the patient, the severity of coronary artery lesions, left ventricular function, and other conditions[221]. Valvuloplasty is the most commonly used technique. In children undergoing valve replacement, mechanical valves, which are more durable than bioprosthetic valves, are commonly used[222].

c. Surgical Treatment of Aortic Aneurysms and Peripheral Aneurysms

In addition to coronary aneurysms, patients with Kawasaki disease may develop aneurysms in the ascending aorta, abdominal aorta, iliac artery, or axillary artery[216]. The use of synthetic grafts has been reported in the treatment of descending aortic aneurysms. Surgical treatment of aneurysms is indicated only for large or progressive lesions.

d. Heart Transplantation

More than ten cases of heart transplantation for the treatment of Kawasaki disease have been reported in the world. It has been reported that they have severe left ventricular dysfunction with a left ventricular fractional shortening (FS) of 5~24%, 16% on average, and that all patients had coronary artery lesions, and many patients (about 40%) had ventricular arrhythmia, ventricular tachycardia, or ventricular fibrillation. Heart transplantation was performed at the age of 8.5years on average, and two children underwent it at the age ≤4months of age[223]. Heart transplantation is beneficial in (1) patients with significant left ventricular dysfunction, and (2) patients who have life-threatening arrhythmia and significant lesions in peripheral segments of the coronary arteries.

3. Summary of Treatment Options (Table 17)

Table 17 summarizes treatment options for coronary artery lesions by severity. As the major causes of death during the remote phase of Kawasaki disease are coronary stenosis due to intimal hyperplasia and ischemic heart disease due to thrombotic coronary occlusion, pharmacotherapy is important in avoiding these cardiac accidents and improving the QOL of patients. For patients not responding to pharmacotherapy who have the progression of stenotic lesions and cannot control the risk of thrombosis, non-pharmacotherapy such as PCI and CABG should be considered proactively.

Table 17 Indications of Treatment by Classification of Severity of Coronary Artery Lesions due to Kawasaki Disease

Antiplatelet drugs (aspirin, dipyridamole, ticlopidine)	
Severity classification IV, V	Class I
Severity classification III	Class II
Severity classification I, II	Class III
Anticoagulant drugs (warfarin)	
Severity classification IV, V	Class I
Severity classification III	Class II
Severity classification I, II	Class III
Coronary vasodilators (e.g., Calcium channel blockers, β-blockers, nitrates)	
Severity classification V	Class I
Severity classification IV	Class II
Severity classification I, II, III	Class III
Drugs for heart failure (ACE inhibitors, ARBs, β-blockers)	
Severity classification V	Class I
Severity classification IV	Class II
Severity classification I, II, III	Class III
PCI	
Severity classification V (b)	Class I
Severity classification V (a)	Class II
Severity classification I, II, III, IV	Class III
CABG	
Severity classification V (b)	Class I
Severity classification V (a)	Class II
Severity classification I, II, III, IV	Class III

ACE, angiotensin converting enzyme; ARBs, angiotensin II receptor blockers; CABG, coronary artery bypass grafting; PCI, percutaneous coronary intervention.

Appropriate decision making is essential in the treatment of cardiovascular sequelae in Kawasaki disease according to careful consideration of the patient's disease status, age, school life (e.g., exercise, school events, and going to university), and social life (e.g., career, job, marriage, and pregnancy/childbirth).

V. Management and Follow-up during Childhood

1. Guidance on Activities of Daily Life and Exercise (Including the School Activity Management Table)

The guidance on activities of daily life and exercise mainly includes management of daily activities in school. The following management is desirable (See School Activity Management Table, the 2011 revision[224]. **Tables 18** and **19**).

Table 18   School Activity Management Table (for Elementary School Children)

Table 18. School Activity Management Table (for Elementary School Children)

[Revised in 2011]

Name   M / F   Birth date   School Activity Management Table (for Elementary School Children)

1. Diagnosis (findings)   (years)   School   Grade   Class   Date

2. Level of management	3. School sport club activity	4. Next visit	
Management needed: A, B, C, D, E	Name of club ( ) Prohibited	___ years ___ months later	Name of institution:
No management needed	Allowed (Note:) or when symptoms develop		Name of physician: (seal)

[Level of management: A - Requires treatment at home or in hospital, B - Goes to school but must avoid exercise, C - Can do mild exercise, D - Can do moderate exercise, E - Can do intense exercise]

Sport activity		Intensity of exercise	Mild exercise (C, D, E - allowed)	Moderate exercise (D, E - allowed)	Intense exercise (E - allowed)
Basic exercise*	Warming-up exercise Exercise-play to improve athletic ability	Grade 1–2	Balance exercise-play (play consists of different body postures such as lying down, sitting up/down, and standing up)	Exercise play using apparatus (grabbing, releasing, rotating, rolling or going through the apparatus)	Exercise-play to change location (crawling, running, jumping, and hopping)
	Warming-up exercise Exercise to improve athletic ability	Grade 3–4	Balance exercise (exercise consists of different body postures such as lying down, sitting up/down, standing up, and hopping)	Exercise using apparatus (grabbing, holding, rotating, and releasing the apparatus, and exercise using a rope)	Strength competition (push or pull the partner, or complete strength, combination of basic movements
	Warming-up exercise Strength-training exercise	Grade 5–6	Exercise to improve flexibility (including stretching), light walking	Exercise to improve techniques (rhythmic exercise and exercise using a ball, hoop or clubs)	Full-body activities within a given time/course (short-rope jumping, long-rope jumping, long-distance running)
Athletics	Running and jumping exercise-play	Grade 1–2	Walking in different ways, rubber rope jumping	Hopscotch	Full-strength foot race, straight-course relay race, relay race with low obstacles
	Running and jumping exercise	Grade 3–4	Walking and light standing broad jump	Slow jogging, light jumping (standing long/high jump)	Full-strength foot race, round-course relay race, low hurdle race, long/high jump with short running start
	Athletics	Grade 5–6	Walking and light standing broad jump		Full-strength sprint, hurdle race, long jump with running start, high jump with running start
Ball sports	Games, ball games, tag (for early grades), games using goals or nets, baseball-type games (for middle grades)	Grade 1–2	Target shooting with ball throwing, bouncing and catching	Target shooting with ball kicking and holding, ball kicking, tag, encampment games	Competition-style exercise
	Ball sports	Grade 3–4	Basic ball handling (passing, catching, kicking, dribbling, shooting, and batting)	Simple games (games with basic exercises with modified rules to fit the place and apparatus used)	
		Grade 5–6			
Type of sport	Exercise-play using apparatus	Grade 1–2	Exercise-play using climbing frames	Exercise-play using monkey bars and wall bars	Exercise-play using mat, horizontal bars and vaulting horse
Apparatus gymnastics	Apparatus gymnastics using mats, vaulting horse or horizontal bars	Grade 3–4 Grade 5–6	Basic exercises Mat exercise (basic movements such as forward roll, backward roll, handstand against wall, and bridging) Vaulting horse (basic movements such as jumping with legs apart) Horizontal bars (basic movements such as forward roll landing)	Basic techniques Mat exercise (e.g., forward/backward rolls, forward/backward rolls with legs apart, handstand against wall, and handstand with support) Vaulting horse (e.g., jumping with legs apart with short running start, jumping with legs folded, and forward roll on the horse) Horizontal bars (e.g., back hip circle with support, forward roll landing with a leg over the bar, front hip circle, and back hip circle)	Combination of gymnastic movements
Swimming	Play with water	Grade 1–2	Play with water (foot race, playing train in swimming pool)	Floating and diving (e.g., prone float with hands against the wall, and paper-rock-scissors or staring game in water)	Relay race in the pool, bobbing, and bobbing
	Floating and swimming	Grade 3–4	Floating (e.g., prone float, back float, jelly fish float)	Floating (e.g., kick and float)	Freestyle and breaststroke with supportive apparatus
	Swimming	Grade 5–6	Swimming movements (flutter kicks, frog kicks)	Swimming (e.g., repeated bobbing)	Freestyle and breaststroke
Dance	Rhythmic play	Grade 1–2	Pretend play (e.g., birds, bugs, dinosaurs, and animals)	Pretend play (e.g., airplane, fun-park rides)	Rhythmic play (e.g., bouncing, whirling, twisting, and skipping)
	Expression movement	Grade 3–4 Grade 5–6	Improvised expression movement	Light rhythmic dance, folk dance, simple Japanese folk dance	Combination of variable movements (e.g., rock and samba dance) Japanese folk dance with strenuous movements
	Outdoor activities such as play in the snow or on the ice, skiing, skating, and waterfront activities		Playing on snow or ice	Walking with ski plates or skates and waterfront activities	Skiing and skating
Cultural activities			Cultural activities without prolonged activities requiring physical strength	Most cultural activities not described in the right column	Playing instruments requiring physical exertion (such as trumpet, trombone, oboe, bassoon, horn), playing or conducting quick rhythmical music, playing in a marching band
School events and other activities			- Follow the above intensity of exercise during athletic festival, during athletic meetings, ball sports competitions, and exercise tests. - Students other than those in Category "E" should consult with their school physician or their attending physicians in determining whether they will participate in other special school activities such as class trips, training camp, school trip, camp schools, and seaside schools. - Consult with their school physician or their attending physicians for the distance of running and swimming (refer to the school curriculum guidelines).		
Remarks					

Definitions

Mild exercise: Physical activities that do not increase respiratory rate in average children at the same age

Moderate exercise: Physical activities that increase respiratory rate without causing shortness of breath in average children at the same age. Players may talk with partners, if any, during exercise.

Intense exercise: Physical activities that increase respiratory rate and cause shortness of breath in average children at the same age.

* Basic exercise: including resistance (isometric) exercise.

Adapted from The Japanese Society of School Health. Guide for the use of the School Activity Management Table for Children with Heart Disease, the 2011 revision. 2013: 3–11[224].

Table 19 School Activity Management Table (for Junior and Senior High School students)

Table 19. School Activity Management Table (for Junior and Senior High School Students)

[Revised in 2011]

Name   M / F   Birth date   (years)   School   Grade   Class

Name of institution: Date

Name of physician: (seal)

1. Diagnosis (findings)

2. Level of management — Management needed: A, B, C, D, E — No management needed

3. School sport club activity — Name of club ( ) Allowed (Note:)-Prohibited

4. Next visit — years,____months later or when symptoms develop

[Level of management: A - Requires treatment at home or in hospital, B - Goes to school but must avoid exercise, C - Can do mild exercise, D - Can do moderate exercise, E - Can do intense exercise]

Sport activity		Intensity of exercise	Mild exercise (C, D, E - allowed)	Moderate exercise (D, E - allowed)	Intense exercise (E - allowed)
Basic exercise*		Warming-up exercise	Light exercise or rhythmic movement to communicate with other students	Exercise to improve flexibility, techniques, high-force movement, and endurance	Exercise with maximum endurance, speed, and muscle strength
		Strength-training exercise	Basic movements (throwing, hitting, catching, kicking, jumping)		
Apparatus gymnastics		(Mat, vaulting horse, horizontal bar, and balance beam)	Calisthenics, light mat exercise, balance exercise, light jumping	Practice of low-grade technique, running start to perform holding, jumping and basic techniques (including rotation)	Performance, competition, combination of actions
Athletics		(racing, jumping, throwing)	Basic motion, standing broad jump, light throwing, light jumping (must avoid running)	Jogging, short run and jump	Long-distance running, sprint race, competition, time race
Swimming		(freestyle, breaststroke, backstroke, butterfly)	Easy movement in water, float, prone float, kick and float, etc.	Slow swimming	Competition, swimming marathon, time race, start and turn
Type of sport	Ball sports	Goal games: Basketball, Handball, Soccer, Rugby	Basic movements (e.g., passing, shooting, dribbling, feinting, lifting, trapping, throwing, kicking, and handling)	Simple games using basic movements (adjust games according to the time, space and apparatus available to practice collaborative playing, and offensive/defensive components)	Competition
		Net games: Volleyball, Table tennis, Tennis, Badminton	Basic movements (e.g., passing, servicing, receiving, tossing, feinting, stroking, and shots)		
		Baseball-type games: Softball, Baseball	Basic movements (e.g., pitching, catching, and batting)		
		Golf	Basic movements (light swinging)	Practicing at golf range	Time race, applied practice, simplified game, game, competition
Martial arts		Judo, kendo, sumo	Etiquette, basic movement (e.g., ukemi, swinging, saboki)	Practicing simple techniques and forms with modest basic movements	Applied practice, competition
Dance		Original dance, folk dance, modern dance	Basic movement (e.g., hand gesture, steps, expressions)	Dance with modest basic movements, etc.	Dance recitals, etc.
Outdoor activity		Play in the snow or on the ice, skiing, skating, camping, climbing, swimming marathon, water-front activities	Playing on water, snow, or ice	Walking with ski plates or skates, slow skiing/skating, hiking on flatlands, playing in the water, etc.	Climbing, swimming marathon, diving, canoeing, boating, surfing, wind surfing, etc.
Cultural activities			Cultural activities not requiring long-term physical activity	Most cultural activities not described in the right column	Playing instruments requiring physical exertion (such as trumpet, trombone, oboe, bassoon, horn), playing or conducting quick rhythmical music, playing in a marching band
School events and other activities				· Follow the above intensity of exercise during athletic festival, during athletic meetings, ball sports competitions, and exercise tests. · Students other than those in Category "E" should consult with their school physician or their attending physicians in determining whether they will participate in other special school activities such as class trips, training camp, school trip, camp schools, and seaside schools.	
Remarks					

Definitions

Mild exercise: Physical activities that do not increase respiratory rate in average students at the same age.

Moderate exercise: Physical activities that increase respiratory rate without causing shortness of breath in average students at the same age. Players may talk with partners, if any, during exercise.

Intense exercise: Physical activities that increase respiratory rate and cause shortness of breath in average students at the same age.

* Basic exercise: including resistance (isometric) exercise.

Adapted from The Japanese Society of School Health. Guide for the use of the School Activity Management Table for Children with Heart Disease, the 2011 revision. 2013: 3–11[224].

1.1 Children without Evidence of Coronary Artery Lesions during the Acute Phase

No restriction of activities of daily life or exercise is needed. In the School Activity Management Table, physicians may indicate "no management needed" for children ≥5years after onset. During the 5-year period after onset, "E-allowed" (i.e., Category E [intense exercise is allowed] in terms of management, with school sport club activities "allowed") should be selected in the table. When a patient is assigned the "no management needed" rating, the attending physician should indicate the termination of follow-up on the existing or newly created "Acute Phase Kawasaki Disease in Summary" (**Figure 5**) of the patient, and provide advice on how to prevent lifestyle-related diseases to the patient and parents.

1.2 Patients not Evaluated for Coronary Artery Lesions during the Acute Phase

1.2.1 Patients in Whom Examination after the Acute Phase Revealed no Coronary Artery Lesions

No restriction of activities of daily life or exercise is needed. Follow the instructions in Section 1.1 "Children without Evidence of Coronary Artery Lesions during the Acute Phase" above.

1.2.2 Patients in Whom Examination after the Acute Phase Revealed Persistent Coronary Artery Lesions According to the Criteria for Severity of Coronary Artery Lesions in This Guideline

a. Patients in Whom Examination after the Acute Phase Revealed no Coronary Artery Lesions (or Revealed Regression of Coronary Artery Lesions)

No restriction of activities of daily life or exercise is needed. Follow the instructions in Section 1.1 "Children without Evidence of Coronary Artery Lesions during the Acute Phase" above.

b. Patients not Evaluated with CAG

Follow the instructions on activities of daily life and exercise in Section 1.3 "Patients Who Have Been Evaluated for Coronary Artery Lesions during and after the Acute Phase" below. Patients should be categorized into the following groups, and provided with instructions accordingly.

(1) Patients in whom echocardiography detected small aneurysms or dilatation
(2) Patients in whom echocardiography detected medium aneurysms

(3) Patients in whom echocardiography detected giant aneurysms

It is desirable that patients in groups (2) and (3) undergo CAG.

c. Patients in Whom CAG Revealed Persistent Coronary Artery Lesions

Follow the instructions on activities of daily life and exercise in Section 1.3 "Patients Who Have Been Evaluated for Coronary Artery Lesions during and after the Acute Phase" below. Patients should be categorized into the following groups, and provided with instructions accordingly.

(1) Patients in whom CAG revealed small aneurysms or dilatation remaining
(2) Patients in whom CAG revealed medium aneurysms remaining
(3) Patients in whom CAG revealed giant aneurysms remaining

1.3 Patients Who Have Been Evaluated for Coronary Artery Lesions during and after the Acute Phase

1.3.1 Patients in Whom Transient Coronary Dilatation Disappeared after the Acute Phase

No restriction of activities of daily life or exercise is needed. Follow the instructions in Section 1.1 "Children without Evidence of Coronary Artery Lesions during the Acute Phase" above.

1.3.2 Patients with Remaining Small Aneurysms or Dilatation

No restriction of activities of daily life or exercise is needed. "E-allowed" should be selected in the School Activity Management Table.

(1) Follow the instructions in Section 1.1 "Children without Evidence of Coronary Artery Lesions during the Acute Phase" above when coronary artery lesions regress.
(2) Patients with remaining coronary artery lesions should be followed up at 2 months, 6 months, and 1 year after onset and annually or later.

1.3.3 Patients with Remaining Medium or Giant Aneurysms

It is desirable that patients of this type be followed by pediatric cardiologists.

a. Patients with no Findings of Stenosis or Myocardial Ischemia

No restriction of activities of daily life or exercise is needed. "E-allowed" should be selected in the School Activity Management Table not including giant aneurysms.

For patients with giant aneurysms, physicians should select "D-prohibited" (Category D [moderate exercise is allowed] in terms of management, with school sport club activities "prohibited") in the School Activity Management Table, in principle. Patients with regressed giant aneurysms should be followed periodically because aneurysms with an internal diameter of ≥6mm may be calcified or progress to stenotic lesions in 10 or 20 years.

b. Patients with Findings of Stenosis or Myocardial Ischemia

Intense exercise should be restricted. The level of allowable exercise should be rated at "D" or more severe category. School sport club activities should be "prohibited".

c. Patients with a History of Myocardial Infarction

Activities of daily life and exercise should be restricted. Patients should be rated as Category "A" to "E" on the basis of their condition. School sport club activities should be "prohibited," in principle.

1.4 Lesions other than Coronary Artery Lesions

1.4.1 Valvular Disease

Pediatric cardiologists should evaluate patients with valvular disease due to Kawasaki disease to determine whether their activities of daily life and exercise should be restricted. Cardiac functions and indications for surgical treatment should be evaluated. Patients exhibiting improvement of echocardiographic findings may be assigned the rating of "no management needed".

1.4.2 Arrhythmia

Pediatric cardiologists should evaluate patients with arrhythmia due to Kawasaki disease to determine whether their activities of daily life and exercise should be restricted. The criteria for management of patients with arrhythmia (Guidelines for management of arrhythmia with no underling diseases, the 2002 revision, published by the School Cardiac Screening Study Committee of the Japanese Society of Pediatric Cardiology and Cardiac Surgery) should be followed when cardiac function is normal and myocardial ischemia can be ruled out[225]. Arrhythmic patients with findings of abnormal cardiac function or myocardial ischemia should be collectively evaluated based on all available data.

1.4.3 Aneurysms other than Coronary Aneurysms

Pediatric cardiologists should manage these lesions individually based on their location and severity.

1.5 Management after Heart Surgery

Pediatric cardiologists should follow patients undergoing heart surgery such as CABG, valvular surgery, and heart transplantation to ensure appropriate follow-up evaluation and patient education.

1.6 Vaccinations

Maternal antibodies play important roles in preventing measles, rubella, mumps and varicella infections[226]. Vaccinations against these diseases should be performed in order at least 6 months after high-dose IVIG therapy.

1.7 Lifestyle Changes to Prevent Arteriosclerosis

Since there is concern that a history of Kawasaki disease may be a risk factor for the development of arteriosclerosis in later life, it is preferable that patients be educated on the prevention of lifestyle-related diseases when they receive their "Acute phase Kawasaki disease in summary" (**Figure 5**).

1.8 Cooperation with Cardiologists

Patients with sequelae in Kawasaki disease should be followed by cardiologists when they grow up. Attending physicians should discuss with patients (or family) the schedule of follow-up by different departments in order to ensure lack of interruption of follow-up evaluation. Careful attention should be paid to avoid discontinuation of follow-up evaluation.

2. Follow-up Evaluation

There are no clearly defined policies on the timing and duration of non-invasive follow-up evaluation of patients with a history of Kawasaki disease in Japan. However, there is an almost complete consensus of opinion that patients with giant aneurysms and patients with regressed medium aneurysms should be followed up for life[35, 146, 148, 227].

The following guidelines are designed for patients who underwent periodic echocardiography during the acute phase of Kawasaki disease. Patients are classified by severity of coronary artery lesions on the basis of echocardiographic findings for the coronary arteries during roughly the first 30 days after onset, and guidance on how to follow up coronary artery lesions by cardiologists is provided based on the severity of echocardiographic coronary findings.

The reader should refer to the "Classification of coronary aneurysms during the acute phase" (**Table 4a**), and the "Severity classification" (**Table 4b**).

2.1 Severity Classification of Coronary Artery Lesions Based on Echocardiographic Findings

Table 20 lists the severity classification of coronary artery lesions based on echocardiographic findings.

Table 20 Criteria for Severity Classification of Coronary Artery Lesions due to Kawasaki Disease

Echocardiographic classification	Severity classification (See **Table 4b**)	Echocardiographic findings
A-1	I	No dilatation of coronary arteries. The coronary arteries tend to be larger during the acute phase than in control children[228, 229], but no localized dilatation is detectable with echocardiography.
A-2	II	Slight and transient dilatation of coronary arteries, which subsides within 30 days after onset.
A-3	Milder cases in Category III	Small aneurysms with an internal diameter of ≤4mm are detectable on day 30 after onset.
A-4	Some cases in Categories III, IV and V	Medium aneurysms are detectable on day 30 after onset.
A-4-1		Medium aneurysms with an internal diameter of >4~<6mm are detectable.
A-4-2		Medium aneurysms with an internal diameter of 6~<8mm are detectable.
A-5	IV, V	Giant aneurysms with an internal diameter of ≥8mm are detectable on day 30 after onset.

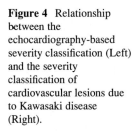 **Figure 4** Relationship between the echocardiography-based severity classification (Left) and the severity classification of cardiovascular lesions due to Kawasaki disease (Right).

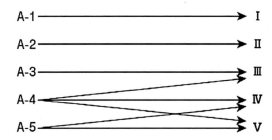

2.2 Relationship between Echocardiography-Based Severity Classification and the Severity Classification of Cardiovascular Lesions due to Kawasaki Disease

The severity of cardiovascular lesions evaluated according to the severity classification of cardiovascular lesions due to Kawasaki disease (**Table 4b**) changes over time depending on the duration after onset. **Figure 4** shows typical relationships between the two classification systems.

2.3 Follow-up Evaluation According to the Echocardiography-Based Severity Classification

2.3.1. Patients in Category A-1

Patients in Category A-1, i.e., patients with no dilatation of coronary arteries, correspond to Category I of the severity classification of cardiovascular lesions due to Kawasaki disease.

Patients in this category should be followed for 5 years, i.e., at 1, 2, and 6 months and 1 and 5 years after the onset of Kawasaki disease. Additional annual follow-up may be scheduled from the second to fifth years through consultation between patients/family and attending physicians. Further follow-up schedules in the sixth year and thereafter should be scheduled individually.

Follow-up evaluation should include ECG, echocardiography, and, if required, chest X-ray. It is desirable that patients be evaluated with exercise ECG at the time of final evaluation.

2.3.2 Patients in Category A-2

This category (patients with slight and transient dilatation of coronary arteries which subsides within 30 days after the onset of Kawasaki disease) corresponds to Category II of the severity classification of cardiovascular lesions due to Kawasaki disease.

It is believed that these patients have no significant problems in terms of coronary artery lesions[37, 38, 148, 166, 227]. Follow-up examination should be performed as specified in the section on Category A-1.

2.3.3 Patients in Category A-3

This category (patients who have small aneurysms at 30 days after the onset of Kawasaki disease) corresponds to relatively mild cases among those classified in Category III of the severity classification of cardiovascular lesions due to Kawasaki disease.

In principle, patients should be followed every 3 months until findings of dilatation disappear and then annually until entry into elementary school (age of 6, 7), then in 4th grade (age 9, 10), at entry into junior high school (age of 12, 13), and at entry into senior high school (age of 15, 16).

Follow-up examination should be performed as specified in the section on Category A-1, and exercise ECG should be added in children at ages when it is feasible. In patients ≥10years after onset, coronary imaging by MDCT or MRCA (the latter is more preferable considering radioactive exposure) should be considered as the final coronary imaging at the time of final follow-up evaluation.

2.3.4 Patients in Category A-4

This category (Patients who have medium aneurysms at 30 days after the onset of Kawasaki disease) corresponds to some cases among those classified in Categories III, IV, and V.

Since long-term prognosis in this category differs significantly among patients, the duration of follow-up should be determined individually according to patient condition. Typically, echocardiographically detected coronary dilatations disappear within one year after onset, and regression of coronary artery lesions detectable by CAG is observed during the two years after onset[146, 230].

According to findings reported by now[35-48, 148, 166, 227], patients in category A-4 are further classified into two categories by the internal diameter of coronary aneurysms on day 30 after onset, A-4-1 (>4~<6mm) and A-4-2 (6~<8mm). The recommended schedules and items of follow-up evaluation are as follows.

a. Patients in Category A-4-1

In this category of patients who have medium aneurysms with an internal diameter of >4~<6mm, thickening of the intima and media is observed, but no progression to stenotic lesions nor calcification of coronary artery lesions is observed in 20 years after onset. Patients should be evaluated once every 1~3 months with ECG, echocardiography, chest X-ray (when necessary), and exercise ECG (when feasible) until dilatation is no longer observed on echocardiography. Following the disappearance of dilatation, patients should be evaluated annually. Patients with aneurysms remaining 1 year after onset should be evaluated once every 3~6 months. Selective CAG may be considered on an individual basis. Although the prognosis of this category of patients is considered relatively good, it is desirable that they undergo MDCT or MRCA every five years to evaluate the coronary arteries until further evidence becomes available.

b. Patients in Category A-4-2

In this category of patients who have medium aneurysms with an internal diameter of 6~<8mm, the incidence rates of stenotic and calcified lesions increase over time, and the progression to arteriosclerotic lesions is also noted. Patients should be followed in a fashion similar to those in Category A-4-1. Patients must undergo follow-up with selective CAG at least once during the early convalescent phase and at the time of disappearance of echocardiographically evident coronary dilatations. Patients with persistent aneurysms should be followed appropriately.

2.3.5 Patients in Category A-5

This category (i.e., patients who have giant aneurysms at 30 days after the onset of Kawasaki disease) corresponds to Categories IV and V of the severity classification of cardiovascular lesions due to Kawasaki disease.

It is believed that aneurysms in patients in this category do not regress completely and may frequently progress to coronary occlusive lesions[146, 230–232]. Patients with persistent giant aneurysms must be followed for life and receive treatment continuously, and should be individually evaluated to design tailor-made treatment.

All patients in this category should undergo initial selective CAG during the early convalescent phase of Kawasaki disease to specify the extent of lesions. As aneurysms outside the coronary arteries may develop in about 2~3% of patients, careful observation should be made[146]. As thrombotic occlusion in giant aneu-rysms in right coronary artery may often develop in the first two years after onset [232], and the incidence of stenotic lesions in giant aneurysms in the left anterior descending artery increases over time[146, 232], patients should be carefully observed for clinical signs/symptoms, and followed with appropriate combinations of ECG, exercise ECG, echocardiography, stress myocardial scintigraphy, selective CAG, MRI, MRCA, MDCT or other appropriate techniques. The duration of follow-up differs among individual patients. In general, patients should be evaluated once every 1~3 months during the first year, and once every 3~6 months or later.

2.4 Acute Phase Kawasaki Disease in Summary

In 2003, the Japan Kawasaki Disease Research Society (currently the Japanese Society of Kawasaki Disease) developed the "Acute phase Kawasaki disease in summary" (**Figure 5**) to encourage patients who had coronary artery lesions during the acute phase of Kawasaki disease as well as those who were treated successfully to carry summarized medical records during the acute phase of this disease (e.g., clinical signs/symptoms, treatment, and cardiac complications)[233]. Because long-term prognosis of this disease after reaching adulthood is still unclear, it is important for individuals with a history of this disease to keep medical information during the acute phase, and provide the information to healthcare professionals whenever necessary.

3. Problems in Shifting from Childhood to Adulthood

3.1 Is a History of Kawasaki Disease a Risk Factor for Arteriosclerosis?

No consistent evidence is available on this matter. The presence of medium aneurysms with an internal diameter of $\geq$6mm during the acute phase is believed a risk factor for arteriosclerosis[227, 231, 234]. In patients with coronary aneurysms with an internal diameter of >4~<6mm during the acute phase, thickening of the intima and media have been noted in some cases during the remote phase[227], and they are considered to be at risk for developing new stenotic or calcified lesions in 30~40 days after onset. Patients with a history of Kawasaki disease, including those who have no coronary artery lesions during the acute phase and those with transient coronary dilatation during the first 30 days after onset of the disease should use the "Acute phase Kawasaki disease in summary" (**Figure 5**) to provide accurate medical information during the acute phase to cardiologists who treat them.

3.2 Collaboration with Cardiologists Providing Healthcare Services to Adult Patients

Pediatricians with expertise in Kawasaki disease cannot cover healthcare services to adult patients with a history of the disease who experience lifestyle-related diseases, pregnancy, childbirth or other adult-onset conditions. There is a need for special clinics for adult patients with a history of Kawasaki disease where patients are managed by cardiologists and supported by obstetricians whenever necessary.

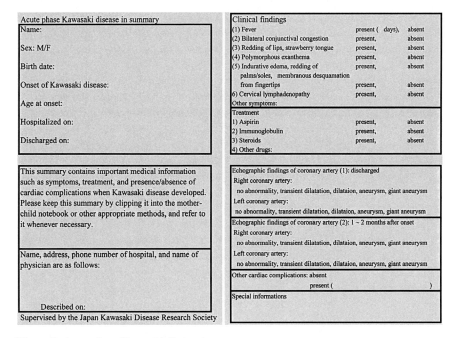

Figure 5 Acute phase Kawasaki disease in summary.

3.3 How to Avoid Dropouts

It has been reported that dropouts, i.e., patients who stop visiting their clinic, occur in a relatively early phase of follow-up[235, 236]. As both patients and pediatric cardiologists should be responsible for continuing follow-up evaluations, healthcare professionals should make every effort to prevent dropout by identifying patients who stop visiting their clinic and encourage them to visit for follow-up.

VI. Problems during Adulthood

1. Progression of Arteriosclerosis: Pathological Features

Cardiovascular sequelae caused by arteritis in Kawasaki disease may be named as arteriosclerosis due to Kawasaki disease, which differs substantially from athero-sclerosis in etiology, pathology and pathophysiology. However, the evidence is limited for the effect of atherosclerosis as a lifestyle-related disease during adult-hood on arteriosclerosis due to Kawasaki disease.

It has been pointed out that endothelial dysfunction and chronic inflammatory reactions may continue during the remote phase in patients with medium or giant aneurysms including those in whom aneurysms have regressed[35, 36, 38, 237]. Because endothelial dysfunction is a precursor of atherosclerosis, it is highly likely that patients with persistent vascular dysfunction and perfusion abnormalities due to sequelae even after the remission of acute-phase inflammation have a high risk for the progression to atherosclerosis. In a study in patients during the remote phase of Kawasaki disease, intravascular echocardiography revealed the presence of intimal hyperplasia at the sites of regressed coronary aneurysms and severe intimal hyperplasia and calcification at the sites of localized stenotic lesions[37].

Although a histopathological study has revealed the active remodeling of the coronary artery lesions due to Kawasaki disease during the remote phase[42], only a few reports have described the relationship between arteriosclerotic lesions due to Kawasaki disease and atherosclerosis. A pathological study of autopsy cases of adult patients with a history of Kawasaki disease has reported that advanced atherosclerotic lesions with microcalcification, necrotic cell debris containing cholesterin crystals, aggregation of foamy cells and hemorrhage are present in the walls of giant aneurisms, while in regressed aneurysms and recanalized aneurysms after thrombotic occlusion, small aggregations of foamy cells and penetration of plasma elements in the thickened intima composed of dense fibrotic tissues[39]. When comparing these findings with autopsy findings of young Japanese patients with atherosclerosis[238], it can be concluded that coronary aneurysms due to Kawasaki disease have more severe atherosclerotic lesions than in coronary artery lesions in patients without a history of the disease. However, the findings noted in regressed aneurysms and recanalized lumen represent initial changes in atherosclerosis, and it is thus difficult to conclude that severe atherosclerosis occurs in coronary sequelae in Kawasaki disease. There is no consensus on the relationship between arteriosclerosis due to Kawasaki disease and atherosclerosis, and further investigation is required.

2. Progression of Arteriosclerosis: Clinical Features

Recent studies have reported findings suggestive of the presence of vascular abnormalities in patients with and without cardiovascular sequelae in Kawasaki disease during the remote phase of vasculitis due to the disease[39, 42, 239–241], which provoked a discussion about what kind of follow-up measures are required for adults with a history of this disease during childhood.

Vascular disorder in patients with a history of Kawasaki disease ranges widely from endothelial cell dysfunction to structural vascular dysfunction. It is believed that persistent endothelial cell dysfunction causes structural vascular dysfunction through complex interactions between inflammation, oxidant stress, different cytokines, among others[242].

Morphological assessment of coronary arteries has been performed with transthoracic echocardiography and X-ray CAG. However, IVUS, a new technique enabling detailed assessment of coronary arteries, has made cardiologists understand the importance of detailed assessment of the coronary arteries as it revealed the presence of intimal hyperplasia in coronary arteries that appeared normal with the conventional procedures[243]. More recently, MDCT and MRCA using the black blood method have become available as less invasive methods of morphological assessment. These new procedures can detect calcification of coronary arteries that develop frequently in the remote phase of Kawasaki disease. In general, calcification of coronary arteries is considered as a risk factor for cardiovascular events[244, 245], but the mechanism of the development of calcification due to Kawasaki disease has not been clarified. Further investigation is necessary.

It is widely known that endothelial cell dysfunction occurs as a precursor of morphological changes such as intimal hyperplasia[246]. Because morphological changes decrease the plasticity of arteries, assessment of vascular function is drawing attention as a procedure to facilitate early intervention. Flow-mediated dilation (FMD), a new measure of vascular function using reactive hyperemia that stimulates the release of nitric oxide (NO) from endothelium, may accurately detect vascular dysfunction. Recent studies have reported a decrease in FMD during the remote phase of Kawasaki disease[241, 247], which suggest that the history of Kawasaki disease is a risk factor for endothelial cell dysfunction.

In the presence of endothelial cell dysfunction, it is likely that the process to atherosclerosis, starting with the expression of adhesion molecules and inflammatory processes, occurs over time. However, atherosclerosis is an entity different from arteriosclerosis due to Kawasaki disease occurring during the remote phase of Kawasaki disease. Although the development of atherosclerosis during the remote phase of Kawasaki disease has not been reported, it has been reported that a high-cholesterol diet induced the development of atherosclerosis developed in an animal model of vasculitis similar to Kawasaki disease[248].

Further investigation is necessary to understand how atherosclerosis develops in coronary arteries affected by arteriosclerosis due to Kawasaki disease. We hope that this question will be solved when patients with a history of Kawasaki disease who have persistent endothelial cell dysfunction become middle age and have a higher risk for atherosclerosis.

VII. Management of Adults with a History of Kawasaki Disease

Currently, there are no data on the actual status and pathological features of adult patients with a history of Kawasaki disease, and no standards are available for the diagnosis and treatment of such patients.

The most important points in the management of adult patients with cardiovascular sequelae in Kawasaki disease are (1) to clarify the accurate status of the cardiovascular sequelae; (2) to control and manage the risk factors for the progression to atherosclerosis; and (3) to administer appropriate drug and non-pharmacotherapies to ensure better prognosis.

1. Diagnosis

In adult patients, correct evaluation of coronary artery lesions is often difficult with transthoracic echocardiography as the lung overlapping the heart may reduce the quality of images. Noninvasive techniques or catheter-based methods of CAG are required for the evaluation of coronary artery lesions.

1.1 Patients without Coronary Aneurysms during Childhood

Family and patients should discuss with attending physicians the need for follow-up evaluation on an individual basis, and patients may undergo noninvasive evaluation once every several years during adulthood if they request it[249].

1.2 Asymptomatic Patients with Coronary Aneurysms Persisting from Childhood

It is desirable that patients should be evaluated with noninvasive techniques 2~3 times each year and that CAG should be performed once every several years.

1.3 Patients with Angina, Myocardial Infarction, Heart Failure, or Severe Arrhythmia in Adulthood

It is desirable that patients should be evaluated with noninvasive techniques 3~4 times each year and CAG as appropriate.

1.4 Adult Patients with Coronary Aneurysms with Unknown History of Kawasaki Disease

Basically, young adults with coronary aneurysms should be followed similarly to patients who had coronary aneurysms in childhood.

2. Treatment

2.1 Pharmacotherapy

No evidence has been obtained on the optimal treatment period and dose of oral aspirin for adult patients with coronary aneurysms due to Kawasaki disease.

2.1.1 Patients without Coronary Aneurysms during Childhood

Patients without coronary aneurysms during childhood may discontinue antiplatelet treatments such as aspirin.

2.1.2 Asymptomatic Patients with Coronary Aneurysms Persisting from Childhood

Asymptomatic patients with coronary aneurysms persisting from childhood must, in principle, continue to take aspirin and other appropriate drugs. In addition to improvements of lifestyle such as weight control and smoking cessation, prevention and appropriate treatment of coronary risk factors such as diabetes mellitus, hyperlipidemia, and hyperuricemia are necessary.

2.1.3 Patients with Angina, Myocardial Infarction, Heart Failure, or Severe Arrhythmia in Adulthood

These patients should be treated in a fashion similar to patients with such conditions associated with etiologies other than Kawasaki disease. In addition to aspirin, antiplatelet drugs, antianginal drugs, diuretics, and other drugs for the treatment of heart failure, or antiarrhythmic drugs may be required. When ischemia is demonstrated on exercise ECG or radionuclide imaging, appropriate coronary intervention should be performed.

2.1.4 Adult Patients with Coronary Aneurysms with Unknown History of Kawasaki Disease

Basically, young adults with coronary aneurysms should be treated as described in Sections 2.1.2 "Asymptomatic Patients with Coronary Aneurysms Persisting from Childhood" and 2.1.3 "Patients with Angina, Myocardial Infarction, Heart Failure, or Severe Arrhythmia in Adulthood" above.

2.2 Non-Pharmacotherapy

Adult patients with a history of Kawasaki disease include those who were diagnosed with Kawasaki disease during childhood and underwent elective PCI during school age for the treatment of angina (coronary aneurysm due to Kawasaki disease, stenosis distal or proximal to a coronary aneurysm), and those who were not diagnosed during childhood but need the treatment for coronary artery disease that developed for the first time during adulthood.

Kokura Memorial Hospital in Kyushu, Japan, has conducted a long-term follow-up survey in 39 patients who underwent the first elective PCI for the treatment of a total of 44 cardiovascular lesions due to Kawasaki disease at the median age of 16 years, and were followed for 13 years. During 5 years after treatment, 35% of the patients underwent repeated PCI for restenosis. Most of these patients underwent repeated PCI in the first year after the initial PCI. No patients received repeated PCI from 5~15 years after the initial PCI. No patients experienced the progression or rupture of coronary aneurysms. The long-term outcome of giant aneurysms was favorable as Suda et al. reported[250]. However, 2 patients (5.6%) had cardiovascular events during adulthood $\geq$ 10years after the initial PCI. These findings indicate that restenosis may occur in some children undergoing PCI at school age during the first year after PCI, but the outcome of repeated PCI is favorable as the lesions are stable with no progression of coronary aneurysms during adulthood. However, these findings also indicate that patients must continue antiplatelet drugs and, for patients with coronary aneurysms, antiplatelet drugs with anticoagulant drugs, and that they tend to develop new coronary artery lesions at an earlier age as compared with people without a history of Kawasaki disease. Patients with a history of Kawasaki disease require more strict medical treatment to prevent arteriosclerosis as compared with people without it[251].

It is not rare that patients in whom Kawasaki disease had been overlooked during childhood present with acute coronary syndrome, which causes more severe symptoms than those observed in children with Kawasaki disease, during adulthood due to coronary artery lesions in Kawasaki disease. Among 3,300 patients who were hospitalized in Kokura Memorial Hospital due to AMI during the period from 2000~2011, 55 patients (1.6%) were hospitalized at the age of less than 40 years, and five of the 55 patients (9.1%) had coronary aneurysms specific to coronary sequelae in Kawasaki disease. None of the five patients had been diagnosed with Kawasaki disease. The prevalence of cardiovascular sequelae in Kawasaki disease is consistent with the findings of Daniels et al. who reported that coronary sequelae in Kawasaki disease are present in 5% of 261 adults less than 40 years of age who were evaluated by angiography for myocardial ischemia[252]. The prevalences of obesity and smokers were significantly lower in these five patients than patients without a history of Kawasaki disease. Many of these five patients did not have known risk factors for arteriosclerosis. PCI was successful in all five patients with a history of Kawasaki disease, but in-hospital mortality was 40%, which was significantly higher than 6% among patients without a history of Kawasaki disease.

3. Guidance on Lifestyle and Exercise

No evidence has been obtained about coronary risk factors that affect the progression and prognosis of coronary artery lesions in adults with a history of Kawasaki disease. However, because they may have additional risk factors for arteriosclerosis during adulthood, patients with a history of Kawasaki disease should be controlled for known coronary risk factors for arteriosclerosis in adults.

Exercise training may favorably affect body weight, sense of well-being, and the use of drugs for the treatment of coronary artery lesions. Exercise therapy should be prescribed according to the results of risk assessment using exercise testing or other appropriate methods.

4. Pregnancy, Labor and Childbirth

4.1 Pregnancy and Labor

Physicians should assess female patients with a history of Kawasaki disease for whether they may maintain normal cardiac function during pregnancy and labor, the risk of drugs during pregnancy including antithrombotic drugs, optimal methods of delivery, and measures for cardiac accidents that may develop during pregnancy or perinatal period[253]. When they reach childbearing age, physicians should assess them for coronary artery lesions, myocardial ischemia or myocardial injury, treat such disorders if present before pregnancy to reduce the risk during delivery, and explain appropriate measures during pregnancy and the risk of childbirth to patients. Pregnant women may undergo cardiac and coronary MRI at week 12 of pregnancy or later[254]. Although the number of women who have a history of Kawasaki disease and had given birth is small and evidence is limited, there have been no serious cardiac accidents reported in this population[255, 256].

4.2 Childbirth

Patients in NYHA Class I without myocardial ischemia may give birth as normal. Women with cardiac dysfunction with a left ventricular ejection fraction (LVEF) of 40~<50% should be monitored carefully during childbirth for the aggravation of cardiac dysfunction due to change in hemodynamics[257]. Patients with normal cardiac function without myocardial ischemia should be assessed using the standard obstetric criteria to determine the method of delivery. When patients with cardiac dysfunction undergo vaginal delivery, the use of forceps or vacuum extractor and epidural anesthesia are beneficial as measures to avoid the risk of cardiac overload due to pain during the second stage of labor[258]. Caesarian section should be considered for women with signs and symptoms of cardiac ischemia.

4.3 Drugs during Pregnancy and Perinatal Period

Physicians should carefully consider the benefits and potential risks of the use of drugs during pregnancy and perinatal period. Drugs used during this period may induce anomaly in the fetus or excessive bleeding during delivery, and may be excreted into the mother's milk[258].

4.3.1 Anticoagulant Drugs and Antiplatelet Drugs

a. Aspirin

When women with coronary artery lesions become pregnant and need the treatment with antiplatelet drugs and anticoagulant drugs during pregnancy, they should be treated with aspirin at a small dose (60~81mg/day) and should be carefully observed. At 34~36 weeks of pregnancy, aspirin should be replaced with continuous intravenous heparin infusion, which should be discontinued 4~6 hours before delivery[258]. When aspirin therapy is continued, patients should be hospitalized and discontinue aspirin therapy one week before delivery[256].

b. Warfarin

It has been reported that the incidence of warfarin fetal complications is dose-dependent, and that the risk of fetal complications is high in patients receiving warfarin at $\geq$5mg/day[259, 260]. Warfarin should be discontinued during the first 12 weeks of pregnancy, when the major organs systems are developing, and weeks 34~36 of pregnancy and thereafter. For patients in whom discontinuation of warfarin increases the risk of thrombogenesis, physicians should consider subcutaneous administration of heparin[258, 261].

4.3.2 Other Drugs

ACE inhibitors should be discontinued during pregnancy, as they are teratogenic. Other drugs should be used only when the benefits overweigh the risk[262, 263].

4.4 Cardiac Accidents

For patients with a risk of cardiac accidents during pregnancy, cardiologists and obstetricians should collaborate closely to prepare for emergency measures according to the individual patient conditions.

4.4.1 AMI

The presence of a giant aneurysm is among the biggest factors that influence the development of AMI[251]. The outcome of myocardial infarction during pregnancy depends on whether the cardiac accident is managed successfully[264, 265]. Women at 20 weeks of pregnancy or thereafter may undergo catheter intervention via the radial artery approach. As the supine position may cause inferior vena cava syndrome, physicians should be careful about the body position of the patient[258].

4.4.2 Arrhythmias

Patients with myocardial injury, cardiac dysfunction or myocardial ischemia may develop ventricular arrhythmias during pregnancy. Physicians should conduct Holter ECG monitoring in such women, and consider treatment when ventricular tachycardia occurs[258].

5. Healthcare System for Adult Patients

As patients with a history of Kawasaki disease are often examined by general internists whose knowledge on this disease is limited. The following problems exist: (1) internists have only limited knowledge and experience in the management of adults with cardiovascular sequelae in Kawasaki disease, and there is only limited information on this matter that is available for physicians and non-physician healthcare professionals; (2) there is only a limited number of specialists who understand the unique pathology and pathophysiology of cardiovascular sequelae in Kawasaki disease during adulthood; and (3) collaborative activities and institutions to ensure effective management through cardiac rehabilitation or other measures have not been fully developed.

5.1 Understanding of Kawasaki Disease by Internists

General internists are not sufficiently aware of the pathophysiology of Kawasaki disease during the acute phase. It is important to foster specialists in this area. Non-physician healthcare professionals should also be educated on cardiovascular sequelae in Kawasaki disease.

5.2 Collaboration between Pediatricians and Cardiologists

Pediatricians and internists must share data on clinical course and laboratory findings obtained from adult patients who had a history of Kawasaki disease.

Collaboration between pediatricians and internists especially cardiologists is essential to diagnose, treat and follow patients with cardiovascular sequelae in Kawasaki disease.

5.3 Coronary Aneurysms and Myocardial Infarction in Young Patients and Kawasaki Disease

Asymptomatic patients with coronary aneurysms due to Kawasaki disease may have ischemic heart disease during adolescence or adulthood. Myocardial infarction is more prevalent than angina among patients with cardiovascular sequelae in Kawasaki disease[266]. There is a need for a nationwide archive to register and disclose childhood medical records of patients with a history of Kawasaki disease.

5.4 Comparison with Adult-Type Myocardial Infarction

In the pathologic evaluation of patients with Kawasaki disease, no severe atherosclerotic lesions are observed although substantial arteriosclerosis is present[267]. Remodeling of coronary artery lesions in patients with sequelae in Kawasaki disease may persist for years after onset, and is associated with intimal hyperplasia and neovascularization[42]. These findings differ from those in juvenile patients with arteriosclerosis not associated with Kawasaki disease.

Because patients with cardiovascular sequelae in Kawasaki disease may have atherosclerosis and may present with more complex lesions in the future, specialists who are fully aware of such condition must be available.

5.5 Cardiac Rehabilitation

Few medical institutions are providing cardiac rehabilitation programs for adults with cardiovascular sequelae in Kawasaki disease. This patient population needs appropriate cardiac rehabilitation programs and facilities where physicians and rehabilitation specialists work together.

VIII. Summary

Table 21 summarizes the pathophysiology, diagnosis, clinical course, treatment, lifestyle management and exercise management for patients with a history of Kawasaki disease by severity.

Table 21 Summarized Guidelines

Severity	Pathophysiology	Diagnosis / clinical course	Treatment	Daily life/exercise management*
I No dilatation	There is no evidence whether or not a history of Kawasaki disease is a factor associated with arteriosclerotic lesion.	Follow up patients for 5 years. Evaluate at 30 days, 60 days, 6 months, 1 year, and 5 year after onset with ECG, echocardiography, and, if necessary, chest X-ray. It is desirable that patients be evaluated with exercise ECG at the final examination.	Basically, no treatment is required during the remote phase. Patients with no coronary aneurysms after the acute phase may discontinue antiplatelet drugs such as aspirin.	No restriction is placed on daily life or exercise.
II Transient dilatation during the acute phase	During the acute phase, histopathologically vasculitis develops in the outer layer of the tunica media and then expands to the intima in coronary arteries. Echocardiography reveals diffuse dilatation of coronary arteries, but these changes subside within 30 days after onset.			Management Table: "No management needed" for children ≥5 years after onset. Consult with parents (or patients) to determine further management. Lifetime prevention of lifestyle-related diseases is important. Junior and senior high school students should be educated on lifestyle-related diseases (e.g., blood lipid measurement, education on smoking cessation, and prevention of obesity).
III Regression	In many cases regression may occur 1~2 years after onset, particularly in small or medium aneurysms. In the segment with regression, decrease in coronary diastolic function, abnormal function of vascular endothelium, and substantial intimal hyperplasia have been reported. Also, it is reported that the occurrence of acute coronary syndrome in adults with a history of Kawasaki	Basically, follow patients annually with ECG, echocardiography, and chest X-ray up to entry into elementary school (age of 6, 7), and then with the same methods and exercise ECG in 4th grade (age 9, 10), at entry into junior high school (age 12, 13), and entry into senior high school (age 15, 16). Follow patients who had coronary aneurysms with a large internal diameter during the	Continue antiplatelet drugs such as aspirin whenever necessary.	No restriction is placed on daily life or exercise. Follow the recommendations for Categories I and II.

(continued)

Table 21 (continued)

Severity	Pathophysiology	Diagnosis / clinical course	Treatment	Daily life/exercise management*
	disease in whom coronary artery lesions were considered regressed after the acute phase of the disease.	acute phase with an appropriate combination of imaging techniques**.		
IV Remaining coronary aneurysms	Aneurysms remaining during the convalescent phase or later are considered sequelae. Histopathologically, progression of inflammation leads to rupture of the internal elastic band, causing panangiitis. The internal and external elastic bands are broken into fragments and ruptured by arterial pressure to form aneurysms. Patients with giant aneurysms must be observed carefully for myocardial ischemia, because in such patients myocardial ischemia may develop even if no significant stenotic lesions are present.	Patients must be followed with exercise ECG and an appropriate combination of imaging techniques**. It is desirable that patients who had coronary aneurysms with a large internal diameter during the acute phase be evaluated with stress myocardial scintigraphy every 2–5 years, since they may have myocardial ischemia.	Continue treatment with antiplatelet drugs such as aspirin. Anticoagulant therapy may be needed in patients with giant aneurysms or thrombi in coronary aneurysms. CABG may be indicated for patients with giant aneurysms not accompanied by significant stenotic lesions when myocardial ischemia has occurred.	No restriction is placed on daily life or exercise. Management Table: "E-allowed". Patients with giant aneurysms: Instruct as "D-prohibited" in the Management Table. In the second year after onset or later, "E-prohibited" is possible when no changes are noted.
V-a Coronary stenotic lesions (no findings of ischemia)	Thrombotic occlusion of medium or giant aneurysms may develop during the relatively early stage after onset. Sudden death may occur, though two-thirds patients with occlusion are asymptomatic.	Patients must be followed for life, and physicians must design the tailor-made management plan for individual patients. Follow-up examination must include exercise ECG and an appropriate combination of	Continue treatment with antiplatelet drugs such as aspirin. Use calcium channel blockers, nitrates, β-blockers, ACE inhibitors, and/or angiotensin receptor II blockers to	No restriction is placed on daily life or exercise. School Activity Management Table: "E-allowed" for patients other than those with giant aneurysms. Explain the importance of pharmacotherapy and

	Patients often show improvement of myocardial ischemia due to the development of recanalized vessels and collateral flow after occlusion. Development/progression of regional stenosis during the	imaging techniques**. Although schedule may differ among individuals, patients are generally evaluated every 3~6 months.	prevent ischemic attacks and treat heart failure.	ensure adherence, as well as symptoms which may occur and actions to be taken when ischemia develops. Patients must be followed at least annually until the stenotic lesions have improved.
V-b Coronary stenotic lesions (with findings of ischemia)	remote phase is more prevalent in the left coronary artery than in the right coronary artery. The segments with greatest prevalence are the proximal segment or the main trunk of the left anterior descending artery. The risk of progression to stenosis/occlusion is higher in larger aneurysms. Stenosis may develop during long-term follow up.		Follow the instructions for pharmacotherapy in Category V-a. Consider CABG or appropriate PCI technique when exercise ECG or stress myocardial scintigraphy reveals ischemia.	Exercise shuld be restricted. Categorize in "D" or higher category based on patient condition. School sport club activities should be "prohibited". Select the most appropriate category from "A" to "D" on the basis of findings of exercise testing and evaluation of severity of myocardial ischemia. Educate patients well about the importance of pharmacotherapy.

*See **Tables 18** and **19**.

**Imaging techniques include echocardiography (including stress echocardiography), stress myocardial scintigraphy, selective CAG, IVUS, MRI, MRA, and MDCT.

ACE, angiotensin converting enzyme; CABG, coronary artery bypass grafting; CAG, coronary angiography; ECG, electrocardiography; IVUS, intravascular ultrasound; MDCT, multi- detector row computed tomography; MRA, magnetic resonance angiography; MRI, magnetic resonance imaging; PCI, percutaneous coronary intervention.

References

1. Kawasaki T. Acute febrile mucocutaneous syndrome with lymphoid involvement with specific desquamation of the fingers and toes in children. *Japanese Journal of Allergology* 1967; 16: 178–222 (in Japanese).
2. Guidelines for Diagnosis and Treatment of Cardiovascular Diseases (2001–2002 Joint Working Groups Report). Guidelines for diagnosis and management of cardiovascular sequelae in Kawasaki disease (JCS 2003). *Circ J* 2003; 67; Suppl IV: 1111–1174 (in Japanese).
3. Guidelines for Diagnosis and Treatment of Cardiovascular Diseases (2007 Joint Working Groups Report). Guidelines for diagnosis and management of cardiovascular sequelae in Kawasaki disease (JCS 2008). http://www.j-circ.or.jp/guideline/pdf/JCS2008_ogawasy_h.pdf (in Japanese) (available January 2013).
4. Nakamura Y, Yashiro M, Uehara R, Sadakane A, Tsuboi S, Aoyama Y, et al. Epidemiologic features of Kawasaki disease in Japan: results of the 2009–2010 nationwide survey. *J Epidemiol* 2012; 22: 216–221.
5. Kawasaki Disease Study Group of the Ministry of Health, Labour and Welfare. Guidelines for the Diagnosis of Kawasaki Disease (MCLS, infantile acute febrile mucocutaneous lymph node syndrome), fifth revision. *J Jpn Pediatr Soc* 2002; 106: 836–837 (in Japanese).
6. Burgner D, Davila S, Breunis WB, Ng SB, Li Y, Bonnard C, et al; International Kawasaki Disease Genetics Consortium. A genome-wide association study identifies novel and functionally related susceptibility Loci for Kawasaki disease. *PLoS Genet* 2009; 5: e1000319, doi: 10.1371/journal.pgen.1000319.
7. Kim JJ, Hong YM, Sohn S, Jang GY, Ha KS, Yun SW, et al; Korean Kawasaki Disease Genetics Consortium. A genome-wide association analysis reveals 1p31 and 2p13.3 as susceptibility loci for Kawasaki disease. *Hum Genet* 2011; 129: 487–495.
8. Tsai FJ, Lee YC, Chang JS, Huang LM, Huang FY, Chiu NC, et al. Identification of novel susceptibility Loci for kawasaki disease in a Han chinese population by a genome-wide association study. *PLoS One* 2011; 6: e16853, doi: 10.1371/journal.pone.0016853.
9. Khor CC, Davila S, Breunis WB, Lee YC, Shimizu C, Wright VJ, et al. Genome-wide association study identifies FCGR2A as a susceptibility locus for Kawasaki disease. *Nat Genet* 2011; 43: 1241–1246.
10. Lee YC, Kuo HC, Chang JS, Chang LY, Huang LM, Chen MR, et al. Two new susceptibility loci for Kawasaki disease identified through genome-wide association analysis. *Nat Genet* 2012; 44: 522–525.
11. Onouchi Y, Ozaki K, Burns JC, Shimizu C, Terai M, Hamada H, et al; Japan Kawasaki Disease Genome Consortium; US Kawasaki Disease Genetics Consortium. A genome-wide association study identifies three new risk loci for Kawasaki disease. *Nat Genet* 2012; 44: 517–521.

12. Onouchi Y, Gunji T, Burns JC, Shimizu C, Newburger JW, Yashiro M, et al. ITPKC functional polymorphism associated with Kawasaki disease susceptibility and formation of coronary artery aneurysms. *Nat Genet* 2008; 40: 35–42.

13. Onouchi Y, Ozaki K, Buns JC, Shimizu C, Hamada H, Honda T, et al. Common variants in CASP3 confer susceptibility to Kawasaki disease. *Hum Mol Genet* 2010; 19: 2898–2906.

14. Khor CC, Davila S, Shimizu C, Sheng S, Matsubara T, Suzuki Y, et al; US and International Kawasaki Disease Genetics Consortia. Genome-wide linkage and association mapping identify susceptibility alleles in ABCC4 for Kawasaki disease. *J Med Genet* 2011; 48: 467–472.

15. Asai T. Severity assessment of Kawasaki disease. *Acta Paediatr Jpn Overseas Ed* 1983; 25: 170–175.

16. Iwasa M, Sugiyama K, Ando T, Nomura H, Katoh T, Wada Y. Selection of high-risk children for immunoglobulin therapy in Kawasaki disease. *Prog Clin Biol Res* 1987; 250: 543–544.

17. Harada K. Intravenous gamma-globulin treatment in Kawasaki disease. *Acta Paediatr Jpn* 1991; 33: 805–810.

18. Kobayashi T, Inoue Y, Takeuchi K, Okada Y, Tamura K, Tomomasa T, et al. Prediction of intravenous immunoglobulin unresponsiveness in patients with Kawasaki disease. *Circulation* 2006; 113: 2606–2612.

19. Egami K, Muta H, Ishii M, Suda K, Sugahara Y, Iemura M, et al. Prediction of resistance to intravenous immunoglobulin treatment in patients with Kawasaki disease. *J Pediatr* 2006; 149: 237–240.

20. Sano T, Kurotobi S, Matsuzaki K, Yamamoto T, Maki I, Miki K, et al. Prediction of nonresponsiveness to standard high-dose gamma-globulin therapy in patients with acute Kawasaki disease before starting initial treatment. *Eur J Pediatr* 2007; 166: 131–137.

21. Kobayashi T, Inoue Y, Tamura K, Morikawa A, Kobayashi T. External validation of a scoring system to predict resistance to intravenous immunoglobulin. *J Pediatr* 2007; 150: e37; author reply e38, doi:10.1016/j.jpeds.2006.12.036.

22. Seki M, Kobayashi T, Kobayashi T, Morikawa A, Otani T, Takeuchi K, et al. External validation of a risk score to predict intravenous immunoglobulin resistance in patients with Kawasaki disease. *Pediatr Infect Dis J* 2011; 30: 145–147.

23. Sleeper LA, Minich LL, McCrindle BM, Li JS, Mason W, Colan SD, et al; Pediatric Heart Network Investigators. Evaluation of Kawasaki disease risk-scoring systems for intravenous immunoglobulin resistance. *J Pediatr* 2011; 158: 831–835. e833.

24. Sudo D, Monobe Y, Yashiro M, Mieno MN, Uehara R, Tsuchiya K, et al. Coronary artery lesions of incomplete Kawasaki disease: a nationwide survey in Japan. *Eur J Pediatr* 2012; 171: 651–656.

25. Manlhiot C, Christie E, McCrindle BW, Rosenberg H, Chahal N, Yeung RS. Complete and incomplete Kawasaki disease: two sides of the same coin. *Eur J Pediatr* 2012; 171: 657–662.

26. Sonobe T, Kiyosawa N, Tsuchiya K, Aso S, Imada Y, Imai Y, et al. Prevalence of coronary artery abnormality in incomplete Kawasaki disease. *Pediatr Int* 2007; 49: 421–426.
27. Ha KS, Jang G, Lee J, Lee K, Hong Y, Son C, et al. Incomplete clinical manifestation as a risk factor for coronary artery abnormalities in Kawasaki disease: a meta-analysis. *Eur J Pediatr* 2013; 172: 343–349.
28. Kuo HC, Yang KD, Juo SH, Liang CD, Chen WC, Wang YS, et al. ITPKC single nucleotide polymorphism associated with the Kawasaki disease in a Taiwanese population. *PLoS One* 2011; 6: e17370, doi: 10.1371/journal. pone.0017370.
29. Lin MT, Wang JK, Yeh JI, Sun LC, Chen PL, Wu JF, et al. Clinical implication of the c allele of the ITPKC gene SNP rs28493229 in Kawasaki disease: Association with disease susceptibility and BCG scar reactivation. *Pediatr Infect Dis J* 2011; 30: 148–152.
30. Kuo HC, Yu HR, Juo SH, Yang KD, Wang YS, Liang CD, et al. CASP3 gene single-nucleotide polymorphism (rs72689236) and Kawasaki disease in Taiwanese children. *J Hum Genet* 2011; 56: 161–165.
31. Takahashi K, Oharaseki T, Naoe S, Wakayama M, Yokouchi Y. Neutrophilic involvement in the damage to coronary arteries in acute stage of Kawasaki disease. *Pediatr Int* 2005; 47: 305–310.
32. Masuda H, Naoe S, Tanaka N. The pathology of coronary arteries in Kawasaki disease (MCLS): A consideration of the relationship between coronary arteritis and the development of aneurysms. *The Journal of Japanese College of Angiology* 1981; 21: 899–912 (in Japanese).
33. Terminology Committee of the Japanese Society of Kawasaki Disease. Draft rules for the terminology of Kawasaki disease. http://www.jskd.jp/info/pdf/yougo201007.pdf (in Japanese)
34. Sasaguri Y, Kato H. Regression of aneurysms in Kawasaki disease: a pathological study. *J Pediatr* 1982; 100: 225–231.
35. Suzuki A, Yamagishi M, Kimura K, Sugiyama H, Arakaki Y, Kamiya T, et al. Functional behavior and morphology of the coronary artery wall in patients with Kawasaki disease assessed by intravascular ultrasound. *J Am Coll Cardiol* 1996; 27: 291–296.
36. Mitani Y, Okuda Y, Shimpo H, Uchida F, Hamanaka K, Aoki K, et al. Impaired endothelial function in epicardial coronary arteries after Kawasaki disease. *Circulation* 1997; 96: 454–461.
37. Sugimura T, Kato H, Inoue O, Fukuda T, Sato N, Ishii M, et al. Intravascular ultrasound of coronary arteries in children. Assessment of the wall morphology and the lumen after Kawasaki disease. *Circulation* 1994; 89: 258–265.
38. Yamakawa R, Ishii M, Sugimura T, Akagi T, Eto G, Iemura M, et al. Coronary endothelial dysfunction after Kawasaki disease: evaluation by intracoronary injection of acetylcholine. *J Am Coll Cardiol* 1998; 31: 1074–1080.
39. Takahashi K, Oharaseki T, Naoe S. Pathological study of postcoronary arteritis in adolescents and young adults: with reference to the relationship between

sequelae of Kawasaki disease and atherosclerosis. *Pediatr Cardiol* 2001; 22: 138–142.

40. Tanaka N, Naoe S, Masuda H, Ueno T. Pathological study of sequelae of Kawasaki disease (MCLS). With special reference to the heart and coronary arterial lesions. *Acta Pathol Jpn* 1986; 36: 1513–1527.

41. Negoro N, Nariyama J, Nakagawa A, Katayama H, Okabe T, Hazui H, et al. Successful catheter interventional therapy for acute coronary syndrome secondary to Kawasaki disease in young adults. *Circ J* 2003; 67: 362–365.

42. Suzuki A, Miyagawa-Tomita S, Komatsu K, Nishikawa T, Sakomura Y, Horie T, et al. Active remodeling of the coronary arterial lesions in the late phase of Kawasaki disease: immunohistochemical study. *Circulation* 2000; 101: 2935–2941.

43. Takahasi K, Shibuya H, Atobe T, Naoe S, Tanaka N. Histopathological study of Kawasaki disease in patients who died of intercurrent diseases. *Prog Med* 1987; 7: 21–25 (in Japanese).

44. Kikuchi F, Mori N, Naoe S, Makita J. A case of death due to bronchial asthma attack in a patient with a history of typical Kawasaki disease who has no evidence of current or previous arteritis at autopsy. *Prog Med* 1987; 7: 131–137 (in Japanese).

45. Harada M, Yokouchi Y, Oharaseki T, Matsui K, Tobayama H, Tanaka N, et al. Histopathological characteristics of myocarditis in acute-phase Kawasaki disease. *Histopathology* 2012; 61: 1156–1167.

46. Yonesaka S, Nakada T, Sunagawa Y, Tomimoto K, Naka S, Takahashi T, et al. Endomyocardial biopsy in children with Kawasaki disease. *Acta Paediatr Jpn* 1989; 31: 706–711.

47. Takahashi K, Shibuya K, Masuda H, Tanaka N. Pathology of cardiac sequelae of Kawasaki disease. *The Journal of Japanese College of Angiology* 1989; 29: 461–469 (in Japanese).

48. Amano S, Hazama F, Kubagawa H, Tasaka K, Haebara H, Hamashima Y. General pathology of Kawasaki disease. On the morphological alterations corresponding to the clinical manifestations. *Acta Pathol Jpn* 1980; 30: 681–694.

49. Landing BH, Larson EJ. Pathological features of Kawasaki disease (mucocutaneous lymph node syndrome). *Am J Cardiovasc Pathol* 1987; 1: 218–229.

50. Takahashi K, Oharaseki T, Yokouchi Y, Hiruta N, Naoe S. Kawasaki disease as a systemic vasculitis in childhood. *Ann Vasc Dis* 2010; 3: 173–181.

51. Takahashi K, Oharaseki T, Yokouchi Y. Aneurysms due to Kawasaki disease during adulthood: Transition from acute phase coronary arteritis to remote phase arteriosclerotic lesions and a consideration of differences from arteriosclerosis in adults without a history of Kawasaki disease. *Vascular Med* 2010; 6: 22–26 (in Japanese).

52. Ogawa S, Ohkubo T, Fukazawa R, Kamisago M, Kuramochi Y, Uchikoba Y, et al. Estimation of myocardial hemodynamics before and after intervention in children with Kawasaki disease. *J Am Coll Cardiol* 2004; 43: 653–661.

53. Donohue TJ, Kern MJ, Aguirre FV, Bach RG, Wolford T, Bell CA, et al. Assessing the hemodynamic significance of coronary artery stenoses: analysis of translesional pressure-flow velocity relations in patients. *J Am Coll Cardiol* 1993; 22: 449–458.

54. Ofili EO, Kern MJ, Labovitz AJ, St Vrain JA, Segal J, Aguirre FV, et al. Analysis of coronary blood flow velocity dynamics in angiographically normal and stenosed arteries before and after endolumen enlargement by angioplasty. *J Am Coll Cardiol* 1993; 21: 308–316.

55. Segal J, Kern MJ, Scott NA, King SB 3rd, Doucette JW, Heuser RR, et al. Alterations of phasic coronary artery flow velocity in humans during percutaneous coronary angioplasty. *J Am Coll Cardiol* 1992; 20: 276–286.

56. Pijls NH, van Son JA, Kirkeeide RL, De Bruyne B, Gould KL. Experimental basis of determining maximum coronary, myocardial, and collateral blood flow by pressure measurements for assessing functional stenosis severity before and after percutaneous transluminal coronary angioplasty. *Circulation* 1993; 87: 1354–1367.

57. Ogawa S. Rheologic and hemodynamic characteristics of coronary arteries. *J Jpn Pediatr Soc* 2009; 113: 1769–1778 (in Japanese).

58. Alpert JS, Thygesen K, Antman E, Bassand JP. Myocardial infarction redefined--a consensus document of The Joint European Society of Cardiology/American College of Cardiology Committee for the redefinition of myocardial infarction. *J Am Coll Cardiol* 2000; 36: 959–969.

59. Braunwald E, Antman EM, Beasley JW, Califf RM, Cheitlin MD, Hochman JS, et al. ACC/AHA guidelines for the management of patients with unstable angina and non-STsegment elevation myocardial infarction. A report of the American College of Cardiology/American Heart Association Task Force on Practice Guidelines (Committee on the Management of Patients With Unstable Angina). *J Am Coll Cardiol* 2000; 36: 970–1062.

60. Okamoto F, Sohmiya K, Ohkaru Y, Kawamura K, Asayama K, Kimura H, et al. Human heart-type cytoplasmic fatty acid-binding protein (H-FABP) for the diagnosis of acute myocardial infarction. Clinical evaluation of H-FABP in comparison with myoglobin and creatine kinase isoenzyme MB. *Clin Chem Lab Med* 2000; 38: 231–238.

61. Lindahl B, Venge P, Wallentin L. Relation between troponin T and the risk of subsequent cardiac events in unstable coronary artery disease. The FRISC study group. *Circulation* 1996; 93: 1651–1657.

62. Ohman EM, Armstrong PW, Christenson RH, Granger CB, Katus HA, Hamm CW, et al. Cardiac troponin T levels for risk stratification in acute myocardial ischemia. GUSTO IIA Investigators. *N Engl J Med* 1996; 335: 1333–1341.

63. Isobe M, Nagai R, Ueda S, Tsuchimochi H, Nakaoka H, Takaku F, et al. Quantitative relationship between left ventricular function and serum cardiac myosin light chain I levels after coronary reperfusion in patients with acute myocardial infarction. *Circulation* 1987; 76: 1251–1261.

64. Khreiss T, József L, Potempa LA, Filep JG. Opposing effects of C-reactive protein isoforms on shear-induced neutrophil-platelet adhesion and neutrophil aggregation in whole blood. *Circulation* 2004; 110: 2713–2720.

65. Mitani Y, Sawada H, Hayakawa H, Aoki K, Ohashi H, Matsumura M, et al. Elevated levels of highsensitivity C-reactive protein and serum amyloid-A late after Kawasaki disease: association between inflammation and late coronary sequelae in Kawasaki disease. *Circulation* 2005; 111: 38–43.

66. Yonesaka S, Takahashi T, Sato T, Eto S, Ohtani K, Kitagawa Y, et al. Ongoing myocardial damage in infants and children with Kawasaki disease. *Respiration & Circulation* 2010; 58: 1273–1279 (in Japanese).

67. Borzutzky A, Gutiérrez M, Talesnik E, Godoy I, Kraus J, Hoyos R, et al. High sensitivity C-reactive protein and endothelial function in Chilean patients with history of Kawasaki disease. *Clin Rheumatol* 2008; 27: 845–850.

68. Berenson GS, Srinivasan SR, Bao W, Newman WP 3rd, Tracy RE, Wattigney WA. Association between multiple cardiovascular risk factors and atherosclerosis in children and young adults. The Bogalusa Heart Study. *N Engl J Med* 1998; 338: 1650–1656.

69. Okada T, Murata M, Yamauchi K, Harada K. New criteria of normal serum lipid levels in Japanese children: the nationwide study. *Pediatr Int* 2002; 44: 596–601.

70. Japan Atherosclerosis Society. Japan Atherosclerosis Society (JAS) Guidelines for Diagnosis and Treatment of Atherosclerotic Cardiovascular Diseases, 2002. 2002: 5–7 (in Japanese).

71. Japan Atherosclerosis Society. Japan Atherosclerosis Society (JAS) Guidelines for Prevention of Atherosclerotic Cardiovascular Diseases, 2007. 2007: 11–13 (in Japanese).

72. Ou CY, Tseng YF, Lee CL, Chiou YH, Hsieh KS. Significant relationship between serum high-sensitivity C-reactive protein, high-density lipoprotein cholesterol levels and children with Kawasaki disease and coronary artery lesions. *J Formos Med Assoc* 2009; 108: 719–724.

73. Boers GH, Smals AG, Trijbels FJ, Fowler B, Bakkeren JA, Schoonderwaldt HC, et al. Heterozygosity for homocystinuria in premature peripheral and cerebral occlusive arterial disease. *N Engl J Med* 1985; 313: 709–715.

74. Welch GN, Loscalzo J. Homocysteine and atherothrombosis. *N Engl J Med* 1998; 338: 1042–1050.

75. Ohzeki T, Nakagawa Y, Nakanishi T, Fujisawa Y, Sai S. Diagnostic criteria for metabolic syndrome in Japanese children. A cohort study to establish the concept, pathophysiology, and diagnostic criteria of metabolic syndrome in children and design effective interventions: An MHLW grant research project for cardiovascular disease and lifestyle-related diseases led by Ohzeki T. A final report in 2005–2007. 2008: 89–91 (in Japanese).

76. Council on Cardiovascular Disease in the Young; Committee on Rheumatic Fever, Endocarditis, and Kawasaki Disease; American Heart Association. Diagnostic guidelines for Kawasaki disease. *Circulation* 2001; 103: 335–336.

77. Ichida F, Fatica NS, O'Loughlin JE, Snyder MS, Ehlers KH, Engle MA. Correlation of electrocardiographic and echocardiographic changes in Kawasaki syndrome. *Am Heart J* 1988; 116: 812–819.

78. Okagawa H, Kondo M, Okuno M, Fujino H, Nishijima S. QT duration in the acute phase of Kawasaki disease. *Prog Med* 1997; 17: 1761–1764 (in Japanese).
79. Onouchi Z, Shimazu S, Tamiya H. The second report on abnormal T waves on ECG in patients with Kawasaki disease: Left ventricular asynergy in short-axis two-dimensional echographic images. *J Jpn Pediatr Soc* 1986; 90: 827–831 (in Japanese).
80. Gravel H, Dahdah N, Fournier A, Mathieu MÈ, Curnier D. Ventricular repolarisation during exercise challenge occurring late after Kawasaki disease. *Pediatr Cardiol* 2012; 33: 728–734.
81. Osada M, Tanaka Y, Komai T, Maeda Y, Kitano M, Komori S, et al. Coronary arterial involvement and QT dispersion in Kawasaki disease. *Am J Cardiol* 1999; 84: 466–468.
82. Okuyama J, Osada M, Sugiyama H, Komori S, Ozaki Y. QT dispersion and its longitudinal change in Kawasaki disease. *Japanese Journal of Electrocardiology* 2001; 21: 800–804 (in Japanese).
83. Nakata T. Premature ventricular contraction in remote-phase Kawasaki disease. *Medical Journal Aomori* 1995; 40: 98–103 (in Japanese).
84. Nakanishi T, Takao A, Kondoh C, Nakazawa M, Hiroe M, Matsumoto Y. ECG findings after myocardial infarction in children after Kawasaki disease. *Am Heart J* 1988; 116: 1028–1033.
85. Hamaoka K, Kamiya Y, Sakata K, Fukumochi Y, Ohmochi Y. Coronary reserve in children of Kawasaki disease with ischemic findings on exercise ECG and myocardial SPECT but angiographically no stenotic lesion. Evaluation of coronary hemodynamics and myocardial metabolism during atrial pacing. *J Jpn Pediatr Soc* 1991; 95: 145–151 (in Japanese).
86. Matsuda M, Shimizu T, Oouchi H, Saito S, Kawade M, Arakaki Y, et al. Diagnosis of myocardial ischemia using body surface electrocardiographic mapping with intravenous dipyridamole in children who have a history of Kawasaki disease. *J Jpn Pediatr Soc* 1995; 99: 1618–1627 (in Japanese).
87. Takechi N, Seki T, Ohkubo T, Ogawa S. Dobutamine stress surface mapping of myocardial ischemia in Kawasaki disease. *Pediatr Int* 2001; 43: 218–225.
88. Seki T, Zhang J, Ogawa S, Hirayama T. Dobutamine stress body surface mapping in Kawasaki disease. *Journal of Nippon Medical School* 1994; 61: 610–619 (in Japanese).
89. Shiono J, Horigome H, Matsui A, Terada Y, Watanabe S, Miyashita T, et al. Evaluation of myocardial ischemia in Kawasaki disease using an isointegral map on magnetocardiogram. *Pacing Clin Electrophysiol* 2002; 25: 915–921.
90. Sumitomo N, Karasawa K, Taniguchi K, Ichikawa R, Fukuhara J, Abe O, et al. Association of sinus node dysfunction, atrioventricular node conduction abnormality and ventricular arrhythmia in patients with Kawasaki disease and coronary involvement. *Circ J* 2008; 72: 274–280.

91. Hamamoto K, Oku I, Yamato K. Evaluation of intracardiac conduction delay in acute phase of Kawasaki disease by signal averaged electrocardiogram. *Heart* 1998; 30: 21–27 (in Japanese).

92. Tsuchida A, Ito S, Oka R, Saito T, Yoshioka, I. Recording by signal-averaged electrocardiogram in patients with Kawasaki disease. *J Jpn Pediatr Soc* 1990; 94: 1168–1173 (in Japanese).

93. Dahdah NS, Jaeggi E, Fournier A. Electrocardiographic depolarization and repolarization: long-term after Kawasaki disease. *Pediatr Cardiol* 2002; 23: 513–517.

94. Kuramochi Y, Takechi N, Ohkubo T, Ogawa S. Longitudinal estimation of signal-averaged electrocardiograms in patients with Kawasaki disease. *Pediatr Int* 2002; 44: 12–17.

95. Takeuchi M, Matsushita A, Tsuda E, Kurotobi S, Kogaki S. Clinical assessment of ventricular late potential in children with Kawasaki disease: Frequency analysis and its clinical significance. *Prog Med* 1994; 14: 1828–1832 (in Japanese).

96. Ogawa S, Nagai Y, Zhang J, Yuge K, Hino Y, Jimbo O, et al. Evaluation of myocardial ischemia and infarction by signal-averaged electrocardiographic late potentials in children with Kawasaki disease. *Am J Cardiol* 1996; 78: 175–181.

97. Genma Y, Ogawa S, Zhang J, Yamamoto M. Evaluation of myocardial ischemia in Kawasaki disease by dobutamine stress signal-averaged ventricular late potentials. *Cardiovasc Res* 1997; 36: 323–329.

98. Tanaka N, Ueno T, Naoe S, Masuda H. Kawasaki disease: Pathological features and sequelae of arteritis. *Japanese Journal of Clinical Medicine* 1983; 41: 2008–2016 (in Japanese).

99. Nakada T, Yonesaka S, Sunagawa Y, Tomimoto K, Takahashi T, Matsubara T, et al. Coronary arterial calcification in Kawasaki disease. *Acta Paediatr Jpn* 1991; 33: 443–449.

100. Fuse S, Kobayashi T, Arakaki Y, Ogawa S, Katoh H, Sakamoto N, et al. Standard method for ultrasound imaging of coronary artery in children. *Pediatr Int* 2010; 52: 876–882.

101. Newburger JW, Sanders SP, Burns JC, Parness IA, Beiser AS, Colan SD. Left ventricular contractility and function in Kawasaki syndrome. Effect of intravenous gamma-globulin. *Circulation* 1989; 79: 1237–1246.

102. Yanagisawa M, Yano S, Shiraishi H, Nakajima Y, Fujimoto T, Itoh K. Coronary aneurysms in Kawasaki disease: follow-up observation by two-dimensional echocardiography. *Pediatr Cardiol* 1985; 6: 11–16.

103. Minich LL, Tani LY, Pagotto LT, Young PC, Etheridge SP, Shaddy RE. Usefulness of echocardiography for detection of coronary artery thrombi in patients with Kawasaki disease. *Am J Cardiol* 1998; 82: 1143–1146, A1110.

104. Miyashita M, Karasawa K, Taniguchi K, Kanamaru H, Ayusawa M, Sumitomo N, et al. Usefulness of real-time 3-dimensional echocardiography for the evaluation of coronary artery morphology in patients with Kawasaki disease. *J Am Soc Echocardiogr* 2007; 20: 930–933.

105. Nakano H, Saito A, Ueda K, Tsuchitani Y. Valvular lesions complicating Kawasaki disease: a Doppler echocardiographic evaluation. *J Cardiogr* 1986; 16: 363–371 (in Japanese).

106. Takeuchi D, Saji T, Takatsuki S, Fujiwara M. Abnormal tissue Doppler images are associated with elevated plasma brain natriuretic peptide and increased oxidative stress in acute Kawasaki disease. *Circ J* 2007; 71: 357–362.

107. Noto N, Ayusawa M, Karasawa K, Yamaguchi H, Sumitomo N, Okada T, et al. Dobutamine stress echocardiography for detection of coronary artery stenosis in children with Kawasaki disease. *J Am Coll Cardiol* 1996; 27: 1251–1256.

108. Ishii M, Himeno W, Sawa M, Iemura M, Furui J, Muta H, et al. Assessment of the ability of myocardial contrast echocardiography with harmonic power Doppler imaging to identify perfusion abnormalities in patients with Kawasaki disease at rest and during dipyridamole stress. *Pediatr Cardiol* 2002; 23: 192–199.

109. Hijazi ZM, Udelson JE, Snapper H, Rhodes J, Marx GR, Schwartz SL, et al. Physiologic significance of chronic coronary aneurysms in patients with Kawasaki disease. *J Am Coll Cardiol* 1994; 24: 1633–1638.

110. Paridon SM, Galioto FM, Vincent JA, Tomassoni TL, Sullivan NM, Bricker JT. Exercise capacity and incidence of myocardial perfusion defects after Kawasaki disease in children and adolescents. *J Am Coll Cardiol* 1995; 25: 1420–1424.

111. Miyagawa M, Mochizuki T, Murase K, Tanada S, Ikezoe J, Sekiya M, et al. Prognostic value of dipyridamole-thallium myocardial scintigraphy in patients with Kawasaki disease. *Circulation* 1998; 98: 990–996.

112. Kondo C, Hiroe M, Nakanishi T, Takao A. Detection of coronary artery stenosis in children with Kawasaki disease. Usefulness of pharmacologic stress 201Tl myocardial tomography. *Circulation* 1989; 80: 615–624.

113. Ogawa S, Fukazawa R, Ohkubo T, Zhang J, Takechi N, Kuramochi Y, et al. Silent myocardial ischemia in Kawasaki disease: evaluation of percutaneous transluminal coronary angioplasty by dobutamine stress testing. *Circulation* 1997; 96: 3384–3389.

114. Karasawa K, Ayusawa M, Noto N, Yamaguchi H, Okada T, Harada K. The dobutamine stress T1-201 myocardial single photon emission computed tomography for coronary artery stenosis caused by Kawasaki disease. *Ped Cardiol Card Surg* 1994; 9: 723–733 (in Japanese).

115. Prabhu AS, Singh TP, Morrow WR, Muzik O, Di Carli MF. Safety and efficacy of intravenous adenosine for pharmacologic stress testing in children with aortic valve disease or Kawasaki disease. *Am J Cardiol* 1999; 83: 284–286, A286.

116. Kinoshita S, Suzuki S, Shindo A, Watanage K, Yamashita S. The accuracy and side effects of pharmacologic stress Thallium myocardial scintigraphy with adenosine triphosphate disodium (ATP) infusion in the diagnosis of coronary artery disease. *The Japanese Journal of Nuclear Medicine* 1994; 31: 935–941 (in Japanese).

117. Germano G, Erel J, Lewin H, Kavanagh PB, Berman DS. Automatic quantitation of regional myocardial wall motion and thickening from gated technetium-99 m sestamibi myocardial perfusion single-photon emission computed tomography. *J Am Coll Cardiol* 1997; 30: 1360–1367.

118. Johnson LL, Verdesca SA, Aude WY, Xavier RC, Nott LT, Campanella MW, et al. Postischemic stunning can affect left ventricular ejection fraction and regional wall motion on post-stress gated sestamibi tomograms. *J Am Coll Cardiol* 1997; 30: 1641–1648.

119. Ishikawa Y, Fujiwara M, Ono Y, Tsuda E, Matsubara T, Furukawa S, et al. Exercise- or dipyridamoleloaded QGS is useful to evaluate myocardial ischemia and viability in the patients with a history of Kawasaki disease. *Pediatr Int* 2005; 47: 505–511.

120. Karasawa K, Miyashita M, Taniguchi K, Kanamaru H, Ayusawa M, Noto N, et al. Detection of myocardial contractile reserve by low-dose dobutamine quantitative gated single-photon emission computed tomography in patients with Kawasaki disease and severe coronary artery lesions. *Am J Cardiol* 2003; 92: 865–868.

121. Karasawa K, Ayusawa M, Noto N, Sumitomo N, Okada T, Harada K. Optimum protocol of technetium-99 m tetrofosmin myocardial perfusion imaging for the detection of coronary stenosis lesions in Kawasaki disease. *J Cardiol* 1997; 30: 331–339 (in Japanese).

122. Monzen H, Hara M, Hirata M, Nakanishi A, Ogasawara M, Suzuki T, et al. Exploring a technique for reducing the influence of scattered rays from surrounding organs to the heart during myocardial perfusion scintigraphy with technetium-99 m sestamibi and technetium-99 m tetrofosmin. *Ann Nucl Med* 2006; 20: 705–710.

123. Karasawa K, Ayusawa M, Ymasita T. Pharmacologic stress myocardial perfusion imaging for the detection of coronary stenotic lesions due to Kawasaki disease: Comparison of dobutamine and adenosine triphosphate disodium. In: Kato H, editor. Kawasaki disease: proceedings of the 5th International Kawasaki Disease Symposium, Fukuoka, Japan, 22–25 May 1995. Elsevier 1995: 472–478.

124. Yamazaki J, Nishimura T, Nishimura S, Kajiya T, Kojima K, Kato K. The Diagnostic Value for Ischemic Heart Disease of Thallium-201 Myocardial Scintigraphy by Intravenous Infusion of SUNY4001 (Adenosine): The Report of Clinical Trial at Multi-Center: Phase III. *The Japanese Journal of Nuclear Medicine* 2004; 41: 133–142 (in Japanese).

125. Subcommittee for Standardization of Radionuclide Imaging, Medical and Pharmaceutical Committee for the Japan Radioisotope Association. Recommendations for a pediatric dose in nuclear imaging. Japan Radioisotope Association. *Radioisotopes* 1988; 37: 627–632 (in Japanese).

126. Guidelines for Diagnosis and Treatment of Cardiovascular Diseases (2010–2011 Joint Working Groups Report). Guidelines for Drug Therapy in Pediatric Patients with Cardiovascular Diseases (JCS 2012). Guidelines for Diagnosis and Treatment of Cardiovascular Diseases 2012: 89–301 (in Japanese).

127. Lassmann M, Biassoni L, Monsieurs M, Franzius C, Jacobs F; EANM Dosimetry and Paediatrics Committees. The new EANM paediatric dosage card. *Eur J Nucl Med Mol Imaging* 2007; 34: 796–798.

128. Pediatric Nuclear Medicine Practice Committee of the Japanese Society of Nuclear Medicine. Consensus guidelines for nuclear medicine procedures for children, 2013 (in Japanese).

129. Kanamaru H, Sato Y, Takayama T, Ayusawa M, Karasawa K, Sumitomo N, et al. Assessment of coronary artery abnormalities by multislice spiral computed tomography in adolescents and young adults with Kawasaki disease. *Am J Cardiol* 2005; 95: 522–525.

130. Kanamaru H, Kimijima T, Mugishima H. Cardiovascular imaging: Cardiac CT. *Journal of Japanese Society of Pediatric Radiology* 2011; 27: 106–117 (in Japanese).

131. Liu X, Zhao X, Huang J, Francois CJ, Tuite D, Bi X, et al. Comparison of 3D free-breathing coronary MR angiography and 64-MDCT angiography for detection of coronary stenosis in patients with high calcium scores. *AJR Am J Roentgenol* 2007; 189: 1326–1332.

132. Ozgun M, Rink M, Hoffmeier A, Botnar RM, Heindel W, Fischbach R, et al. Intraindividual comparison of 3D coronary MR angiography and coronary CT angiography. *Acad Radiol* 2007; 14: 910–916.

133. Kanamaru H, Karasawa K, Ichikawa R, Abe O, Miyashita M, Taniguchi K, et al. Advantages of multislice spiral computed tomography for evaluation of serious coronary complications after Kawasaki disease. *J Cardiol* 2007; 50: 21–27 (in Japanese).

134. Suzuki A, Takemura A, Inaba R, Sonobe T, Tsuchiya K, Korenaga T. Magnetic resonance coronary angiography to evaluate coronary arterial lesions in patients with Kawasaki disease. *Cardiol Young* 2006; 16: 563–571.

135. Takemura A, Suzuki A, Inaba R, Sonobe T, Tsuchiya K, Omuro M, et al. Utility of coronary MR angiography in children with Kawasaki disease. *AJR Am J Roentgenol* 2007; 188: W534–W539.

136. Botnar RM, Kim WY, Börnert P, Stuber M, Spuentrup E, Manning WJ. 3D coronary vessel wall imaging utilizing a local inversion technique with spiral image acquisition. *Magn Reson Med* 2001; 46: 848–854.

137. Fayad ZA, Fuster V, Fallon JT, Jayasundera T, Worthley SG, Helft G, et al. Noninvasive in vivo human coronary artery lumen and wall imaging using black-blood magnetic resonance imaging. *Circulation* 2000; 102: 506–510.

138. Kim RJ, Wu E, Rafael A, Chen EL, Parker MA, Simonetti O, et al. The use of contrast-enhanced magnetic resonance imaging to identify reversible myocardial dysfunction. *N Engl J Med* 2000; 343: 1445–1453.

139. Katsumata N, Suzuki A, Takemura A, Kitatsume T, Inaba R, Korenaga T, et al. Imaging of recanalized vessels and evaluation of myocardial disorder with MR coronary angiography. *Prog Med* 2007; 27: 1574–1578 (in Japanese).

140. Kato H, Ichinose E, Kawasaki T. Myocardial infarction in Kawasaki disease: clinical analyses in 195 cases. *J Pediatr* 1986; 108: 923–927.

141. Suzuki A, Kamiya T, Tsuda E, Tsukano S. Natural history of coronary arterial lesions in Kawasaki disease. *Prog Pediatr Cardiol* 1997; 6: 211–218.

142. Ino T, Akimoto K, Ohkubo M, Nishimoto K, Yabuta K, Takaya J, et al. Application of percutaneous transluminal coronary angioplasty to coronary arterial stenosis in Kawasaki disease. *Circulation* 1996; 93: 1709–1715.

143. Sugimura T, Yokoi H, Sato N, Akagi T, Kimura T, Iemura M, et al. Interventional treatment for children with severe coronary artery stenosis with calcification after long-term Kawasaki disease. *Circulation* 1997; 96: 3928–3933.

144. Kato H, Ichinose E, Yoshioka F, Takechi T, Matsunaga S, Suzuki K, et al. Fate of coronary aneurysms in Kawasaki disease: serial coronary angiography and long-term followup study. *Am J Cardiol* 1982; 49: 1758–1766.

145. Tahara M, Waki C, Honda A, Shimozono A, Sato T. Comparative study of various methods of assessing Kawasaki disease-related stenotic lesions in coronary artery aneurysms: ultrasonic cardiography, multi-detector row computed tomography, magnetic resonance imaging, coronary angiography, and intravascular ultrasonography. *Japanese Journal of Pediatrics* 2010; 63: 450–456 (in Japanese).

146. Kato H, Sugimura T, Akagi T, Sato N, Hashino K, Maeno Y, et al. Long-term consequences of Kawasaki disease. A 10- to 21-year follow-up study of 594 patients. *Circulation* 1996; 94: 1379–1385.

147. Suzuki A, Kamiya T, Arakaki Y, Kinoshita Y, Kimura K. Fate of coronary arterial aneurysms in Kawasaki disease. *Am J Cardiol* 1994; 74: 822–824.

148. Iemura M, Ishii M, Sugimura T, Akagi T, Kato H. Long term consequences of regressed coronary aneurysms after Kawasaki disease: vascular wall morphology and function. *Heart* 2000; 83: 307–311.

149. Suzuki A, Kamiya T, Ono Y, Okuno M, Yagihara T. Aortocoronary bypass surgery for coronary arterial lesions resulting from Kawasaki disease. *J Pediatr* 1990; 116: 567–573.

150. Fukuda T, Akagi T, Ishibashi M, Inoue O, Sugimura T, Kato H. Noninvasive evaluation of myocardial ischemia in Kawasaki disease: comparison between dipyridamole stress thallium imaging and exercise stress testing. *Am Heart J* 1998; 135: 482–487.

151. Suzuki A, Kamiya T, Ono Y, Kinoshita Y, Kawamura S, Kimura K. Clinical significance of morphologic classification of coronary arterial segmental stenosis due to Kawasaki disease. *Am J Cardiol* 1993; 71: 1169–1173.

152. Ishii M, Ueno T, Akagi T, Baba K, Harada K, Hamaoka K, et al; Research Committee of Ministry of Health, Labour and Welfare--"Study of treatment and long-term management in Kawasaki disease". Guidelines for catheter intervention in coronary artery lesion in Kawasaki disease. *Pediatr Int* 2001; 43: 558–562.

153. Ishii M, Ueno T, Ikeda H, Iemura M, Sugimura T, Furui J, et al. Sequential follow-up results of catheter intervention for coronary artery lesions after Kawasaki disease: quantitative coronary artery angiography and intravascular ultrasound imaging study. *Circulation* 2002; 105: 3004–3010.

154. Takahashi K, Hirota A, Naoe S, Tsukada T, Masuda H, Tanaka N. A morphological study of intimal thickening in sequelae of coronary arterial lesions of Kawasaki disease (1). *The Journal of Japanese College of Angiology* 1991; 31: 17–25 (in Japanese).

155. Guidelines for Diagnosis and Treatment of Cardiovascular Diseases (1998–1999 Joint Working Groups Report). Guidelines for Secondary Prevention of Myocardial Infarction. *Jpn Circ J* 2000; 64 (Suppl. IV): 1081–1127 (in Japanese).

156. Ogawa S, Fukazawa R, Kamisago M, Uchikoba Y, Ikegam E, Watanabe M, et al. Angiotensin ii type 1 receptor blockers inhibit significant coronary stenosis in patients with coronary aneurysm after Kawasaki disease. *Circulation* 2004; 110 (Suppl): 707.

157. Li Z, Iwai M, Wu L, Liu HW, Chen R, Jinno T, et al. Fluvastatin enhances the inhibitory effects of a selective AT1 receptor blocker, valsartan, on atherosclerosis. *Hypertension* 2004; 44: 758–763.

158. Yamada K, Fukumoto T, Shinkai A, Shirahata A, Meguro T. The platelet functions in acute febrile mucocutaneous lymph node syndrome and a trial of prevention for thrombosis by antiplatelet agent. *Nihon Ketsueki Gakkai Zasshi* 1978; 41: 791–802.

159. Shirahata A, Nakamura T, Ariyoshi N. Blood coagulation status in patients beyond 1 year after the onset of Kawasaki disease. *J Jpn Pediatr Soc* 1990; 94: 2608–2613 (in Japanese).

160. Shirahata A, Nakamura T, Asakura A. Optimal aspirin therapy for Kawasaki disease: Discussion of antithrombotic therapy. *J Jpn Pediatr Soc* 1985; 89: 2207–2214 (in Japanese).

161. Deleted in proof.

162. Onouchi Z, Hamaoka K, Sakata K, Ozawa S, Shiraishi I, Itoi T, et al. Long-term changes in coronary artery aneurysms in patients with Kawasaki disease: comparison of therapeutic regimens. *Circ J* 2005; 69: 265–272.

163. Suzuki A, Kamiya T, Ono Y, Kinoshita Y. Thrombolysis in the treatment of patients with Kawasaki disease. *Cardiol Young* 1993; 3: 207–215.

164. Tsuda E, Yasuda T, Naito H. Vasospastic angina in Kawasaki disease. *J Cardiol* 2008; 51: 65–69.

165. Flynn JT. Pediatric use of antihypertensive medications: Much more to learn. *Curr Ther Res Clin Exp* 2001; 62: 314–328.

166. Sugimura T, Kato H, Inoue O, Takagi J, Fukuda T, Sato N. Vasodilatory response of the coronary arteries after Kawasaki disease: evaluation by intracoronary injection of isosorbide dinitrate. *J Pediatr* 1992; 121: 684–688.

167. Ishikita T, Umezawa T, Saji T, Matsuo N, Yabe Y. Functional abnormality of coronary arteries in children after Kawasaki disease: Distensibility of coronary arterial wall by isosorbide dinitrate. *Ped Cardiol Card Surg* 1992; 8: 265–270 (in Japanese).

168. Guidelines for Diagnosis and Treatment of Cardiovascular Diseases (2009 Joint Working Groups Report). Guidelines for Diagnostic Evaluation of Patients with Chronic Ischemic Heart Disease (JCS 2010). http://www.j-circ.or.jp/guideline/pdf/JCS2010_yamagishi_h.pdf (in Japanese)(available January 2013).

169. Guidelines for Diagnosis and Treatment of Cardiovascular Diseases (2008 Joint Working Groups Report). Guidelines for management of anticoagulant and antiplatelet therapy in cardiovascular disease (JCS 2009) http://www.j-circ.or.jp/guideline/pdf/JCS2009_hori_h.pdf (in Japanese)(available January 2013).

170. Guidelines for Diagnosis and Treatment of Cardiovascular Diseases (2005 Joint Working Groups Report). Guidelines for the primary prevention of ischemic heart disease revised version (JCS 2006). http://www.j-circ.or.jp/guideline/pdf/JCS2006_kitabatake_h.pdf (in Japanese)(available January 2013).

171. Guidelines for Diagnosis and Treatment of Cardiovascular Diseases (2006 Joint Working Groups Report). Guidelines for Management of Acute Coronary Syndrome without Persistent ST Segment Elevation (JCS 2007). http://www.j-circ.or.jp/guideline/pdf/JCS2007_yamaguchi_h.pdf (in Japanese) (available January 2013).

172. Guidelines for Diagnosis and Treatment of Cardiovascular Diseases (2009 Joint Working Groups Report). Guidelines for Treatment of Chronic Heart Failure (JCS 2010). http://www.j-circ.or.jp/guideline/pdf/JCS2010_matsuzaki_h.pdf (in Japanese)(available January 2013).

173. Guidelines for Diagnosis and Treatment of Cardiovascular Diseases (2010 Joint Working Groups Report). Guidelines for Treatment of Acute Heart Failure (JCS 2011). http://www.j-circ.or.jp/guideline/pdf/JCS2011_izumi_h.pdf (in Japanese)(available January 2013).

174. Scientific Committee for the Japanese Society of Pediatric Cardiology and Cardiac Surgery. Guidelines for pharmacotherapy of heart failure in children. *Ped Cardiol Card Surg* 2001; 17: 501–512 (in Japanese).

175. Newburger JW, Takahashi M, Gerber MA, Gewitz MH, Tani LY, Burns JC, et al. Diagnosis, treatment, and long-term management of Kawasaki disease: a statement for health professionals from the Committee on Rheumatic Fever, Endocarditis and Kawasaki Disease, Council on Cardiovascular Disease in the Young, American Heart Association. *Circulation* 2004; 110: 2747–2771.

176. Smith SC Jr, Allen J, Blair SN, Bonow RO, Brass LM, Fonarow GC, et al. AHA/ACC guidelines for secondary prevention for patients with coronary and other atherosclerotic vascular disease: 2006 update: endorsed by the National Heart, Lung, and Blood Institute. *Circulation* 2006; 113: 2363–2372.

177. Monagle P, Chalmers E, Chan A, DeVeber G, Kirkham F, Massicotte P, et al. Antithrombotic therapy in neonates and children: American College of Chest Physicians Evidence-Based Clinical Practice Guidelines (8th Edition). *Chest* 2008; 133 (6 Suppl): 887S–968S.

177a. Smith SC Jr, Feldman TE, Hirshfeld JW Jr, Jacobs AK, Kern MJ, King SB 3rd, et al. ACC/AHA/SCAI 2005 guideline update for percutaneous coronary intervention: a report of the American College of Cardiology/American Heart Association Task Force on Practice Guidelines (ACC/AHA/SCAI Writing Committee to Update 2001 Guidelines for Percutaneous Coronary Intervention). *Circulation* 2006; 113: e166–e286, Doi:10.1161/CIRCULATIONAHA.106.173220.

178. Kato H, Inoue O, Ichinose E, Akagi T, Sato N. Intracoronary urokinase in Kawasaki disease: treatment and prevention of myocardial infarction. *Acta Paediatr Jpn* 1991; 33: 27–35.

179. Nakagawa M, Watanabe N, Okuno M, Okamoto N, Fujino H. Effects of intracoronary tissue-type plasminogen activator treatment in Kawasaki disease and acute myocardial infarction. *Cardiology* 2000; 94: 52–57.

180. Shiraishi J, Sawada T, Tatsumi T, Azuma A, Nakagawa M. Acute myocardial infarction due to a regressed giant coronary aneurysm as possible sequela of Kawasaki disease. *J Invasive Cardiol* 2001; 13: 569–572.

181. Tsubata S, Ichida F, Hamamichi Y, Miyazaki A, Hashimoto I, Okada T. Successful thrombolytic therapy using tissue-type plasminogen activator in Kawasaki disease. *Pediatr Cardiol* 1995; 16: 186–189.

182. Sato Y, Nishi T. A case of acute myocardial infarction developing following Kawasaki disease in whom PTCR · PTCA proved effective. *Ped Cardiol Card Surg* 1996; 12: 777–782 (in Japanese).

183. Ohkubo M, Ino T, Shimazaki S, Akimoto K, Nishimoto K, Matsubara K, et al. Successful percutaneous transluminal coronary recanalization with tissue plasminogen activator in Kawasaki disease. *J Jpn Pediatr Soc* 1994; 98: 1758–1765 (in Japanese).

184. Effectiveness of intravenous thrombolytic treatment in acute myocardial infarction. Gruppo Italiano per lo Studio della Streptochinasi nell'Infarto Miocardico (GISSI). *Lancet* 1986; 1: 397–402.

185. Randomised trial of intravenous streptokinase, oral aspirin, both, or neither among 17,187 cases of suspected acute myocardial infarction: ISIS-2. ISIS-2 (Second International Study of Infarct Survival) Collaborative Group. *Lancet* 1988; 2: 349–360.

186. Guidelines for Diagnosis and Treatment of Cardiovascular Diseases (2006–2007 Joint Working Groups Report). Guidelines for the management of patients with ST-elevation myocardial infarction (JCS 2008). *Circ J* 2008; 72 (Suppl. IV): 1347–1464 (in Japanese).

187. Ino T, Nishimoto K, Akimoto K, Park I, Shimazaki S, Yabuta K, et al. Percutaneous transluminal coronary angioplasty for Kawasaki disease: a case report and literature review. *Pediatr Cardiol* 1991; 12: 33–35.

188. Satler LF, Leon MB, Kent KM, Pichard AD, Martin GR. Angioplasty in a child with Kawasaki disease. *Am Heart J* 1992; 124: 216–219.

189. Nishimura H, Sawada T, Azuma A, Kohno Y, Katsume H, Nakagawa M, et al. Percutaneous transluminal coronary angioplasty in a patient with Kawasaki disease. A case report of an unsuccessful angioplasty. *Jpn Heart J* 1992; 33: 869–873.

190. Kawata T, Hasegawa J, Yoshida Y, Yoshikawa Y, Kawachi K, Kitamura S. Percutaneous transluminal coronary angioplasty of the left internal thoracic artery graft: a case report in a child. *Cathet Cardiovasc Diagn* 1994; 32: 340–342.

191. Hijazi ZM, Smith JJ, Fulton DR. Stent implantation for coronary artery stenosis after Kawasaki disease. *J Invasive Cardiol* 1997; 9: 534–536.

192. Hijazi ZM. Coronary arterial stenosis after Kawasaki disease: role of catheter intervention. *Catheter Cardiovasc Interv* 1999; 46: 337.

193. Ueno T, Kai H, Ikeda H, Ichiki K, Hashino T, Imaizumi T. Coronary stent deployment in a young adult with Kawasaki disease and recurrent myocardial infarction. *Clin Cardiol* 1999; 22: 147–149.

194. Hashmi A, Lazzam C, McCrindle BW, Benson LN. Stenting of coronary artery stenosis in Kawasaki disease. *Catheter Cardiovasc Interv* 1999; 46: 333–336.

195. Akagi T, Ogawa S, Ino T, Iwasa M, Echigo S, Kishida K, et al. Catheter interventional treatment in Kawasaki disease: A report from the Japanese Pediatric Interventional Cardiology Investigation group. *J Pediatr* 2000; 137: 181–186.

196. Misumi K, Taniguchi Y. The 34th Kinki-district meeting on Kawasaki disease: Cardiologists' view of coronary lesions and coronary events associated with Kawasaki disease -- On current practices of cardiac intervention with rotablators, excimer laser angioplasty, and drug-eluting stents. *Prog Med* 2010; 30: 1899–1904 (in Japanese).

197. Kato H, Ishii M, Akagi T, Eto G, Iemura M, Tsutsumi T, et al. Interventional catheterization in Kawasaki disease. *J Interv Cardiol* 1998; 11: 355–361.

198. Oda H, Miida T, Ochiai Y, Toeda T, Higuma N, Ito E. Successful stent implantation in acute myocardial infarction and successful directional coronary atherectomy of a stenotic lesion involving an aneurysm in a woman with Kawasaki disease of adult onset. *J Interv Cardiol* 1997; 10: 375–380.

199. Miyazaki A, Tsuda E, Miyazaki S, Kitamura S, Tomita H, Echigo S. Percutaneous transluminal coronary angioplasty for anastomotic stenosis after coronary arterial bypass grafting in Kawasaki disease. *Cardiol Young* 2003; 13: 284–289.

200. Tsuda E, Miyazaki S, Takamuro M, Fuse S, Tsuji Y, Echigo S. Strategy for localized stenosis caused by Kawasaki disease: midterm results of percutaneous transluminal coronary balloon angioplasty in two infants. *Pediatr Cardiol* 2006; 27: 272–275.

201. Tsuda E, Miyazaki S, Yamada O, Takamuro M, Takekawa T, Echigo S. Percutaneous transluminal coronary rotational atherectomy for localized stenosis caused by Kawasaki disease. *Pediatr Cardiol* 2006; 27: 447–453.

202. Muta H, Ishii M. Percutaneous coronary intervention versus coronary artery bypass grafting for stenotic lesions after Kawasaki disease. *J Pediatr* 2010; 157: 120–126.

203. Ariyoshi M, Shiraishi J, Kimura M, Matsui A, Takeda M, Arihara M, et al. Primary percutaneous coronary intervention for acute myocardial

infarction due to possible sequelae of Kawasaki disease in young adults: a case series. *Heart Vessels* 2011; 26: 117–124.

204. Kitamura S, Kawachi K, Oyama C, Miyagi Y, Morita R, Koh Y, et al. Severe Kawasaki heart disease treated with an internal mammary artery graft in pediatric patients. A first successful report. *J Thorac Cardiovasc Surg* 1985; 89: 860–866.

205. D' Amico TA, Sabiston DC. Kawasaki's disease. In: Surgery of the chest. Sabiston DC, Spencer FC, editors. Philadelphia: Saunders, 1990: 1759–1766.

206. Mavroudis C, Backer CL, Muster AJ, Pahl E, Sanders JH, Zales VR, et al. Expanding indications for pediatric coronary artery bypass. *J Thorac Cardiovasc Surg* 1996; 111: 181–189.

207. Kitamura S, Tsuda E, Wakisaka Y. Pediatric coronary artery bypass grafting for Kawasaki disease: 20-years' outcome. *Japanese Journal of Clinical Medicine* 2008; 66: 380–386 (in Japanese).

208. Tsuda E, Kitamura S, Kimura K, Kobayashi J, Miyazaki S, Echigo S, et al. Long-term patency of internal thoracic artery grafts for coronary artery stenosis due to Kawasaki disease: comparison of early with recent results in small children. *Am Heart J* 2007; 153: 995–1000.

209. Kitamura S, Kawasaki T, Kato H, Asai T, Yanagawa H, Hamashima Y, et al. Surgical treatment subcommittee for the Ministry of Health and Welfare research project on mental and physical disorders. Research on disorders of unknown cause in infants and young children, Book 2: Study on Kawasaki disease. A study report in 1985. 1986: 39–42 (in Japanese).

210. Tsuda E, Kitamura S; Cooperative Study Group of Japan. National survey of coronary artery bypass grafting for coronary stenosis caused by Kawasaki disease in Japan. *Circulation* 2004; 110: II61–II66.

211. Yamauchi H, Ochi M, Akaishi J, Ohmori H, Hinokiyama K, Saji Y, et al. Surgical therapy in patients with giant coronary artery aneurysms due to Kawasaki disease. *Ped Cardiol Card Surg* 2004; 20: 94–99 (in Japanese).

212. Ozkan S, Saritas B, Aslim E, Akay TH, Aslamaci S. Coronary bypass surgery in Kawasaki disease in a four-year-old patient: case report. *J Card Surg* 2007; 22: 511–513.

213. Kitamura S, Seki T, Kawachi K, Morita R, Kawata T, Mizuguchi K, et al. Excellent patency and growth potential of internal mammary artery grafts in pediatric coronary artery bypass surgery. New evidence for a "live" conduit. *Circulation* 1988; 78: I129–I139.

214. Kitamura S, Kawachi K, Seki T, Morita R, Nishii T, Mizuguchi K, et al. Bilateral internal mammary artery grafts for coronary artery bypass operations in children. *J Thorac Cardiovasc Surg* 1990; 99: 708–715.

215. Takeuchi Y, Gomi A, Okamura Y, Mori H, Nagashima M. Coronary revascularization in a child with Kawasaki disease: use of right gastroepiploic artery. *Ann Thorac Surg* 1990; 50: 294–296.

216. Kitamura S. Surgical management for cardiovascular lesions in Kawasaki disease. *Cardiol Young* 1991; 1: 240–253.

217. Kitamura S, Tsuda E, Kobayashi J, Nakajima H, Yoshikawa Y, Yagihara T, et al. Twenty-five-year outcome of pediatric coronary artery bypass surgery for Kawasaki disease. *Circulation* 2009; 120: 60–68.

218. Fukazawa R, Ikegam E, Watanabe M, Hajikano M, Kamisago M, Katsube Y, et al. Coronary artery aneurysm induced by Kawasaki disease in children show features typical senescence. *Circ J* 2007; 71: 709–715.

219. Kuramochi Y, Ohkubo T, Takechi N, Fukumi D, Uchikoba Y, Ogawa S. Hemodynamic factors of thrombus formation in coronary aneurysms associated with Kawasaki disease. *Pediatr Int* 2000; 42: 470–475.

220. Ogawa S. Issues in healthcare in adults: Current medical and surgical treatment of cardiovascular sequelae of Kawasaki disease. *Yamabiko Tsushin* 2006; 142: 2–7 (in Japanese).

221. Kitamura S, Kawashima Y, Kawachi K, Harima R, Ihara K, Nakano S, et al. Severe mitral regurgitation due to coronary arteritis of mucocutaneous lymph node syndrome. A new surgical entity. *J Thorac Cardiovasc Surg* 1980; 80: 629–636.

222. Endo M. Surgical treatment of Kawasaki disease in the future. *Prog Med* 1991; 11: 97–99 (in Japanese).

223. Travaline JM, Hamilton SM, Ringel RE, Laschinger JC, Ziskind AA. Cardiac transplantation for giant coronary artery aneurysms complicating Kawasaki disease. *Am J Cardiol* 1991; 68: 560–561.

224. Guide for the use of the School Activity Management Table for Children with Heart Disease; Guide for the use of the School Activity Management Table for Children with Renal Disease – For schools and school physicians, the 2011 revision. The Japanese Society of School Health. 2013: 3–11 (in Japanese).

225. School Cardiac Screening Study Committee for the Japanese Society of Pediatric Cardiology and Cardiac Surgery. Guidelines for management of arrhythmia with no underling diseases, the 2002 revision. *Ped Cardiol Card Surg* 2002; 18: 610–611 (in Japanese).

226. Sonobe T. Practice of immunization: High-dose gamma-globulin therapy and immunization. *Japanese Journal of Pediatric Medicine* 1994; 26: 1929–1933 (in Japanese).

227. Tsuda E, Kamiya T, Kimura K, Ono Y, Echigo S. Coronary artery dilatation exceeding 4.0mm during acute Kawasaki disease predicts a high probability of subsequent late intima-medial thickening. *Pediatr Cardiol* 2002; 23: 9–14.

228. Kurotobi S, Nagai T, Kawakami N, Sano T. Coronary diameter in normal infants, children and patients with Kawasaki disease. *Pediatr Int* 2002; 44: 1–4.

229. de Zorzi A, Colan SD, Gauvreau K, Baker AL, Sundel RP, Newburger JW. Coronary artery dimensions may be misclassified as normal in Kawasaki disease. *J Pediatr* 1998; 133: 254–258.

230. Akagi T, Rose V, Benson LN, Newman A, Freedom RM. Outcome of coronary artery aneurysms after Kawasaki disease. *J Pediatr* 1992; 121: 689–694.

231. Tsuda E, Kamiya T, Ono Y, Kimura K, Kurosaki K, Echigo S. Incidence of stenotic lesions predicted by acute phase changes in coronary arterial diameter during Kawasaki disease. *Pediatr Cardiol* 2005; 26: 73–79.

232. Suzuki A. Long-term prognosis of coronary artery disorder. In: Kamiya T, editor. Diagnosis and treatment of Kawasaki disease: With special emphasis on cardiovascular disorders. Osaka: Nippon Rinsho Sha, 1994; 266–275 (in Japanese).

233. Ogino H. Introduction of the Kawasaki disease patient card –Development of the "acute phase Kawasaki disease in summary" supervised by the Japan Kawasaki Disease Research Society. *Prog Med* 2003; 23: 1806–1811 (in Japanese).

234. Kaichi S, Tsuda E, Fujita H, Kurosaki K, Tanaka R, Naito H, et al. Acute coronary artery dilation due to Kawasaki disease and subsequent late calcification as detected by electron beam computed tomography. *Pediatr Cardiol* 2008; 29: 568–573.

235. Shinohara T. Clinical study of dorp out cases in Kawasaki disease with cardiovascular lesions. Proceedings for the 32nd meeting of the Japanese Society of Kawasaki Disease. 2012: 86 (in Japanese).

236. Abe O, Sumitomo N, Kamiyama H, Nakajima S, Kawamura K, Watanabe H, et al. Investigation neglecting medical examination among Kawasaki Disease with reference myocardial perfusion imaging. Proceedings for the 32nd meeting of the Japanese Society of Kawasaki Disease. 2012: 88 (In Japanese).

237. Gordon JB, Kahn AM, Burns JC. When children with Kawasaki disease grow up: Myocardial and vascular complications in adulthood. *J Am Coll Cardiol* 2009; 54: 1911–1920.

238. Imakita M, Yutani C, Strong JP, Sakurai I, Sumiyoshi A, Watanabe T, et al. Second nation-wide study of atherosclerosis in infants, children and young adults in Japan. *Atherosclerosis* 2001; 155: 487–497.

239. Sakata K, Onouchi Z. Plasma Thrombomodulin levels in patients with Kawasaki disease in long-term periods. *J Jpn Pediatr Soc* 1993; 97: 93–96 (in Japanese).

240. Dhillon R, Clarkson P, Donald AE, Powe AJ, Nash M, Novelli V, et al. Endothelial dysfunction late after Kawasaki disease. *Circulation* 1996; 94: 2103–2106.

241. Niboshi A, Hamaoka K, Sakata K, Yamaguchi N. Endothelial dysfunction in adult patients with a history of Kawasaki disease. *Eur J Pediatr* 2008; 167: 189–196.

242. Schober A, Zernecke A. Chemokines in vascular remodeling. *Thromb Haemost* 2007; 97: 730–737.

243. Suzuki A, Tsuda E, Fujiwara M, Arakaki Y, Onn Y, Kamiya T. Intravascular echographic findings of artery lesions of remote-phase Kawasaki disease. *Prog Med* 1996; 16: 1797–1800 (in Japanese).

244. Vliegenthart R, Hollander M, Breteler MM, van der Kuip DA, Hofman A, Oudkerk M, et al. Stroke is associated with coronary calcification as detected by electron-beam CT: the Rotterdam Coronary Calcification Study. *Stroke* 2002; 33: 462–465.

245. Kondos GT, Hoff JA, Sevrukov A, Daviglus ML, Garside DB, Devries SS, et al. Electron-beam tomography coronary artery calcium and cardiac events: a 37-month follow-up of 5635 initially asymptomatic low- to intermediate-risk adults. *Circulation* 2003; 107: 2571–2576.

246. Ross R. Atherosclerosis--an inflammatory disease. *N Engl J Med* 1999; 340: 115–126.

247. Gaenzer H, Neumayr G, Marschang P, Sturm W, Kirchmair R, Patsch JR. - Flow-mediated vasodilation of the femoral and brachial artery induced by exercise in healthy nonsmoking and smoking men. *J Am Coll Cardiol* 2001; 38: 1313–1319.

248. Liu Y, Onouchi Z, Sakata K, Ikuta K. An experimental study on the role of smooth muscle cells in the pathogenesis of atherosclerosis of the coronary arteritis. *J Jpn Pediatr Soc* 1996; 100: 1453–1458 (in Japanese).

249. Ohni S, Goto S, Nakamura H, Yamada T, Hirano M, Sakurai I. Adult multiple coronary aneurysms of Kawasaki's disease's sequelae; two autopsy cases. *The Official Journal of Japanese Society of Laboratory Medicine* 1998; 46: 177–181 (in Japanese).

250. Suda K, Iemura M, Nishiono H, Teramachi Y, Koteda Y, Kishimoto S, et al. Long-term prognosis of patients with Kawasaki disease complicated by giant coronary aneurysms: a single-institution experience. *Circulation* 2011; 123: 1836–1842.

251. Tsuda E, Hirata T, Matsuo O, Abe T, Sugiyama H, Yamada O. The 30-year outcome for patients after myocardial infarction due to coronary artery lesions caused by Kawasaki disease. *Pediatr Cardiol* 2011; 32: 176–182.

252. Daniels LB, Tjajadi MS, Walford HH, Jimenez-Fernandez S, Trofimenko V, Fick DB Jr, et al. Prevalence of Kawasaki disease in young adults with suspected myocardial ischemia. *Circulation* 2012; 125: 2447–2453.

253. Tsuda E. Pregnancy and delivery in patients with a history of Kawasaki disease. *Cardioangiology* 2011; 69: 341–345 (in Japanese).

254. De Wilde JP, Rivers AW, Price DL. A review of the current use of magnetic resonance imaging in pregnancy and safety implications for the fetus. *Prog Biophys Mol Biol* 2005; 87: 335–353.

255. Nolan TE, Savage RW. Peripartum myocardial infarction from presumed Kawasaki's disease. *South Med J* 1990; 83: 1360–1361.

256. Tsuda E, Kawamata K, Neki R, Echigo S, Chiba Y. Nationwide survey of pregnancy and delivery in patients with coronary arterial lesions caused by Kawasaki disease in Japan. *Cardiol Young* 2006; 16: 173–178.

257. Perloff JK, Koos B. Pregnancy and congenital heart disease: The mother and the fetus. In: Perloff JK, Child JS, editors. Congenital heart disease in adults. 2nd edn. Philadelphia: W.B. Saunders, 1998; 144–164.

258. Guidelines for Diagnosis and Treatment of Cardiovascular Diseases (2009 Joint Working Groups Report). Guidelines for Indication and Management of Pregnancy and Delivery in Women with Heart Disease (JCS 2010). http://www.j-circ.or.jp/guideline/pdf/JCS2010niwa.h.pdf (in Japanese)(available January 2013).

259. Chong MK, Harvey D, de Swiet M. Follow-up study of children whose mothers were treated with warfarin during pregnancy. *Br J Obstet Gynaecol* 1984; 91: 1070–1073.

260. Vitale N, De Feo M, De Santo LS, Pollice A, Tedesco N, Cotrufo M. Dose-dependent fetal complications of warfarin in pregnant women with mechanical heart valves. *J Am Coll Cardiol* 1999; 33: 1637–1641.

261. Arakawa K, Akita T, Nishizawa K, Kurita A, Nakamura H, Yoshida T, et al. Anticoagulant therapy during successful pregnancy and delivery in a Kawasaki disease patient with coronary aneurysm--a case report. *Jpn Circ J* 1997; 61: 197–200.

262. Buttar HS. An overview of the influence of ACE inhibitors on fetal-placental circulation and perinatal development. *Mol Cell Biochem* 1997; 176: 61–71.

263. Cooper WO, Hernandez-Diaz S, Arbogast PG, Dudley JA, Dyer S, Gideon PS, et al. Major congenital malformations after first-trimester exposure to ACE inhibitors. *N Engl J Med* 2006; 354: 2443–2451.

264. Badui E, Valdespino A, Lepe L, Rangel A, Campos A, Leon F. Acute myocardial infarction with normal coronary arteries in a patient with dermatomyositis. Case report. *Angiology* 1996; 47: 815–818.

265. Regitz-Zagrosek V, Blomstrom Lundqvist C, Borghi C, Cifkova R, Ferreira R, Foidart JM, et al. ESC Guidelines on the management of cardiovascular diseases during pregnancy: the Task Force on the Management of Cardiovascular Diseases during Pregnancy of the European Society of Cardiology (ESC). *Eur Heart J* 2011; 32: 3147–3197.

266. Pongratz G, Gansser R, Bachmann K, Singer H, Worth H. Myocardial infarction in an adult resulting from coronary aneurysms previously documented in childhood after an acute episode of Kawasaki's disease. *Eur Heart J* 1994; 15: 1002–1004.

267. Fujiwara H. Sequelae of Kawasaki disease in adults. In: Kawasaki T, Hamashima Y, Kato H, Shigematsu I, Yanagawa H, editors. Kawasaki disease. Tokyo: Nankodo Co., Ltd., 1988; 235–240 (in Japanese).

Appendix. Disclosure of Potential Conflicts of Interest (COI): Guidelines for Diagnosis and Management of Cardiovascular Sequelae in Kawasaki Disease (JCS 2013)

Author	Employer/leadership position (private company)	Stakeholder	Patent royalty	Honorarium	Payment for manuscripts	Research grant	Scholarship (educational) grant/ endowed chair	Other rewards	Potential COI of the marital partner, first-degree family members, or those who share income and property.
Members: Kazuhiko Nishigaki				Shionogi Boehringer Ingelheim Japan Mochida Pharmaceutical					
Members: Masami Ochi							St. Jude Medical Japan Senko Medical Instrument Manufacturing Edwards Lifesciences Corporation		

Companies are listed only by name. The following members have no COI to disclose.

Members with no COI to disclose.

Chair: Shunichi Ogawa, None

Members: Mamoru Ayusawa, None

Members: Masahiro Ishii, None

Members: Hirotarou Ogino, None

Members: Tsutomu Saji, None

Members: Kenji Hamaoka, None

Members: Ryuji Fukazawa, None

Collaborators: Hiroshi Kamiyama, None

Collaborators: Kei Takahashi, None

Collaborators: Etsuko Tsuda, None

Collaborators: Hiroyoshi Yokoi, None

Index

© Springer Japan 2017
B.T. Saji et al. (eds.), *Kawasaki Disease*, DOI 10.1007/978-4-431-56039-5